Stimuli-Responsive Biomaterials for Inflammatory Diseases

This book reviews the use of stimuli-responsive biomaterials in the diagnosis, treatment, and management of inflammatory diseases. It begins by providing a foundational understanding of inflammatory diseases and presents fundamental principles of stimuli-responsive biomaterials. This book provides insights into the characteristics of ideal biomaterials and the chemical principles that enable stimuli-responsive drug delivery systems to function effectively. A detailed classification of these advanced materials is presented based on their responsive triggers, such as pH, temperature, light, and biological signals. The application of stimuli-responsive biomaterials in cancer therapeutics is discussed, as is their use in addressing autoimmune disorders, including lupus and rheumatoid arthritis, through targeted treatment strategies. The book also covers the innovative uses of these materials in managing inflammatory arthritis and various bone disorders, focusing on targeted drug delivery and improved patient outcomes. Further, it examines the potential of these smart materials in treating neuroinflammatory and neurological disorders, cardiovascular and cerebrovascular diseases, and in managing diabetes and obesity. The book highlights the development and application of injectable hydrogels that respond to various stimuli and presents the role of artificial intelligence and machine learning in the design of smart drug delivery systems. This book is intended for researchers working in biomedical engineering, drug delivery, and pharmaceutical sciences.

Key Features:

- Provides an in-depth review of stimuli-responsive biomaterials and their applications in the diagnosis, treatment, and management of inflammatory diseases
- Presents classification of advanced biomaterials based on their responsive triggers, such as pH, temperature, light, and biological signals
- Highlights the use of stimuli-responsive biomaterials in cancer theranostics, autoimmune disorders, and targeted treatment strategies
- Emphasizes the development and application of injectable hydrogels and the integration of artificial intelligence in designing smart drug delivery systems
- Examines in-depth explanations of the chemical principles and mechanisms that enable stimuli-responsive drug delivery systems

Stimuli-Responsive Biomaterials for Inflammatory Diseases

Advances in Research and Clinical Applications

Edited by
Mohammed Gulzar Ahmed, Vetriselvan Subramaniyan,
Sagnik Nag, and Sourav Mohanto

CRC Press
Taylor & Francis Group
Boca Raton London New York

CRC Press is an imprint of the
Taylor & Francis Group, an **informa** business

Designed cover image: Shutterstock Image Id: 1956436417

First edition published 2026
by CRC Press
2385 NW Executive Center Drive, Suite 320, Boca Raton FL 33431

and by CRC Press
4 Park Square, Milton Park, Abingdon, Oxon, OX14 4RN

CRC Press is an imprint of Taylor & Francis Group, LLC

ISBN: 978-1-032-90811-3 (hbk)
ISBN: 978-1-032-90863-2 (pbk)
ISBN: 978-1-003-56020-3 (ebk)

DOI: 10.1201/9781003560203

Typeset in Times
by KnowledgeWorks Global Ltd.

Contents

Preface

Inflammation continues to be a prominent cause of disease worldwide. Inflammatory disorders include but are not limited to diseases of joints, the nervous system, the cardiovascular system, metabolic regulation, and skin. The conventional therapeutic regimens often fail to provide an accurate and sustainable treatment approach. Therefore, exploring an alternative approach is the need of the hour. Stimuli-responsive biomaterials are considered as a promising strategy that can be designed to respond to biological or extrinsic signals in a controlled manner. This feature exhibits high applicability for drug delivery, diagnosis, imaging, and regenerative medicine in inflammation-associated diseases. This book, *Stimuli-Responsive Biomaterials for Inflammatory Diseases: Advances in Research and Clinical Applications*, is designed to offer fundamental theories as well as translational research insights. The first few chapters present the burden of inflammatory diseases, the development of stimuli-responsive biomaterials, and the chemistry behind the design and manufacturing of these biomaterials. The next chapters classify these materials and their applications into disease domains such as cancer, arthritis, neurological disorders, diabetes, obesity, cardiovascular diseases, autoimmune diseases, and chronic wound management. It also covers the applications in other domains of science, technology, and medicine, including the diagnostics and imaging of the materials. Besides disease-related uses, the book also discusses such cutting-edge areas as nanotechnology and intelligent or smart materials. The specialized sections cover emerging applications of artificial intelligence (AI) and machine learning (ML) in drug delivery systems and 3D and 4D bioprinting in the development and fabrication of highly tunable patient-centric smart materials for drug delivery. In concert, these chapters show how material science, computing methods, and translational medicine intersect to manage the unmet challenges in inflammatory diseases. This collection compiles contributions of basic researchers and clinicians in the fields of chemistry, materials science, drug delivery science, biomaterials, pharmacology, and medicine. Their corroborative expertise enlightens the emerging scope in the sensory biomaterial research as well as its limitations and directs the future frontier of material science toward a brighter direction. We would like to acknowledge all the authors for their work and reviewers for providing constructive comments that helped to improve the chapters. We hope that this book will provide advantageous information for graduate students, early-career researchers, and clinicians who would like to explore or investigate the stimuli-responsive biomaterials and their clinical application for inflammatory diseases.

Mohammed Gulzar Ahmed
Vetriselvan Subramaniyan
Sagnik Nag
Sourav Mohanto

Editorial Note

Inflammation and inflammatory disorders are among the most pressing health problems faced by mankind at this point in history. They impact millions of people around the world in several forms (from arthritis and autoimmune diseases to heart disease, diabetes, and stroke). Although there are decades of research and improvement in understanding the pathophysiology and therapeutic areas, treatment is still limited, and relapses or side effects can complicate management. In recent years, researchers and clinicians have begun to explore novel approaches to address inflammatory conditions. An area that has been rapidly growing is the field of "stimuli-responsive biomaterials." Unlike conventionally marketed therapeutic molecules or materials, these are materials meant for sensing the changes in their environment rapidly and responding in a smarter way. These smart biomaterials can release the drug upon change in pH and respond to oxidative stress, temperature change, and enzymatic changes. For inflammatory diseases, the body's internal environment is highly dynamic; the approach could open the floodgate of therapeutic possibilities that are more targeted, less invasive, and more appropriate and tailored to patients' needs.

The genesis of this book stemmed from a fundamental question, i.e., how do we consolidate and directly link this expanding knowledge on these materials with inflammatory diseases? Though a lot of reviews and papers exist, they are in distinct journals and fields. We really needed to create a reference that is organized, comprehensive, useful, and approachable for experts and freshers in the field. The beginning of the book introduces inflammatory diseases and covers the current scenario and the challenges they pose to conventional therapy; the second part focuses on the role of biomaterials in shaping a variety of therapeutic strategies. Initial chapters provide an overview of how so-called stimuli-responsive biomaterials have been developed, the chemistry that underpins their fabrication mechanism, and the classification of biomaterials based on their material and function. These chapters discuss the fundamentals that will cater to the curiosity of the fresh minds who want to initiate their research in these fields. From there, the book escalates into sections on specific diseases. Each chapter discusses and fills the gap between the knowledge of the structure of these biomaterials and the conditions in which they can be used therapeutically. These structure–function bridges help us to embark on a common mechanistic understanding to tackle diverse medical problems employing the same underlying fundamentals. More importantly, the chapters do not simply discuss the theoretical nuances of the materials but call attention to their potential in preclinical and clinical applications.

We also decided to incorporate a chapter focusing on imaging and theranostic applications that may explore artificial intelligence (AI), machine learning (ML), and 3D/4D bioprinting. These topics highlight the rapid progress of stimuli-responsive biomaterial research by bringing together classic biological and medical research with more advanced methods and approaches, inculcating an interdisciplinary approach. Together, they provide a sense of where the field is heading and how future collaborations between engineers, material scientists, and clinicians will be the key to overcoming the challenges. Besides showcasing progress, the book also does not deny the limitations and challenges in current research perspectives. There are also unresolved issues about long-term safety, scalability, and regulatory approval. For these materials to move from bench to bedside, researchers must collaborate closely with industry, clinicians, and policymakers. We hope that this book serves as a reminder of what has been accomplished, as well as a starting point for discussions on what we still need to achieve.

The culmination of this project was possible only due to the dedicated effort and time of many contributors from myriads of academic and clinical backgrounds. Therefore, every author brings the opinion from different viewpoints, such as from a chemical, a biological, and an engineering aspect, converging into clinical application. The collective contributions of these individuals are the sources of the strength of this book, and we express our appreciation for the time and energy they invested in their respective research and systematically penning down the acquired information in the respective fields. We also expect that readers from different segments will like this book for diverse reasons. For experienced researchers, it may be used as a reference for the ongoing research progress. For students and young scientists, it could pave their way into an interesting, result-oriented, fast-progressing field. For clinicians, it could provide clues about where the next generation therapies might head.

In the end, this book is a testament to a collective endeavor to confront some of the most challenging issues in healthcare. Inflammatory conditions are complicated; there is no one-size-fits-all answer. But in our consideration of how new biomaterials can be applied in diverse conditions, we think we are closer to therapies that work better, are accurate, and are more patient-oriented. We are truly grateful to everyone who has contributed to this volume, including reviewers and supportive colleagues. We hope that it will not just expand knowledge but also inspire further progress ahead.

Acknowledgments

Sourav Mohanto dedicates this book to his late mother, Mrs. Smriti Mohanto, in gratitude for her unwavering support and love from the universe. He would also like to express his gratitude to his wife, Mrs. Adrija Bhunia, for her steadfast intellectual support, understanding, and love throughout his academic journey. He would like to acknowledge the Anusandhan National Research Foundation, Department of Science and Technology, Government of India, and Yenepoya (Deemed to be University), India, for providing the research fellowship, resources, and intellectual support to complete this book.

Sagnik Nag would like to sincerely acknowledge his parents, Shri Gobinda Nag and Srimati Sutapa Nag, for their unconditional support and guidance throughout his journey. He is also grateful for the opportunities that life and faith have given him at the right time, which have helped him move forward in meaningful ways. His heartfelt thanks go to his teachers, mentors, friends, and collaborators, each of whom has played an important role in shaping his path and contributing to his growth. Sagnik also extends his gratitude to the Jeffrey Cheah School of Medicine and Health Sciences, Monash University Malaysia, for providing him with the platform, support, and encouragement to pursue his aspirations.

Editor Biographies

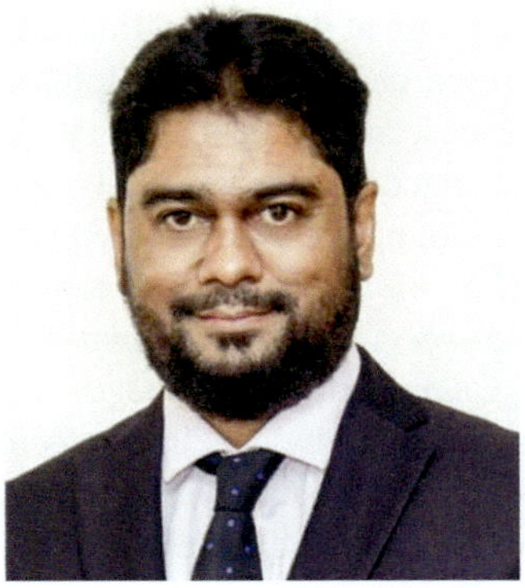

Mohammed Gulzar Ahmed is currently serving as Professor and Dean at Yenepoya Pharmacy College & Research Centre, which is a part of Yenepoya (Deemed to be University), India. He obtained his Master's degree from Manipal College of Pharmaceutical Sciences (MCOPS), India, and completed his Doctorate from Rajiv Gandhi University of Health Sciences, Karnataka, India. He has a strong academic and research record with the witnessed publication of 170+ research and review articles in national and international journals, 12 book chapters, six books, and seven patents to his credit. During his academic career, he has presented over 50 research papers at national and international conferences. He is a reviewer for several highly reputable national and international journals. He has successfully guided more than 25 postgraduate students and supervises 9+ PhD students. Additionally, he has secured research grants from Rajiv Gandhi University of Health Sciences, Yenepoya (Deemed to be University), Vision Group of Science and Technology, Government of Karnataka, and the Anusandhan National Research Foundation, Department of Science and Technology, Government of India.

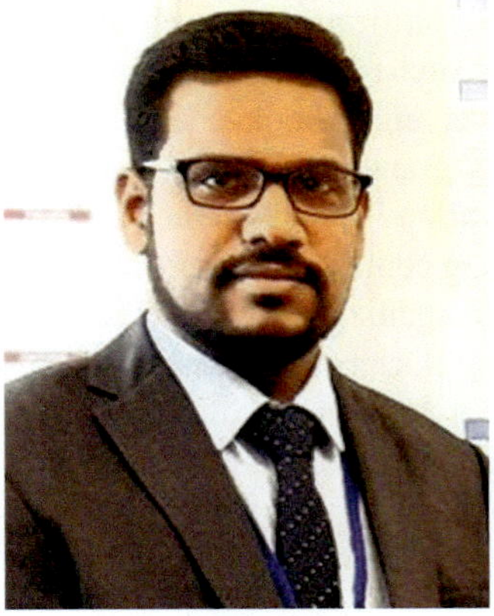

Vetriselvan Subramaniyan is currently serving as Professor of Pharmacology in the Sir Jeffrey Cheah Sunway Medical School at Sunway University. He graduated from Annamalai University, India, and began his academic journey in 2008 at Rajiv Gandhi University of Health Sciences, India. Over his career, he has accumulated more than 15 years of teaching and research experience at prestigious institutions such as Arba Minch University in Ethiopia, MAHSA University in Malaysia, among others. A prolific researcher, Prof. Vetriselvan has authored over 350 papers with a cumulative impact factor exceeding 1000, filed eight patents internationally, and contributed to over six book chapters. His expertise is widely recognized, as evidenced by numerous grants, including a Monash University Research Travel Grant and an FRGS grant from Malaysia's Ministry of Higher Education. He is also ranked among the Top 2% of Scientists in the World according to Stanford University and is Fellow of the Malaysian Scientific Association. Professor Vetriselvan has held prominent academic leadership roles, including serving as Acting Dean, Deputy Dean at MAHSA University, and held visiting and adjunct professorships at institutions in China, Cambodia, and India. His supervisory work is extensive, with 28 completed student research projects and ongoing PhD supervision at multiple international universities. He is an active member of several professional organizations, including the British Pharmacological Society, the Indian Pharmacological Society, the Obesity Society, and the Malaysian Scientific Association. His research focuses on advancing drug development and pharmacology, and he has delivered keynote addresses at over 30 conferences worldwide.

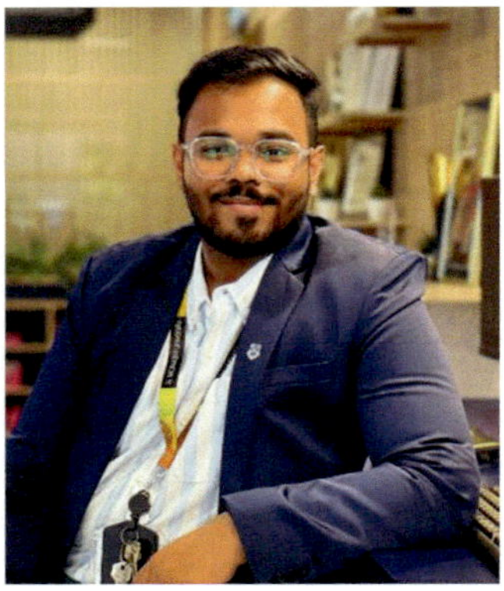

Sagnik Nag is an active nano-biomaterials researcher at Jeffrey Cheah School of Medicine and Health Sciences (JCSMHS), Monash University, Malaysia. He completed his postgraduate studies in the domain of Biotechnology in 2023 with record academic scores from Vellore Institute of Technology (VIT), Tamil Nadu, India. Priorly, he was closely associated with NanoBios Lab at the Indian Institute of Technology, Bombay (IIT-B) as a research trainee in the domain of Biomaterials, Pharmaceutical Sciences, and Drug Delivery. At the budding stage of his career, he managed to obtain 1500+ citations and more than 50 Scopus-indexed publications in reputed high-impact factor journals like *ACS Biomaterials Science & Engineering*, *International Journal of Surgery*, *Travel Medicine and Infectious Disease*, *Materials Today Chemistry*, *ACS Omega*, and *Frontiers in Immunology*. Sagnik's academic pursuits have been characterized by excellence from the outset. With a voracious appetite for knowledge, he embarked on his educational journey, acquiring a strong foundation in pharmaceutical sciences. He was recently conferred and elected as Associate at the Royal Society of Biology.

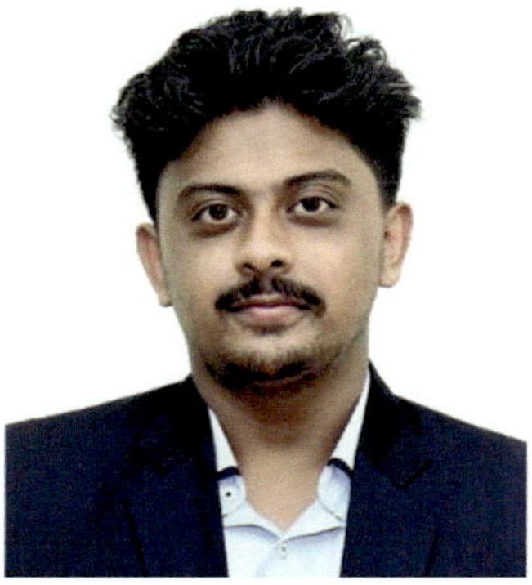

Sourav Mohanto is an active academician and researcher at Yenepoya Pharmacy College & Research Centre, Yenepoya (Deemed to be University), Karnataka, India, and has completed his postgraduate study in the domain of Pharmaceutics from Central University of Sikkim, India. He is closely associated with various research projects related to biomaterials development and utilization, as well as drug-delivery science. As an early career researcher, he obtained numerous high-impact indexed publications, over eight book chapters, over four national and international patents granted/published, and three design patents granted. He has guided various students at the university level and was nominated as an organizing committee member for multiple conference bodies and professional organizations across the globe. He has also been a member of the Royal Society of Chemistry (RSC), the American Chemical Society (ACS), the Controlled Release Society-Indian Local Chapter, the Association of Pharmaceutical Teachers of India (APTI), and many more. Sourav has also been associated with various journals as an editorial board member and reviewer and actively participated in international and national conferences across the globe.

1 Introduction to Inflammatory Diseases

Gaps and Prospects

Anuj Kumar Borah and Chongtham Sovachandra Singh
Department of Biotechnology, Royal School of Biosciences, The Assam Royal Global University, Guwahati, Assam, India

Jiwasmika Baishya
Department of Microbiology, Royal School of Biosciences, The Assam Royal Global University, Guwahati, Assam, India

Sthiti Porna Dutta
Department of Forensic Science, Royal School of Life Sciences, The Assam Royal Global University, Guwahati, Assam, India

Taranga Jyoti Baruah
Department of Microbiology, Royal School of Biosciences, The Assam Royal Global University, Guwahati, Assam, India

Anupam Chatterjee
Department of Biotechnology, Royal School of Biosciences, The Assam Royal Global University, Guwahati, Assam, India

Debabrata Ghoshdastidar
Department of Pharmaceutics, Guru Nanak Institute of Pharmaceutical Science & Technology, Kolkata, West Bengal, India

Amlan Das
Department of Microbiology, Royal School of Biosciences, The Assam Royal Global University, Guwahati, Assam, India

1.1 INTRODUCTION TO INFLAMMATION

1.1.1 Basic Insight into Inflammation: Characteristics and Types

An intricate biological reaction, inflammation, is the response of the immune system to various stimuli, including infections, damaged cells, or irritants. It is an essential system that the body uses to start the healing process and defend against more damage. Inflammation serves to remove the original source of cell damage, remove necrotic cells and tissues that were harmed by the initial shock, and start the healing process. An essential and advantageous process, inflammation aids in

DOI: 10.1201/9781003560203-1

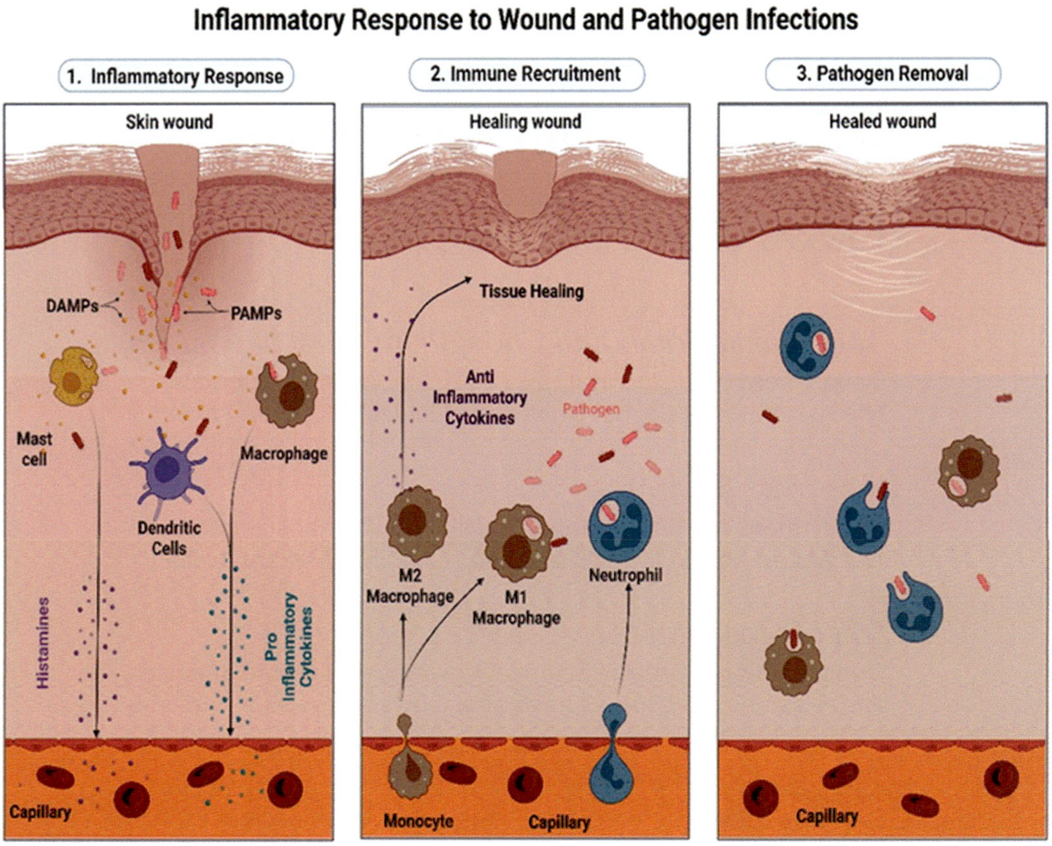

FIGURE 1.1 The inflammatory response to wound healing and pathogen invasion involves inflammatory cells like mast cells, dendritic cells, and macrophages, which recognize DAMPs and PAMPs through PRRs. This triggers the inflammatory response and its resolution, ultimately leading to wound closure, pathogen removal, and tissue repair, ensuring proper healing. (Created with BioRender.com.)

the body's defense against infection and aids in the healing process (Figure 1.1). Inflammation can be broadly categorized into acute and chronic forms. Acute inflammation is the body's immediate defense response to injury or infection, typically resolving within a few days. It is marked by classical signs such as redness, swelling, warmth, pain, and impaired function, with neutrophils being the predominant immune cells involved [1]. The redness (erythema) in acute inflammation results from heightened blood circulation to the affected area due to vasodilation, which is facilitated by factors like histamine acting on vascular smooth muscle. This process begins in the arterioles and extends to open additional capillary beds in the inflamed region. Both blood vessels and lymphatic vessels are essential in acute inflammation. Increased vascular permeability leads to edema, while lymphatic vessels work to drain excess fluid, transporting leukocytes, cell debris, and microbes. These vessels may proliferate during inflammation to manage the increased workload. Finally, the acute inflammatory regulatory mechanisms involving specific chemical mediators and immune cells conclude the response to prevent collateral damage [2].

Chronic inflammation develops gradually, often taking days to manifest, and persists for an extended period, sometimes lasting years. Unlike acute inflammation, its classical signs and symptoms are less evident. The cellular composition typically includes monocytes, macrophages, and lymphocytes [3]. This type of chronic inflammation can occur due to ongoing infections by pathogens like mycobacteria, fungi, viruses, and parasites, which are difficult to eradicate. These infections can trigger delayed hypersensitivity reactions, leading to a granulomatous response or an unresolved acute inflammation transitioning into a chronic phase [4]. Additionally, chronic inflammation can arise due to long-term exposure to harmful substances. Exogenous toxins, such as silica dust causing silicosis, and endogenous factors, like high cholesterol leading to atherosclerosis, are common examples [5]. It is also implicated in non-traditional inflammatory disorders, such as Alzheimer's disease, type 2 diabetes, metabolic syndrome, and certain cancers, where inflammatory mechanisms support disease progression and tumor development.

1.1.2 Inflammatory Diseases Due to Acute and Chronic Inflammatory Responses

Inflammatory diseases occur as a result of imbalanced acute or chronic inflammatory responses, which are essential biological processes activated in response to tissue damage, infections, or detrimental stimuli. Inflammation has a twofold function; it acts as an essential protective mechanism that aids immune responses, yet it can also lead to considerable tissue damage if it becomes excessive [2]. The inflammatory response begins when pattern recognition receptors (PRRs), including toll-like receptors (TLRs) found on immune cells such as macrophages and dendritic cells identify pathogen-associated molecular patterns (PAMPs) or damage-associated molecular patterns (DAMPs). The acknowledgment activates intracellular signaling pathways, including the nuclear factor kappa B (NF-κB) pathway, which ultimately leads to the generation of pro-inflammatory cytokines, chemokines, and lipid mediators [6].

Acute inflammation is a rapid and short-term response marked by enhanced vascular permeability, the infiltration of leukocytes, and the secretion of inflammatory products like prostaglandins (PGs), leukotrienes (LTs), and histamines. Neutrophils are crucial during this stage as they move to the injury location via chemotaxis, influenced by signals like interleukin-8 (IL-8) and complement proteins. These cells remove pathogens and cellular debris through processes such as phagocytosis, degranulation, and the secretion of neutrophil extracellular traps (NETs) [7]. However, the overactivation of neutrophils may result in unintended harm to surrounding tissues due to the discharge of proteolytic enzymes and reactive oxygen species (ROS). Under normal circumstances, acute inflammation resolves through the action of specialized pro-resolving lipid mediators such as lipoxins, resolvins, and protectins, which promote macrophage-mediated clearance of apoptotic cells and restoration of tissue homeostasis [8, 9].

Chronic inflammation occurs when the process of resolution does not succeed, resulting in prolonged immune activation and damage to tissues. In contrast to acute inflammation, which mainly features neutrophils, chronic inflammation is driven by monocytes, macrophages, and lymphocytes [2]. The ongoing activation of macrophages leads to a steady release of cytokines that promote inflammation, such as tumor necrosis factor-alpha (TNF-α), interleukin-1 beta (IL-1β), and interleukin-6 (IL-6). This process maintains the inflammatory response and contributes to tissue remodeling and fibrosis by activating fibroblasts and promoting excessive deposition of extracellular matrix. The adaptive immune system is crucial, particularly T-helper cells (Th1 and Th17), which enhance sustained inflammation by releasing interferon-gamma (IFN-γ) and interleukin-17 (IL-17). This process aids in the recruitment and activation of additional immune cells [10].

The extended existence of inflammatory substances in chronic inflammation is fundamental to numerous diseases. In cases of autoimmune disorders, an abnormal immune reaction directed at self-antigens results in ongoing inflammation and damage to tissues. In conditions such as rheumatoid arthritis, inflammatory cytokines contribute to synovial hyperplasia and the breakdown of cartilage, while in multiple sclerosis, immune-mediated harm to the myelin sheath disrupts neuronal function. Chronic intestinal inflammation characterizes inflammatory bowel diseases (IBDs), such as Crohn's disease and ulcerative colitis, which are influenced by imbalanced immune reactions to gut microbiota.

In different situations, ongoing inflammation plays a role in metabolic and cardiovascular conditions. Atherosclerosis begins with the buildup of oxidized low-density lipoproteins (LDL) within the walls of arteries, which results in the infiltration of macrophages and the creation of foam cells. The persistent secretion of inflammatory substances like TNF-α and IL-1β contributes to endothelial impairment and plaque instability, heightening the likelihood of thrombosis and cardiovascular incidents. In a similar manner, chronic obstructive pulmonary disease (COPD) results from extended exposure to irritants such as cigarette smoke, which triggers ongoing activation of macrophages and neutrophils. This process contributes to airway remodeling and ongoing lung damage due to the overproduction of matrix metalloproteinases (MMPs) and proteolytic enzymes [4].

Neuroinflammation is crucial in the context of neurodegenerative diseases like Alzheimer's disease, where the persistent activation of microglia results in continuous cytokine release and oxidative stress, which in turn worsens neuronal loss and the buildup of amyloid-beta plaques. This ongoing inflammatory condition interferes with synaptic activity and plays a role in cognitive deterioration, demonstrating that inflammation affects neurological well-being in ways that go beyond the immune system [11]. Overall, inflammatory diseases result from intricate immune processes that, while initially protective, can become detrimental when dysregulated. Grasping the processes at the molecular and cellular level that control inflammation offers essential knowledge for developing therapeutic approaches designed to adjust immune responses and avert significant tissue harm. Strategies aimed at inflammatory cytokines, immune cell signaling pathways, and resolution mechanisms show the potential to reduce the effects of chronic inflammatory diseases and enhance patient outcomes.

1.2 PATHOPHYSIOLOGY AND MOLECULAR SIGNATURES OF INFLAMMATORY DISEASES

1.2.1 Immune Cells and Inflammation

The inflammatory response varies depending on the nature and location of the initiating stimulus. However, all the responses follow a general mechanism that can be outlined as: (1) activation of PRRs; (2) initiation of inflammatory signaling pathways; (3) secretion of inflammatory mediators, including chemical mediators like cytokines and chemokines; and (4) recruitment of immune cells to the site of inflammation. This coordinated response aims to eliminate the stimulus and initiate tissue repair [2] (Figure 1.1).

1.2.2 Activation of Pattern-Recognition Receptors

The PRRs expressed on the cell surface of both immune and nonimmune recognize microbial structures called PAMPs. Similarly, some PRRs can also recognize various endogenous DAMPs and host biomolecules activated during tissue or cell damage. DAMPs are essential in triggering and sustaining inflammation that does not involve infection. In the event that cells are disrupted, they release DAMPs, which can draw innate immune cells to the site of damage even in the absence of pathogens. PRR protein families include TLRs, C-type lectin receptors (CLRs), retinoic acid-inducible gene (RIG) I-like receptors (RLRs), and nucleotide-binding oligomerization domain (NOD)-like receptors (NLRs) [12]. Transduction of signals triggered by PAMPs and DAMPs are mediated by myeloid differentiation factors-88 (MyD88) in conjunction with TLRs, initiating a cascade of intracellular signaling processes that eventually result in the translocation of key transcription factors to the nucleus, including AP-1, NF-κB, and IRF3 [13].

1.2.3 Initiation of Inflammatory Signaling Pathways

Inflammatory pathways play a significant role in the development of several chronic diseases, involving key mediators and regulatory mechanisms. These pathways are activated by various stimuli, including microbial components and cytokines such as IL-1β, IL-6, and TNF-α. These inflammatory signals interact with receptors such as the TLRs, IL-1R, IL-6R, and TNFR. The activation of these receptors' triggers key signaling cascades, such as the MAPK, NF-κB, and JAK-STAT pathways, which regulate the inflammatory response and contribute to the advancement of the disease [14].

1.2.4 Release of Inflammatory Mediators

In response to stimuli, immune cells like macrophages and adipocytes are activated, leading to the release of inflammatory cytokines, including ILs, TNFs, IFNs, chemokines, and TGFs, alongside other inflammatory proteins and enzymes. Cytokines, primarily secreted by monocytes, macrophages, and lymphocytes, are crucial in regulating inflammation. These molecules can either exacerbate (pro-inflammatory) or alleviate (anti-inflammatory) inflammation, largely by attracting leukocytes to the site of injury or infection to aid in defense or repair. The intricate cytokine network also manages the immune response to infection and inflammation. However, excessive production of cytokine can lead to harmful outcomes, such as tissue damage, disrupted blood flow, organ failure, or even death. In addition, inflammatory proteins like C-reactive protein (CRP), haptoglobin, serum amyloid A, fibrinogen, and alpha-1-acid glycoprotein assist in tissue repair and the defense against infection. These proteins support homeostasis during stress, trauma, or infection, acting alongside the immune system to restore balance [15].

1.2.5 Immune Cells Response

The inflammatory response involves coordinated interaction of various immune cells, such as activated macrophages, monocytes, and neutrophils. At the injured tissue, epithelial and endothelial cells secrete signaling factors, triggering an inflammatory signaling cascade that attracts neutrophils, monocytes, mast cells, and lymphocytes [2]. Neutrophils are the first responders, targeting pathogens, but they can also damage host tissues [16]. Monocytes migrate into injured tissue and differentiate into macrophages or dendritic cells. Macrophages play key roles in inflammation, from initiation and maintenance to resolution, by presenting antigens, phagocytosing pathogens, and releasing cytokines. Mast cells, present in connective tissue and epithelial surfaces, release mediators like histamine and cytokines, driving inflammation [17]. Platelets also influence inflammation, with their interactions with immune cells affecting conditions like atherosclerosis and infection. The acute phase response (APR), triggered by infection or injury, is amplified by immune cells releasing inflammatory mediators, sustaining the inflammatory process [18].

To prevent the progression from acute to chronic inflammation, it is essential to suppress the inflammatory response to avoid further tissue damage. Inflammation resolution is a tightly controlled process involving mediator production, during which chemokine gradients diminish over time. Eventually, white blood cells no longer detect these gradients, stopping their recruitment to the injury site. Dysregulation of this process can result in uncontrolled chronic inflammation. The key processes in inflammation resolution include the reduction of neutrophil infiltration, neutrophil apoptosis, counter-regulation of cytokines, macrophage polarization, and the initiation of healing [19]. Chronic inflammation arises when acute inflammation fails to resolve tissue injury, contributing to diseases such as cardiovascular issues, atherosclerosis, type 2 diabetes, rheumatoid arthritis, and cancer. Understanding the mechanisms behind this dysfunction can aid in developing more effective targeted therapies.

1.2.6 Cytokines and Chemokines in Inflammation

Cytokines and chemokines are small proteins that act as critical regulators of inflammation and immunity. They facilitate cell-to-cell communication, modulating immune responses to ensure homeostasis and protect against pathogens. They have low molecular weight and serve as messengers that influence the behavior of either the cell producing them (autocrine), nearby cells (paracrine), or distant cells (endocrine). Their involvement is crucial in both acute and chronic inflammatory processes, as well as in tissue repair and immune surveillance. Cytokines exert their effects by binding to specific receptors on the surface of target cells or, in soluble form, by circulating in plasma. This interaction initiates intracellular signaling pathways that regulate a range of cellular processes, including activation, proliferation, migration, differentiation, and apoptosis. These signaling cascades play a crucial role in maintaining immune balance but can also contribute to pathological conditions when dysregulated. For instance, excessive cytokine activity is often observed in autoimmune diseases and chronic inflammatory disorders. Cytokines are categorized based on their structure, origin, or function. Key functional groups include the following:

- *Interleukins (ILs)*: Mediators produced by leukocytes that act on other immune cells, facilitating communication and coordination within the immune system.
- *Interferons (IFNs)*: Known for their antiviral activity and regulatory roles in the immune response.
- *Colony-Stimulating Factors (CSFs)*: Essential for the differentiation and proliferation of hematopoietic stem cells.
- *TNFs*: Central to the regulation of immune responses and inflammation.
- *Transforming Growth Factors (TGFs)*: Involved in tissue remodeling and immune suppression.

Cytokines are further classified as pro-inflammatory or anti-inflammatory, depending on their effects on immune activity. Pro-inflammatory cytokines, such as IL-1, TNF-α, and IL-6, promote inflammation and mobilize immune cells to sites of injury or infection. Conversely, anti-inflammatory cytokines like IL-10 and TGF-β counteract these effects, preventing excessive immune activation and tissue damage. Pro-inflammatory cytokines are heavily implicated in the pathogenesis of various diseases. They are crucial during the early phases of infection or injury, helping to recruit immune cells and initiate tissue repair. However, their overproduction or prolonged activity can lead to chronic inflammation and tissue damage, contributing to diseases like asthma, rheumatoid arthritis, psoriasis, and cancer. IL-1 is a potent pro-inflammatory cytokine composed of two forms: IL-1α and IL-1β. IL-1α is released by necrotic cells and acts as a DAMP to signal tissue injury. IL-1β, on the other hand, is primarily produced by activated macrophages and plays a pivotal role in acute and chronic inflammation. IL-1β recruits granulocytes, promotes the production of PGs, and facilitates the activation of adaptive immunity through T-helper cells. TNF is another critical pro-inflammatory cytokine divided into TNF-α and TNF-β (lymphotoxin-α). TNF-α, produced by macrophages, T cells, and other immune cells, induces the expression of inflammatory genes, stimulates immune responses, and contributes to cell death in infected or damaged tissues. Overactivation of TNF-α is associated with chronic inflammatory diseases like Crohn's disease, rheumatoid arthritis, and psoriasis. Targeting TNF-α through inhibitors has become a cornerstone in the treatment of autoimmune diseases.

Chemokines, a subclass of cytokines, specialize in guiding the migration and positioning of immune cells to specific locations in response to infection, injury, or inflammation. These small, structurally conserved molecules bind to G protein-coupled receptors (GPCRs) on leukocytes, initiating intracellular signaling pathways that regulate cellular adhesion, migration, and activation. The chemokine system is a finely tuned network categorized into homeostatic and inflammatory chemokines. Homeostatic chemokines maintain normal immune surveillance and lymphoid tissue architecture, while inflammatory chemokines are upregulated during immune responses to recruit leukocytes like neutrophils, monocytes, and lymphocytes to affected sites. Chemokines such as CXCL8 (IL-8) and CCL2 (monocyte chemoattractant protein-1) play pivotal roles in early inflammation. CXCL8 recruits neutrophils to sites of infection, facilitating pathogen clearance, while CCL2 attracts monocytes that differentiate into macrophages to amplify immune responses.

However, in chronic inflammatory diseases, this system often becomes dysregulated, leading to persistent inflammation and tissue damage. For instance, in rheumatoid arthritis, synovial tissues show elevated levels of chemokines like CCL2 and CXCL10, which attract monocytes and T cells, perpetuating local inflammation and cartilage destruction. Similarly, in IBD, chemokines such as CXCL8 exacerbate epithelial damage and immune cell infiltration, disrupting gut homeostasis.

Chronic inflammation involves sustained cytokine activity, often contributing to the progression of autoimmune and allergic diseases. Cytokines like IL-4, IL-5, and IL-13 are heavily implicated in asthma, where they drive mucus overproduction, eosinophilic inflammation, and bronchial hyperreactivity. IL-6, a multifunctional cytokine, is involved in immune regulation, acute phase responses, and hematopoiesis. However, its excessive production is linked to diseases such as multiple myeloma, rheumatoid arthritis, and Castleman's disease [20]. The dual-edged nature of chemokines becomes evident in conditions such as asthma, multiple sclerosis, and cancer. In asthma, CCL11 (eotaxin) recruits' eosinophils to the airway, driving inflammation and tissue remodeling. In multiple sclerosis, chemokines like CXCL10 mediate the migration of autoreactive T cells into the central nervous system, causing demyelination and neuronal damage. In cancer, the tumor microenvironment leverages chemokines such as CXCL12 to recruit immunosuppressive cells, enhance angiogenesis, and facilitate metastasis.

Fibrosis also underscores the pathological potential of chemokines. Chronic chemokine activity, particularly through CCL2 and CCL13, stimulates fibroblast activation and extracellular matrix deposition, leading to tissue scarring and organ dysfunction. In systemic sclerosis, a fibrotic disease, aberrant chemokine expression is implicated in vascular damage and collagen overproduction. IL-6 is produced by a variety of cells, including T cells, macrophages, and endothelial cells. While essential for normal immune function and hematopoiesis, excessive IL-6 levels can lead to severe inflammatory responses. IL-6 inhibitors, such as tocilizumab, have shown therapeutic efficacy in autoimmune diseases and cytokine-release syndromes [20]. Understanding the roles of cytokines in inflammation has paved the way for targeted therapies. Blocking specific cytokines or their receptors has proven effective in managing autoimmune diseases, chronic inflammation, and even some cancers. Examples include the following:

- *Anti-TNF Therapies*: Widely used in rheumatoid arthritis and IBDs.
- *IL-4 and IL-13 Inhibitors*: Effective in treating asthma and other allergic conditions.
- *IL-6 Inhibitors*: Used in cytokine release syndromes and autoimmune disorders.
- *IL-7 Therapy*: Promising in restoring immune function in conditions like sepsis and COVID-19.

The central role of chemokines in inflammation has made them attractive targets for therapeutic intervention. Strategies include chemokine receptor antagonists, neutralizing antibodies, and small-molecule inhibitors. For example, maraviroc, a CCR5 antagonist, has shown promise in inflammatory and fibrotic diseases. Similarly, CXCR4 inhibitors like plerixafor disrupt chemokine-mediated tumor progression and metastasis. These advances underscore the potential of chemokine-targeted therapies in managing autoimmune diseases, chronic inflammation, and cancer. Cytokines and chemokines are indispensable components of the immune system, orchestrating the complex interplay between inflammation, tissue repair, and immune regulation. Their roles in mediating both protective and pathological processes highlight their dual-edged nature. A deeper understanding of cytokine biology not only elucidates the mechanisms underlying inflammatory diseases but also opens avenues for innovative therapeutic strategies aimed at restoring immune balance and mitigating disease progression.

1.2.7 Prostaglandin and Leukotriene as Modulator of Inflammation

Eicosanoids, derived from arachidonic acids, are lipid mediators that play significant roles in inflammation and various biological functions. The two main families of eicosanoids are PGs and LTs. Arachidonic acid is released from cell membrane phospholipids by phospholipase A2 in response to stimuli and undergoes oxidation through the cyclooxygenase (COX) or 5-lipoxygenase (5-LO) pathways [21]. These pathways then generate the bioactive lipid mediators—PGs and LTs—essential for homeostasis and pivotal in inflammatory processes [22]. The COX pathway converts arachidonic acid into PGs and thromboxanes, which are involved in critical processes like platelet aggregation and smooth muscle contraction. COX-1 and COX-2 produce PGs, which regulate inflammation, vascular tone, and labor. Some of the major proteins are PTGE2 (engaged in vasodilation and vascular leakage), PTGD2 (related to mast cell maturation and eosinophil recruitment), PTGF2 (involved in smooth muscle contraction), and PTGI2 (connected with platelet aggregation inhibition). LTs, which are generated by 5-LO, are crucial in illnesses such as asthma and allergies. LTB4 attracts neutrophils and activates leukocytes to start inflammation, whereas cysteinyl LTs (CysLTs- LTC4, LTD4, and LTE4) cause bronchoconstriction and vascular leakage, which impact smooth muscle and vascular permeability. The LO pathway generates hydroperoxy acids including 12-HETE and 5-HETE, which are precursors to LTs. Both PGs and LTs function by binding to specific GPCRs [23]. PGs interact with receptors such as PTGFR, PTGIR, and TXA2R, whereas LTs bind to BLTR1, BLTR2, CysLTR1, and CysLTR2. NSAIDs and LT modifiers inhibit COX enzymes, which reduces PG production and LT levels, respectively. NSAIDs can also direct arachidonic acid metabolism to the LO pathway, potentially boosting LT synthesis and worsening asthma or urticaria. Genetic differences, such as single nucleotide polymorphisms in the PG and LT receptor genes, can affect receptor function, disease risk, and medication responses. Understanding these genetic markers sheds light on disorders such as NSAID hypersensitivity, which is the most frequent drug-related hypersensitivity [24]. Exploring eicosanoid biosynthesis and its precise enzymatic regulation, emphasizing PGs' local action and LTs' role in immune responses, will lead to advances in this field by informing about the therapeutic strategies for inflammatory diseases and disorders.

1.3 CONVENTIONAL DIAGNOSIS AND THERAPY FOR VARIOUS INFLAMMATORY DISEASES

The inflammatory reaction is not possible without PGs and LTs. Recent research underlines the importance of genetic variants in PG and leukotriene receptors related to disease sensitivity and treatment responses (Table 1.1). Variations in PTGFR, PTGI2, and related genes have been linked to glaucoma, asthma, and several cardiovascular illnesses. While PTGI2 polymorphisms including A984C increase platelet aggregation and the risk of cerebral infarction, PTGFR influences the efficacy of latanoprost in glaucoma patients. Though the results are often contradictory, polymorphisms in the PTGDR gene—more especially, −441C>T and −197T>C—have been associated with allergy disorders and asthma in several populations. Asthma is linked to CRTH2 variations including rs11571288 and rs545659; functional tests show higher Th2 cytokine production and enhanced mRNA stability [25]. Preterm birth, asthma, and hypertension are associated with variants in PTGER2 and PTGER3. By their impact on transcription factor binding and gene expression, polymorphisms in PTGER4—including rs77208—are also linked to Crohn's disease and inflammation. PGE2 causes nociception, edema, and erythema; LTB4 is implicated in leukocyte recruitment. Rat studies show that eicosapentaenoic acid (EPA) reduces PGE2 and TXB2 levels in inflammatory exudates and lowers paw edema; it has little effect on LTB4 levels or leukocyte numbers. By restricting PG synthesis, EPA reduces inflammation and offers a non-toxic method free of interference with leukocyte recruitment or triene PG synthesis [24]. Variants of TBXA2R, including V80E and rs76896, affect thrombosis and risk of atherosclerosis as well as platelet function. Furthermore, associated with the severity of asthma and NSAID-exacerbated respiratory illness (NERD) are TBXA2R SNPs including rs133060 and 924C>T. Through changes in gene expression and ligand potency, variants in CYSLTR1 and CYSLTR2—such as −634C>T and 601A>G—affect asthma, atopy, and NSAID-induced diseases [22].

TABLE 1.1
Summary of the Diseases and Disorders Caused by Different Variations of PGs and LTs Receptors

Variants of PGs and LTs	Associated Disease and Disorder	References
PTGFR	Latanoprost in glaucoma patients	[23]
PTGI2 variants like A984C	Platelet aggregation and cerebral infarction	[23]
PTGDR polymorphisms such as −441C>T and −197T>C	Asthma and allergies	[25]
CRTH2 variants including rs11571288 and rs545659	Asthma, increased mRNA stability and enhanced Th2 cytokine expression	[25]
Variants in PTGER2 and PTGER3	Asthma, hypertension and preterm birth	[24]
PTGER4 polymorphisms such as rs7720838	Crohn's disease and inflammation	[24]
PGE2	promotes edema, redness, and pain,	[24]
TBXA2R variants like rs768963 and V80E	Atherosclerosis, thrombosis, platelet function	[22]
TBXA2R SNPs such as rs13306046 and 924C>T	Severe asthma and NSAID-exacerbated respiratory disease (NERD)	[22]
Variants in CYSLTR1 and CYSLTR2, including −634C>T and 601A>G	Asthma, atopy, and NSAID-induced conditions	[22, 24]
LTB4	Recruitment of leukocytes	[24]

Although many genetic associations are population-specific, advancements in genomics, including next-generation sequencing and integrative omics, deepen our understanding of these pathways by predicting the functional effects of SNPs, providing insights into protein structures and functions, *etc.* Additionally, population-specific genetic findings highlight the importance of larger, ethnically diverse cohorts and advanced genomic technologies. Integrating transcriptomics, metabolomics, and bioinformatics is expected to refine our understanding of genetic contributions to inflammation, paving the way for personalized medicine.

1.4 TREATMENT OF INFLAMMATORY DISEASES—GAPS AND CHALLENGES

Significant progress has been made in addressing the severe consequences of chronic inflammation, yet an effective treatment regimen for inflammatory diseases remains elusive. This is largely due to several key challenges in inflammation research, including the lack of robust biomarkers, limited mechanistic understanding, difficulties in developing personalized therapies, resistance to conventional treatments, and the complex transition from acute to chronic inflammation. These gaps continue to hinder the development of more effective and targeted interventions.

1.4.1 Biomarkers

In response to damage, illness, or trauma, the immune system releases specific proteins and substances into the bloodstream during inflammation. These proteins, referred to as acute phase reactants, function as inflammatory biomarkers, indicating the body's immunological reaction. Inflammation is a multifaceted process involving numerous interacting pathways, as evidenced by the diverse array of measurable biomarkers. Common biomarkers encompass CRP, procalcitonin (PCT), neopterin, PG E2 (PGE2), serum amyloid A, cytokines (such as IL-1β), alpha-1-acid glycoprotein, mannose-binding lectin, ceruloplasmin, hepcidin, and haptoglobin. Furthermore, parameters such as the erythrocyte sedimentation rate (ESR), leukocyte count, and the leukocyte–monocyte ratio are utilized to assess inflammation levels. Biomarkers facilitate early diagnosis, elucidate disease progression, and inform therapy options.

Although other biomarkers exist, ESR, CRP, and PCT are predominantly utilized in clinical practice owing to various limitations associated with alternative indicators. A major concern is the absence of uniformity. Current biomarkers lack globally agreed reference values, complicating accurate inflammation assessment and potentially hindering clinical decision-making and patient care [26]. Even the most often utilized biomarkers—ESR, CRP, and PCT—have no consistent ranges to fairly evaluate the degree of inflammation. Furthermore, many of these indicators need repeated testing to guarantee consistent findings. The expression and release of acute phase reactants depend on age and sex, hence, reference values particular to age and sex become even more important. An adult's "normal" degree of inflammation, for instance, can be different for a youngster or an elderly person. Although some more recent biomarkers—like NF-κB—show promise as markers of inflammation—they also provide difficulties. Tissue- and time-specific NF-κB levels hamper interpretation [27]. Another promising marker, GlycA, found in plasma or serum, could offer useful information; however, measuring it requires an expensive method known as nuclear magnetic resonance (NMR) [27]. Additionally, markers like ICAM-1 and VCAM-1 are not direct indicators of inflammation but may provide supporting information [28]. Given these challenges, it is recommended that at least two complementary markers be used to assess inflammation accurately, such as combining a cytokine with an acute phase protein (APP), to provide a more complete picture of the body's inflammatory response [27].

Inflammation is an intricate biological process essential for the body's response to injury, infection, or harmful stimuli. Infectious agents, non-infectious agents, and cellular damage are the primary triggers of numerous interactions among various cytokines, immune cells, and a range of other proteinaceous and non-proteinaceous factors. Acute inflammation serves as a crucial and advantageous response; however, chronic inflammation may lead to tissue damage and contribute to the onset of various diseases. Comprehending the mechanisms that drive inflammation is essential for formulating effective treatment strategies [29]. The inflammatory process is complex, involving a sequence of events, including the activation of specialized immune cells, the release of various cytokines, and the initiation of multiple signaling pathways. This makes it particularly challenging to identify the root mechanism that mediates acute to chronic transformation of inflammation. While NF-κB, MAPK, and JAK-STAT signaling are classically recognized contributors to inflammation, their cross-talk with other signaling molecules and pathways worsen the problem [2]. Further, with the progressive understanding of inflammation, newer and robust inflammation hubs such as NRLP3 inflammasome are being discovered, necessitating novel therapeutic interventions.

A further limitation in our comprehension is the organ-specific characteristics of inflammatory processes. Inflammation exhibits varying effects and consequences contingent upon the specific organ or tissue affected. Neuroinflammation, characterized by inflammation in the nervous system, can be detrimental and play a significant role in the onset of various neurological disorders. The role of the gut microbiome in inflammation contributes to the complexity of the issue. Gut microbial dysbiosis leads to intestinal barrier impairment, pathogen colonization, and inflammation in metabolic disorders. Infectious agents, non-infectious agents, and cellular damage are primary triggers of numerous interactions among various cytokines, immune cells, and a range of proteinaceous and non-proteinaceous factors. The microbiota is also connected to the release of various cytokines, pro- and anti-inflammatory from immune cells such as T-reg cells and Th17 cells. For instance, *Lactobacillus rhamnosus* and *Lactobacillus reuteri* influence T-reg cell production of IL-10 which is anti-inflammatory in action [30]. Gut microbial changes-reduction in beneficial bacterium such as *Bifidobacterium* and *Lactobacillus* and increased colonization of detrimental species such as *Firmicutes*, *Streptococcus*, and *Staphylococcus* are reportedly connected to enhanced expression of inflammatory cytokines (e.g., IL-6, IL-1β, and TNF-α) and reduced expression of anti-inflammatory cytokines (e.g., IL-10) [31]. Considering the involvement of multiple players, multiple routes to inflammation, and tissue and time-dependent course of inflammation, the precise mechanistic insights often remain unmet complicating treatment regimens.

1.4.2 Personalized Medicine

While a range of pathological signatures and signaling pathways have been understood, the underlying mechanism of inflammation may vary from person to person. Genetic predisposition remains a common observation in inflammation and inflammation-driven disease. Genetic signatures for different inflammatory disease phenotypes are now known to provide substantial inputs in the development of personalized treatment programs that are customized to the individual patient's unique characteristics, ultimately enhancing the efficacy of the interventions [32]. A promising framework for treating inflammatory conditions is also the idea of "4P medicine"—personalization, prediction, prevention, and participation—which emphasizes actively involving patients in their own care and giving them the power to make treatment decisions [33].

The first hurdle in personalized or precision medicine is a unique, patient-specific robust biomarker. Generally, *diagnostic*, *prognostic*, or *predictive* biomarkers are at the heart of precision medicine. A diagnostic biomarker, such as serum prostate-specific antigen (PSA), would enable early diagnosis of a disease way before the symptoms arise. A prognostic marker is a sound indicator of progression, remission, and clinical events that may arise in due course of time, whereas a predictive biomarker can reveal whether a person would respond to a particular drug or not. This is particularly because of genetic variants [34]. Personalized medicines can be stratified to provide matching therapy for a precise set of patient populations with unique clinical biomarkers [35]. For an effective treatment regimen, however, biomarker combinations may be utilized. While personalized medicine sounds promising, many other hurdles are there. Apart from individual genotypes, epigenetic modifications, lifestyle, and environment many times are the central controller of the strength of inflammation. Further, the gut microbial profile also changes with individuals, making it hard to understand disease biology. Thus, integration of omics-based approaches such as genomics, transcriptomics, proteomics, epigenomics, metabolomics, phenomics, and microbiomics are of high demand and value in personalized medicine [34]. While rodent systems are used for pharmacogenomics and pharmacogenetics analysis, there is a lack of variability in such systems, which is a prerequisite for basic and translation research in precision medicine [36]. Various organoid models and machine-learning approaches are being considered currently to fill these gaps. Bioelectronic therapy is another area envisaged to augment precision medicine in controlling inflammation.

1.4.3 Conventional Treatment Resistance

Inflammation, a vital cascade of events including the detection and elimination of infection and anomalies in tissue damage, is a double-edged sword. When it becomes chronic and unresolved, inflammation becomes detrimental. For a resolution to be successful, endogenous programs must be activated, pro-inflammatory molecules must be switched to pro-resolving ones, such as annexin-A1 and certain lipid mediators, and granulocytes must be eliminated by apoptosis, which is then removed by nearby macrophages [37]. Current anti-inflammatory treatments, such as nonsteroidal anti-inflammatory medications, glucocorticoid (GC) receptor agonists, and antibodies for pro-inflammatory cytokines, particularly aim to reduce or neutralize the concentration of pro-inflammatory mediators and prevent leukocyte recruitment and activation. Short-term inflammation can be efficiently reduced by these treatments, but they frequently do not address the root causes of chronic inflammation, which can lead to treatment resistance and a recurrence of the inflammatory illness. On the other hand, pro-resolution-based strategies can tackle multiple inflammatory conditions [37]. Nevertheless, treatment resistance over time has been a vital challenge. Out of the many factors correlated with treatment resistance in inflammation, the genetic factor remains the central one. Mutation in genes of cytokine receptors such as TNF receptor or IL-1 receptor are associated with diversified responses to anti-TNF biologics to tackle inflammation [38]. Similarly, the metabolism of drugs and immune cell signaling may also change with genetic changes contributing to treatment resistance. As discussed in earlier sections of this state of art, inflammation is an intricate interplay between several signaling pathways, and thus, blocking one signaling pathway is not going to fully shut down the inflammatory cascade of events. Immune tolerance to therapeutics is another cause of treatment resistance. Gut microbial dysbiosis can change immune responses, impacting how inflammation develops and how well a treatment works [39]. Extant pieces of evidence reveal that changes in gut microbiota may lead to reduced response to treatments like GCs or TNF inhibitors [40]. Furthermore, some gut microbes may directly worsen inflammation, which would make treatment results much more challenging. Further, variability in drug metabolism, cellular heterogeneity, and tissue-specific responses to anti-inflammatory biologics may exaggerate treatment resistance.

The unique beauty of predictive biomarkers can be utilized to tackle treatment resistance, which provides informed decisions to avoid ineffective therapeutics [34]. Further, newer robust signaling proteins and pathways, which are the central hubs to several signaling pathways linked to inflammation, can be targeted. Selective immunomodulation is also thought to be a sound means to tackle treatment resilience. Apart from these, targeted drug delivery and theragnostic measures may be developed to tackle the issues with conventional treatments.

1.4.4 Chronic Inflammation and Immune Response to Acute Challenges

The immune system's reaction to acute challenges that include infection and cellular insults is vital to neutralize the threat and initiate the healing process. This is particularly achieved through activation of immune cells and production of various cytokines which are pro-inflammatory in nature. However, such inflammation is immediate, localized, and self-limiting. And also serves as a mechanism to prevent future damage. Acute responses often restore the equilibrium if it is resolved promptly. On the other hand, chronic inflammation is a result of persistent inflammation that arises due to multiple reasons including long-term exposure to infections, environmental influence, and lifestyle. Chronic inflammation is represented by continued immunological activation, elevated and sustained cytokines, and ROS which in due course of time lead to tissue damage [41]. Despite the significant advancements in understanding inflammation, the shift from acute to chronic status still needs to be decoded. Nevertheless, a number of variables, including genetic predisposition and environmental effects, are known to be the key players [32]. Early detection of inflammation (at the asymptotic state) and understanding possible progression and remission through biomarkers may provide a measure to tackle inflammation and avoid chronicity [34]. SPMs, or specialized pro-resolving mediators, aid in tissue healing and the cessation of the inflammatory response [42]. Nowadays, it is well acknowledged that acute responses are essential for rapid defense, but acute-to-chronicity needs intervention and resolution.

1.5 SCOPE OF STIMULI-RESPONSIVE BIOMATERIALS AND NANOMEDICINE

Conventional treatments for inflammatory conditions, such as NSAIDs and corticosteroids, often provide temporary relief and cause adverse effects due to their systemic nature and inability to precisely target inflammation sites. This has driven research into more effective and targeted therapies using biomaterials and nanotechnology. Biomaterials, engineered from natural or synthetic sources, offer several advantages for drug delivery, including biocompatibility, biodegradability, and the ability to be modified for specific purposes (Figure 1.2). These materials can deliver therapeutic agents directly to inflamed tissues while minimizing side effects. Nanoparticles can penetrate biological barriers more effectively due to their small size and enable the controlled release of drugs. They also offer the potential to modulate the immune response, enhancing therapeutic outcomes. The combination of stimuli-responsive biomaterials and nanoparticles creates a powerful platform for targeted, controlled drug delivery. This innovative approach overcomes the limitations of traditional treatments, offering promising solutions for inflammatory disease management. The ability to deliver therapeutic agents

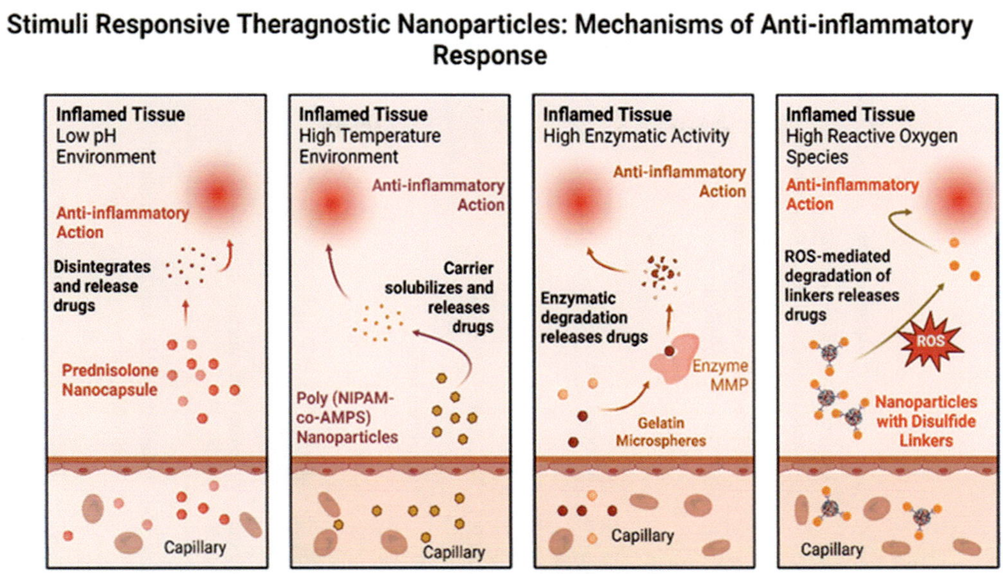

	Stimuli Responsive Theragnostic Nanoparticles for Inflammatory Diseases			
Stimuli	Low pH environment surrounding the inflamed tissue	High Temperature environment surrounding the inflamed tissue, hyperthermia treatment may also cause high Temperature	Increased Enzyme activity such as Metalloproteinase (MMP) and Cathepsin	Increased levels of Reactive Oxygen Species (ROS) and Reduced Glutathione
Examples	Prednisolone Nanocapsules, Nanoparticles of budesonide, etc.	Poly(NIPAM-co-AMPS) Nanoparticles, NGPEGSS Nanoparticle system incorporating NIPAM, etc.	Gelatin Microspheres, Extracellular HNE-responsive PEG-hydrogel, etc.	Disulfide-containing PEG-PLGA Nanoparticles

FIGURE 1.2 Mechanisms of action of various stimuli-responsive theragnostic nanoparticles used in drug delivery and therapy. These nanoparticles are designed to release their payloads (drugs) in response to specific environmental stimuli, enhancing therapeutic efficacy while minimizing side effects. (Created with BioRender.com.)

precisely to inflamed tissues and release them in a controlled manner is a cornerstone of effective inflammatory disease treatment. Stimuli-responsive biomaterials, designed to respond to specific cues present at the inflammation site, have emerged as a powerful delivery system for achieving this goal. These materials undergo physicochemical changes in response to stimuli, such as pH, temperature, enzymatic activity, or redox environment, enabling targeted delivery and controlled release of therapeutic payloads.

1.5.1 pH-Responsive Materials

Inflamed tissues often exhibit a lower pH compared to healthy tissues. This acidic microenvironment, caused by increased metabolic activity and the production of lactic acid, provides a unique trigger for pH-responsive biomaterials. These materials are designed to remain stable at physiological pH but degrade or release their cargo upon encountering the acidic conditions of inflamed tissues. Prednisolone nanocapsule, dual pH- and time-dependent polymeric NPS of budesonide, polyketal nanoparticles, polyketal microparticles, acetal-modified cyclodextrin and poly(cyclodextrin) nanoparticles, polymer–drug conjugates (PDCs), and acid-sensitive sheddable PEGylated PLGA nanoparticles are some of the pH-responsive biomaterials investigated for role in management of inflammation (Table 1.2; Figure 1.2) [43–47].

TABLE 1.2
Stimuli-Responsive Biomaterial for Tackling Inflammation

Stimuli-Responsive Biomaterials	Nanomaterials	Composition and Mechanisms of Action	Applications	References
pH-responsive	Prednisolone nanocapsule	Prednisolone in a polymer wall surrounding an oily core and coated with a pH-responsive enteric polymer (Eudragit S100).	Designed for oral administration and release of prednisolone in the colon to tackle inflammatory bowel diseases (IBD) or other colonic diseases.	[43]
	Dual pH- and time-dependent polymeric NPS of budesonide	Eudragit FS30D (pH-sensitive polymer) and Eudragit RS100 (controlled-release polymer) are designed for oral administration and release budesonide in the colon, minimizing early drug release and activity in the stomach and small intestine.	IBD or other colonic diseases.	[54]
	Polyketal nanoparticles	Fabricated from a hydrophobic polymer, poly(1,4-phenylene-acetone dimethylene ketal) (PPADK) that undergoes acid-accelerated degradation into low MW and non-acidic products, releasing the encapsulated therapeutic agent (e.g., dexamethasone) in acidic microenvironments.	Myocardial infarction	[44]
	Polyketal microparticles	Fabricated from Poly-(cyclohexane-1,4-diyl acetone dimethylene ketal) (PCADK), are designed to deliver p38 inhibitor (SB239063)	Myocardial infarction	[45]
	Acetal-modified cyclodextrin and poly(cyclodextrin) nanoparticles	Synthesized with pH-actuated degradability and exhibits hydrophobic-to-hydrophilic switching and dissociation upon contact with acidic environments, releasing the encapsulated drug (e.g., Rapamycin).	Atherosclerosis	[46]
	Polymer–drug conjugates (PDCs)	These conjugates are designed with acidic pH-labile acyl hydrazone linkages and release the drug (e.g., dexamethasone) upon triggering by an acidic milieu.	Rheumatoid arthritis	[47]
	Acid-sensitive sheddable PEGylated PLGA nanoparticles	They undergo dePEGylation at the target site due to the acidic pH, enhancing the distribution and retention of nanoparticles at the pathological lesion.	Chronic inflammation	[55]
Thermo-responsive	Poly(NIPAM-co-AMPS) nanoparticles	N-isopropyl acrylamide (NIPAM) and 2-acrylamido-2-methylpropane sulfonic acid (AMPS) monomers are thermo-sensitive and release the encapsulated anti-inflammatory peptides such as KAFAK in response to temperature changes.	Inflamed cartilage explants and reduced pro-inflammatory cytokine production.	[47]
	NGPEGSS NPs system incorporating NIPAM, AMPS, BAC, and PEG polymers	Based on poly(NIPAM) nanoparticles with degradable disulfide crosslinks. It is thermo-sensitive and releases the encapsulated anti-inflammatory peptide KAFAK in response to temperature changes.	This approach aims to target inflamed cartilage explants and suppress IL-6 production.	

	PNIPA hydrogel	This hydrogel is thermo-responsive and releases the loaded antigen while acting as an adjuvant due to its inherent properties.	Treatment of rheumatoid arthritis.	[48]
Enzyme-responsive	Enzyme-degradable gelatin microspheres	Designed to release anti-inflammatory cytokines (IL-4 and IL-13) in response to proteolytic enzymes (e.g., collagenase) that are overexpressed in arthritic flares.	Spatiotemporally controlled release of anti-inflammatory agents for cartilage preservation and repair in osteoarthritis.	[49]
	Azoreductase-responsive supramolecular hydrogels	Self-assembling tripeptide derivatives conjugated with Olsalazine that undergo a gel-to-sol transition and releases bioactive 5-aminosalicylic acid upon azoreductase-catalyzed reduction.	Targeted drug delivery for the treatment of IBD.	
	Esterase-responsive hydrogel microfibers	Generated from amphipathic Ascorbyl-palmitate containing an esterase-cleavable ester linkage that releases the encapsulated anti-inflammatory drug dexamethasone (Dex) upon enzymatic cleavage.	Targeted drug delivery for the treatment of IBD.	[50]
	MMP-responsive supramolecular hydrogels	Formed by self-assembling triglycerol monostearate (TG-18), which encapsulates the corticosteroid triamcinolone acetonide (TA). They release TA upon contact with enzymes (esterase or MMPs) or synovial fluid from patients with RA.	Flare-responsive drug delivery for the treatment of RA.	[51]
Redox-responsive	Disulfide-containing PEG–PLGA nanoparticles	These nanoparticles employ disulfide bonds in their structure, which are cleavable by glutathione (GSH), a reducing agent found in higher concentrations in inflamed tissues. Upon reaching an inflamed site, the disulfide bonds break, releasing the encapsulated anti-inflammatory drug dexamethasone (Dex).	This novel approach has been researched for treating inflammatory bowel disease (IBD), leveraging the high GSH concentration in the inflamed gut as an effective trigger for drug release.	[56]
	Extracellular HNE-responsive PEG hydrogel	This hydrogel incorporates an immobilized sidechain containing a human neutrophil elastase (HNE)-cleavable substrate, designed to degrade in response to HNE activity and release the encapsulated drug. HNE, an enzyme released by neutrophils during inflammation, serves as the trigger for this mechanism.	This novel hydrogel system has been researched for treating various inflammatory conditions, including arthritis and wound healing, where HNE plays a significant role in the inflammatory cascade.	[52]
	HNE-responsive nanoparticle-in-microgel delivery platform	This platform consists of microgels encapsulating nanoparticles containing therapeutic agents, designed to de-crosslink in response to human neutrophil elastase (HNE) activity, thereby releasing the encapsulated nanoparticles.	This novel platform has been studied for treating various inflammatory conditions where HNE is present, such as arthritis and lung inflammation, and demonstrates versatility in its ability to be loaded with diverse therapeutic agents, including anti-inflammatory drugs, cytokines, and other bioactive molecules.	[53]

(Continued)

TABLE 1.2 (*Continued*)
Stimuli-Responsive Biomaterial for Tackling Inflammation

Stimuli-Responsive Biomaterials	Nanomaterials	Composition and Mechanisms of Action	Applications	References
	Enzyme/redox dual-responsive nanoparticles	These nanoparticles are engineered to release growth factors or other therapeutic agents in response to both the presence of specific enzymes (e.g., matrix metalloproteinases, MMPs) and the reducing environment found in wounds. Researchers exemplified this approach by developing nanoparticles composed of poly(ethylene glycol) (PEG) and poly(lactic-co-glycolic acid) (PLGA) crosslinked with disulfide bonds, loaded with fibroblast growth factor-2 (FGF-2), and further modified with MMP-cleavable peptides. This design aimed to release FGF-2 specifically at wound sites where MMPs are elevated, and the redox environment is reducing.	This dual-responsive approach highlights the potential for enhancing targeted drug delivery in wound healing applications by leveraging both enzymatic activity and redox sensitivity to achieve more precise and effective treatment.	[57]
	pH/enzyme/redox triple-responsive microparticles	These microparticles are engineered to release anti-cancer drugs in response to the acidic pH of the tumor microenvironment, the presence of tumor-associated enzymes (e.g., cathepsins), and the reducing environment within tumor cells. Researchers exemplified this approach by developing microparticles composed of poly(lactic acid) (PLA) and poly(glycolic acid) (PGA) crosslinked with disulfide bonds, loaded with the anti-cancer drug doxorubicin (DOX), and further modified with pH-sensitive linkers and cathepsin-cleavable peptides.	These multi-stimuli-responsive materials are utilized for targeted drug delivery for cancer treatment.	[58]

1.5.2 Thermo-Responsive Materials

The body's temperature provides another valuable stimulus for controlled drug delivery. Thermo-responsive materials undergo a phase transition in response to temperature changes, altering their properties, such as solubility or viscosity. This allows for the triggered release of therapeutic agents at specific temperatures, such as the increased temperature that occurs in inflamed tissues or during hyperthermia treatments. Poly(NIPAM-co-AMPS) nanoparticles, NGPEGSS NPs system incorporating NIPAM, AMPS, BAC, and PEG polymers, and PNIPA hydrogel are examples of thermo-responsive materials noted for modulation of inflammatory cascades (Table 1.2) [48].

1.5.3 Enzyme-Responsive Materials

Inflamed tissues often show increased levels of enzymes like MMPs and cathepsins. Enzyme-responsive materials take advantage of this enzymatic activity to trigger controlled drug release. These materials contain enzyme-sensitive linkers that are specifically degraded by target enzymes, releasing the therapeutic payload. Key design factors include enzyme specificity for inflammation sites, careful control of cleavage rates to optimize drug release, and ensuring biocompatibility to avoid toxicity. Stability in physiological conditions is also essential for effective targeting and maintaining therapeutic efficacy. Together, these factors enable precise, safe drug delivery, and improved treatment outcomes. Enzyme-degradable gelatin microspheres, extracellular HNE-responsive PEG hydrogel, HNE-responsive nanoparticle-in-microgel delivery platform, azoreductase-responsive supramolecular hydrogels, esterase-responsive hydrogel microfibers, and MMP-responsive supramolecular hydrogels are some of the enzyme-responsive inventions envisaged as modulators of inflammation in various diseases (Table 1.2) [49–53].

1.5.4 Redox-Responsive Materials

Inflamed tissues often exhibit a shift in the redox balance, with increased levels of ROS and a reduced glutathione (GSH) concentration. Redox-responsive materials leverage this imbalance to trigger drug release. These materials incorporate redox-sensitive linkers that are cleaved by ROS or reduced by GSH, leading to the release of the therapeutic payload. Disulfide-containing PEG–PLGA nanoparticles, Extracellular HNE-responsive PEG hydrogel, HNE-responsive nanoparticle-in-microgel delivery platform, and azoreductase-responsive supramolecular hydrogels are notable examples of redox-responsive materials (Table 1.2) [52, 53, 56].

1.6 CONCLUSION

The development of stimuli-responsive biomaterials and nanoparticles for inflammatory disease treatment represents a significant advancement in the field of nanomedicine, offering a promising approach to overcome the limitations of conventional therapies. By leveraging the unique properties of these materials, researchers can achieve targeted delivery, controlled release, and even modulation of the immune response at the site of inflammation. Despite the challenges associated with clinical translation, safety, and a comprehensive understanding of immune interactions, continued research and development hold immense promise for realizing the full potential of these innovative technologies. With ongoing efforts to address these challenges and explore new frontiers in stimuli-responsive nanomedicine, we can anticipate the emergence of novel and effective therapies that will improve patient outcomes and quality of life for individuals suffering from inflammatory diseases.

Declaration of AI and AI-Assisted Technologies

During the preparation of this work, the authors used QuillBot AI in order to paraphrase the sentences. After using this tool, the authors reviewed and edited the content as needed and take full responsibility for the content of the publication.

REFERENCES

1. Hannoodee, S. and D.N. Nasuruddin, Acute Inflammatory Response, in StatPearls. 2024, StatPearls Publishing Copyright © 2024, StatPearls Publishing LLC.: Treasure Island (FL).
2. Chen, L., et al., Inflammatory responses and inflammation-associated diseases in organs. Oncotarget, 2018. 9(6): p. 7204–7218.
3. Pahwa, R., A. Goyal and I. Jialal, Chronic Inflammation, in StatPearls. 2024, StatPearls Publishing Copyright © 2024, StatPearls Publishing LLC.: Treasure Island (FL). Available from: https://www.ncbi.nlm.nih.gov/books/NBK493173/
4. Furman, D., et al., Chronic inflammation in the etiology of disease across the life span. Nature Medicine, 2019. 25(12): p. 1822–1832.
5. Parke, D.V. and A.L. Parke, Chemical-induced inflammation and inflammatory diseases. International Journal of Occupational Medicine and Environmental Health, 1996. 9(3): p. 211–217.
6. Li, D. and M. Wu, Pattern recognition receptors in health and diseases. Signal Transduction and Targeted Therapy, 2021. 6(1): p. 291.
7. Soliman, A.M. and D.R. Barreda, Acute inflammation in tissue healing. International Journal of Molecular Sciences, 2022. 24(1).
8. Kohli, P. and B.D. Levy, Resolvins and protectins: Mediating solutions to inflammation. British Journal of Pharmacology, 2009. 158(4): p. 960–971.
9. Chandrasekharan, J.A. and N. Sharma-Walia, Lipoxins: nature's way to resolve inflammation. Journal of Inflammation Research, 2015. 8: p. 181–192.
10. Kany, S., J.T. Vollrath and B. Relja, Cytokines in inflammatory disease. International Journal of Molecular Sciences, 2019. 20(23).
11. Zhang, W., et al., Role of neuroinflammation in neurodegeneration development. Signal Transduction and Targeted Therapy, 2023. 8(1): p. 267.
12. Takeuchi, O. and S. Akira, Pattern recognition receptors and inflammation. Cell, 2010. 140(6): p. 805–820.
13. Rubartelli, A. and M.T. Lotze, Inside, outside, upside down: Damage-associated molecular-pattern molecules (DAMPs) and redox. Trends in Immunology, 2007. 28(10): p. 429–436.
14. Henríquez-Olguín, C., et al., Altered ROS production, NF-κB activation and interleukin-6 gene expression induced by electrical stimulation in dystrophic mdx skeletal muscle cells. Biochimica et Biophysica Acta, 2015. 1852(7): p. 1410–1419.
15. Murata, H., N. Shimada and M. Yoshioka, Current research on acute phase proteins in veterinary diagnosis: An overview. The Veterinary Journal, 2004. 168(1): p. 28–40.
16. Jabbour, H.N., et al., Inflammatory pathways in female reproductive health and disease. Reproduction, 2009. 138(6): p. 903–919.
17. Huang, C., A. Sali and R.L. Stevens, Regulation and function of mast cell proteases in inflammation. Journal of Clinical Immunology, 1998. 18(3): p. 169–183.
18. Aggrey, A.A., et al., Platelet induction of the acute-phase response is protective in murine experimental cerebral malaria. Journal of Immunology, 2013. 190(9): p. 4685–4691.
19. Headland, S.E. and L.V. Norling, The resolution of inflammation: Principles and challenges. Seminars in Immunology, 2015. 27(3): p. 149–160.
20. Nicholas, C. and G.B. Lesinski, Immunomodulatory cytokines as therapeutic agents for melanoma. Immunotherapy, 2011. 3(5): p. 673–690.
21. Malmsten, C.L., Prostaglandins, thromboxanes, and leukotrienes in inflammation. The American Journal of Medicine, 1986. 80(4): p. 11–17.
22. Cornejo-García, J.A., et al., Pharmacogenomics of prostaglandin and leukotriene receptors. Frontiers in Pharmacology, 2016. 7: p. 316.
23. Thompson, M.D., et al., Pharmacogenetics of the G protein-coupled receptors. Pharmacogenomics in Drug Discovery and Development, 2014: p. 189–242.
24. Funk, C.D., Prostaglandins and leukotrienes: Advances in eicosanoid biology. Science, 2001. 294(5548): p. 1871–1875.
25. Huang, J.-L., et al., Sequence variants of the gene encoding chemoattractant receptor expressed on Th2 cells (CRTH2) are associated with asthma and differentially influence mRNA stability. Human Molecular Genetics, 2004. 13(21): p. 2691–2697.
26. Singh, G., Re: C-reactive protein versus erythrocyte sedimentation rate: Implications among patients with no known inflammatory conditions. The Journal of the American Board of Family Medicine, 2022. 35(1): p. 209–209.

27. Menzel, A., et al., Common and novel markers for measuring inflammation and oxidative stress ex vivo in research and clinical practice—Which to use regarding disease outcomes? Antioxidants, 2021. 10(3): p. 414.
28. Qiu, S., et al., Association between circulating cell adhesion molecules and risk of type 2 diabetes: A meta-analysis. Atherosclerosis, 2019. 287: p. 147–154.
29. Hasturk, H. and A. Kantarci, Activation and resolution of periodontal inflammation and its systemic impact. Periodontology 2000, 2015. 69(1): p. 255–273.
30. Liu, Y., et al., *Lactobacillus reuteri* strains reduce incidence and severity of experimental necrotizing enterocolitis via modulation of TLR4 and NF-κB signaling in the intestine. American Journal of Physiology-Gastrointestinal and Liver Physiology, 2012. 302(6): p. G608–G617.
31. Chu, J., et al., Immunological mechanisms of inflammatory diseases caused by gut microbiota dysbiosis: A review. Biomedicine & Pharmacotherapy, 2023. 164: p. 114985.
32. Zittan, E., I.M. Gralnek and M.S. Berns, The new proactive approach and precision medicine in Crohn's disease. Biomedicines, 2020. 8(7): p. 193.
33. Spindel, S. and K.E. Sapsford, Evaluation of optical detection platforms for multiplexed detection of proteins and the need for point-of-care biosensors for clinical use. Sensors, 2014. 14(12): p. 22313–22341.
34. Litman, T., Personalized medicine—Concepts, technologies, and applications in inflammatory skin diseases. Apmis, 2019. 127(5): p. 386–424.
35. Trusheim, M.R., E.R. Berndt and F.L. Douglas, Stratified medicine: Strategic and economic implications of combining drugs and clinical biomarkers. Nature Reviews Drug Discovery, 2007. 6(4): p. 287–293.
36. Kasprick, A., K. Bieber and R.J. Ludwig, Drug discovery for pemphigoid diseases. Current Protocols in Pharmacology, 2019. 84(1): p. e55.
37. Alessandri, A.L., et al., Resolution of inflammation: Mechanisms and opportunity for drug development. Pharmacology & Therapeutics, 2013. 139(2): p. 189–212.
38. Prieto-Pérez, R., et al., Association between genetic polymorphisms and response to anti-TNFs in patients with inflammatory bowel disease. International Journal of Molecular Sciences, 2016. 17(2): p. 225.
39. Forbes, J.D., G. Van Domselaar and C.N. Bernstein, The gut microbiota in immune-mediated inflammatory diseases. Frontiers in Microbiology, 2016. 7: p. 1081.
40. Franzin, M., et al., Microbiota and drug response in inflammatory bowel disease. Pathogens, 2021. 10(2): p. 211.
41. Germolec, D.R., et al., Markers of inflammation. Immunotoxicity Testing: Methods and Protocols, 2018: p. 57–79.
42. Rasquel-Oliveira, F.S., et al., Specialized pro-resolving lipid mediators: Endogenous roles and pharmacological activities in infections. Molecules, 2023. 28(13): p. 5032.
43. Katzer, T., et al., Prednisolone-loaded nanocapsules as ocular drug delivery system: Development, in vitro drug release and eye toxicity. Journal of Microencapsulation, 2014. 31(6): p. 519–528.
44. Heffernan, M.J. and N. Murthy, Polyketal nanoparticles: A new pH-sensitive biodegradable drug delivery vehicle. Bioconjugate Chemistry, 2005. 16(6): p. 1340–1342.
45. Fiore, V.F., et al., Polyketal microparticles for therapeutic delivery to the lung. Biomaterials, 2010. 31(5): p. 810–817.
46. Gadade, D.D. and S.S. Pekamwar, Cyclodextrin based nanoparticles for drug delivery and theranostics. Advanced Pharmaceutical Bulletin, 2020. 10(2): p. 166–183.
47. Junyaprasert, V.B. and P. Thummarati, Innovative design of targeted nanoparticles: Polymer-drug conjugates for enhanced cancer therapy. Pharmaceutics, 2023. 15(9).
48. Liu, K., T.C. Ovaert and J.J. Mason, Preparation and mechanical characterization of a PNIPA hydrogel composite. Journal of Materials Science: Materials in Medicine, 2008. 19(4): p. 1815–1821.
49. Solorio, L., et al., Gelatin microspheres crosslinked with genipin for local delivery of growth factors. Journal of Tissue Engineering and Regenerative Medicine, 2010. 4(7): p. 514–523.
50. Qiao, J., et al., Construction of esterase-responsive hyperbranched polyprodrug micelles and their antitumor activity in vitro. e-Polymers, 2022. 22(1): p. 513–521.
51. Noddeland, H.K., et al., Design and characterization of matrix metalloproteinase-responsive hydrogels for the treatment of inflammatory skin diseases. Acta Biomaterialia, 2023. 157: p. 149–161.
52. Aimetti, A.A., A.J. Machen and K.S. Anseth, Poly(ethylene glycol) hydrogels formed by thiol-ene photopolymerization for enzyme-responsive protein delivery. Biomaterials, 2009. 30(30): p. 6048–6054.
53. Aimetti, A.A., M.W. Tibbitt and K.S. Anseth, Human neutrophil elastase responsive delivery from poly(ethylene glycol) hydrogels. Biomacromolecules, 2009. 10(6): p. 1484–1489.

54. Guo, X., et al., PLGA-based Micro/Nanoparticles: An overview of their applications in respiratory diseases. International Journal of Molecular Sciences, 2023. 24(5).
55. Potestà, P., Eudragit FS 30 D: A new pH-sensitive polymer covering for mesalamine. European Review for Medical and Pharmacological Sciences, 2001. 5(1): p. 30.
56. Aldayel, A.M., et al., Acid-sensitive sheddable PEGylated PLGA nanoparticles increase the delivery of TNF-α siRNA in chronic inflammation sites. Molecular Therapy Nucleic Acids, 2016. 5(7): p. e340.
57. Zhang, S., et al., pH and redox dual-responsive nanoparticles based on disulfide-containing poly(β-amino ester) for combining chemotherapy and COX-2 inhibitor to overcome drug resistance in breast cancer. Journal of Nanobiotechnology, 2019. 17(1): p. 109.
58. Liang, Y., et al., pH/redox/α-amylase triple responsive metal-organic framework composites for pest management and plant growth promotion. Microporous and Mesoporous Materials, 2022. 344: p. 112230.

2 Evolution and General Overview of Stimuli-Responsive Biomaterials

Ayush Madan
Department of Biotechnology, School of Research & Technology, People's University, Bhopal, Madhya Pradesh, India

Ramandeep Saini
Chandigarh College of Technology, Chandigarh Group of Colleges, Landran, Greater Mohali, Punjab, India

Mantosh Kumar Satapathy
Department of Pharmacology, School of Medicine, College of Medicine, Taipei Medical University, Taipei, Taiwan

Department of Medical Research, Cathay General Hospital, Taipei, Taiwan

Graduate Institute of Biomedical Materials and Tissue Engineering; and International Ph.D. Program in Biomedical Engineering, College of Biomedical Engineering, Taipei Medical University, Taipei, Taiwan

Neetu Panwar
School of Applied Sciences, Shri Venkateshwara University, Gajraula, Uttar Pradesh, India

Pranshul Sethi
Department of Pharmacology, College of Pharmacy, Shri Venkateshwara University, Gajraula, Uttar Pradesh, India

Chitkara College of Pharmacy, Chitkara University, Rajpura, Punjab, India

Sonali Rastogi
Chitkara College of Pharmacy, Chitkara University, Rajpura, Punjab, India

Department of Pharmacy, Venkateshwara Group of Institutions, Roorkee, Uttarakhand, India

Urvee Dave
Department of Pharmacy, Bhupal Noble's University, Udaipur, Rajasthan, India

DOI: 10.1201/9781003560203-2

2.1 INTRODUCTION

Stimuli-responsive biomaterials are defined as specialized materials that demonstrate considerable alterations in their properties after being exposed to certain environmental stimuli [1]. Stimuli-responsive biomaterials have become crucial in biomedical applications because they can react to physiological conditions and deliver targeted, controlled delivery systems and responsive tissue engineering scaffolds. Stimuli-responsive biomaterials have shifted from facilitated to highly advanced materials created to react to dynamic changes in stimuli such as pH, temperature, enzymes, light, and electric or magnetic fields [2]. These materials were developed by investigating synthetic polymers that can be made temperature sensitive, e.g., poly(N-isopropylacrylamide) (PNIPAM), which experiences a drastic solubility shift at a critical temperature [3]. Gradually, biologically responsive materials sensitive to biological stimuli like pH and enzymes were invented with the idea of the dynamic nature of the body and the necessity of a specific drug delivery system. Cellular and molecular biology knowledge has also improved the design of these materials to be able to replicate biological processes to make them more advanced in their therapeutic application [4]. Current research in stimuli-responsive biomaterials aims to develop materials that can react to multiple stimuli at once, which provides greater control over the release of drug kinetics and site-specificity. For instance, pH-sensitive biomaterials, developed for drug delivery to the acidic tumor microenvironment, have transitioned to multi-responsive systems, whereby they typically are pH-sensitive and redox-sensitive, providing greater control and efficacy [5]. Innovations in nanotechnology have advanced the field even more, with nanoscale stimuli-responsive biomaterials now leading the way for targeted therapies, regenerative medicine, and diagnostics [6]. These advancements represent a move from conventional therapies to more personalized and adaptive health care. The field still faces barriers, especially in regard to clinical application and the pathway to regulatory approval of these biomaterials. New advances in stimuli-responsive biomaterials are continuously changing the paradigm of treatment to achieve notable improvements in therapeutic outcomes using intelligent, adaptive biomaterials [7]. This book chapter will look into the evolution, classification, mechanisms, and application of stimuli-responsive biomaterials and expand on their design considerations, challenges, and outlooks for the future.

2.2 OVERVIEW OF STIMULI-RESPONSIVE BIOMATERIALS

Stimuli-responsive biomaterials are made to alter their physical or chemical characteristics in response to certain environmental triggers in a controllable and targeted manner for biomedical applications [8]. Stimuli-responsive biomaterials can be categorized according to the types of stimuli they respond or react to (physical (e.g., temperature, light), chemical (pH and redox state), and biological (e.g., enzymes), each with different applications (e.g., drug delivery, tissue engineering, and diagnostics). Temperature-sensitive materials are among the most often researched, with PNIPAM being a classic example that undergoes a sharp change in solubility close to physiological temperature [9]. Thermo-responsive materials can be used for applications such as controlled drug delivery and intelligent hydrogels for tissue engineering. Light-responsive materials, such as those containing photo-responsive groups, can be precisely controlled using external light sources, allowing for spatial and temporal drug release and cell adhesion [10]. pH-responsive biomaterials, particularly useful for targeting tumor environments (which tend to be more acidic), undergo structural changes in reaction to fluctuations in pH, thus controlling drug release in acidic regions [11]. Redox-responsive biomaterials utilize intracellular redox gradients for selective drug release, exploiting the higher concentrations of glutathione in tumor cells to achieve site-specific release. Enzyme-responsive biomaterials, designed to degrade or alter their structure under the influence of certain enzymes, are particularly promising for focusing on certain disease locations or tissues. Multi-stimuli-responsive biomaterials, designed to respond to two or more stimuli simultaneously, have recently drawn notice because of their enhanced precision and adaptability in complex biological environments [12]. These materials improve therapeutic outcomes by incorporating dual or multi-trigger responses, such as combining pH and temperature sensitivity or redox and enzyme sensitivity, for better-controlled drug delivery systems. Stimuli-responsive biomaterials are an advance in biomedical materials. They are changing from static, simple passive materials to dynamic and active systems, which possess complex responses for personalized and specific applications, as shown in Table 2.1. Their potential capabilities for enhancing treatment efficacy and outcomes will sustain active research in a stimulating field.

2.3 HISTORICAL EVOLUTION OF BIOMATERIALS

Development in biomaterials has been revolutionized over the last few decades with advances in chemistry, biology, and materials science. Biomaterials, which were developed from simple and biocompatible materials, were first designed to restore or fix organs and tissues that have been damaged. Early biomaterials were primarily metals and ceramics and were used widely for dental implants, joint replacement, and bone plates because of their biocompatibility and strength. The main limitation with biomaterials was that they were not functional because they lacked adaptive functionalities, as they were designed to provide structural support and not interact with dynamic biological systems.

2.3.1 Early Developments in Biomaterials

During the mid-20th century, the first generation of biomaterials was developed, which were distinguished by their biocompatibility and ability to prevent adverse reactions with tissue. There were metals, such as cobalt–chromium alloys and stainless steel, and alumina ceramics that were effective at providing mechanical support, but did not allow tissue integration. Then, biomaterials based on polymers emerged in the 1970s, opening a new area of the field for applications with soft tissues such as contact lenses and sutures. The synthetic polymers they developed (e.g., polyethylene, polymethyl methacrylate) were chosen for their inertness and durability but had limitations, including flexibility and degradation [31]. The late 20th century marked the 'second generation' of biomaterials, with an emphasis on bioactivity and tissue compatibility. In the 1980s and 1990s, researchers developed bioactive ceramics, including hydroxyapatite, that could form direct chemical bonds with bone tissue, allowing osseointegration. Last, this period introduced bioresorbable polymers such as polylactic acid (PLA) and polyglycolic acid (PGA) that fully degraded in the body for temporary mechanical support with tissue regeneration applications [32]. The journey continued with the emergence of a third generation of biomaterials that are inherently designed to actively engage with biological systems. This generation included: tissue-engineered scaffolds, drug-delivery vehicles, and stimuli-responsive materials that act to replicate the natural extracellular matrix (ECM) as well as support cellular growth. Hydrogels were developed as extremely soft tissue analogs with high-water content, prominent as biocompatible materials, allowing for controlled drug release and cellular encapsulation [33]. The field of biomaterials today includes multifunctional materials that have tunable properties. Investigators in the field of biomaterials still study intelligent systems that could dynamically interact with biological tissues, using the advances being made in nanotechnology, regenerative medicine, and responsive drug delivery. Today's biocompatible and intelligent biomaterials can now respond to cellular cues, working to expand the limits of traditional use and moving toward personalized health care solutions.

2.3.2 Evolution of Stimuli-Responsive Biomaterials

The transition of passive materials to a dynamic system that responds to environmental stimuli is a significant step forward in biomaterial science. The early stimuli-responsive materials were often derived from processes that occur in nature, such as protein folding or cell membranes, to support

TABLE 2.1
Summary of the Various Types of Stimuli-Responsive Materials

Stimuli Type	Responsive Materials	Mechanism of Responsiveness	Biomedical Applications	References
		Physical Stimuli		
Temperature	Poly(N-isopropylacrylamide) (PNIPAM)	Phase transition at LCST (e.g., hydrophilic to hydrophobic)	• Controlled drug release (e.g., cancer therapy) • Injectable hydrogels for tissue scaffolding	[13]
	Polyethylene glycol (PEG)-based copolymers	Sol-gel transition	• Drug carriers for temperature-sensitive therapies	[14]
	Poloxamers (pluronics)	Micellar formation above critical micelle temperature	• Drug solubilization and sustained release	[15]
Light	Azobenzene-functionalized polymers	Cis-trans isomerization	• Optically controlled drug delivery • Light-triggered actuators	[16]
	Spiropyran-incorporated hydrogels	Photocleavage or isomerization	• Photoresponsive biosensors • Controlled release systems	[17]
	Gold nanoparticles (AuNPs)	Plasmonic photothermal effect	• Photothermal therapy (e.g., cancer ablation)	[18]
Magnetic field	Superparamagnetic iron oxide nanoparticles (SPIONs)	Magnetic alignment and hyperthermia	• Hyperthermia cancer therapy • Targeted drug delivery • MRI contrast agents	[19]
	Magnetite (Fe_3O_4) nanoparticles	Magnetic dipole interactions	• Magnetically guided tissue engineering scaffolds	[20]
		Chemical Stimuli		
pH	Chitosan	Protonation/deprotonation	• pH-sensitive drug release in acidic tumor microenvironments	[5]
	Poly(β-amino ester)-based hydrogels	pH-dependent degradation	• Controlled release in inflamed tissues	[21]
Ionic strength	Alginate	Ionic cross-linking or dissociation	• Injectable gels for wound healing	[22]
	Polyelectrolyte multilayers	Electrostatic interactions	• Biosensors and drug reservoirs	[23]
Redox potential	Glutathione-sensitive disulfide-linked polymers	Cleavage of disulfide bonds	• Intracellular drug release (e.g., anticancer agents in redox-rich cytoplasm)	[24]
	Selenium-containing nanomaterials	Redox-responsive degradation	• Antioxidant delivery	[25]
		Biological Stimuli		
Enzymes	Collagenase-sensitive hydrogels	Enzymatic degradation	• Targeted drug release in collagen-rich tumor environments	[26]
	Hyaluronidase-responsive scaffolds	Cleavage of hyaluronic acid	• Controlled release for tissue regeneration • Tumor-specific drug delivery	[27]
	Matrix metalloproteinase (MMP)-sensitive polymers	Enzymatic cleavage	• Cancer therapy targeting MMP-overexpressing tumors	[28]
Biomolecules	Glucose-responsive hydrogels	Swelling based on glucose levels	• Insulin delivery systems for diabetes	[29]
	Antibody-functionalized nanoparticles	Binding-induced conformational change	• Targeted drug delivery and imaging	[30]

the development of synthetic polymers that could replicate the functions in nature. The first wave of stimuli-responsive biomaterials came in the 1960s with the discovery of polymers that react to temperature, particularly PNIPAM. These materials undergo repeatable sharp phase transitions near physiological temperature, making them useful for tissue engineering and drug delivery applications. Next came pH-responsive polymers in the 1980s, developed for drug release in response to the acidic environments of tumors and inflamed tissues. These early advancements of temperature and pH-responsive materials provided a new mechanism of controlled drug delivery and mitigated the shortcomings of traditional drug delivery systems. In the 1990s, the materials moved to being multi-responsive, responding to multiple stimuli simultaneously. The light-sensitive materials allowed for more spatial and temporal control over drug release, while redox-responsive materials utilized the intracellular redox gradients found within cancer cells for site-specific drug delivery. The advent of enzyme-responsive systems during this time also allowed for the specificity of biomaterials by targeting tissue-specific enzymatic activity. During the 2000s, the interest in nanotechnology led to the usage of nanoscale stimuli-responsive systems like nanogels, micelles, and dendrimers. This new approach of drug delivery and imaging modalities allowed for more precision and smaller therapeutic doses, especially for cancer therapy, as shown in Figure 2.1. Additionally, there were also dual-stimuli-responsive systems, like pH and temperature-sensitive nanoparticles, which improved the therapy and reduced off-target effects [34]. Recent developments in material science and biotechnology have enabled the use of smart biomaterials with programmable responses. Many of these materials are inspired by natural systems, with elements that can dynamically adapt and respond to environmental changes, allowing for personalized treatments. Ongoing work is employing artificial intelligence (AI) and machine learning (ML) to develop more advanced and predictive stimuli-responsive materials to use clinically. The development of stimuli-responsive biomaterials is part of an ongoing shift toward intelligent, multifunctional systems that adhere to the tenets of personalized medicine. Change is on the horizon for healthcare, including more effective therapies with targeted outcomes and fewer side effects [35].

2.3.3 Physicochemical Characteristics of Stimuli-Responsive Biomaterials

Stimuli-responsive biomaterials represent an advanced class of materials that exhibit unique physicochemical properties, enabling them to change their behavior in response to external stimuli. These characteristics make them highly effective in applications such as drug delivery, tissue engineering, and diagnostics, as shown in Table 2.2.

2.3.3.1 Responsiveness to External Stimuli

Stimuli-responsive biomaterials change dynamically in response to environmental stimuli, facilitating targeted biomedical applications. Temperature-sensitive polymers such as PNIPAM have a lower critical solution temperature (LCST), which changes from hydrophilic to hydrophobic phases, potentially useful for thermo-sensitive drug delivery. pH-responsive materials swell or are broken down in acidic conditions, such as tumor environments, which provide for site-specific delivery. Light-responsive biomaterials, such as azobenzene-based polymers, undergo structure modification under certain wavelengths, making controlled localized therapy possible. Redox-responsive systems take advantage of intracellular gradients, e.g., excess glutathione in cancer cells, to initiate drug release. Enzyme-responsive materials disintegrate in response to disease-related enzymes, providing high specificity for targeted therapy [37].

2.3.3.2 Swelling and Degradation

Swelling is a critical characteristic of hydrogels, enabling controlled drug release. Stimuli-responsive hydrogels swell in response to changes in temperature, pH, or ionic strength, releasing encapsulated drugs or biomolecules. Biodegradable polymers, including PLA and PGA, degrade under physiological conditions, making them ideal for tissue engineering and controlled release applications [37].

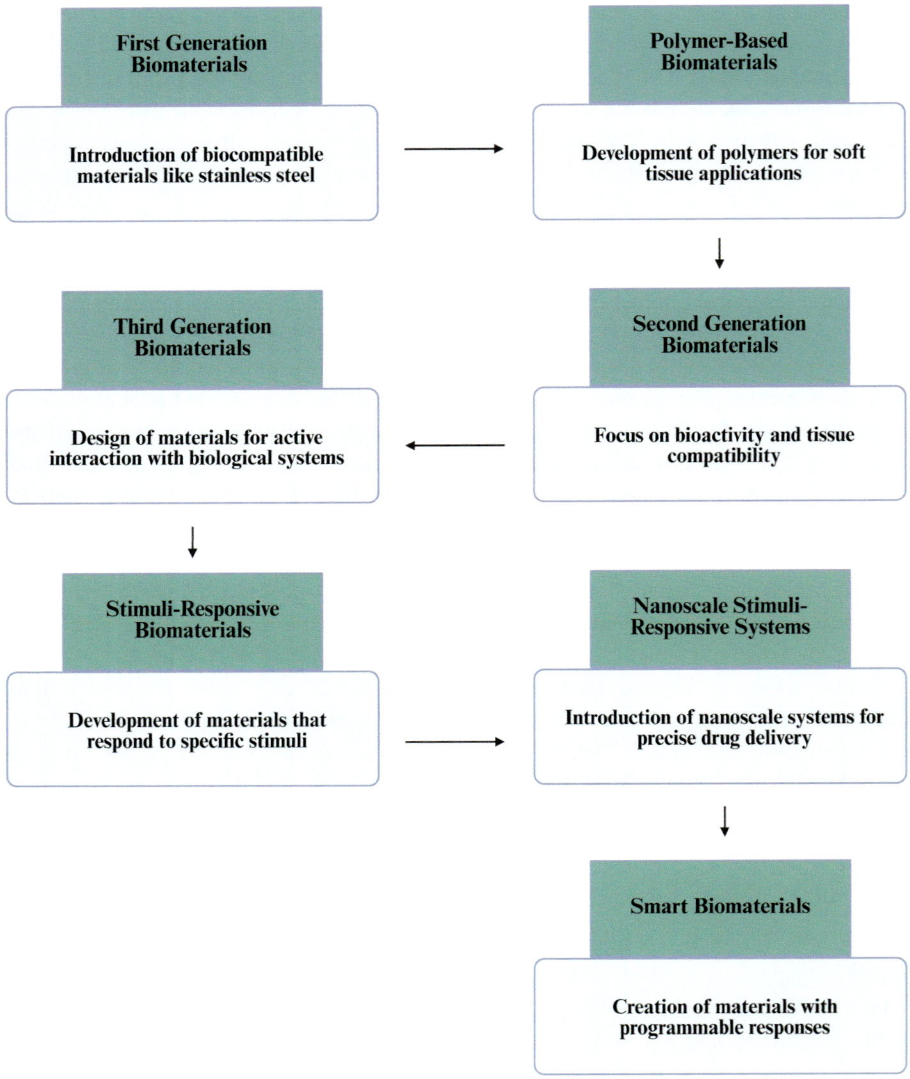

FIGURE 2.1 The evolution of biomaterials from first-generation to smart responsive systems. This figure depicts the progressive development of biomaterials, from first-generation biocompatible metals to smart biomaterials with programmable responses. Key milestones include polymer-based materials, bioactive systems, stimuli-responsive designs, and nanoscale drug delivery platforms.

2.3.3.3 Self-Assembly

Self-assembly is an essential feature of nanostructured stimuli-responsive biomaterials. Nanoparticles, micelles, and liposomes spontaneously form in response to environmental stimuli. These self-assembled systems exhibit enhanced stability, controlled drug encapsulation, and targeted delivery. Dual- or multi-stimuli-responsive self-assembled systems have shown improved therapeutic efficacy by integrating multiple response mechanisms.

2.3.3.4 Surface Properties and Functionalization

Surface functionalization improves the biocompatibility and targeting ability of stimuli-responsive biomaterials. Tailored functional groups enhance tissue interaction, cell adhesion, and immune evasion, while hydrophobic-to-hydrophilic transitions aid dispersion and controlled drug release [38].

TABLE 2.2
Physicochemical Properties of Stimuli-Responsive Materials

Properties	Responsive Mechanism	Examples of Materials	Biomedical Applications	References
Temperature sensitivity	These materials undergo phase transitions at specific temperatures, such as the lower critical solution temperature (LCST) or upper critical solution temperature (UCST). Below the LCST, they are hydrophilic and swollen, while above it, they collapse into a hydrophobic state.	• Poly(N-isopropylacrylamide) (PNIPAM): Hydrogels that shrink above LCST. • Polyethylene glycol (PEG)-based copolymers: Exhibit reversible sol-gel transitions. • Poloxamers (pluronic): Form micelles at elevated temperatures.	• Controlled drug delivery, such as temperature-triggered release for localized cancer therapy. • Injectable hydrogels for minimally invasive procedures, forming scaffolds in situ.	[14, 15]
pH responsiveness	Materials respond to changes in environmental pH through protonation or deprotonation of functional groups, such as carboxyl (–COOH) or amino (–NH_2) groups. This alters their solubility, swelling, or structural integrity.	• Chitosan: Becomes positively charged in acidic environments, facilitating drug release. • Poly(acrylic acid): Swells in basic pH environments. • Poly(β-amino ester): Degrades in acidic conditions, enabling controlled release.	• Targeted drug release in acidic tumor microenvironments. • Controlled delivery in inflamed tissues with abnormal pH levels. • Oral drug delivery systems for stomach or intestinal targeting.	[22, 23]
Swelling capacity	These materials absorb water and swell in response to external stimuli such as pH, temperature, or ionic strength. This property is determined by the cross-link density and the hydrophilic nature of the polymer.	• Alginate: Swells due to ionic interactions, forming gels in the presence of calcium ions. • Poly(vinyl alcohol): Swells under hydrated conditions, providing mechanical support. • pH-sensitive polyacrylamide derivatives: Swell or shrink based on environmental pH.	• Wound healing hydrogels for sustained release of antimicrobial agents. • Scaffolds for tissue engineering, mimicking the extracellular matrix (ECM). • Biosensors for detecting environmental changes.	[22, 25]
Degradation behavior	These materials are designed to degrade in response to specific triggers, such as enzymatic activity, pH, or redox conditions. Degradation often releases therapeutic agents or allows scaffold remodeling.	• Collagenase-sensitive hydrogels: Degrade in collagen-rich environments, ideal for wound healing. • Glutathione-sensitive disulfide-linked polymers: Cleave in high redox environments, such as inside tumor cells. • Hyaluronic acid-based scaffolds: Enzymatically degraded by hyaluronidase.	• Tumor-specific drug release where enzyme levels are elevated. • Regenerative medicine with biodegradable scaffolds that degrade as tissue regenerates. • Drug delivery systems with timed release profiles.	[26, 27]

(Continued)

TABLE 2.2 (*Continued*)
Physicochemical Properties of Stimuli-Responsive Materials

Properties	Responsive Mechanism	Examples of Materials	Biomedical Applications	References
Hydrophilicity/ hydrophobicity	Materials alter their surface properties, switching between hydrophilic and hydrophobic states in response to external stimuli, such as temperature or light. This enables precise control of interactions with water or biological molecules.	• PNIPAM: Exhibits hydrophobicity above its LCST, leading to material shrinkage. • Azobenzene-functionalized hydrogels: Undergo reversible cis-trans isomerization in response to UV or visible light. • Poly(vinylidene fluoride) copolymers: Transition between hydrophobic and hydrophilic phases.	• Smart coatings for biosensors, enhancing sensitivity and specificity. • Optically controlled drug delivery systems for spatial precision. • Surface modification for anti-fouling and antimicrobial applications.	[13, 17]
Mechanical properties	Materials exhibit changes in mechanical properties, such as stiffness or elasticity, in response to external stimuli. This is crucial for materials mimicking dynamic biological tissues.	• MMP-sensitive hydrogels: Gradually lose stiffness as they degrade enzymatically. • Thermo-responsive elastomers: Become more flexible or rigid with temperature changes. • Cross-linked alginate hydrogels: Modulate elasticity with ionic cross-linking.	• Dynamic tissue scaffolds that adapt to cellular activity. • Shape-memory biomaterials for implants that respond to environmental triggers. • Flexible electronics integrated with biological systems.	[19, 31]
Optical properties	Changes in optical characteristics, such as transparency, fluorescence, or color, occur in response to stimuli, such as light or pH. These changes are often used for monitoring or therapeutic applications.	• Gold nanoparticles (AuNPs): Exhibit plasmonic effects for light absorption and heat generation. • Spiropyran-incorporated hydrogels: Change color upon exposure to UV light. • Quantum dots: Emit fluorescence in response to external conditions.	• Photothermal therapy for cancer by converting light to heat. • Real-time biosensors for detecting physiological changes. • Imaging agents for diagnostics and intraoperative guidance.	[36]

2.3.3.5 Mechanical Properties

The mechanical characteristics of stimuli-responsive biomaterials, including elasticity, tensile strength, and viscosity, are crucial for tissue engineering and biomedical applications. For instance, hydrogels with tunable stiffness mimic the ECM, promoting cell attachment, proliferation, and differentiation.

2.3.3.6 Biocompatibility and Toxicity

Biocompatibility is a fundamental requirement for stimuli-responsive biomaterials. These materials must be non-toxic and non-immunogenic while maintaining high functionality. Advances in polymer chemistry have reduced the cytotoxicity of these materials, making them safer for in vivo applications. Biodegradable materials, including polycaprolactone (PCL), minimize long-term risks by degrading into non-toxic by-products.

2.3.3.7 Programmable and Multifunctional Properties

Modern stimuli-responsive biomaterials are designed to integrate multiple stimuli-responsiveness into a single system. Multi-stimuli-responsive materials (e.g., pH- and temperature-responsive systems) provide enhanced control in complex environments, aligning with the goals of personalized medicine and next-generation therapeutic strategies.

2.4 CLASSIFICATION OF STIMULI-RESPONSIVE BIOMATERIALS

Stimuli-responsive biomaterials are classified based on different categories, such as the type of stimuli they respond to, which include physical, chemical, and biological stimuli and the types of material. This classification reflects their diverse applications in controlled drug delivery, tissue engineering, diagnostics, and regenerative medicine.

2.4.1 Classification Based on Stimuli Type

Stimuli-responsive biomaterials are categorized based on the type of stimulus they respond to. These stimuli are broadly divided into physical, chemical, and biological types, with each offering unique mechanisms of action and applications in biomedical fields. Table 2.1 summarizes the types of stimuli, examples of responsive materials, their mechanisms, and specific biomedical applications.

2.4.1.1 Physical Stimuli

Physical stimuli-responsive biomaterials are engineered to respond to external stimuli such as temperature, light, or magnetic fields, providing non-invasive and targeted therapeutic solutions. Temperature-responsive materials, for example, PNIPAM, exhibit phase transitions at specific temperatures, transitioning from hydrophilic to hydrophobic states near body temperature, which allows for controlled drug delivery. Light-responsive biomaterials, incorporating groups, such as azobenzene or spiropyran, change structure when exposed to specific light wavelengths and are used in systems for ultraviolet (UV)- or near-infrared-triggered drug release and photodynamic cancer therapy. Magnetic field-responsive materials, including nanoparticles, such as Fe_3O_4, respond to magnetic fields for applications such as hyperthermia treatment and targeted drug delivery, allowing therapeutic agents to be directed precisely while minimizing side effects.

2.4.1.2 Chemical Stimuli

Chemical stimuli-responsive biomaterials are designed to respond to variations in the chemical environment, including changes in pH, ionic strength, and the presence of specific molecules. pH-responsive materials swell, shrink, or degrade in acidic conditions commonly found in tumor tissues or inflamed sites, making them ideal for targeted drug delivery. Ionic strength-sensitive biomaterials alter their structural properties with the changing salt concentration, which is advantageous for drug release in physiological fluids [39]. Some systems respond uniquely to specific molecules, such as glucose-sensitive hydrogels. These are designed to release therapeutic agents in the presence of target molecules that are specifically tuned, such as glucose or reactive oxygen species (ROS). Therefore, systems that could release therapeutic agents as a function of specific molecules are highly desirable, especially in applications, like insulin delivery to diabetic patients.

2.4.1.3 Biological Stimuli

Biological stimuli-responsive biomaterials are designed to respond to specific biomolecules or biological events, providing the highest specificity and precision of function. Enzyme-responsive materials respond to enzymes, such as matrix metalloproteinases (MMPs) or hyaluronidase [40]. These enzymes are typically overexpressed under pathological conditions, such as cancer or inflammation. This makes enzyme-responsive biomaterials well-suited for application in targeted drug delivery systems or tissue regeneration applications. Similarly, biomolecule-responsive systems react to specific biological signals, such as antibodies or growth factors, enabling the development of advanced biosensors and precision drug delivery platforms. For instance, materials responsive to disease-specific antigens facilitate highly selective therapeutic targeting, minimizing systemic side effects and improving treatment outcomes.

2.4.2 Classification Based on Type of Material

Stimuli-responsive biomaterials can also be classified based on the type of material used in their design and construction. Each material type, polymers, lipid-based materials, and inorganic materials, offers unique properties and advantages for specific biomedical applications as shown in Table 2.3.

2.4.2.1 Polymers

Polymers represent the most extensively utilized class of materials in stimuli-responsive systems due to their structural versatility and ease of functional modification. Polymers are either synthetic or natural, both of which have different advantages for biomedical applications. Synthetic polymers, such as PNIPAM and polyethylene glycol (PEG), are commonly used; PNIPAM is temperature-sensitive and suitable for drug delivery and tissue engineering, and PEG increases hydrophilicity and decreases immunogenicity, enhancing biocompatibility in therapeutic systems. Natural polymers, including alginate, chitosan, and hyaluronic acid, offer excellent biocompatibility and biodegradability, making them ideal for wound healing and site-specific drug delivery, particularly in acidic tumor environments, where pH-responsive behavior is advantageous. These polymers are often formulated into hydrogels for controlled drug release, tissue scaffolding, and biosensing. Emerging multi-responsive polymeric systems that respond to multiple stimuli, such as temperature and pH, further enhance precision and adaptability in therapeutic applications.

2.4.2.2 Lipid-Based Materials

Due to their structural similarity to biological membranes and excellent biocompatibility, lipid-based materials are emerging as attractive platforms to develop stimuli-responsive systems. They are particularly useful for the delivery of hydrophobic drugs and for targeted tissue delivery. Liposomes are vesicles made up of phospholipid bilayers that can carry hydrophilic and hydrophobic agents, and they can be manipulated to release drugs based on pH, temperature, or enzymatic stimuli. For example, pH-sensitive liposomes can release targeted drugs in acidic tumor microenvironments. Solid lipid nanoparticles (SLNs) and nanostructured lipid carriers (NLCs) offer increased structural stability and controlled drug release. SLNs consist only of solid lipids, while NLCs utilize a combination of solid and liquid lipids to increase flexibility and drug loading capacity. Lipid-based materials are well documented for their applications in cancer therapy, gene delivery, and immunotherapy, as they are highly selective, have low toxicity, have high encapsulation efficiency, and can enhance the bioavailability of drugs [41].

TABLE 2.3
Material Types and Their Stimuli-Responsiveness

Material Type	Examples	Advantages	Limitations	Biomedical Applications	References
Polymers	• Poly(N-isopropylacrylamide) (PNIPAM): A thermo-responsive polymer with LCST properties. • Polyethylene glycol (PEG): Widely used for surface functionalization to reduce immunogenicity. • Chitosan: A pH-sensitive natural polymer derived from chitin.	• Highly biocompatible, making them suitable for clinical applications. • Easily tunable chemical and physical properties through functionalization. • Exhibit low toxicity when natural or appropriately synthesized. • Provide versatility in responsiveness (temperature, pH, enzymatic).	• Synthetic polymers, including PNIPAM, may leave residual toxic monomers. • Limited mechanical strength, particularly in hydrogels. • Potential immunogenicity of synthetic derivatives may require additional modification.	• Drug Delivery: Controlled and targeted delivery of drugs in response to stimuli. • Tissue Engineering: Formation of scaffolds mimicking the extracellular matrix (ECM). • Hydrogels: Used in wound healing and as injectable matrices.	[15, 21]
Lipids	• Phospholipids: Key components of liposomes, forming bilayer structures. • Solid lipid nanoparticles (SLNs): Provide controlled drug release and high stability. • Liposomes: Versatile carriers for both hydrophilic and lipophilic drugs.	• High biocompatibility with minimal immunogenic response. • Ability to encapsulate both hydrophilic and hydrophobic drugs. • Efficient drug encapsulation and targeted delivery. • Natural phospholipids are generally safe and biodegradable.	• Stability issues, such as oxidation of unsaturated lipids or aggregation under storage conditions. • Limited inherent responsiveness; requires integration with other stimuli-responsive materials. • Production at an industrial scale can be challenging.	• Drug delivery: Used for encapsulating small molecules, proteins, and vaccines. • Vaccine Adjuvants: Enhance immunogenicity and improve the stability of antigens. • Cancer Therapy: Targeted drug delivery to tumor sites using liposomes.	[22, 23]
Inorganic materials	• Gold nanoparticles (AuNPs): Used in photothermal therapy and imaging due to their plasmonic properties. • Superparamagnetic iron oxide nanoparticles (SPIONs): Responsive to magnetic fields for drug targeting and hyperthermia. • Quantum dots: Fluorescent nanocrystals for imaging and diagnostics.	• High chemical and thermal stability compared to organic materials. • Exhibit unique stimuli-specific responsiveness (e.g., magnetic or optical properties). • Suitable for dual-functionality, combining imaging and therapy (theranostics).	• Potential cytotoxicity due to ion release or reactive oxygen species (ROS) generation. • Complex synthesis procedures and functionalization challenges. • Risk of long-term accumulation in tissues due to limited biodegradability.	• Imaging and diagnostics: Quantum dots and AuNPs are widely used in real-time imaging. • Hyperthermia therapy: SPIONs used in tumor-specific heating. • Theranostics: Dual-use systems for therapy and diagnostics in personalized medicine.	[26, 27]

2.4.2.3 Inorganic Materials

The use of inorganic materials in stimuli-responsive biomedical systems has been growing, as they often possess inherent characteristics such as thermal stability, the ability to respond to magnetic fields, and optical tunability. For example, metal nanoparticles, including gold and silver, exhibit plasmonic behavior, making them an effective candidate for use in platforms such as photothermal therapy and biomedical imaging, and can exploit various surface functionalities that enable responsiveness to light, pH, etc., to allow for greater control over therapeutic interventions. Magnetic nanoparticles, frequently iron oxide-based nanoparticle systems, can respond to external magnetic fields and have consequently gained use in hyperthermia therapy, site-specific drug delivery, and diagnostic imaging, as they are capable of being localized by guiding magnetic fields for therapeutic interventions. Also, mesoporous silica nanoparticles (MSNs) are another promising inorganic system, as they have a high surface area and tunable pore sizes that further offer increased surface bonding reaction capability for high drug loading and controlled release through triggering environmental changes (pH, redox potential, or enzyme content) [42]. Together, these inorganic platforms have considerable potential for various prosecutable uses, including theranostic uses, where diagnostics and therapy can be integrated to provide personalized treatments in real time.

2.5 MECHANISMS OF STIMULI-RESPONSIVENESS

Stimuli-responsive biomaterials exhibit dynamic changes in their physicochemical properties when exposed to specific external or internal stimuli. These mechanisms are driven by molecular-level interactions or macroscopic phase transitions, which are finely tuned to achieve precise biomedical outcomes.

2.5.1 Thermo-Responsive Mechanisms

Thermo-responsive biomaterials undergo structural or solubility changes in response to temperature variations, particularly around physiological temperatures (~37°C). These transitions are primarily governed by two mechanisms: the LCST and the upper critical solution temperature (UCST). Polymers such as PNIPAM exhibit an LCST near 32°C, below which they remain hydrophilic and swollen due to hydrogen bonding with water molecules. Above this threshold, these bonds are disrupted, leading to polymer collapse and a shift to a hydrophobic state. In contrast, materials exhibiting UCST behavior become soluble above a certain temperature due to the breakdown of inter-chain interactions. These phase transitions are thermodynamically driven by entropy changes in water molecules, promoting polymer aggregation at higher temperatures. Thermo-responsive biomaterials are widely applied in drug delivery, where hydrogels release therapeutic agents upon heating above the LCST for localized treatment, and in tissue engineering, where injectable thermogels form in situ scaffolds that conform to physiological conditions [43].

2.5.2 Photo-Responsive Mechanisms

Photo-responsive biomaterials leverage light as an external trigger to induce molecular transformations such as isomerization, bond cleavage, or conformational changes. A key mechanism involves reversible isomerization, exemplified by azobenzene-containing polymers that switch between trans and cis configurations upon exposure to visible and UV light, respectively. This dynamic alteration modulates properties, such as solubility, mechanical strength, and optical behavior. Another mechanism is photo-cleavage, where materials such as spiropyran and coumarin undergo irreversible bond dissociation upon UV irradiation, leading to controlled drug release or activation of therapeutic agents. The photothermal effect observed in materials, including gold nanoparticles, enables the conversion of absorbed light into heat, which can initiate localized drug release or ablate pathological tissues [44]. These processes are driven by photon-induced excitation of chromophores or nanoparticle surfaces, resulting in structural or thermal responses. Applications include light-triggered drug delivery using photosensitive hydrogels and photodynamic therapy (PDT), wherein photosensitizers generate cytotoxic ROS under light exposure to selectively destroy tumor cells.

2.5.3 Magneto-Responsive Mechanisms

Magneto-responsive biomaterials are engineered to react to external magnetic fields, offering spatial and temporal control over their behavior and localization. Two principal mechanisms drive their functionality. First, magnetic alignment involves superparamagnetic nanoparticles, such as iron oxide (Fe_3O_4), aligning with applied magnetic fields to exert mechanical forces, guide movement, or concentrate drug-loaded carriers at specific anatomical sites. Second, magnetic hyperthermia leverages alternating magnetic fields to induce localized heating through hysteresis losses and Neel or Brownian relaxation processes. This heat generation disrupts cellular membranes or denatures proteins, effectively inducing apoptosis in cancer cells. At the molecular level, these responses are mediated by magnetic dipole–dipole interactions and nanoscale energy dissipation. These mechanisms underpin applications such as targeted drug delivery, where functionalized magnetic nanoparticles are directed precisely to diseased tissues, and cancer therapy, where localized hyperthermia selectively eradicates tumor cells while sparing healthy surrounding tissues.

2.5.4 pH-Responsive Mechanisms

pH-responsive biomaterials are engineered to undergo structural or functional transformations in response to changes in environmental pH, making them highly effective for targeted drug delivery in pathophysiological conditions. The process primarily involves the protonation and deprotonation of some ionizable functional groups, such as carboxylic acids or amines. For example, in an acid environment, these groups become protonated, increasing the hydrophilicity of the material, eventually leading to swelling or dissolution of the material while allowing for controlled release of the drug. Changes in pH alter electrostatic interactions within the polymeric environment, which causes a reversible change in drug permeability and mechanical properties. In addition, some materials also exhibit a hydrophobic to hydrophilic transition due to pH changes, which will affect how quickly the drug can be released from those materials. Changes in charge density and hydration states drive the pH-responsive behavior, so this type of polymer system is useful in tumor therapy because the acidic tumor microenvironments can be used to stimulate localized drug release, and in inflammation therapy, topical acidic conditions can promote the targeted delivery of topical anti-inflammatories.

2.5.5 Enzyme-Responsive Mechanisms

Enzyme-Responsive Biomaterials utilize the specificity and spatiotemporal control afforded by enzymes engineered to degrade or modulate their material structure. A central mechanism of degradation or material change is enzymatic cleavage, whereby a cross-linker or polymer backbone is specific to enzymes, such as MMPs, elastase, or hyaluronidase, and furnishes a release of drug or allows for cellular infiltration and scaffold remodeling. Enzyme-activated responses are triggered by the incorporation or attachment of cleavable peptide motifs, or functional groups released only by the catalytic activity of the enzyme on target substrate or polymer backbone [45]. These two mechanisms are augmented by each scaffold being subjected to structural remodeling expressed as dynamic changes dependent on enzymatic activity, and mimicking the architectural topology of the tissue microenvironment, which promotes cell adhesion, proliferation, and differentiation. These two mechanisms are primarily governed by enzyme-substrate recognition coupled with the specificity of the enzyme and substrate, which enables a precise localized response of the material system. Applications for enzyme-responsive biomaterials include smart drug delivery systems, which use enzyme-sensitive hydrogels to release therapeutics at pathological sites with increased levels of degradation by enzymes, and tissue engineering, wherein scaffold degradation is controlled to facilitate tissue regeneration and healing.

2.6 FUNCTIONALIZATION OF BIOMATERIALS FOR BIOMEDICAL AND TISSUE ENGINEERING APPLICATIONS

Functionalization is a key step in the biomaterials design process that seeks to improve the interaction of materials with biological systems and modify the properties of the material to meet specific biomedical and tissue engineering needs. By incorporating functional groups, bioactive molecules, or nanostructures, the biomaterials can achieve improvements in biocompatibility, controlled drug delivery, tissue integration, and regeneration. The following has been summarized in Table 2.4.

2.6.1 Importance of Functionalization

Functionalization of biomaterials is critical in improving their properties and applicability in biomedical applications. Functionalizing the biomaterial by adding specific chemical groups or bioactive moieties will improve its biocompatibility by reducing the immune rejection, while increasing integration with host tissues. It will also facilitate targeted drug delivery by having specific targeted interaction with diseased cells and ultimately increase the therapeutic benefit and limit the systemic toxicity. In tissue engineering, functionalized scaffolds can provide structural and biochemical cues similar to biological ECM to promote cellular adhesion, proliferation, and differentiation. Functionalization allows for precise control over drug release kinetics, enabling both on-demand and sustained delivery tailored to specific clinical needs, ultimately improving treatment outcomes.

2.6.2 Techniques for Functionalization

2.6.2.1 Surface Functionalization

Surface functionalization involves modifying the outermost layer of biomaterials to enhance their interaction with biological environments and is extensively applied in implants, scaffolds, and drug delivery systems. Physical adsorption is a simple yet effective method where biomolecules such as proteins, peptides, or growth factors are non-covalently bound to the surface, preserving their biological activity, e.g., fibrin or fibronectin coatings facilitate cellular adhesion and migration [46, 47]. Chemical grafting provides more stable modification through the covalent attachment of functional groups such as carboxyl, amino, or thiol groups, allowing precise immobilization of bioactive agents. A notable example is PEGylation, where grafting PEG reduces protein adsorption and immune recognition, enhancing biocompatibility. Plasma surface modification introduces reactive functional groups via ionized gas exposure, significantly improving hydrophilicity, surface wettability, and cellular adhesion, particularly on polymeric substrates. Layer-by-layer (LbL) assembly enables the creation of multilayered films through sequential deposition of oppositely charged polyelectrolytes, allowing incorporation of bioactive molecules for controlled release applications. Finally, biomimetic coatings such as calcium phosphate or hydroxyapatite replicate the mineral composition of bone, enhancing osseointegration and supporting osteoconductivity in orthopedic implants [48].

2.6.2.2 Bulk Functionalization

Bulk functionalization involves modifying the internal composition of biomaterials to impart desired mechanical, thermal, or biological properties critical for advanced biomedical applications. One prominent strategy is the incorporation of nanostructures, where nanoparticles such as gold, silver, or magnetic entities are embedded within the biomaterial matrix. These nanostructures endow the material with specialized functionalities, including antimicrobial activity, imaging contrast, and

TABLE 2.4
Functionalization Techniques and Applications

Functionalization Type	Techniques	Examples	Biomedical Relevance	References
Surface functionalization	PEGylation	• PEG-coated nanoparticles • PEGylated liposomes	• Immune evasion: PEG chains prevent protein adsorption and immune recognition. • Circulation time: Extends half-life in the bloodstream. • Improved biocompatibility: Reduces systemic side effects of therapeutics.	[46]
	Plasma treatment	• Plasma-treated polyethylene • Surface-activated polystyrene	• Reactive surface generation: Introduces functional groups (e.g., carboxyl or amine) for biomolecule binding. • Enhanced wettability: Improves hydrophilicity for cell adhesion and tissue integration.	[47]
	Layer-by-layer (LbL) assembly	• Polyelectrolyte multilayers • Protein-functionalized films	• Controlled drug release: Multilayers allow sustained release profiles. • Customizable surfaces: Enables functional films for biosensors or implants.	[48]
	Biomimetic coatings	• Hydroxyapatite coatings • Calcium phosphate layers	• Bone integration: Mimics the natural mineralized structure of bone. • Tissue regeneration: Enhances osteoblast attachment and proliferation.	[49]
	Electrochemical deposition	• Conductive polymer films • Gold-coated surfaces	• Biosensor development: Deposited layers facilitate bio-electronic interactions. • Electrode modifications: Improved electrical conductivity for neural stimulation and diagnostics.	[50]
Bulk functionalization	Nanoparticle incorporation	• Gold nanoparticles in hydrogels • Iron oxide in polymers	• Imaging and targeting: Adds magnetic or optical properties for precision therapy and diagnostics. • Thermal stability: Enhances mechanical and thermal robustness.	[51]
	Cross-linking	• Enzyme-sensitive hydrogels • Redox-sensitive polymers	• Stimuli-responsiveness: Cross-links break under specific triggers (e.g., enzymatic or redox). • Mechanical stability: Improves the structural integrity of scaffolds.	[52]
	Blending of polymers	• PLA-PEG blends • Chitosan-alginate composites	• Synergistic properties: Combines flexibility, biodegradability, and responsiveness. • Tunable features: Adjusts degradation rates and mechanical strength.	[53]
	Incorporation of bioactive molecules	• Growth factors (VEGF, BMPs) in scaffolds • Enzyme-loaded matrices	• Tissue healing: Promotes angiogenesis and tissue repair. • Targeted responses: Activates cell signaling pathways in regenerative medicine.	[54]
	Functional nanofibers	• Electrospun nanofibers with drugs • Collagen-coated nanofibers	• ECM mimicry: Replicates extracellular matrix structure for cell adhesion and proliferation. • Controlled release: Delivers drugs or biomolecules over time.	[55]

magneto-responsiveness. For example, gold nanoparticles conjugated with antibodies have shown promise in targeted cancer imaging and therapy. Another widely adopted method is polymer blending and cross-linking, which involves combining polymers to modulate flexibility, hydrophilicity, and degradation profiles. Cross-linking further enhances the mechanical integrity of hydrogels and scaffolds, and enzyme-sensitive cross-linkers enable site-specific degradation aligned with biological cues. Functional nanofibers fabricated through electrospinning are increasingly employed for their ability to deliver bioactive agents in a controlled manner while mimicking the ECM. These nanofibrous scaffolds facilitate cell adhesion, proliferation, and tissue integration, making them highly suitable for regenerative medicine applications [49].

2.6.3 Applications of Functionalized Biomaterials in Biomedical and Tissue Engineering

2.6.3.1 Functionalization for Drug Delivery Systems

Functionalization of biomaterials has significantly advanced drug delivery by enabling precise, controlled, and site-specific therapeutic release. One widely adopted strategy is ligand-targeted delivery, wherein biomaterials are functionalized with ligands such as folic acid or antibodies to recognize and bind to overexpressed receptors on diseased cells, including cancerous tissues. This approach enhances therapeutic specificity and minimizes systemic toxicity. For instance, antibody-functionalized liposomes have demonstrated selective delivery of chemotherapeutic agents to HER2-positive breast cancer cells. In addition, stimuli-responsive delivery systems incorporate functional groups sensitive to environmental cues, such as pH, temperature, or redox potential—to enable localized drug release. Tumor-targeted formulations often exploit the acidic microenvironment of cancer tissues to trigger drug release precisely at the site of pathology. Hydrophilic surface coatings, such as PEGylation play a crucial role in improving systemic circulation time by preventing opsonization and clearance by immune cells. These strategies collectively enhance the therapeutic efficacy, safety, and bioavailability of advanced drug delivery platforms [56].

2.6.3.2 Functionalization for Tissue Engineering

Functionalization is a unique property of tissue engineering, with the specific ability to provide scaffolds with improved biological performance, which enables scaffolds to directly participate in tissue repair or regeneration. For example, with traditional bioactive scaffolds, bioactive growth factors, such as vascular endothelial growth factor (VEGF) and bone morphogenic proteins (BMPs), provide the ability to induce angiogenesis and osteogenesis. For example, collagen scaffolds functionalized with BMP-2 have demonstrated in vitro and in vivo effectiveness for stimulating bone regeneration as part of the fracture healing process. Another important type of functionalization includes mimicking the ECM in scaffolds using natural materials such as collagen, elastin, or glycosaminoglycans, which naturally have ECM biochemical and structural characteristics that provide the capability for cellular adhesion, proliferation, and differentiation. With the emergence of fabrication technologies like additive manufacturing, scaffolds can be designed with functional groups or bioactive molecules, while maintaining control over architecture, and enabling the opportunity for individualized regenerative engineered solutions on an as-needed basis. When inventive procedures like functionalization and bioactivity are both utilized in tissue engineering, scaffold performance and therapeutic relevance are enhanced.

2.6.3.3 Functionalization for Infection Prevention

Functionalization of biomaterials with antimicrobial properties represents an essential strategy for reducing the incidence of infection and biofilm formation, particularly in clinical contexts involving implants and wound care. Silver nanoparticles are an efficient functionalization agent; incorporating silver nanoparticles into the surfaces of biomaterials provides a sustained antimicrobial activity by releasing silver ions that can alter the bacterial membrane and disrupt their metabolic processes. There are commercial devices, such as silver-coated catheters, that have demonstrated this functionalization approach by considerably reducing the rate of urinary tract infections (UTIs) despite being the most common hospital-acquired infections. Zwitterionic coatings are another emerging non-leaching option. Zwitterionic surfaces demonstrate a resistance to bacterial adhesion by preventing nonspecific protein binding that can result in biofilm formation. Zwitterionic surfaces, which are hydrophilic, may be particularly beneficial for long-term implantable devices (i.e., cardiovascular and orthopedic implants) where infection resistance is vital for continued use. These functionalization examples demonstrated here represent properties that enhance the sterility and safety of biomaterials in biomedical applications.

2.7 CURRENT CHALLENGES AND FUTURE DIRECTIONS

Even with substantial progress made in the field of stimuli-responsive biomaterials, there are still challenges in their development, characterization, and clinical use. These challenges are primarily associated with biocompatibility, biodegradability, minimizing toxicity, and the complex synthesis and characterization processes. It is important to closely examine these challenges for the continued evolution of this developing research area.

2.7.1 Biocompatibility, Biodegradability, and Toxicity

2.7.1.1 Biocompatibility Challenges and Solutions

Biocompatibility is still a basic requirement of any biomaterial for biomedical applications, as undesirable interactions with the host immune system can result in inflammation, fibrosis, or implant rejection. Synthetic polymers like PNIPAM are attractive because of their stimuli-responsive behavior, but raise concerns for biocompatibility due to unreacted monomer or degradation by-products that may lead to local irritation and inflammation. Synthetic scaffolds and biosensors result in a foreign body reaction characterized by immune cell infiltration and fibrotic encapsulation. There have been various strategies to reduce the foreign body response. Surface functionalization with hydrophilic polymers, such as PEGylation, is one approach to reduce protein adsorption and immune cell activation, leading to systemic tolerance and biocompatibility. The use of hybrid biomaterials with both natural components, such as chitosan or collagen, and synthetic matrix is an attractive option to balance mechanical functional performance and improved biological acceptance [57]. All of these solutions can lead to safer and more effective biomaterial-based therapeutics.

2.7.1.2 Biodegradability Challenges and Solutions

Biodegradability of biomaterials is one of many design parameters that should be precisely tuned with therapeutic or regenerative timelines in mind. If degradation is too quick, there can be a loss of structural or functional material before it has been used therapeutically, while if the degradation time is too long, residual material can remain and pose risks of chronic toxicity or fibrotic encapsulation. Some biodegradable polymers, such as PLA, lead to the generation of acidic by-products when they degrade, which can lower local pH and cause damage to surrounding tissues, and consequently limit their long-term utility in implants and drug delivery systems. To address these issues, a variety of strategies have been utilized to achieve controlled degradation profiles, including modifying cross-link density in both hydrogel and scaffold systems. Incorporating enzyme-sensitive cross-linkers further enables degradation that is spatially and temporally regulated in response to pathological cues. Blending synthetic polymers with natural biopolymers, such as alginate or gelatin, has proven effective in balancing degradation kinetics and minimizing the release of harmful by-products, enhancing the safety and efficacy of degradable biomaterial systems [58].

2.7.1.3 Toxicity from Degradation Products and Mitigation Strategies

Toxicity arising from the degradation products of biomaterials, particularly in nanoparticle and polymer-based systems, presents a significant concern in clinical translation. Metal-based nanoparticles, such as silver and gold, are known to release ions that can disrupt cellular signaling pathways, induce oxidative stress, and lead to cytotoxic effects. Nanoparticles lacking biocompatible surface modifications are prone to bioaccumulation in vital organs such as the liver and spleen, potentially resulting in long-term toxicity and systemic side effects. To address these challenges, surface coating with biocompatible materials such as PEG or albumin has been shown to reduce ion leaching, enhance systemic circulation, and promote renal or hepatic clearance. Functionalization with antioxidant moieties has emerged as an effective strategy to neutralize ROS, minimizing oxidative tissue damage. These approaches collectively enhance the safety profile of degradable nanomaterials, making them more suitable for long-term biomedical applications.

2.7.2 Challenges in Synthesis and Characterization

2.7.2.1 Complex Synthesis Processes and Optimization Strategies

The development of stimuli-responsive biomaterials frequently involves multi-step and highly controlled chemical synthesis, particularly when designing systems responsive to multiple environmental cues. These complex procedures introduce significant challenges in reproducibility, scalability, and cost-effectiveness. For instance, dual- or multi-stimuli-responsive materials often require intricate polymerization and functionalization protocols, increasing susceptibility to batch-to-batch variability and synthesis errors. The use of toxic solvents or hazardous reagents in traditional synthesis routes poses substantial barriers to clinical translation due to regulatory and safety concerns. To overcome these limitations, one-pot synthesis methods and green chemistry approaches have been developed to simplify production workflows and reduce environmental impact. The automation of synthesis using high-throughput robotic platforms offers improved consistency, scalability, and process control, making industrial-scale fabrication of complex biomaterials more feasible and reliable, as illustrated in Figure 2.2.

2.7.2.2 Scalability for Industrial Production

Translating laboratory-scale synthesis of stimuli-responsive biomaterials into industrial-scale production remains a formidable challenge due to high operational costs and the need for specialized equipment. Techniques such as photo-crosslinking and UV irradiation, commonly employed in the synthesis of light-responsive hydrogels, are particularly difficult to scale due to energy-intensive requirements and limited throughput, impeding commercial viability. Batch-to-batch variability in nanoparticle synthesis presents a critical obstacle, compromising product uniformity, reproducibility, and therapeutic efficacy. To address these issues, scalable fabrication techniques such as spray drying, extrusion, and electrospinning have been adopted, enabling the large-scale production of nanoparticles and scaffolds while preserving functional integrity. Process optimization and efficient reagent utilization contribute to cost reduction and enhance the feasibility of manufacturing stimuli-responsive biomaterials at an industrial scale, accelerating their clinical and commercial deployment [59].

2.7.2.3 Characterization Limitations and Advanced Analytical Approaches

Comprehensive characterization of stimuli-responsive biomaterials is vital for evaluating their performance and reliability; their dynamic and multi-dimensional responsiveness poses significant analytical challenges. Conventional techniques often fall short in capturing real-time behavior and complex interactions triggered by environmental stimuli such as pH, temperature, or light. This limitation becomes more pronounced in systems exhibiting multi-stimuli-responsiveness, such as nanoparticles or hydrogels that require synchronized evaluation of multiple response mechanisms. To address these challenges, in situ characterization techniques, including live-cell imaging and

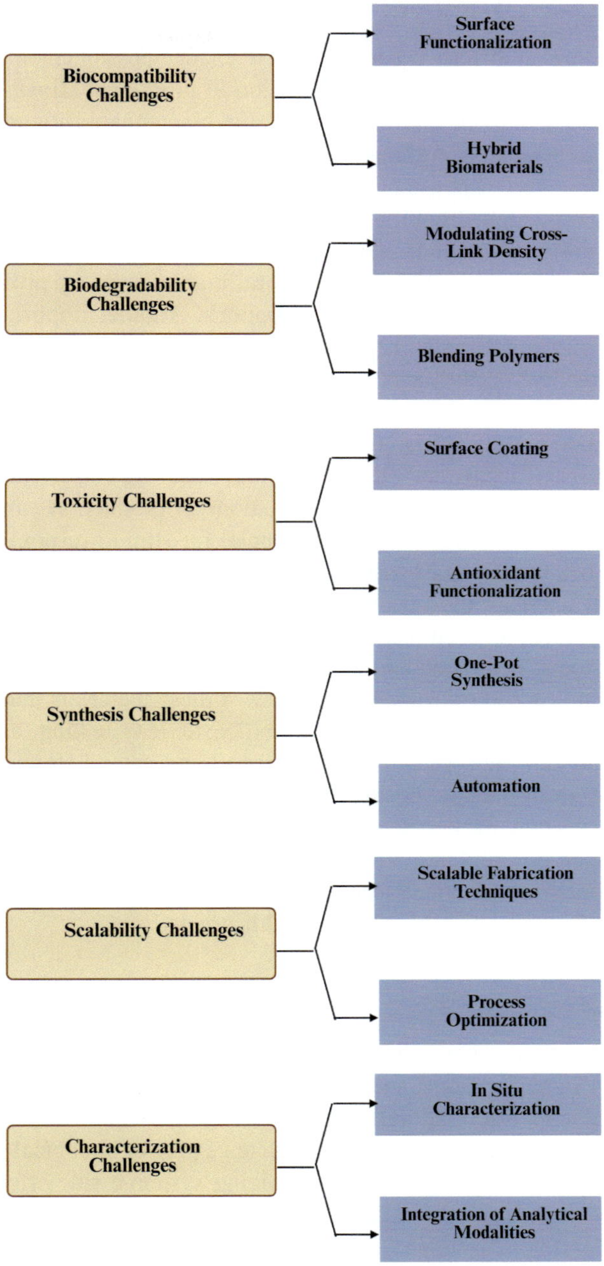

FIGURE 2.2 Key challenges in biomaterials research, including biocompatibility, biodegradability, toxicity, synthesis, scalability, and characterization, and corresponding strategies, such as surface functionalization, hybrid biomaterials, automation, and in situ analytical integration, to address these limitations and advance the field.

real-time spectroscopy, have emerged as powerful tools for observing biomaterial behavior under physiological conditions. The integration of multiple analytical modalities, such as combining thermal analysis with fluorescence imaging, enables a more holistic assessment of material structure, function, and responsiveness. These advanced methodologies are essential for optimizing material design and ensuring consistent performance in complex biomedical environments.

2.8 CURRENT STATE-OF-THE-ART AND PERSPECTIVES

Stimuli-responsive biomaterials have great potential to change possible biomedical and tissue engineering applications, but in order for them to function in prominent clinical and industrial applications, several key issues must be addressed. First, the biocompatibility and biosecurity of these biomaterials must be re-evaluated. Although advances have been made, many synthetic biomaterials can still elicit an immune response or toxic degradation products due to polymer degradation. Surface functionalization with hydrophilic polymers such as PEG, alongside the integration of natural polymers, such as collagen or chitosan, may reduce the risks associated with synthetic biomaterials. Hybrid materials with both synthetic and natural ingredients may provide useful, functional possibilities, while also providing biocompatible options. Another important requirement is the manufacturing scalability and affordability of biomaterials. While many stimuli-responsive biomaterials demonstrate excellent performance at the laboratory scale, their production at the industrial scale is often limited due to the cost and complexity of synthesis processes. Some strategies to mitigate this include one-pot synthesis, green chemistry approaches, and scalable manufacturing techniques, including spray drying and electrospinning. Ensuring consistent quality through minimizing batch-to-batch variation and exploring variations in production parameters is critical for further biomaterial use at industrial scales. It is crucial for stimuli-responsive biomaterials to be integrated with advanced technologies such as 3D bioprinting and AI [60]. By combining the engineering and biological sciences, the various approaches and fields that arise provide opportunities for personalized and precision-based medical solutions, just like patient-specific implants or adaptive drug delivery systems. Efforts should also characterize how regulations and standardizations should be developed in order to translate the delivery of these materials into the clinical space. In addition, creating global standards for biocompatibility, toxicity testing, and safety assessments will increase the speed at which we can attain approval and extend strategies into clinical practices. At last, there is an immediate need to tackle unmet medical challenges. The development of stimuli-responsive systems for unplaced or understudied areas, such as rare genetic conditions, neurodegenerative conditions, and individualized oncology, will broaden the range of these materials. Biomaterials responding to patient-specific biomarkers or that dynamically adapt respiratory physiological processes can drastically improve healthcare delivery.

2.9 CONCLUSION

Stimuli-responsive biomaterials have changed the paradigm of biomedical science through unique accuracy and efficacy in applications, such as drug delivery, tissue engineering, and regenerative medicine. The adaptable nature of stimuli-responsive biomaterials in response to physical stimuli (e.g., temperature or light exposure), chemical stimuli (e.g., pH), or biological stimuli (e.g., enzymes) allows localized therapeutic delivery, while minimizing systemic side effects. The versatility of these materials has been showcased in many different applications. From controlled drug delivery systems to bioactive scaffolds for tissue regeneration, stimuli-responsive biomaterials have become critical tools in modern medicine. The ability of stimuli-responsive biomaterials to adapt to complex and dynamic biological settings uniquely differentiates them from conventional biomaterials, allowing them to successfully address a variety of medical needs. Despite these advancements, there are also major challenges, especially with respect to biocompatibility, biodegradability, and scalability. Overcoming these challenges will require new materials design, new synthesis protocols, and even multidisciplinary collaboration. Simplifying these complex processes and a green, sustainable process may facilitate scale-up and translate to improved accessibility. In the future, the collaboration of stimuli-responsive biomaterials and new technologies will define the next version of a biomedical application. The opportunity for multifunctional systems, combining cubes that would embed stimuli-responsiveness with self-healing, real-time, and bioimaging, will prospectively represent future innovations. The field of personalized and precision medicine will also rely on designed biomaterials that target individual patient needs, for better therapeutic outcomes with more efficacy and safety. Although stimuli-responsive biomaterials present unique challenges, their potential to have a significant impact on healthcare makes them extremely promising. Continued research and innovation, as well as collaboration among material scientists, engineers, and clinicians, will ensure that these materials will not only solve existing healthcare needs but will also anticipate every new healthcare challenge and ultimately improve patient care and quality of life.

Declaration of AI and AI-Assisted Technologies

During the preparation of this work, the authors used QuillBot AI in order to paraphrase the sentences. After using this tool, the authors reviewed and edited the content as needed and take full responsibility for the content of the publication.

REFERENCES

1. Gelmi A, Schutt CE. Stimuli-responsive biomaterials: Scaffolds for stem cell control. Advanced Healthcare Materials. 2021 Jan;10(1):2001125.
2. Wei H, Cui J, Lin K, Xie J, Wang X. Recent advances in smart stimuli-responsive biomaterials for bone therapeutics and regeneration. Bone Research. 2022 Feb 23;10(1):17.
3. Protsak IS, Morozov YM. Fundamentals and advances in stimuli-responsive hydrogels and their applications: A review. Gels. 2025 Jan 2;11(1):30.
4. Liao Z, Liu T, Yao Z, Hu T, Ji X, Yao B. Harnessing stimuli-responsive biomaterials for advanced biomedical applications. Exploration. 2025 Feb;5(1):20230133.
5. Wang Y, Deng T, Liu X, Fang X, Mo Y, Xie N, Nie G, Zhang B, Fan X. Smart nanoplatforms responding to the tumor microenvironment for precise drug delivery in cancer therapy. International Journal of Nanomedicine. 2024 Dec 31:6253–77.
6. Jayabal R. Nanomaterials in regenerative medicine: Advancing the future of tissue engineering. Regenerative Engineering and Translational Medicine. 2025 May 6;11:1–9.
7. Gao Q, Lee JS, Kim BS, Gao G. Three-dimensional printing of smart constructs using stimuli-responsive biomaterials: A future direction of precision medicine. International Journal of Bioprinting. 2022 Nov 9;9(1):638.
8. Khizar S, Zine N, Errachid A, Elaissari A. Introduction to stimuli-responsive materials and their biomedical applications. In Stimuli-Responsive Materials for Biomedical Applications 2023 (pp. 1–30). American Chemical Society.
9. Ansari MJ, Rajendran RR, Mohanto S, Agarwal U, Panda K, Dhotre K, Manne R, Deepak A, Zafar A, Yasir M, Pramanik S. Poly(N-isopropylacrylamide)-based hydrogels for biomedical applications: A review of the state-of-the-art. Gels. 2022 Jul 20;8(7):454.
10. Pokharel M, Park K. Light mediated drug delivery systems: A review. Journal of Drug Targeting. 2022 Apr 21;30(4):368–80.
11. Ding H, Tan P, Fu S, Tian X, Zhang H, Ma X, Gu Z, Luo K. Preparation and application of pH-responsive drug delivery systems. Journal of Controlled Release. 2022 Aug 1;348:206–38.
12. Jia R, Teng L, Gao L, Su T, Fu L, Qiu Z, Bi Y. Advances in multiple stimuli-responsive drug-delivery systems for cancer therapy. International Journal of Nanomedicine. 2021 Feb 25;16:1525–51.
13. Throat S, Bhattacharya S. Macromolecular poly(N-isopropylacrylamide) (PNIPAM) in cancer treatment and beyond: Applications in drug delivery, photothermal therapy, gene delivery and biomedical imaging. Advances in Polymer Technology. 2024;2024(1):1444990.
14. Dethe MR, Prabakaran A, Ahmed H, Agrawal M, Roy U, Alexander A. PCL-PEG copolymer based injectable thermosensitive hydrogels. Journal of Controlled Release. 2022 Mar 1;343:217–36.
15. Mod Razif MR, Chan SY, Widodo RT, Chew YL, Hassan M, Hisham SA, Rahman SA, Ming LC, Tan CS, Lee SK, Liew KB. Optimization of a luteolin-loaded TPGS/Poloxamer 407 nanomicelle: The effects of copolymers, hydration temperature and duration, and freezing temperature on encapsulation efficiency, particle size, and solubility. Cancers. 2023 Jul 24;15(14):3741.
16. Samui AB. Photoresponsive polymers. In Smart Polymers 2022 Apr 26 (pp. 15–40). CRC Press.
17. Hu C. Light-triggered stimuli-responsive microgels (Doctoral dissertation, RWTH Aachen University, 2021).

18. Pontico M, Conte M, Petronella F, Frantellizzi V, De Feo MS, Di Luzio D, Pani R, De Vincentis G, De Sio L. 18F-fluorodeoxyglucose (18F-FDG) functionalized gold nanoparticles (GNPs) for plasmonic photothermal ablation of cancer: A review. Pharmaceutics. 2023 Jan 18;15(2):319.
19. Rahman M. Magnetic resonance imaging and iron-oxide nanoparticles in the era of personalized medicine. Nanotheranostics. 2023 Aug 21;7(4):424.
20. Dasari A, Xue J, Deb S. Magnetic nanoparticles in bone tissue engineering. Nanomaterials. 2022 Feb 24;12(5):757.
21. Bakirdogen G, Selcuk E, Kahveci EL, Ozbek T, Derman S, Kahveci MU. Fabrication of poly(β-amino ester) and hyaluronic acid based pH responsive nanocomplex as an antibiotic release system. International Journal of Biological Macromolecules. 2024 Feb 1;258:129060.
22. Man E, Lamprou D, Easdon C, McLellan I, Yiu HH, Hoskins C. Exploration of dual ionic cross-linked alginate hydrogels via cations of varying valences towards wound healing. Polymers. 2022 Nov 29;14(23):5192.
23. Petrila LM, Bucatariu F, Mihai M, Teodosiu C. Polyelectrolyte multilayers: An overview on fabrication, properties, and biomedical and environmental applications. Materials. 2021 Jul 26;14(15):4152.
24. Bawa KK. Development of dual stimuli-responsive degradable polylactide-based multifunctional materials for drug delivery (Doctoral dissertation, Concordia University), 2021.
25. Birhan YS, Tsai HC. Recent developments in selenium-containing polymeric micelles: Prospective stimuli, drug-release behaviors, and intrinsic anticancer activity. Journal of Materials Chemistry B. 2021;9(34):6770–801.
26. Radman BA, Alhameed AM, Shu G, Yin G, Wang M. Cellular elasticity in cancer: A review of altered biomechanical features. Journal of Materials Chemistry B. 2024;12(22):5299–324.
27. Abbasi YF, Bera H, Cun D, Yang M. Recent advances in pH/enzyme-responsive polysaccharide-small-molecule drug conjugates as nanotherapeutics. Carbohydrate Polymers. 2023 Jul 15;312:120797.
28. Ghafari Y, Asefnejad A, Ogbemudia DO. Gold nanoparticles in biomedicine: Advancements in cancer therapy, drug delivery, diagnostics, and tissue regeneration. Scientific Hypotheses. 2024 Feb 18;1:21–35.
29. Mohanty AR, Ravikumar A, Peppas NA. Recent advances in glucose-responsive insulin delivery systems: Novel hydrogels and future applications. Regenerative Biomaterials. 2022 Jan 1;9:rbac056.
30. Arshavsky-Graham S, Heuer C, Jiang X, Segal E. Aptasensors versus immunosensors—Which will prevail? Engineering in Life Sciences. 2022 Mar;22(3–4):319–33.
31. Mukherjee C, Varghese D, Krishna JS, Boominathan T, Rakeshkumar R, Dineshkumar S, Rao CB, Sivaramakrishna A. Recent advances in biodegradable polymers–properties, applications and future prospects. European Polymer Journal. 2023 Jun 23;192:112068.
32. Hajebi S, Mohammadi Nasr S, Rabiee N, Bagherzadeh M, Ahmadi S, Rabiee M, Tahriri M, Tayebi L, Hamblin MR. Bioresorbable composite polymeric materials for tissue engineering applications. International Journal of Polymeric Materials and Polymeric Biomaterials. 2021 Sep 2;70(13):926–40.
33. Radulescu DM, Neacsu IA, Grumezescu AM, Andronescu E. New insights of scaffolds based on hydrogels in tissue engineering. Polymers. 2022 Feb 18;14(4):799.
34. Park D, Lee SJ, Park JW. Aptamer-based smart targeting and spatial trigger–response drug-delivery systems for anticancer therapy. Biomedicines. 2024 Jan 15;12(1):187.
35. Sadraei A, Naghib SM. 4D printing of physical stimuli-responsive hydrogels for localized drug delivery and tissue engineering. Polymer Reviews. 2025 Jan 2;65(1):104–68.
36. Sharma A, Sengupta S, Kumar L, Upadhyay T, Kabra A, Lalhlenmawia H, Kumar D, Singh J. Recent advancements in photodynamic therapy and cancer biosensor using natural products. Talanta Open. 2023 Dec 1;8:100261.
37. Joshi G, Sharma V, Saxena R, Yadav KS. Polylactic coglycolic acid (PLGA)-based green materials for drug delivery. In Applications of Advanced Green Materials 2021 Jan 1 (pp. 425–440). Woodhead Publishing.
38. Giridhar S, Anandamurthy HC. Advances in controlled drug delivery using grafted copolymer. In Graft Copolymers of Polysaccharides for Drug Delivery Systems 2025 Jul 15 (pp. 201–235). Apple Academic Press.
39. Kanjilal B, Zhu Y, Krishnadoss V, Unagolla JM, Saemian P, Caci A, Cheraghali D, Dehzangi I, Khademhosseini A, Noshadi I. Bioionic liquids: Enabling a paradigm shift toward advanced and smart biomedical applications. Advanced Intelligent Systems. 2023 May;5(5):2200306.
40. Singhai H, Rathee S, Sahu A, Patil UK, Jain SK. Enzyme-responsive vesicular carriers as an emerging approach for tumor targeting. In Tumor-Targeting with Stimuli-Responsive Vesicular Nanocarriers 2025 Jan 1 (pp. 111–135). Academic Press.

41. Zhang Z, Yao S, Hu Y, Zhao X, Lee RJ. Application of lipid-based nanoparticles in cancer immunotherapy. Frontiers in Immunology. 2022 Aug 8;13:967505.
42. Fatima R, Katiyar P, Kushwaha K. Recent advances in mesoporous silica nanoparticle: Synthesis, drug loading, release mechanisms, and diverse applications. Frontiers in Nanotechnology. 2025 Mar 18;7:1564188.
43. Castillo-Henríquez L, Castro-Alpízar J, Lopretti-Correa M, Vega-Baudrit J. Exploration of bioengineered scaffolds composed of thermo-responsive polymers for drug delivery in wound healing. International Journal of Molecular Sciences. 2021 Jan 30;22(3):1408.
44. Georgeous J, AlSawaftah N, Abuwatfa WH, Husseini GA. Review of gold nanoparticles: Synthesis, properties, shapes, cellular uptake, targeting, release mechanisms and applications in drug delivery and therapy. Pharmaceutics. 2024 Oct 16;16(10):1332.
45. Yousefiasl S, Zare I, Ghovvati M, Ghomi M. Enzyme-responsive materials: Properties, design, and applications. In Stimuli-Responsive Materials for Biomedical Applications 2023 (pp. 203–229). American Chemical Society.
46. Ben Mabrouk A. The Role of Physical Barrier Functions of Polyethylene Glycol Modified Nanoparticles in Modulating Their Blood Circulation.
47. Nitti P, Narayanan A, Pellegrino R, Villani S, Madaghiele M, Demitri C. Cell-tissue interaction: The biomimetic approach to design tissue engineered biomaterials. Bioengineering. 2023 Sep 25;10(10):1122.
48. Yu M, Ren TX, Jin XG, Tang X, Tang MM, Ma XH, Xu ZL. Theoretical and experimental research of polyelectrolyte multilayer membrane prepared by layer by layer self-assembly. Desalination. 2024 Jul 1;580:117561.
49. Berger MB, Slosar P, Schwartz Z, Cohen DJ, Goodman SB, Anderson PA, Boyan BD. A review of biomimetic topographies and their role in promoting bone formation and osseointegration: Implications for clinical use. Biomimetics. 2022 Apr 16;7(2):46.
50. Qin C, Yue Z, Wallace GG, Chen J. Bipolar electrochemical stimulation using conducting polymers for wireless electroceuticals and future directions. ACS Applied Bio Materials. 2022 Oct 19;5(11):5041–56.
51. Singh P, Pandit S, Balusamy SR, Madhusudanan M, Singh H, Amsath Haseef HM, Mijakovic I. Advanced nanomaterials for cancer therapy: Gold, silver, and iron oxide nanoparticles in oncological applications. Advanced Healthcare Materials. 2025 Feb;14(4):2403059.
52. Davari N, Bakhtiary N, Khajehmohammadi M, Sarkari S, Tolabi H, Ghorbani F, Ghalandari B. Protein-based hydrogels: Promising materials for tissue engineering. Polymers. 2022 Feb 28;14(5):986.
53. Ghasemiyeh P, Mohammadi-Samani S. Polymers blending as release modulating tool in drug delivery. Frontiers in Materials. 2021 Nov 9;8:752813.
54. Hwang HS, Lee CS. Nanoclay-composite hydrogels for bone tissue engineering. Gels. 2024 Aug 3;10(8):513.
55. Verma AK. An insight into collagen-based nano biomaterials for drug delivery applications. In Engineered Biomaterials: Synthesis and Applications 2023 Nov 27 (pp. 397–428). Springer Nature Singapore.
56. Tenchov R, Sasso JM, Zhou QA. PEGylated lipid nanoparticle formulations: Immunological safety and efficiency perspective. Bioconjugate Chemistry. 2023 May 10;34(6):941–60.
57. Amiryaghoubi N, Fathi M, Adibkia K, Barar J, Omidian H, Omidi Y. Chitosan-based biomaterials: Their interaction with natural and synthetic materials for cartilage, bone, cardiac, vascular, and neural tissue engineering. In Sheikh, F.A. (eds.), Engineering Materials for Stem Cell Regeneration 2021 (pp. 619–50). Springer. https://doi.org/10.1007/978-981-16-4420-7_22
58. Maitra J, Bhardwaj N. Development of bio-based polymeric blends–a comprehensive review. Journal of Biomaterials Science, Polymer Edition. 2025 Jan 2;36(1):102–36.
59. Siebenmorgen C. Stimuli-Responsive Polymeric Composites for Advanced Controllable Biomaterials.
60. Jaafari A, Rahmani Z, Zolfagharizadeh A, Amoozegar H. Innovations in Biomedical Engineering: A Comprehensive Review of Emerging Trends and Technologies.

3 Ideal Biomaterials and Chemistry Underlying Stimuli-Responsive Drug Delivery

Mehuli Das, Yashaswi Dutta Gupta, Sayani Bhattacharya, and Suman Bhandary
Department of Biological Sciences, School of Life Science and Biotechnology, Adamas University, Kolkata, West Bengal, India

3.1 INTRODUCTION

The evolution of drug delivery systems (DDS) can be seen in the early 20th century, establishing a noteworthy turning point in pharmaceutical advancements when the first attempts were made to boost the therapeutic efficacy of drugs through controlled release mechanisms [1]. Initially, these systems focused on improving bioavailability and reducing side effects by using simple formulations such as liposomes and microspheres. The emergence of sophisticated technologies in the latter half of the 20th and early 21st centuries has facilitated the improvement of advanced DDS able to react quickly to specific external and internal stimuli [2]. This evolution has led to the advent of stimuli-responsive DDS, which offer significant improvements in targeted therapy by releasing drugs in response to physiological changes or external triggers. Despite the advancements in DDS, there are still several obstacles that prevent its clinical application and efficacy. One of the primary issues is the lack of specificity in drug delivery, which often results in systemic side effects and diminished therapeutic consequences [3]. Conventional drug delivery methods typically dispense therapeutic agents consistently throughout the body, leading to off-target effects that can be detrimental, particularly in cancer therapy, where healthy tissues may also be affected [4]. Furthermore, many conventional DDS struggle with premature drug release, which can compromise treatment efficiency and lead to suboptimal drug concentrations at target sites of interest. The complexity of biological environments adds another layer of difficulty; factors such as pH variations, enzymatic activity, and tumor microenvironments can significantly affect drug release profiles, making it challenging to achieve precise control over therapeutic delivery [5].

Moreover, the immunogenicity of certain carriers poses a significant barrier to their effectiveness. Many materials used in DDS can provoke immune responses, leading to fast clearance from circulation and reduced therapeutic efficacy [6]. The intricate chemistry involved in designing stimuli-responsive carriers further complicates their pharmaceutical development. Investigators must circumnavigate a myriad of parameters, including carrier size, surface charge, and nanomaterial composition, to optimize performance while ensuring biocompatibility and biodegradability [7, 8]. These challenges highlight the pressing need for inventive approaches that boost the accuracy and efficacy of DDS. The rationale for advancing research in stimuli-responsive DDS is multifaceted. First, these systems hold promise for achieving targeted therapy, which is particularly crucial in cases of oncology where localized treatment can minimize damage to healthy tissues while maximizing therapeutic impact on tumors. By designing carriers that respond specifically to tumor microenvironments—such as acidic pH or elevated enzyme levels—researchers aim to improve

DOI: 10.1201/9781003560203-3

drug accumulation at target sites while reducing systemic exposure [9]. Additionally, stimuli-responsive systems can facilitate on-demand drug release, allowing for greater control over pharmacokinetics and pharmacodynamics [10]. This capability especially benefits chronic diseases that require sustained drug action without continuous administration.

Investigators are increasingly focusing on identifying optimal biomaterials that not only meet the basic requirements of biocompatibility and biodegradability but also exhibit tailored responsiveness to several stimuli, including changes in pH, temperature, redox conditions, light exposure, and ultrasound [11]. Advanced materials science, combined with nanotechnology, has led significant innovations in carrier design, enabling the engineering of polymers, lipids, and inorganic nanoparticles (NPs) for specific applications. Multidisciplinary synthesis and functionalization approaches highlight the potential for creating next-generation DDS capable of overcoming existing limitations while addressing specific clinical needs [12].

This chapter aims to present an in-depth exploration of ideal biomaterials and the underlying chemistry that enable effective stimuli-responsive DDS. We will explore fundamental requirements for biomaterials used in DDS, including their mechanical properties and interactions with biological environments. Additionally, we will delve into various types of stimuli—such as pH changes, temperature fluctuations, redox reactions, magnetic fields, light exposure, and ultrasound—and examine how these factors influence drug release mechanisms. We aim to elucidate how polymers, lipids, inorganic NPs, and hydrogels can be tailored for precise responsiveness by analyzing a range of these materials. Ultimately, this chapter seeks to contribute valuable insights into the design and application of stimuli-responsive DDS while emphasizing the importance of a multidisciplinary approach in advancing this innovative field.

3.2 FUNDAMENTAL REQUIREMENTS OF BIOMATERIALS IN DDS

Although the discovery of drugs targeting a broad spectrum of diseases has been extensive, the method of drug delivery determines the efficacy of the specific drug. The pharmacokinetic properties of a drug, absorption, distribution, metabolism, and excretion, are highly dependent on the mode of delivery of the drug [13]. For almost 60 years, biomaterials have been developed and utilized in sophisticated DDS through collaborative efforts. Using some of the biomaterials as carriers for drug delivery into biological systems has proven to increase the efficacy of the drugs. Key considerations for employing biomaterials in DDS encompass the following.

3.2.1 Biocompatibility and Toxicity

Researchers must use biocompatible materials for drug delivery, meaning these materials must perform their specific function without causing any harmful reactions in the body. It must be such that once it enters the body, it can surpass the immune system without activating it. Metals such as titanium are frequently utilized in orthopedic implants because of their superior mechanical strength and outstanding biocompatibility, which allow osseointegration without significant immune response, e.g., a bioceramics (hydroxyapatite) can mimic the mineral component of bone and allow adhesion of cells and allows their growth; they are often used in bone grafts for implants, because of their biocompatibility and non-toxicity [14].

3.2.2 Biodegradability

It is possible to encapsulate drugs in biodegradable polymers and release them into the environment under controlled conditions. These biodegradable polymers facilitate accurate dose and long-lasting therapeutic benefits, both of which are advantageous for the management of chronic illnesses. Biodegradable materials can be engineered to reduce the likelihood of toxicity and inflammation by minimizing off-target effects. Biodegradable biomaterials for drug delivery offer a more environmentally friendly solution, as they naturally degrade in the body, eliminating the need for surgical removal of residual materials and reducing waste. This approach promotes sustainability and minimizes the ecological footprint of medical interventions. Scientists formulate biodegradable materials into NPs, hydrogels, and other delivery systems to enhance the bioavailability of a specific drug. In ocular drug delivery, biodegradable materials enhance the drug's bioavailability within the eye [15].

3.2.3 Targeting Ability

In order to ensure targeted drug distribution to the intended place, biomaterials for tumor treatment are made to bind particular receptors on tumor cells selectively. Synthetic biomaterials are essential for delivering proteins, small molecules, and macromolecules in their native forms, preserving their biological activity and preventing degradation. Scientists observed that silicone rubbers could release drugs like histamine, atropine, and steroids over several days to months [15].

3.2.4 Release of Therapeutics from Stimuli-Dependent DDS

In diseased, inflamed, and infected tissues, pH levels often decrease due to metabolic dysregulation or abnormal angiogenesis, leading to oxygen and nutrient shortages. This triggers a shift toward glycolytic metabolism. Such pH variations across organs, tissues, and cellular compartments are key considerations when designing nanomaterials for site-specific therapeutic release. Materials that respond to temperature changes by altering their physical structure or properties are gaining prominence in biomedical applications, particularly in controlled drug release and tissue regeneration. Similarly, light-responsive biomaterials enable precise control of cellular behavior and compound release for tissue regeneration, leveraging light's non-invasive, spatial, and temporal precision. Notably, investigators can combine these responsive materials to create sophisticated systems. Polymers that react to oxidative or reductive stimuli, as well as external electrical signals, owe their responsiveness to specific chemical moieties, including disulfide linkages, metal-containing complexes, and electron-rich compounds like viologens and tetrathiafulvalene. These materials hold significant potential for biomedical applications, which will be discussed further in the following sections [16].

3.3 DESIGN AND ENGINEERING OF STIMULI-RESPONSIVE DDS

Smart DDS are designed to release medications in a controlled manner, triggered by specific physiological or environmental cues. The design of these systems heavily relies on the incorporation of various chemical bonds that can undergo reversible or irreversible changes upon stimulation (Table 3.1). Below is an overview of the key types of chemical bonds utilized in ideal stimuli-responsive DDS, along with recent references highlighting their applications.

3.3.1 Dynamic Covalent Bonds

Dynamic covalent bonds, characterized by their reversible nature, have been instrumental in advancing adaptive DDS. Recent studies have highlighted the potential of imine bonds, disulfide bonds, and boronic ester linkages in creating responsive DDS that adapt to environmental changes. Imine bonds, formed between amines and aldehydes or ketones, are pH-sensitive and hydrolyze under acidic conditions (Figure 3.1A). This property makes them suitable for tumor-targeted drug release, as the tumor microenvironment often exhibits lower pH levels. Recent research has demonstrated the incorporation of imine bonds into polymeric drug carriers, enabling controlled drug release in acidic tumor environments. Disulfide linkages exhibit redox sensitivity, making them susceptible

TABLE 3.1
Detailed Tabular Representation of Various Types of Chemical Bonds Commonly Utilized in Stimuli-Responsive Ideal DDS

Bond Type	Mechanism/Trigger	Characteristics	Applications	References
Covalent bonds	Cleavage by specific stimuli	Strong and stable under normal conditions but cleavable under specific triggers.	pH-sensitive bonds (e.g., hydrazone, imine, acetal bonds in acidic microenvironments of tumors)	[17]
Disulfide bonds	Redox-responsive	Stable in oxidizing environments, cleaved by reducing agents (e.g., glutathione in cancer cells).	Controlled drug release in tumor microenvironments rich in glutathione	[17]
Ionic bonds	pH-sensitive dissociation	Reversible, dependent on ionic strength and pH changes.	Electrostatic interactions in polyelectrolyte complexes for gene or drug delivery	[18]
Hydrogen bonds	Temperature or solvent-dependent disruption	Reversible and sensitive to environmental conditions such as temperature, pH, or hydration.	Self-assembled hydrogels or micelles for thermo-responsive drug delivery	[19]
Hydrophobic interactions	Temperature, solvent, or pH-responsive	Non-covalent interactions stabilized by hydrophobic domains, responsive to solvent polarity or temperature changes.	Formation of micelles or nanoparticles for encapsulating hydrophobic drugs	[20]
π–π stacking interactions	Chemical or light-responsive changes	Reversible interactions between aromatic rings are sensitive to chemical environment or external stimuli.	Stabilizing nanocarriers or controlling release via light-triggered conformational changes	[21]
Dynamic covalent bonds	Stimuli-triggered dynamic breaking/forming	Reversible under specific stimuli such as light, pH, or redox conditions.	Schiff base linkages for pH-responsive or glucose-responsive drug delivery systems	[17]
Metal-coordination bonds	pH- or ion concentration-sensitive dissociation	Formed between metal ions and ligands, often reversible under pH or redox changes.	Metal-polymer complexes in drug delivery for anticancer or antibacterial applications (e.g., cisplatin release)	[22]
Enzyme-cleavable Bonds	Biological stimuli (enzyme activity)	Bonds engineered for selective cleavage by enzymes highly expressed in diseased tissues.	Peptide bonds cleaved by proteases in cancer or inflammatory environments	[23]
Host–guest interactions	Environmental-responsive reversible binding	Inclusion complexes sensitive to environmental stimuli like pH or temperature.	Cyclodextrin-based systems for stimuli-responsive drug loading and release	[24]
Cleavable ester bonds	Covalent bonds are susceptible to hydrolysis	Ester-based prodrugs for pH-responsive release.	pH-responsive drug delivery system (HMSNs-β-CD/Ada-PEG@DOX) for tumor therapy, featuring accelerated hydrolysis in acidic and basic environments, mimicking the tumor microenvironment cascade	[17]
Thioether bonds	Covalent bonds between sulfur and carbon atoms	Oxidation-sensitive polymers for reactive oxygen species (ROS)-responsive drug release.	Oxidative cleavage under high ROS conditions	[17]
Ferroptosis-responsive bonds	Bonds responding to lipid peroxidation or oxidative stress	Lipid-based nanoparticles targeting ferroptotic pathways in cancer therapy.	Oxidation-induced drug release	[25]
Photo-cleavable bonds	Bonds that break upon light exposure	Coumarin or nitrobenzyl-based systems for light-triggered drug release.	UV or visible light cleaves the bond	[26]

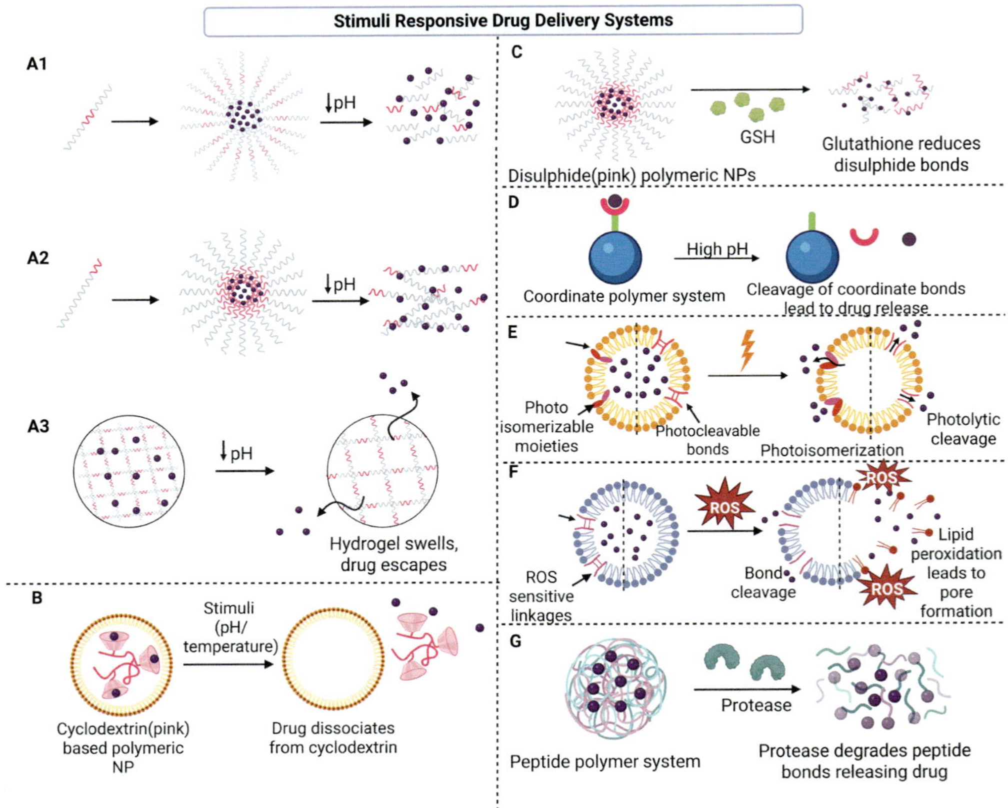

FIGURE 3.1 Stimuli-responsive drug delivery systems. (A) Acid-labile linkers (pink), such as acetal, imine, hydrazone, ester, or Schiff's base bonds, connect nanoparticle components (1) or the drug to the matrix (2). These linkages break in the acidic tumor microenvironment, releasing the drug. They can also be incorporated into hydrogels that swell in acidic pH, facilitating drug release (3). (B) β-cyclodextrin-based polymeric NPs enable environmental stimuli-responsive drug delivery. (C) Disulfide-cross-linked polymeric NPs degrade in the presence of glutathione, releasing the drug. (D) Coordinate polymer systems, with NP functional groups (green) and metal ions (pink), release the drug under acidic conditions as the coordinate bonds break. (E) NPs functionalized with photoisomerizable moieties (azobenzene) or photolabile bonds (coumarin, nitrobenzyl) trigger light-responsive drug release via isomerization (trans–cis) or bond cleavage, respectively. (F) ROS-sensitive bonds (thioether) or lipid peroxidation of liposomes (red) cause NP degradation and drug release via bond cleavage and pore formation, respectively. (G) Enzyme-responsive systems, with substrate-functionalized polymers (peptide bonds in blue), degrade upon protease exposure, releasing the drug.

to breakdown by reductive molecules such as glutathione (GSH), a naturally occurring antioxidant found in high concentrations within cells. This feature facilitates controlled drug release within cells. Recent advancements have shown that NPs with disulfide bonds can enhance the stability of drug carriers and confirm the release of therapeutics in response to the intracellular reducing environment. Boronic ester bonds are responsive to pH and glucose levels, making them valuable in designing glucose-responsive insulin delivery systems. Advances in dynamic covalent boronate chemistry have showcased the versatility of boronic ester linkages in the design of adaptive DDS. By leveraging these reversible bonds, investigators can rapidly optimize polymeric vectors for gene delivery, paving the way for the development of responsive DDS that adapt to specific physiological cues. This approach holds promise for enhancing treatment outcomes while mitigating adverse effects [17].

3.3.2 Supramolecular Interactions

Investigators have advanced intelligent DDS that enable precise, targeted release of therapeutic agents by developing stimuli-responsive host–guest complexes. By harnessing non-covalent binding interactions between molecular hosts, such as cyclodextrins, and guest molecules, these systems can be engineered to respond to specific environmental cues, including shifts in pH, temperature fluctuations, or exposure to light (Figure 3.1B). One prominent illustration of this concept is the combination of β-cyclodextrin (β-CD) as the host molecule and azobenzene-based compounds as the guest. Upon irradiation with light of specific wavelengths, azobenzene undergoes a reversible configurational switch between trans and cis configurations, enabling dynamic control over the host–guest interaction [27]. Scientists have leveraged the photoresponsive properties of azobenzene to design supramolecular assemblies that selectively release therapeutic agents in response to light cues. These multifunctional systems enable precise temporal and spatial control over drug delivery, ultimately leading to improved treatment outcomes and reduced adverse reactions. Another advancement in this field is the development of supramolecular polymers that incorporate stimuli-responsive host–guest interactions. These polymers can self-assemble into nanostructures capable of encapsulating therapeutic agents. Upon encountering specific triggers, such as shifts in pH or temperature, the supramolecular forces governing these nanostructures can be selectively disrupted, prompting their disintegration and the controlled liberation of the sequestered therapeutic agents. This approach allows for the design of DDS that are responsive to the unique microenvironments of diseased tissues, such as the acidic environment of tumor sites [24]. While synthetic polymers utilized in nanomedicine development generally exhibit biodegradable and biocompatible properties, their breakdown is often hindered by their substantial molecular mass and robust covalent linkages between constituent monomers, resulting in prolonged degradation periods spanning weeks or months. The limited metabolic and elimination efficiency of these exogenous nanomaterials frequently leads to interactions with various immune system components. Significant adverse effects and potential immunotoxicity can result from this, potentially hindering the treatment process or diminishing the effectiveness of anticancer therapies. Yu et al. designed nanotheranostics based on supramolecular polymers using β-CD-GSH-responsive disulfide bond-camptothecin (CPT) as a supramolecular monomer [28].

In this system, β-CD served as the host, and CPT acted as the guest, linked via a GSH-sensitive disulfide (SS) bond (Figure 3.1C). A strategically positioned β-CD moiety served as a molecular gatekeeper on the surface, forming selective host–guest complexes with adamantane (Ada) moieties that were covalently attached to the hybrid framework via a reducible disulfide bond. This configuration enabled the GSH-responsive release of doxorubicin (DOX) loaded within the system. The nanomedicine, administered through intraperitoneal injection, demonstrated adequate enrichment in metastatic tumors, outperforming intravenous delivery and resulting in significantly improved therapeutic outcomes *in vivo*. Preclinical evaluations, encompassing both in vitro and in vivo investigations, have consistently demonstrated that this supramolecular nanomedicine exhibits potent anticancer efficacy, significantly impeding metastatic progression. Moreover, its safety profile is characterized by negligible systemic toxicity and long-term immunological tolerance, underscoring the synergistic advantages afforded by the convergence of nanotechnology and supramolecular chemistry [28].

Furthermore, the integration of host–guest chemistry into supramolecular theranostics has been explored. By designing host–guest systems that respond to specific stimuli, investigators have developed nanomedicines that combine therapeutic and diagnostic functions. These supramolecular nanomedicines can release drugs in response to stimuli present in the tumor microenvironment, such as acidic pH or overexpressed enzymes, while simultaneously providing imaging capabilities for monitoring treatment progress [22].

Coordination polymers (CPs) are hybrid materials constructed from metal ions linked to organic ligands, yielding architectures with one, two, or three dimensions. In the context of drug delivery, investigators can tailor CPs to liberate therapeutic payloads in response to specific environmental cues, such as the acidic conditions prevalent in tumor microenvironments or within cellular compartments like lysosomes. Under physiological conditions, the coordination bonds between metal ions and ligands in CPs remain stable, effectively encapsulating the drug molecules. Under acidic conditions, these bonds can undergo cleavage, triggering the disintegration of the polymer framework and the concomitant liberation of the entrapped therapeutic agent. This pH-dependent behavior confers a distinct advantage for selectively targeting acidic tumor microenvironments or intracellular compartments, thereby ensuring site-specific drug release and enhancing therapeutic precision. Scientists have developed nanoscale coordination polymers (NCPs) that exhibit efficient drug loading and pH-triggered release. For instance, a study demonstrated that DOX, a common chemotherapeutic agent, could be effectively loaded onto NPs composed of coordination polymers or NCPs [22].

In the acidic environment of lysosomes, NCPs disintegrated, triggering the release of DOX and concurrent recovery of fluorescence, enabling real-time monitoring of drug release within tumor cells [29]. Investigators have developed a novel pH-responsive coordination polymer sphere for targeted anticancer drug delivery [30]. These spheres exhibit prolonged drug release over multiple days due to their enhanced stability and responsiveness to external pH fluctuations. Notably, drug release is accelerated under mildly acidic conditions compared to physiological pH (Figure 3.1D). Investigators have successfully achieved selective internalization by cancer cells via receptor-mediated endocytosis by functionalizing the surface of these spheres with folic acid.

NPs functionalized with photoresponsive moieties such as azobenzene, coumarin, and o-nitrobenzyl have garnered significant attention for their ability to achieve controlled drug release upon light activation. These advanced delivery systems enable precise spatial and temporal control over therapeutic administration, thereby augmenting efficacy while mitigating adverse effects. The incorporation of azobenzene, which undergoes reversible photoisomerization between its trans and cis configurations in response to specific light wavelengths, allows for dynamic modulation of NP properties. This light-induced conformational shift can alter the NP's physicochemical characteristics, such as its hydrophobicity or structural arrangement, thereby triggering the controlled release of encapsulated therapeutic agents (Figure 3.1E). Recent research has explored the potential of azobenzene-functionalized hydrogels for tailored drug delivery. Notably, scientists have leveraged light-sensitive azobenzene-β-CD host–guest interactions to modulate drug release from hydrogels in response to light stimuli, paving the way for innovative applications in wound management and tissue repair [31]. Light-responsive polyurethanes incorporating coumarin and o-nitrobenzyl groups have been developed, enabling controlled drug release upon light-induced bond cleavage. These platforms provide the benefit of adjustable degradation kinetics, making them attractive candidates for a wide range of biomedical uses, from tissue engineering to controlled drug delivery [26].

Investigators highly value stimuli-responsive DDS for their ability to release therapeutic agents in response to physiological triggers, using key mechanisms such as reactive oxygen species (ROS)-sensitive bonds and enzyme-responsive systems. In environments characterized by elevated levels of ROS, such as inflamed tissues or tumor microenvironments, ROS-labile linkages like thioethers are susceptible to oxidative cleavage, triggering the degradation of NPs and the concomitant liberation of encapsulated therapeutic agents (Figure 3.1F). Recent studies have focused on developing ROS-responsive polymers incorporating thioether groups. For instance, thioether-based ROS-responsive bifunctional monomers have been synthesized to create smart hydrogels suitable for four-dimensional (4D) printing applications. These hydrogels degrade in the presence of ROS, facilitating controlled drug release [32]. Furthermore, researchers have engineered ROS-sensitive hyper-branched polymers incorporating thioether moieties, which have shown promise for tailored drug delivery applications, leveraging the oxidative degradation of these polymers to trigger controlled release. These polymers degrade upon exposure to ROS, enabling targeted drug release in oxidative environments [33].

Enzyme-responsive DDS utilize substrate-functionalized polymers that degrade upon exposure to specific enzymes, releasing the encapsulated drug (Figure 3.1G). These systems commonly employ peptide bonds, particularly to target proteases overexpressed in certain pathological conditions. Recent breakthroughs have led to the creation of enzyme-sensitive nanomaterials, which offer a promising strategy for precision drug delivery, where enzymatic activity triggers the selective release of therapeutic agents. These systems are designed to release therapeutic agents upon enzymatic cleavage, ensuring targeted and efficient drug delivery [34]. Moreover, scientists have investigated the potential of in situ-forming enzyme-responsive peptide–peptide hydrogels as innovative drug delivery vehicles. Upon exposure to specific enzymes, these hydrogels undergo selective degradation, enabling the precise and controlled liberation of encapsulated therapeutic agents [23].

3.4 STIMULI-RESPONSIVE POLYMERS

Innovative DDS rely on polymers that can adapt to external cues through physical or chemical transformations. Self-immolative polymers (SIPs) provide a notable example, as investigators design them to disintegrate completely in response to specific triggers, making them exceptionally well-suited for precision applications in targeted drug delivery and molecular imaging. Scientists commonly construct SIPs with a robust backbone and a triggerable end-cap. Upon activation by a stimulus—such as pH change, light, or the presence of specific ions—the end-cap is cleaved, initiating a domino-like depolymerization of the polymer chain. This triggered disintegration enables the precise and controlled liberation of therapeutic payloads or diagnostic probes, offering a highly tailored approach to drug delivery and molecular imaging. Polymers like poly (phthalaldehyde) (PPA) are notable for their rapid depolymerization into non-toxic monomers, minimizing adverse biological effects [35].

3.4.1 Click Chemistry and Free Radical Initiation for Capturing and Releasing Payloads

Click chemistry serves as a crucial mechanism in the development of stimuli-responsive DDS. Introduced by K Barry Sharpless in 2001, click chemistry encompasses efficient and selective reactions that facilitate the rapid and reliable assembly of complex molecules from smaller units, typically using heteroatom linkages (C-X-C) to join modular components. This methodology has proven particularly advantageous in the field of drug delivery, where it enhances the formulation of nanoscale delivery vehicles and the attachment of therapeutic agents and targeting moieties to these carriers. Integrating click chemistry into multi-stage drug delivery platforms enables the sequential and orthogonal delivery of targeting ligands and therapeutic cargoes, enhancing the precision and efficacy of treatment [36].

Click chemistry facilitates the attachment of stimuli-responsive elements to drug carriers, enabling controlled release in response to specific triggers such as pH, temperature, light, ultrasound, or enzymes. Investigators have pioneered the development of stimuli-responsive silanol conjugates, offering a groundbreaking approach to conjugate, deliver, and release therapeutic agents in a controlled and on-demand manner, thereby optimizing treatment outcomes (Figure 3.2A) [37]. Recent breakthroughs have utilized bioorthogonal chemistry to develop active targeting DDSs aimed at tumors, immune systems, or bacteria, thereby increasing the specificity and effectiveness of treatments (Figure 3.2B). Interdisciplinary researchers and innovators will revolutionize the development of intelligent drug delivery platforms by harnessing efficient and biocompatible bioorthogonal chemistry and cutting-edge solutions to transform healthcare outcomes [38].

Investigators anticipate utilizing this approach in CAR-T and similar therapies to enhance their retention within tumor sites, thereby increasing the overall effectiveness of cell-based treatments.

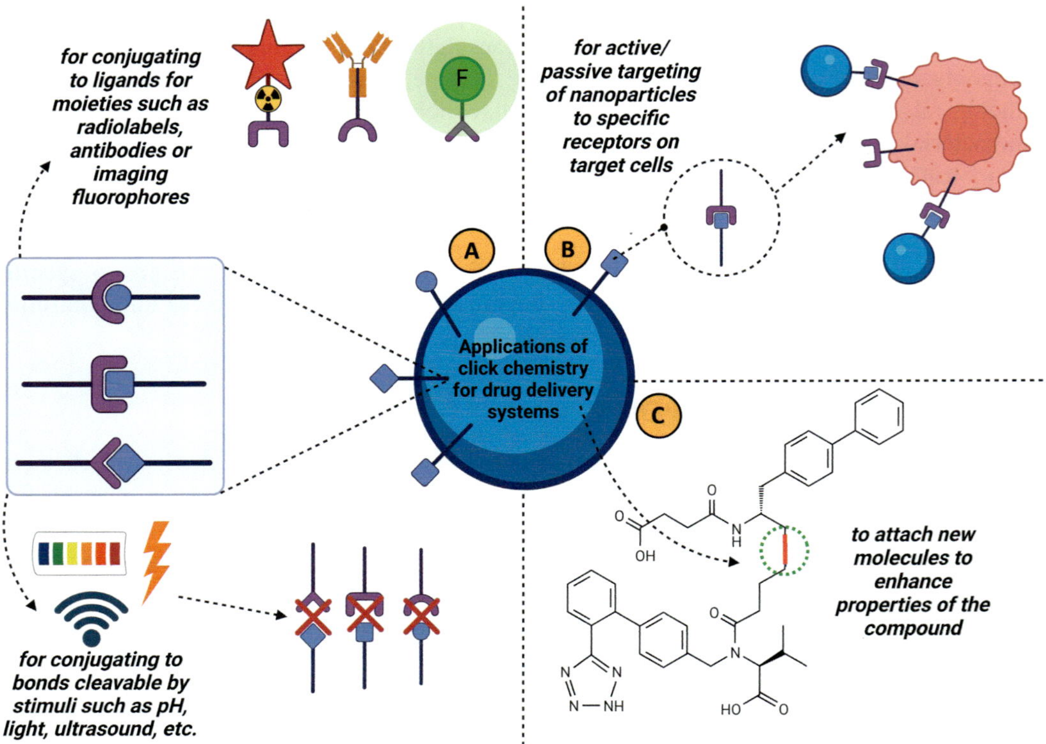

FIGURE 3.2 Applications of click chemistry to enhance capabilities of DDS by (A) conjugating stimuli-sensitive therapeutic/diagnostic moieties, (B) enhancing active/passive cell targeting capabilities, and (C) conjugating molecules to enhance efficacy of functionalized compounds.

Click chemistry has been utilized to link therapeutic agents with polymers or other compounds, improving their chemical stability, water solubility, and therapeutic performance. For instance, its application in bioconjugation has facilitated the creation of precisely engineered antibody-drug conjugates (ADCs) [39]. These ADCs exhibit greater uniformity and targeted binding, resulting in enhanced therapeutic efficiency and reduced off-target effects (Figure 3.2C).

A recent investigation presented a novel two-stage capture-and-release mechanism leveraging azide-dibenzocyclooctyne (DBCO) click chemistry. This innovative system successfully demonstrated the sequestration and subsequent liberation of a fluorescent cargo, facilitated by the formation of a polyethylene glycol diacrylate (PEGDA)-based capturing matrix. The release mechanism was activated by oxidative stress, highlighting the potential of combining click chemistry with free radical initiation for stimuli-responsive drug delivery. This approach leverages the specificity of click chemistry for payload attachment and the responsiveness of free radical initiation for controlled release, offering a promising strategy for targeted therapeutic and diagnostic applications. Breakthroughs in stimuli-responsive biomaterials have given rise to pioneering drug delivery platforms that harness click chemistry and enzymatic degradation to exert exquisite control over therapeutic cargo capture and release. A prominent illustration of this concept is a dual-phase, capture-and-release system that synergistically combines azide–DBCO click chemistry with matrix metalloproteinase (MMP)-cleavable peptides. This responsive and clickable biomaterial system holds significant potential for treating conditions characterized by high oxidative stress and upregulated MMP activity, such as cancer and inflammatory diseases. The ability to control payload capture and release both temporally and spatially enhances therapeutic efficacy while minimizing off-target effects [40] (Figure 3.3).

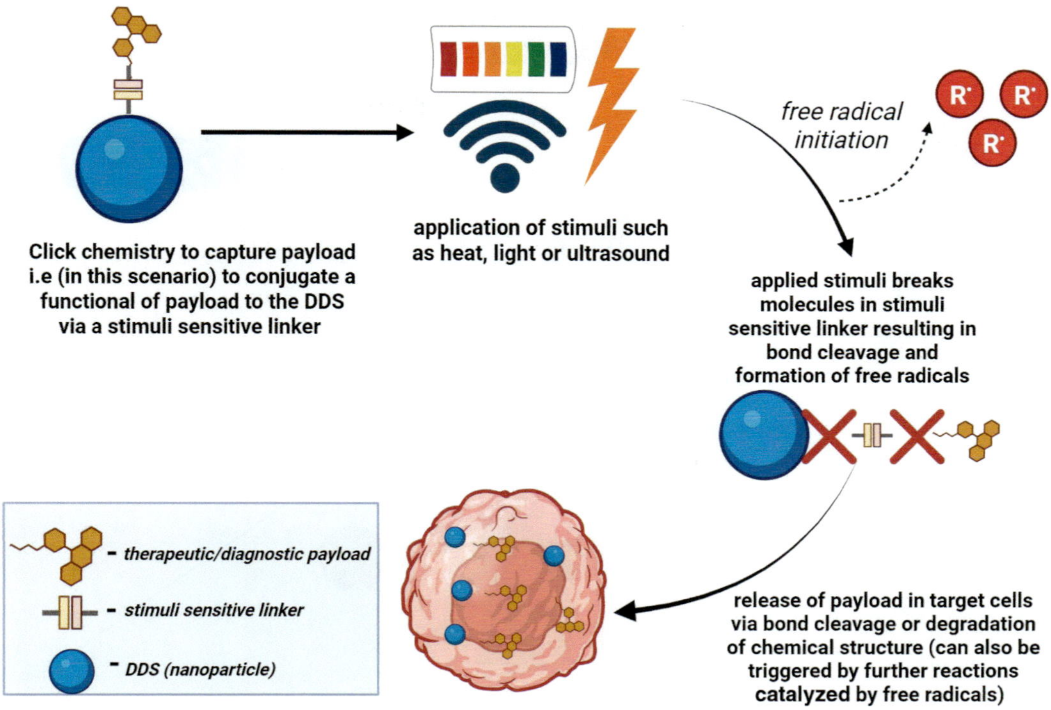

FIGURE 3.3 The schematic generically represents how researchers use click chemistry and free radical initiation to capture and release therapeutic or diagnostic payloads in response to stimuli.

3.5 DIFFERENT TYPES OF STIMULI-RESPONSIVE BIOMATERIALS

Advancements in science and technology have made it challenging for conventional bio-based materials to meet the evolving needs of society. Consequently, there is growing interest among investigators in developing bio-based polymer materials with stimuli-responsive properties. Investigators design these adaptive materials to transform their structural and chemical properties in response to specific environmental cues, enabling them to interact dynamically with their surroundings. To achieve desired functionalities, various types of bio-based stimuli-responsive materials are being developed and explored.

3.5.1 Natural Polymers

3.5.1.1 Chitosan

Crustaceans and fungi naturally provide chitosan through their exoskeletons and chitin-based cell walls. Although scientists consider chitosan a cellulose derivative, organisms that produce cellulose do not produce it. It has a structural similarity to that of cellulose, but at the C2 position, there is the presence of an acetamide group (Figure 3.4A). The amino groups in chitosan's polymer chain impart key properties by accepting protons and forming positively charged ammonium derivatives. These features, along with their natural origin and biodegradability, make chitosan and its derivatives ideal for use in stimuli-responsive DDS. The biodegradability of chitosan depends on its degree of deacetylation, with higher deacetylation increasing water interactions and enhancing hydrolysis, thereby promoting biodegradation [41]. Chitosan NPs, being cationic, form strong ionic interactions with negatively charged drug molecules, allowing them to adhere to mucosal surfaces and improve drug encapsulation. Cross-linking through amino group interactions enhances

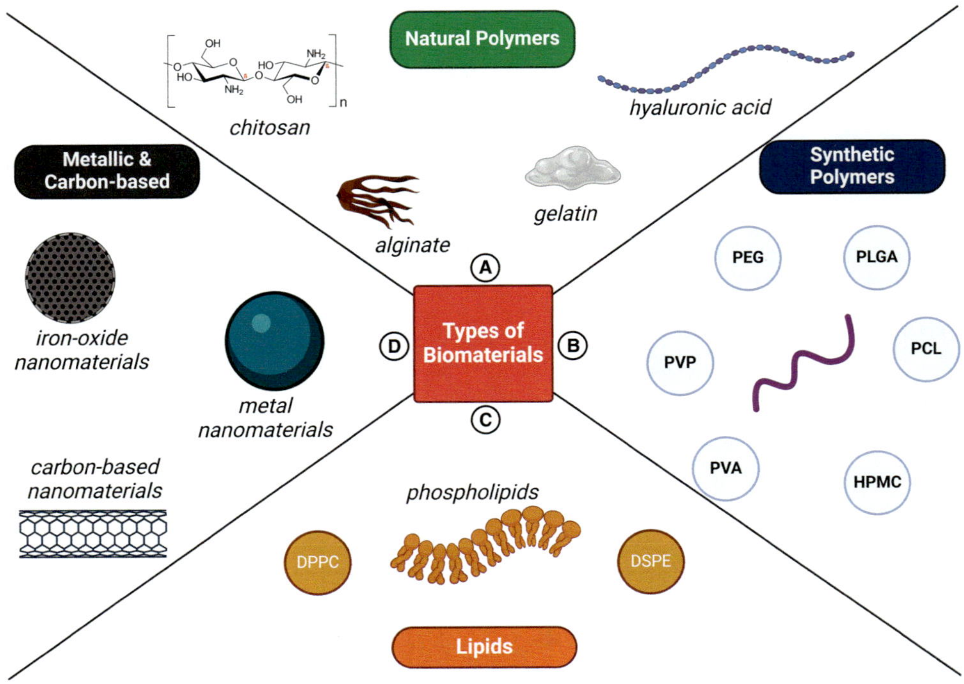

FIGURE 3.4 Types of biomaterials used in DDS, such as (A) natural polymers, (B) synthetic polymers, (C) phospholipids, and (D) metal NPs.

stability, but positively charged particles face higher immune clearance and toxicity risks compared to anionic or neutral ones. Surface modification using charged polysaccharide derivatives reduces opsonization and prolongs circulation time, with polyethylene glycol (PEG) encapsulation further increasing retention time [42].

In acidic environments, chitosan's amine groups become protonated to NH_3^+, increasing its solubility and reducing aggregation in the body. However, at higher pH levels, deprotonation occurs, raising the risk of aggregation. Acidic conditions facilitate gel formation for drug encapsulation, but the chitosan structure breaks down, causing rapid drug release. Chitosan, along with thermoresponsive polymers, can lead to the formation. The drugs arrive as a liquid at room temperature into injectable drug delivery devices, where they form a gel depot in the body that can release the drug gradually. At body temperature, the drug is entrapped in a gel matrix, and the drug gets released slowly [43]. The amino groups in chitosan get protonated in acidic environments and can interact with superoxide radicals, which is one of its antioxidant characteristics, thereby neutralizing the oxidative stress. This property further enhances chitosan-based biomaterials' ability to deliver drugs within cells with high oxidative stress efficiently. It is often possible to design chitosan-encapsulated drugs so that they only release the drug molecules when exposed to a particular wavelength of light. Ultrasound waves can induce pore formation within the cells, allowing pores to form in them. This pore formation can allow the entry of chitosan-encapsulated drug more efficiently within the cells [44].

3.5.1.2 Alginate

Alginate, a linear biopolymer, is extracted from brown algae using alkaline solutions like NaOH (Figure 3.4A). Two uronic acid monomers, α-L-guluronic acid and β-D-mannuronic acid, form it by joining through 1,4-glycosidic bonds. These monomers can organize themselves homogeneously (M block) or heterogeneously (G block). The G block enables gel formation by binding with divalent cations, such as calcium ions, through carboxyl groups at the C6 position. This interaction creates a mesh structure that entraps water, forming a gel and enabling controlled drug release. The M/G block ratio influences gel stiffness, with higher G block content and length promoting stronger calcium binding and firmer gels [45, 46]. Naturally sourced alginate contains impurities that may provoke an immunogenic response, triggering cytokine release and inflammation at the injection site [47]. In contrast, gels made from highly purified commercial alginate are biocompatible and do not induce such responses. After drug delivery, alginate lyase biodegrades alginate by cleaving the glycosidic bonds between monomers, resulting in smaller oligosaccharides that the body rapidly eliminates [46].

By functionalizing alginate's surface with peptides, antibodies, or specific ligands, researchers can ensure precise drug delivery, leveraging the affinity of these molecules for cell receptors to trigger the release of therapeutic agents exclusively upon binding to target cells. Alginate's mucoadhesive properties help it remain on mucosal surfaces, protecting encapsulated drugs from enzymatic degradation and reducing clearance, thereby extending circulation time. Under acidic conditions, alginate's carboxyl groups become protonated, decreasing its ability to form cross-links and leading to gel disintegration, which may result in uncontrolled drug release. In contrast, under basic conditions, deprotonation stabilizes the gel, facilitating controlled drug delivery [45].

Alginate can also carry drugs at different temperatures without structural changes, and its retention as poly (N-isopropyl acrylamide) (PNIPAM), the gel undergoes a phase transition from hydrophilic to hydrophobic, allowing for controlled drug release and localized heating [48, 49]. Redox-active environments, such as tumors, can trigger the release of alginate-coated drugs, and thiol surface modification can further enhance this release. Additionally, alginate can be combined with magnetic NPs, making it responsive to alternating magnetic fields, which generate localized heat for targeted drug release. Alginate, if modified, can contain light-responsive components that, in the presence of a specific wavelength of light, can cause the sol–gel transition of alginate, which can cause drug release. At low-intensity ultrasound, the ultrasound breaks the linkage between Ca^{2+} and the carboxyl group, triggering a gel-to-sol transition that allows drug release. By applying ultrasound externally at the target areas, the encapsulated drug can be released at the target site [50, 51].

3.5.1.3 Hyaluronic Acid

Hyaluronic acid (HA), a naturally occurring non-sulfated glycosaminoglycan, is characterized by its repeating structural motif, comprising alternating units of D-glucuronic acid and N-acetyl-D-glucosamine, linked through specific β-glycosidic bonds (Figure 3.4A). It often forms aggregates with proteoglycans and has excellent moisture retention, viscoelasticity, and hygroscopic properties, making it suitable as a lubricant and shock absorber, even at low concentrations (as low as 0.1%). Hyaluronan synthase produces HA inside the inner plasma membrane and transports it outside [52].

The biodegradability of HA, particularly when chemically modified (e.g., oxidation at the C6 position of N-acetyl-D-glucosamine), can be influenced by the presence of compounds like nicotinic acid, which enhance biodegradability. As a biomaterial, HA offers advantages such as high biocompatibility and minimal immunogenicity, as it naturally exists in the body and is recognized as a self-molecule, reducing the risk of immune response when used in stimuli-dependent DDS. Carbodiimide-mediated cross-linking is a common strategy for modifying HA, wherein the reagent facilitates the formation of ester linkages between the carboxylic acid and alcohol functionalities of adjacent HA chains. The carbodiimide activates the carboxyl group, enabling it to react with the hydroxyl group on another HA molecule. To prolong the duration of drug circulation encapsulated in HA, lysine methyl esters can be incorporated during the cross-linking process, helping maintain HA integrity for a longer timespan [53]. Due to its high hydrophilicity, HA efficiently transports water-based drugs to target organs. Since cancer cells often overexpress CD44, HA binds to CD44 receptors on cancer cells, enabling targeted drug release.

Additionally, light-activated nanocarriers conjugated with HA can release drugs upon exposure to specific wavelengths. Enzymes like hyaluronidases also cleave HA, facilitating gradual drug release over time. HA is susceptible to breakage at higher temperatures, and when they are injected in a fluid state into the body at the body's physiological temperature, it tends to form gels. These gels tend to entrap drug molecules and allow controlled release of the drug within the body. Often for easy administration, HA is conjugated with PNIPAM, which allows HA-based hydrogel to remain in a fluid state at room temperature [54]. Under acidic conditions, carboxyl groups in the HA structure undergo protonation and result in lower solubility in aqueous solutions. They tend to be less stable under these conditions. However, under neutral to basic conditions, they remain more stable, and pH-susceptible degradation occurs gradually, thus increasing the circulation time of the drug. In cancer cells, pH is low, so drug release occurs very quickly [55]. HA can undergo oxidation in the presence of hydrogen peroxide, and this can alter its functionality. Thus, HA can be modified to form thiolated hydrogels, which are more stable and compact, are hyaluronidase-resistant, and can perform controlled drug release. Exposure to high oxidative environments triggers the cleavage of disulfide bonds, inducing a controlled degradation process that enables the precise and targeted release of encapsulated therapeutic agents [43].

By integrating HA with magnetic NPs, investigators can create targeted DDS that leverage magnetic guidance to direct therapeutic agents to specific tissues or organs within the body. Investigators can apply alternating magnetic fields to guide the magnetic NP-bound HA-encapsulated drug to the target site, where the generated localized heat might alter the structure of the complex, thereby triggering drug release [56]. Specific linkers might be attached to the HA-encapsulated drug; these linkers can undergo cleavage by light, thus releasing the drug. Sometimes, certain NP-bound HA-encapsulated drugs may undergo localized heating due to light exposure, which can also cause drug release at a controlled level. Ultrasound waves can cause small cavity formation, and this can lead to the production of mechanical forces that can disrupt HA-encapsulated drug molecule. Heating can cause phase transition, thus causing drug release, and it can also guide proper drug localization [31].

3.5.1.4 Gelatin

Gelatin, derived from collagen through acid, alkali, or thermal denaturation, consists of a mix of proteins and polypeptides, resulting from the breakdown of collagen's tertiary structure (Figure 3.4A). There are two types: Type A, which is cationic and obtained via acid hydrolysis, and Type B, which is anionic and produced by alkali treatment. Type A gelatin has more carboxyl groups, while Type B contains more carboxyl groups due to the removal of amide groups. Gelatin's amino acid sequence features a repeating pattern of glycine (one-third) and proline (two-thirds). Gelatin is biodegradable and broken down by gelatinases, a subset of MMPs, and can also undergo hydrolysis in water. It can be cross-linked chemically or physically to improve stability and manage deterioration. The development of gelatin-based matrices enables the creation of stimuli-responsive systems that react to temperature, pH fluctuations, or enzymatic activity, facilitating precise control over drug release at desired locations. Furthermore, gelatin's inherent biocompatibility and low immunogenic potential make it an attractive candidate for targeted therapeutic delivery applications. It remains stable at lower temperatures but transitions from gel to sol state at temperatures above 30°C, leading to drug release via thermal degradation [57, 58].

Gelatin is amphoteric, and pH changes influence its solubility. It aggregates near its isoelectric point and is more soluble at higher pH levels. By engineering gelatin to remain steady at physiological pH and degrade in acidic tumor environments, scientists can target drug release to tumors [58]. Redox-sensitive gelatin systems, containing disulfide bonds, can release drugs in response to intracellular GSH levels, facilitating drug delivery to cytoplasm or intracellular compartments [43]. Additionally, researchers can combine gelatin with superparamagnetic iron oxide NPs to enable controlled drug release through magnetic fields, where they regulate the release rate by adjusting the field's frequency and strength. Photocross-linkable gelatin, such as gelatin methacryloyl, becomes more permeable when exposed to specific wavelengths of light, releasing encapsulated drugs. Gold NPs also convert light to heat, further promoting gelatin denaturation and drug release. Finally, ultrasound can disrupt gelatin's triple helix structure, reducing viscosity and improving drug delivery through mechanical stress [56, 57, 59].

3.5.2 Synthetic Polymers

3.5.2.1 Poly (Lactic-Co-Glycolic Acid)

Poly (lactic-co-glycolic acid) (PLGA) stands out as a versatile, biodegradable, and biocompatible polymer, widely utilized in tissue engineering and pharmaceutical applications. Its appeal stems from its tunable degradation kinetics, excellent biocompatibility profile, and regulatory approval, making it an attractive material for various biomedical applications (Figure 3.4B). Researchers can tailor the properties of PLGA to suit specific therapeutic needs by adjusting its lactide-to-glycolide ratio, molecular weight, and drug loading [60]. This biodegradable polymer is composed of ester linkages between lactic acid and glycolic acid, which hydrolyze in aqueous environments. The degradation rate of PLGA is influenced by its monomeric composition, with higher glycolic acid content leading to faster breakdown. A commonly employed 75:25 lactide-to-glycolide ratio enables sustained drug release. PLGA's molecular weight typically ranges from 5 to 40 kDa, and its glass transition temperature falls between 40°C and 60°C. This polymer is soluble in various organic solvents, including acetone, dichloromethane, and benzyl alcohol. Its versatility allows for conjugation with specific targeting moieties, including peptides and antibodies, enabling precise delivery to desired sites. Moreover, its encapsulation capabilities accommodate a broad spectrum of therapeutic agents, making it a valuable platform for diverse biomedical applications. Drug release is pH and temperature-dependent, with acidic environments promoting faster hydrolysis and drug release. Modifying PLGA with PEG enhances its hydrophilicity, improving water absorption, degradation rate, circulation time, and drug release kinetics [61]. The surface charge of PLGA NPs (positive, negative, or neutral) influences their cellular uptake, with anionic particles often showing different efficiencies than neutral or cationic ones. Investigators can engineer PLGA to facilitate redox-sensitive drug delivery, where increased levels of ROS, commonly associated with inflamed tissues, trigger the polymer's degradation and the subsequent release of the therapeutic agent. Additionally, esterases in the body can break down PLGA to enhance drug release. Magnetic NPs incorporated into PLGA carriers allow external magnetic fields to target specific tissues, while light-sensitive components enable controlled release upon exposure to specific wavelengths of light. Finally, PLGA formulations can respond to ultrasound, enhancing localized drug release through heating or cavitation effects [62].

3.5.2.2 Polyethylene Glycol

PEG is synthesized through the polymerization of ethylene oxide and water, resulting in a molecule with the general formula $C_{2n}H_{4n+2}O_{n+1}$, where "n" denotes the number of repeating ethylene glycol units (Figure 3.4B). Scientists widely use PEG in biomedical applications due to its hydrophilicity, low viscosity, biocompatibility, and minimal immunogenicity. The polymerization process can occur in either the gas or liquid phase, with the liquid phase being more common in industry, typically using sodium hydroxide as a catalyst. PEG can be monofunctional or bifunctional, and PEGylation is often employed to enhance a drug's pharmacokinetic properties by improving its stability and circulation time [63].

PEG is commonly used to enhance the circulation time of therapeutic molecules by coating their surface, improving their solubility in bodily fluids due to its hydrophilic nature [64]. It is non-toxic, elicits minimal immune responses, and is predominantly excreted via the kidneys, though its metabolism by enzymes like alcohol dehydrogenase and cytochrome P-450 is still under study. Despite being slowly digested in the body, PEG accumulation in cells, particularly macrophages, has raised concerns about long-term exposure. PEG's low immunogenicity makes it ideal for drug formulations, providing a "stealth" feature that prevents immune detection and prolongs circulation time [65].

PEGylation imparts "stealth" properties to NPs, reducing immune detection and enhancing circulation time. By exploiting the enhanced permeability and retention (EPR) effect in tumor tissues, PLGA enhances therapeutic efficacy while minimizing clearance by the reticuloendothelial system (RES). Nevertheless, the presence of pre-existing anti-PEG antibodies in specific individuals can potentially hasten drug elimination, compromising treatment outcomes. Overall, PEGylation improves drug delivery by lowering immunological recognition and prolonging treatment impact. Its hydrophilic nature forms a protective barrier around therapeutic agents, reducing immune recognition by creating steric hindrance. The immune system does not significantly activate it in its native form, so researchers consider it minimally immunogenic. Although PEGylated proteins or NPs may trigger some antibody production, the response is generally lower compared to other polymers. PEGylation serves as a cloaking mechanism, evading rapid elimination by the RES and prolonging bloodstream circulation. This stealthy approach minimizes immune recognition, allowing therapeutic agents to remain undetected for an extended period [66].

The pH changes can alter the ionization of functional groups on PEG or PEGylated substances, influencing their stability and interactions with other biomolecules. PEG's physical qualities, such as viscosity and solubility, can change with temperature, and this could impact its efficiency in DDS, especially in formulations requiring specific heat conditions for peak performance. The concentration of PEG in a formulation has a considerable impact on its behavior. Higher concentrations may cause higher viscosity and changed release profiles of encapsulated medicines as the polymer's structure and interactions with surrounding molecules change. The surface density of PEG chains on NPs influences their interaction with biological fluids. A dense PEG layer enhances steric repulsion, reducing protein binding and improving biocompatibility, while lower densities may alter protein and cell interactions. PEG is adaptable for redox-responsive systems, where it can release drugs in oxidative environments, such as inflamed tissues with elevated ROS. For instance, modifying PEG with redox-sensitive elements allows PLGA-based carriers to degrade under high ROS, triggering drug release [67]. PEG can also be infused with magnetic NPs to enable targeted delivery using an external magnetic field. Additionally, light-sensitive modifications to PEG enable controlled drug release upon exposure to specific wavelengths. PEG-based systems can further incorporate ultrasound-responsive materials, facilitating localized drug release through heating or cavitation effects [68].

3.5.2.3 Polycaprolactone (PCL)

Polycaprolactone (PCL) comprises repeated ε-caprolactone units linked by ester bonds and typically synthesized through ring-opening polymerization or polycondensation of 6-hydroxycaproic acid (Figure 3.4B). These ester linkages contribute to its biodegradability and mechanical strength [69]. Its versatility in functionalization enables the incorporation of various drugs, enhancing compatibility and effectiveness. It is helpful for chronic inflammatory diseases because it allows drug release in response to inflammation-related stimuli such as pH changes or enzymes, ensuring targeted delivery to inflamed tissues and reducing systemic adverse effects [70]. The Food and Drug Administration (FDA) approved PCL for several biological uses due to its low toxicity and biocompatibility. Its breakdown products are safe, and the body naturally breaks them down. Beyond leveraging the EPR effect for tumor-specific accumulation, PCL NPs can be further modified with targeted ligands, enabling precise and selective delivery of therapeutic agents to desired sites. Furthermore, PCL is appropriate for long-term treatments in chronic disorders, as we can change its disintegration rate by simply modifying its molecular weight or combining it with other polymers [69].

PCL is a biocompatible, biodegradable polymer with a low melting point, making it suitable for thermoplastic processing. Elevated temperatures increase polymer chain mobility, allowing enzymes like lipases and esterases to access ester linkages, accelerating breakdown. In thermophilic environments, enzymatic activity is enhanced, further promoting PCL degradation. Additionally, acidic or basic conditions affect the hydrolysis of ester bonds, altering degradation rates [71]. Incorporating redox-sensitive links allows PCL to respond to high ROS levels in tumors or inflamed tissues, releasing drugs at the target site. Similarly, embedding magnetic NPs in PCL matrices creates magnetically responsive systems. An external magnetic field can direct these systems to specific body locations, enabling localized drug delivery [72]. Photodegradable compounds or light-sensitive molecules can also be introduced into PCL to achieve light-triggered drug release, allowing controlled, site-specific drug delivery.

Furthermore, ultrasound can enhance drug release from PCL-based formulations by inducing mechanical stress, heat, or cavitation. This non-invasive method provides precise targeting with minimal side effects. In particular, PCL is a perfect material for localized therapy in inflammatory illnesses and cancer because of its mechanical strength, low toxicity, biodegradability, and capacity to maintain drug release [73].

3.5.2.4 Hydroxypropyl Methylcellulose (HPMC)

Among others, hydroxypropyl methylcellulose (HPMC) is a commonly used polymer in pharmaceutical formulations due to its unique properties (Figure 3.4B). It forms a gel-like layer upon hydration, enabling sustained drug release, making it ideal for controlled-release tablets and capsules. Its high bioadhesive nature allows it to adhere to mucosal surfaces, enhancing drug concentration at absorption sites and improving the bioavailability of buccal, sublingual, nasal, or rectally administered medications. Produced by treating cellulose with an alkaline solution, followed by methyl chloride and propylene oxide treatment, HPMC is chemically modified to include hydroxypropyl and methyl groups. This non-ionic, biocompatible polymer is known for its low toxicity and inert behavior under physiological conditions. Although not biodegradable, its swelling and gel-forming abilities allow controlled drug diffusion, and it can be incorporated into NPs or liposomes for targeted delivery to specific tissues [74]. Its formulation versatility extends to various DDS, including transdermal patches and injectables. HPMC offers controlled drug release in response to inflammation-related triggers, such as pH shifts or enzymatic activity, making it ideal for targeted anti-inflammatory therapy. Its mucoadhesive nature boosts drug absorption through mucosal barriers, while its stability minimizes adverse biological interactions. These properties make HPMC a versatile and reliable excipient in advanced DDS [75].

HPMC shows pH-dependent viscosity and gel formation, influencing drug release rates. It remains stable between pH 3 and 11, forming thinner gels under acidic conditions that accelerate drug release, while alkaline environments increase viscosity, slowing release. Salts impact HPMC gelation by altering the sol–gel transition through salting-in or salting-out effects. Some salts promote gelation at lower temperatures, enhancing controlled release, while others impede gel formation, delaying drug release [76]. HPMC demonstrates thermo-reversible gelation, where temperature changes affect viscosity and gel behavior. This property supports controlled drug release, particularly for mucosal adhesion. HPMC combines with redox-sensitive materials to enable targeted drug delivery in inflamed tissues with high ROS, even though HPMC is not inherently redox-sensitive [77]. Incorporating magnetic NPs into HPMC formulations enables site-specific drug delivery under an external magnetic field.

Additionally, HPMC systems can respond to ultrasound, causing localized heating or cavitation that enhances drug release, making it suitable for non-invasive therapies. Integrating HPMC with photodegradable materials enables light-sensitive drug release. Enzymatic degradation, such as by lipase, also accelerates drug release, and HPMC can be modified to target specific pathological conditions using enzyme-sensitive formulations [78].

3.5.2.5 Polyvinyl Alcohol

The water-soluble synthetic polymer, polyvinyl alcohol (PVA), is composed of polymerizing vinyl acetate and then hydrolyzing it to add hydroxyl (–OH) groups (Figure 3.4B). PVA's non-toxicity, biocompatibility, and capacity to form a hydrogel make it an attractive material for DDS. PVA's biocompatibility is further highlighted by its lack of significant immune response, making it safe for biomedical applications. Factors like temperature and pH influence the degradation of PVA; however, it is not naturally biodegradable. Chemical modifications can control its breakdown. Functionalization with ligands or peptides enhances PVA's potential for targeted drug delivery, especially in cancer therapy. The solubility of PVA is pH-sensitive, affecting the swelling of hydrogels and the release of encapsulated drugs. Temperature also impacts its solubility, with increased temperatures promoting hydrogel formation at room temperature and improving drug release. PVA combines with redox-responsive materials for drug delivery in inflamed tissues with elevated ROS, even though it is not inherently redox-sensitive. Enzymes produced by certain microorganisms can degrade PVA, triggering drug release from the matrix. Furthermore, incorporating PVA into magnetic NPs enables magnetically guided drug delivery using external magnetic fields to target specific tissues or organs. Additionally, PVA combines with photodegradable compounds for controlled drug release under specific light wavelengths [79].

3.5.2.6 Polyvinylpyrrolidone

Polyvinylpyrrolidone (PVP) is a synthetic polymer derived from acetylene, with the molecular formula (C6H9NO)n (Figure 3.4B). It is tasteless, odorless, non-toxic and exhibits excellent biocompatibility, making it suitable for pharmaceutical applications. The polymer's molecular weight varies based on its degree of polymerization, influencing its properties. PVP is highly soluble in both hydrophilic and hydrophobic environments, thermally stable, and maintains stability when heated to 100°C for extended periods. However, prolonged heating can cause a slight yellowing of its aqueous solution [80].

PVP enhances the solubility and stability of both lipophilic and hydrophilic drugs, improving bioavailability and therapeutic efficacy. Its high LD_{50} value indicates low toxicity, and it does not break down into harmful byproducts or accumulate in the body. Higher molecular weight PVP remains non-toxic, while lower molecular weight PVP is excreted easily from the body. PVP-based DDS can respond to environmental factors like pH and temperature, enabling precise drug targeting. PVP remains stable across various pH levels, but pH changes can influence drug ionization, affecting solubility and release rates. The polymer's behavior can also vary with temperature, as increased temperatures enhance PVP chain mobility, accelerating drug release. Specific formulations can form temperature-sensitive gels for controlled release [80, 81]. Though not inherently redox-sensitive, PVP can be combined with materials that respond to ROS, facilitating targeted drug release in inflamed or diseased tissues.

Additionally, PVP can interact with enzymes that modify its matrix, impacting degradation and release profiles. By incorporating magnetic NPs, PVP formulations can achieve magnetically guided drug delivery, while photodegradable polymers enable controlled release upon exposure to specific light wavelengths. Ultrasound-responsive PVP formulations offer non-invasive drug release through localized heating or cavitation effects, enhancing therapeutic delivery. Overall, PVP's versatile properties, including its stability, biocompatibility, and responsiveness to environmental stimuli, make it a valuable component in advanced DDS [82].

3.5.3 Lipids

Lipids have emerged as a popular choice for designing stimuli-responsive drug delivery platforms, leveraging their inherent biocompatibility, adaptability, and capacity to self-assemble into diverse structures, such as liposomes and lipid NPs. These lipid-based systems can be engineered to respond to a range of triggers, including changes in pH, temperature, light exposure, redox potential, and enzymatic activity, thereby enabling precise spatiotemporal control over drug release. Phospholipids are fundamental components of plasma membranes in both prokaryotic and eukaryotic cells. They consist of glycerol-3-phosphate derivatives with a glycerol backbone. One end of the glycerol binds to an organic alcoholic group and an esterified phosphate group, while the other end connects to two fatty acids. These fatty acyl chains differ in carbon length and saturation levels, influencing membrane fluidity and flexibility. Phospholipids exhibit an amphiphilic nature due to their bilayer arrangement, with hydrophilic polar heads exposed to water and hydrophobic tails facing inward. The hydrophilic heads contain polar groups that form hydrogen bonds or electrostatic interactions with water, enabling solubility.

In contrast, the hydrophobic tails resist water interaction. This unique arrangement minimizes free energy by reducing water reorganization around dispersed phospholipids. Specific phospholipids, like phosphatidylcholine, possess zwitterionic properties that lower the risk of triggering immune responses when introduced into the body (Figure 3.4C). Phospholipids are easily broken down by endogenous phospholipases into non-toxic forms, facilitating their metabolism and excretion. In DDS, liposomes, composed of lipid bilayers, are employed to encapsulate and transport drugs. These structures exhibit low immunogenicity and can degrade under varying pH and temperature conditions. Saturated phospholipids, such as dipalmitoylphosphatidylcholine (DPPC), form rigid and impermeable bilayers, enhancing liposome stability. The unique encapsulation properties of liposomes, which can accommodate both hydrophilic and lipophilic compounds, provide a protective environment for therapeutic molecules, shielding them from degradation and enabling controlled, targeted release. Liposomes' dual drug-carrying capabilities, low toxicity, and biodegradability make them a valuable tool for targeted drug delivery [83].

DSPE (1,2-Distearoyl-sn-Glycero-3-Phosphoethanolamine) consists of two C18 stearic acid chains attached to a phosphoethanolamine head, giving it amphiphilic properties (Figure 3.4C). When exposed to aqueous conditions, lipids spontaneously organize into bilayer structures and vesicular assemblies, facilitating the encapsulation of therapeutic agents with diverse solubility profiles, including both water-soluble and water-insoluble drugs. Its high melting point ensures liposomal stability at body temperature, and its biocompatibility reduces immune reactions, making it ideal for biomedical use. Liposomal Encapsulation Technology (LET) enhances drug delivery by protecting therapeutic agents from degradation and oxidation within liposomes. PEGylation of liposomes extends circulation time by minimizing immune detection, ensuring controlled release. The liposomal membrane remains in a gel phase at low temperatures, reducing permeability, while heating induces a phase transition that increases membrane fluidity and facilitates drug release. DPPC stabilizes liposomal membranes at physiological temperatures and facilitates drug release above its melting point of 41.3°C [84].

Phospholipid head groups can gain or lose protons based on pH. At neutral pH, zwitterionic phospholipids carry no net charge, while at acidic pH, they become positively charged. Acidic conditions, like those in tumor microenvironments, promote membrane fusion and drug release into target cells, enhancing delivery efficacy. When exposed to acidic conditions, pH-sensitive liposomes release drugs while remaining stable at physiological pH [85]. Under oxidative stress, polyunsaturated phospholipids may undergo lipid peroxidation, disrupt membrane integrity, and increase permeability. Engineered liposomes remain stable under normal conditions and release drugs under high oxidative stress. Iron oxide NP-containing phospholipids react to external magnetic fields, changing the shape of the membrane and promoting the release of drugs. Unsaturated phospholipids undergo oxidation due to ROS generation upon light exposure, which may result in the production of oxidized phospholipids (OxPL), potentially compromising the integrity of the membrane. Liposomes that have photosensitive phospholipids can lead to the release of drugs upon specific light exposure [86]. Ultrasound waves can cause mechanical stress on phospholipid bilayers, thus leading to the disruption of liposomes, releasing their encapsulated drugs. DPPC shows greater sensitivity to ultrasound than that of higher melting point phospholipids—DPPE. The intensity and frequency of ultrasound can further influence the disruption [52].

3.5.4 Metallic Nanoparticles and Carbon-Based Materials

The emergence of metallic NPs and carbon-based materials, which offer distinct properties enabling stimuli-responsive behavior, has significantly enhanced the development of advanced DDS. Specifically, metallic NPs, including those composed of gold, silver, and iron oxide, exhibit remarkable versatility and can be tailored to respond to a range of triggers, such as changes in pH, temperature, light exposure, and magnetic fields, allowing for precise control over therapeutic release.

3.5.4.1 Metal Oxide Nanoparticles

Metal oxide nanoparticles (MONPs) commonly use hydrophilic biocompatible coating to improve its stability (Figure 3.4D). MONPs' optical, magnetic, and catalytic characteristics can change depending on their size since smaller particles have a higher surface-to-volume ratio. Because of their increased surface area, tunable surface properties, and ease of functionalization, they interact better with biocompatible materials, increasing their sensor efficacy [87]. Their nanoscale size and large surface area enhance stability, bioavailability, and barrier-crossing capabilities, such as through the blood–brain barrier and into the pulmonary system. MONPs integrate into both hydrophilic and hydrophobic systems, offering customizable size, shape, and porosity. Their negatively charged surface allows efficient attachment of diverse functional molecules, making them versatile in biomedical applications [88].

In contrast, positively charged NPs, which attract blood plasma proteins, tend to be more toxic due to their stronger interaction with cell surfaces, leading to potential cellular damage. Positively charged NPs are taken up quickly by macrophages, whereas negatively charged NPs have less macrophage clearance. To guide the NPs to reach their target sites, these NPs are often coated with specific natural polymers like polyethylene glycol, which increases their biocompatibility and allows them to reach the target tissue or organ and perform controlled drug release [89]. MONPs release encapsulated drugs when exposed to high temperatures, enabling targeted drug delivery and phase transitions. They exhibit agglomeration in acidic conditions but show better stability and reduced agglomeration in alkaline environments due to increased electrokinetic stability and negative surface charge. At acidic pH, the surface becomes positively charged, enhancing interactions with negatively charged cellular components, while at alkaline pH, the negative charge increases, causing repulsion from charged biological surfaces. MONPs can also respond to redox conditions, facilitating controlled drug release in tumor microenvironments with high ROS levels, thus reducing side effects on healthy tissues. Upon photoexcitation, the NPs generate heat, triggering drug release [90]. It is possible to functionalize their surface with light-responsive targeted ligands, which produce electron-hole pairs that improve catalytic and redox reactivity when exposed to light. Ultrasound induces structural changes, reduces agglomeration, and enhances NP dispersion in biological systems, improving drug delivery. Additionally, ultrasound increases cell membrane permeability, promoting greater uptake of drug-loaded MONPs at target sites [91].

3.5.4.2 Carbon-Based Nanoparticle

Carbon-based nanoparticles (CBNs) have emerged as promising vectors for targeted therapeutic delivery, owing to their distinctive characteristics. Notably, CBNs can be engineered to respond to various external cues, such as thermal fluctuations, pH variations, light exposure, magnetic forces, and humidity changes—thereby enabling precise spatiotemporal control over the release of therapeutic agents (Figure 3.4D). CBNs are effective carriers for targeted drug and gene delivery due to their unique properties, including responsiveness to external stimuli like temperature, pH, light, magnetic fields, and humidity. This responsiveness enhances their conductivity and allows for chemical modifications, improving compatibility, particularly in cancer therapy. CNTs, hollow and tubular with hemispherical fullerene caps, are primarily produced by methods such as laser ablation, arc discharge, and chemical vapor deposition (CVD), with CVD being the most efficient and cost-effective [92]. Single-walled carbon nanotubes (SWCNTs) are characterized by their small size (1.4 nm diameter, 2–5 μm length) and excellent electrical conductivity, but their hydrophobic sidewalls make them poorly dispersible in liquids. Functionalization with PEG or aromatic compounds can improve their dispersibility and pH-responsiveness. Shape memory materials, combined with CNTs, can respond to heat and light, offering opportunities for low-temperature electroactive applications. Oxidized SWCNTs can be covalently combined with hydrophilic PEG to functionalize the sidewall. SWCNTs are pretty versatile as they can be non-covalently coupled to various aromatic compounds and are pH-stimulated [93].

Porous carbon nanospheres, often functionalized with drugs like DOX, show excellent chemical loading capabilities and pH-responsive properties. However, multi-walled carbon nanotubes (MWCNTs) can induce cytotoxicity, generate ROS, and cause mitochondrial dysfunction, lysosomal damage, and cell death. CBNs can also be modified with ligands or antibodies for targeted drug delivery, improving therapeutic precision and minimizing off-target effects. For example, CNTs can be used in gene delivery by binding to DNA [94]. Temperature-sensitive CNTs, functionalized with thermosensitive polymers like PNIPAM, release encapsulated drugs at elevated temperatures, making them useful for cancer therapy. This approach allows for stimulus-dependent drug release, ensuring that only tumor cells are targeted while sparing healthy cells. Additionally, functionalizing CBNs with specific ligands or antibodies enables targeted drug delivery to receptor-specific cells, ensuring controlled and efficient treatment [95].

3.6 CHALLENGES RELATED TO THE USE OF STIMULI-RESPONSIVE BIOMATERIALS IN CONTROLLED DDS

Stimuli-responsive biomaterials have demonstrated promising efficacy in preclinical studies; however, their successful clinical application faces several challenges. The effectiveness of DDS hinges on their ability to target specific sites with sustained kinetics while avoiding toxicity. In inflammatory arthritis, intricate physiological barriers like high-density extracellular matrix (ECM) and an inflammatory microenvironment can impair therapeutic efficacy and drug bioavailability. Designing precise drug carriers remains a critical bottleneck in managing inflammatory arthritis, as factors such as material type, size, shape, surface charge, and hydrophobicity/hydrophilicity significantly influence performance [96]. Negligible delivery vehicles risk toxicity due to their ability to cross biological membranes and evade immune clearance. Polymeric materials may aggregate or elicit toxic responses, with stabilizers potentially exacerbating toxicity at high doses. Similarly, positively charged carriers are prone to phagocytic uptake, leading to pulmonary toxicity, while certain surface modifications may provoke inflammatory responses [97]. Physicochemical properties of delivery vehicles impact drug behavior at the target site, dosing regimens, and administration frequency, requiring rigorous optimization for stability and controlled drug release.

Although dynamic covalent macromolecular networks offer numerous benefits, challenges persist in areas such as scalability, biocompatibility, and long-term stability. Nevertheless, these networks present significant promise for transforming drug delivery, providing improved control, precision, and therapeutic effectiveness in addressing complex medical conditions like cancer and chronic diseases. While liposomes are widely used due to their ease of synthesis and surface modification capabilities, they face limitations like burst release and poor shelf life, necessitating extensive modifications. Polymeric biomaterials offer sustained release and high drug encapsulation efficiency but lack sufficient functional groups for tailoring stimuli-responsive delivery. Moreover, varying levels of inflammation and oxidative stress during different disease stages affect stimuli responsiveness, making therapeutic predictability challenging [98].

Most preclinical studies rely on murine models, which often fail to mimic the complexities of human inflammatory microenvironments. This discrepancy underscores the need for models that accurately simulate human conditions to evaluate efficacy and safety. Toxicity concerns remain significant, with side effects influenced by delivery vehicle composition, dose, administration route, and differences between animal and human pathophysiology. Some biomaterials may induce allergic reactions, disrupt cell integrity, or produce excessive ROS, compromising biocompatibility. Non-biodegradable carriers further complicate clinical translation due to potential long-term biocompatibility issues. Compliance with regulatory standards from agencies like the FDA and European Medicines Agency (EMA) is essential, and the patients must be informed about the risks, benefits, and long-term safety of these biomaterials.

Additionally, large-scale production poses significant challenges [99]. The multistep synthesis of biomaterials often complicates mass production, increases costs, and affects batch-to-batch reproducibility, despite advancements in techniques like microfluidics. Addressing these challenges requires a multidisciplinary approach to optimize design, ensure safety, and streamline manufacturing, paving the way for the clinical translation of stimuli-responsive biomaterials.

3.7 CONCLUSION AND FUTURE DIRECTIONS

The creation of advanced biomaterials has become a pivotal frontier, converging materials science, biology, and engineering. These cutting-edge materials are distinguished by their capacity to adaptively respond to external cues, exhibiting dynamic shifts in their properties or behavior. This responsiveness enables precise interactions with biological systems, driving innovation in medical research and clinical applications. Material selection is crucial for the functionality and responsiveness of adaptive biomaterials. Scientists have explored a diverse array of material classes, each offering distinct benefits. Adaptive polymers, nanomaterials, and biomimetic constructs exemplify the innovative spirit of this field, allowing for the precise tuning of properties to address specific biomedical needs, from controlled drug delivery to tissue regeneration. Notably, adaptive biomaterials have been engineered to selectively modulate immune responses, suppressing pro-inflammatory signals while promoting anti-inflammatory pathways. This capability renders them essential components in immunomodulation therapies, where their dynamic behavior can optimize therapeutic efficacy by releasing agents in response to disease-specific triggers, unlocking new avenues for personalized medicine. The future of stimuli-responsive biomaterials is inherently interdisciplinary, combining cutting-edge material science, advanced manufacturing, and computational intelligence. These innovations promise to enhance the precision and personalization of medical treatments, particularly for chronic inflammatory conditions. The ability to dynamically adapt to the inflammatory microenvironment and leverage artificial intelligence (AI)-driven insights will redefine therapeutic strategies, offering new hope for patients worldwide.

The application of AI and machine learning (ML) further amplifies the potential of stimuli-responsive biomaterials. These technologies can process vast datasets, including patient clinical data, genetic profiles, imaging results, and material characteristics, to uncover patterns and biomarkers critical for disease management. AI and ML algorithms can optimize the design parameters of biomaterials, such as composition, geometry, and release kinetics, ensuring tailored therapeutic responses. For example, these tools can identify optimal configurations for drug release profiles, degradation rates, and mechanical properties, streamlining the development of next-generation biomaterials [100]. By embracing these advancements, researchers and clinicians can pave the way for a new era in biomedicine, where "ideal" biomaterials play a central role in achieving optimal therapeutic outcomes. The integration of stimuli-responsive biomaterials with AI, ML, and bioprinting technologies holds unparalleled potential to address complex biomedical challenges, ultimately improving patient care.

Declaration of AI and AI-Assisted Technologies

During the preparation of this work the authors used QuillBot AI in order to paraphrase the sentences. After using this tool, the authors reviewed and edited the content as needed and take full responsibility for the content of the publication.

LIST OF ABBREVIATIONS

β-CD: β-cyclodextrin; ADC: Antibody-drug conjugate; AI: Artificial intelligence; DDS: Drug delivery system; DOX: Doxorubicin; ECM: Extracellular matrix; EPR: Enhanced permeability and retention; FDA: Food and Drug Administration; HA: Hyaluronic acid; ML: Machine learning; MMP: Matrix metalloproteinase; MWCNT: Multi-walled carbon nanotube; PEG: Polyethylene glycol; PLGA: Poly (lactic-co-glycolic acid); RES: Reticuloendothelial system; ROS: Reactive oxygen species.

REFERENCES

1. Khan MI, Hossain MI, Hossain MK, Rubel MHK, Hossain KM, Mahfuz AMUB, et al. Recent progress in nanostructured smart drug delivery systems for cancer therapy: A review. ACS Appl Bio Mater. 2022 Mar 21;5(3):971–1012.
2. Asrorov AM, Fang Y, Wang H, Mirzaakhmedov SY, Huang Y. Chapter 14 – Stimuli-responsive systems for smart drug delivery systems. In: Nayak AK, Hasnain MS, Laha B, Maiti S, editors. Advanced and Modern Approaches for Drug Delivery [Internet]. Academic Press; 2023 [cited 2025 Jan 3]. p. 389–420. Available from: https://www.sciencedirect.com/science/article/pii/B9780323916684000265
3. Nel J, Elkhoury K, Velot É, Bianchi A, Acherar S, Francius G, et al. Functionalized liposomes for targeted breast cancer drug delivery. Bioact Mater. 2023 Jun 1;24:401–37.
4. Ahmad A, Imran M, Sharma N. Precision nanotoxicology in drug development: Current trends and challenges in safety and toxicity implications of customized multifunctional nanocarriers for drug-delivery applications. Pharmaceutics. 2022 Nov;14(11):2463.
5. Zhou W, Jia Y, Liu Y, Chen Y, Zhao P. Tumor microenvironment-based stimuli-responsive nanoparticles for controlled release of drugs in cancer therapy. Pharmaceutics. 2022 Nov;14(11):2346.
6. Deshmukh R, Sethi P, Singh B, Shiekmydeen J, Salave S, Patel RJ, et al. Recent review on biological barriers and host–material interfaces in precision drug delivery: Advancement in biomaterial engineering for better treatment therapies. Pharmaceutics. 2024 Aug;16(8):1076.
7. Abbasi R, Shineh G, Mobaraki M, Doughty S, Tayebi L. Structural parameters of nanoparticles affecting their toxicity for biomedical applications: A review. J Nanopart Res. 2023 Feb 27;25(3):43.
8. Oladipo AO, Lebelo SL, Msagati TAM. Nanocarrier design–function relationship: The prodigious role of properties in regulating biocompatibility for drug delivery applications. Chem-Biol Interact. 2023 May 25;377:110466.
9. Wang Y, Deng T, Liu X, Fang X, Mo Y, Xie N, et al. Smart nanoplatforms responding to the tumor microenvironment for precise drug delivery in cancer therapy. Int J Nanomed. 2024 Jun 19;19:6253–77.
10. Fatima M, Almalki WH, Khan T, Sahebkar A, Kesharwani P. Harnessing the power of stimuli-responsive nanoparticles as an effective therapeutic drug delivery system. Adv Mater. 2024;36(24):2312939.
11. Alavi SE, Alharthi S, Alavi SZ, Raza A, Ebrahimi Shahmabadi H. Bioresponsive drug delivery systems. Drug Discov Today. 2024 Jan 1;29(1):103849.
12. Ezike TC, Okpala US, Onoja UL, Nwike CP, Ezeako EC, Okpara OJ, et al. Advances in drug delivery systems, challenges and future directions. Heliyon [Internet]. 2023 Jun 1 [cited 2025 Jan 3];9(6). Available from: https://www.cell.com/heliyon/abstract/S2405-8440(23)04696-0
13. Glassman PM, Muzykantov VR. Pharmacokinetic and pharmacodynamic properties of drug delivery systems. J Pharmacol Exp Ther. 2019 Sep 1;370(3):570–80.
14. Quinn J, McFadden R, Chan CW, Carson L Titanium for orthopedic applications: An overview of surface modification to improve biocompatibility and prevent bacterial biofilm formation. iScience [Internet]. 2020 Nov 20 [cited 2025 Jan 3];23(11). Available from: https://www.cell.com/iscience/abstract/S2589-0042(20)30942-1
15. Tsung TH, Tsai YC, Lee HP, Chen YH, Lu DW. Biodegradable polymer-based drug-delivery systems for ocular diseases. Int J Mol Sci. 2023 Jan;24(16):12976.
16. Hajjar S, Zhou X. pH sensing at the intersection of tissue homeostasis and inflammation. Trends Immunol. 2023 Oct 1;44(10):807–25.
17. Chu S, Shi X, Tian Y, Gao F. pH-responsive polymer nanomaterials for tumor therapy. Front Oncol [Internet]. 2022 Mar 22 [cited 2025 Jan 7];12. Available from: https://www.frontiersin.org/journals/oncology/articles/10.3389/fonc.2022.855019/full
18. Kruk T, Chojnacka-Górka K, Kolasińska-Sojka M, Zapotoczny S. Stimuli-responsive polyelectrolyte multilayer films and microcapsules. Adv Colloid Interface Sci. 2022 Dec 1;310:102773.

19. Sun Y, Davis E. Nanoplatforms for targeted stimuli-responsive drug delivery: A review of platform materials and stimuli-responsive release and targeting mechanisms. Nanomaterials. 2021 Mar;11(3):746.
20. Ristroph KD, Prud'homme RK. Hydrophobic ion pairing: Encapsulating small molecules, peptides, and proteins into nanocarriers. Nanoscale Adv. 2019 Nov 5;1(11):4207–37.
21. Zhao M, Wan S, Peng X, Zhang B, Pan Q, Li S, et al. Leveraging a polycationic polymer to direct tunable loading of an anticancer agent and photosensitizer with opposite charges for chemo–photodynamic therapy. J Mater Chem B. 2020 Feb 12;8(6):1235–44.
22. Adhikari S, Nath P, Das A, Datta A, Baildya N, Duttaroy AK, et al. A review on metal complexes and its anti-cancer activities: Recent updates from *in vivo* studies. Biomed Pharmacother. 2024 Feb 1;171:116211.
23. Coulter SM, Pentlavalli S, An Y, Vora LK, Cross ER, Moore JV, et al. In situ forming, enzyme-responsive peptoid-peptide hydrogels: An advanced long-acting injectable drug delivery system. J Am Chem Soc. 2024 Aug 7;146(31):21401–16.
24. Martínez-Orts M, Pujals S. Responsive supramolecular polymers for diagnosis and treatment. Int J Mol Sci. 2024 Jan;25(7):4077.
25. Hassannia B, Vandenabeele P, Berghe TV. Targeting ferroptosis to iron out cancer. Cancer Cell. 2019 Jun 10;35(6):830–49.
26. Lam KY, Lee CS, Pichika MR, Cheng SF, Tan RYH. Light-responsive polyurethanes: Classification of light-responsive moieties, light-responsive reactions, and their applications. RSC Adv. 2022 May 17;12(24):15261–83.
27. Zhang J, Zhou ZH, Li L, Luo YL, Xu F, Chen Y. Dual stimuli-responsive supramolecular self-assemblies based on the host–guest interaction between β-cyclodextrin and azobenzene for cellular drug release. Mol Pharm. 2020 Apr 6;17(4):1100–13.
28. Yu G, Zhao X, Zhou J, Mao Z, Huang X, Wang Z, et al. Supramolecular polymer-based nanomedicine: High therapeutic performance and negligible long-term immunotoxicity. J Am Chem Soc. 2018 Jun 27;140(25):8005–19.
29. Han K, Zhang WY, Zhang J, Ma ZY, Han HY. pH-responsive nanoscale coordination polymer for efficient drug delivery and real-time release monitoring. Adv Healthc Mater. 2017;6(19):1700470.
30. Gao PF, Zheng LL, Liang LJ, Yang XX, Li YF, Huang CZ. A new type of pH-responsive coordination polymer sphere as a vehicle for targeted anticancer drug delivery and sustained release. J Mater Chem B. 2013 Jun 5;1(25):3202–8.
31. Xing Y, Zeng B, Yang W. Light responsive hydrogels for controlled drug delivery. Front Bioeng Biotechnol [Internet]. 2022 Dec 16 [cited 2025 Jan 3];10. Available from: https://www.frontiersin.org/journals/bioengineering-and-biotechnology/articles/10.3389/fbioe.2022.1075670/full
32. Regato-Herbella M, Morhenn I, Mantione D, Pascuzzi G, Gallastegui A, Caribé dos Santos Valle AB, et al. ROS-responsive 4D printable acrylic thioether-based hydrogels for smart drug release. Chem Mater. 2024 Feb 13;36(3):1262–72.
33. Wang G, Huang P, Wang L, Chen X, Zhou Y, Huang W, et al. ROS-responsive thioether-containing hyperbranched polymer micelles for light-triggered drug release. SmartMat. 2022;3(3):522–31.
34. Hu Q, Katti PS, Gu Z. Enzyme-responsive nanomaterials for controlled drug delivery. Nanoscale. 2014 Oct 10;6(21):12273–86.
35. Gambles MT, Fan B, Borecki A, Gillies ER. Hybrid polyester self-immolative polymer nanoparticles for controlled drug release. ACS Omega. 2018 May 31;3(5):5002–11.
36. Khodadadi Yazdi M, Sajadi SM, Seidi F, Rabiee N, Fatahi Y, Rabiee M, et al. Clickable polysaccharides for biomedical applications: A comprehensive review. Progress in Polymer Science. 2022 Oct 1;133:101590.
37. Mohanan S, Guan X, Liang M, Karakoti A, Vinu A. Stimuli-responsive silica silanol conjugates: Strategic nanoarchitectonics in targeted drug delivery. Small. 2024;20(39):2301113.
38. Yi W, Xiao P, Liu X, Zhao Z, Sun X, Wang J, et al. Recent advances in developing active targeting and multi-functional drug delivery systems via bioorthogonal chemistry. Signal Transduct Target Ther. 2022 Dec 2;7(1):1–25.
39. Chio TI, Bane SL. Click chemistry conjugations. In: Tumey LN, editor. Antibody-Drug Conjugates: Methods and Protocols [Internet]. New York, NY: Springer US; 2020 [cited 2025 Jan 3]. p. 83–97. Available from: https://doi.org/10.1007/978-1-4939-9929-3_6
40. DiMartini ET, Kyker-Snowman K, Shreiber DI. A click chemistry-based, free radical-initiated delivery system for the capture and release of payloads. Drug Deliv. 2023 Dec 31;30(1):2232952.
41. Sabourian P, Tavakolian M, Yazdani H, Frounchi M, Van De Ven TGM, Maysinger D, et al. Stimuli-responsive chitosan as an advantageous platform for efficient delivery of bioactive agents. J Contr Release. 2020 Jan 10;317:216–31.

42. Grewal AK, Salar RK. Chitosan nanoparticle delivery systems: An effective approach to enhancing efficacy and safety of anticancer drugs. Nano TransMed. 2024 Dec 1;3:100040.
43. Chatterjee S, Chi-leung HUI P. Review of stimuli-responsive polymers in drug delivery and textile application. Molecules. 2019 Jan;24(14):2547.
44. Londoño-Berrío M, Pérez-Buitrago S, Ortiz-Trujillo IC, Hoyos-Palacio LM, Orozco LY, López L, et al. Cytotoxicity and genotoxicity of azobenzene-based polymeric nanocarriers for phototriggered drug release and biomedical applications. Polymers. 2022 Jan;14(15):3119.
45. Tan J, Luo Y, Guo Y, Zhou Y, Liao X, Li D, et al. Development of alginate-based hydrogels: Crosslinking strategies and biomedical applications. Int J Biol Macromol. 2023 Jun 1;239:124275.
46. Lakkakula JR, Gujarathi P, Pansare P, Tripathi S. A comprehensive review on alginate-based delivery systems for the delivery of chemotherapeutic agent: Doxorubicin. Carbohydr Polym. 2021 May 1;259:117696.
47. He L, Shang Z, Liu H, Yuan Z X. Alginate-based platforms for cancer-targeted drug delivery. BioMed Res Int. 2020;2020(1):1487259.
48. Cao Y, Cheng Y, Zhao G. Near-infrared light-, magneto-, and pH-responsive GO–Fe_3O_4/Poly(N-isopropylacrylamide)/alginate nanocomposite hydrogel microcapsules for controlled drug release. Langmuir. 2021 May 11;37(18):5522–30.
49. Mirrahimi M, Alamzadeh Z, Beik J, Sarikhani A, Mousavi M, Irajirad R, et al. A 2D nanotheranostic platform based on graphene oxide and phase-change materials for bimodal CT/MR imaging, NIR-activated drug release, and synergistic thermo-chemotherapy. Nanotheranostics. 2022 May 24;6(4):350–64.
50. Baghbani F, Moztarzadeh F. Bypassing multidrug resistant ovarian cancer using ultrasound responsive doxorubicin/curcumin co-deliver alginate nanodroplets. Colloids Surf B: Biointerfaces. 2017 May 1;153:132–40.
51. Li X, Wang Z, Xia H. Ultrasound reversible response nanocarrier based on sodium alginate modified mesoporous silica nanoparticles. Front Chem [Internet]. 2019 Feb 11 [cited 2025 Jan 3];7. Available from: https://www.frontiersin.org/journals/chemistry/articles/10.3389/fchem.2019.00059/full
52. Awad NS, Paul V, AlSawaftah NM, ter Haar G, Allen TM, Pitt WG, et al. Ultrasound-responsive nanocarriers in cancer treatment: A review. ACS Pharmacol Transl Sci. 2021 Apr 9;4(2):589–612.
53. Zhai Y, Zhou X, Jia L, Ma C, Song R, Deng Y, et al. Acetal-linked paclitaxel polymeric prodrug based on functionalized mPEG-PCL diblock polymer for pH-triggered drug delivery. Polymers. 2017 Dec;9(12):698.
54. Trombino S, Servidio C, Curcio F, Cassano R. Strategies for hyaluronic acid-based hydrogel design in drug delivery. Pharmaceutics. 2019 Aug;11(8):407.
55. Tao Y, Chan HF, Shi B, Li M, Leong KW. Light: A magical tool for controlled drug delivery. Adv Funct Mater. 2020;30(49):2005029.
56. Jahanbekam S, Mozafari N, Bagheri-Alamooti A, Mohammadi-Samani S, Daneshamouz S, Heidari R, et al. Ultrasound-responsive hyaluronic acid hydrogel of hydrocortisone to treat osteoarthritis. Int J Biol Macromol. 2023 Jun 15;240:124449.
57. Ambrósio JAR, Pinto BCS, Marmo VLM, Santos KWD, Junior MB, Pinto JG, et al. Synthesis and characterization of photosensitive gelatin-based hydrogels for photodynamic therapy in HeLa-CCL2 cell line. Photodiagnosis Photodyn Ther. 2022 Jun 1;38:102818.
58. Jiang X, Du Z, Zhang X, Zaman F, Song Z, Guan Y, et al. Gelatin-based anticancer drug delivery nanosystems: A mini review. Front Bioeng Biotechnol [Internet]. 2023 Mar 21 [cited 2025 Jan 3];11. Available from: https://www.frontiersin.org/journals/bioengineering-and-biotechnology/articles/10.3389/fbioe.2023.1158749/full
59. Khodashenas B, Ardjmand M, Rad AS, Esfahani MR. Gelatin-coated gold nanoparticles as an effective pH-sensitive methotrexate drug delivery system for breast cancer treatment. Mater Today Chem. 2021 Jun 1;20:100474.
60. Rocha CV, Gonçalves V, da Silva MC, Bañobre-López M, Gallo J. PLGA-based composites for various biomedical applications. Int J Mol Sci. 2022 Jan;23(4):2034.
61. Lu Y, Cheng D, Niu B, Wang X, Wu X, Wang A. Properties of poly (lactic-co-glycolic acid) and progress of poly (lactic-co-glycolic acid)-based biodegradable materials in biomedical research. Pharmaceuticals. 2023 Mar;16(3):454.
62. Guo X, Zuo X, Zhou Z, Gu Y, Zheng H, Wang X, et al. PLGA-based Micro/Nanoparticles: An overview of their applications in respiratory diseases. Int J Mol Sci. 2023 Jan;24(5):4333.
63. Bento C, Katz M, Santos MMM, Afonso CAM. Striving for uniformity: A review on advances and challenges to achieve uniform polyethylene glycol. Org Process Res Dev. 2024 Apr 19;28(4):860–90.
64. Hoffmann MM, Too MD, Paddock NA, Horstmann R, Kloth S, Vogel M, et al. On the behavior of the ethylene glycol components of polydisperse polyethylene glycol PEG200. J Phys Chem B. 2023 Feb 9;127(5):1178–96.

65. Padín-González E, Lancaster P, Bottini M, Gasco P, Tran L, Fadeel B, et al. Understanding the role and impact of poly (ethylene glycol) (PEG) on nanoparticle formulation: Implications for COVID-19 vaccines. Front Bioeng Biotechnol [Internet]. 2022 Jun 7 [cited 2025 Jan 3];10. Available from: https://www.frontiersin.org/journals/bioengineering-and-biotechnology/articles/10.3389/fbioe.2022.882363/full
66. Hoang Thi TT, Pilkington EH, Nguyen DH, Lee JS, Park KD, Truong NP. The importance of poly(ethylene glycol) alternatives for overcoming PEG immunogenicity in drug delivery and bioconjugation. Polymers. 2020 Feb;12(2):298.
67. Li C, Li T, Tian X, An W, Wang Z, Han B, et al. Research progress on the PEGylation of therapeutic proteins and peptides (TPPs). Front Pharmacol [Internet]. 2024 Mar 8 [cited 2025 Jan 3];15. Available from: https://www.frontiersin.org/journals/pharmacology/articles/10.3389/fphar.2024.1353626/full
68. Mannu R, Karthikeyan V, Velu N, Arumugam C, Roy VAL, Gopalan AI, et al. Polyethylene glycol coated magnetic nanoparticles: Hybrid nanofluid formulation, properties and drug delivery prospects. Nanomaterials. 2021 Feb;11(2):440.
69. Bhadran A, Shah T, Babanyinah GK, Polara H, Taslimy S, Biewer MC, et al. Recent advances in polycaprolactones for anticancer drug delivery. Pharmaceutics. 2023 Jul;15(7):1977.
70. Chen F, Liu Q, Xiong Y, Xu L. Current strategies and potential prospects of nanomedicine-mediated therapy in inflammatory bowel disease. Int J Nanomed. 2021 Jun 23;16:4225–37.
71. Cai Z, Li M, Zhu Z, Wang X, Huang Y, Li T, et al. Biological degradation of plastics and microplastics: A recent perspective on associated mechanisms and influencing factors. Microorganisms. 2023 Jul;11(7):1661.
72. Materón EM, Miyazaki CM, Carr O, Joshi N, Picciani PHS, Dalmaschio CJ, et al. Magnetic nanoparticles in biomedical applications: A review. Applied Surface Science Advances. 2021 Dec 1;6:100163.
73. Perolina E, Meissner S, Raos B, Harland B, Thakur S, Svirskis D. Translating ultrasound-mediated drug delivery technologies for CNS applications. Advanced Drug Delivery Reviews. 2024 May 1;208:115274.
74. Kaur G, Grewal J, Jyoti K, Jain UK, Chandra R, Madan J. Chapter 15 – Oral controlled and sustained drug delivery systems: Concepts, advances, preclinical, and clinical status. In: Grumezescu AM, editor. Drug Targeting and Stimuli Sensitive Drug Delivery Systems [Internet]. William Andrew Publishing; 2018 [cited 2025 Jan 3]. p. 567–626. Available from: https://www.sciencedirect.com/science/article/pii/B978012813689800015X
75. Mady OY, Dewedar O, Abdine N, Zaytoon H, Haggag Y. Bioadhesive behaviors of HPMC E5: Comparative analysis of various techniques, histological and human radiological evidence. Sci Rep. 2024 Jan 22;14(1):1840.
76. Mašková E, Kubová K, Raimi-Abraham BT, Vllasaliu D, Vohlídalová E, Turánek J, et al. Hypromellose – A traditional pharmaceutical excipient with modern applications in oral and oromucosal drug delivery. J Contr Release. 2020 Aug 10;324:695–727.
77. Perez-Robles S, Carotenuto C, Minale M. HPMC hydrogel formation mechanisms unveiled by the evaluation of the activation energy. Polymers. 2022 Jan;14(3):635.
78. Rivero Berti I, Rodenak-Kladniew BE, Katz SF, Arrua EC, Alvarez VA, Duran N, et al. Enzymatic active release of violacein present in nanostructured lipid carrier by lipase encapsulated in 3D-bioprinted chitosan-hydroxypropyl methylcellulose matrix with anticancer activity. Front Chem [Internet]. 2022 Jul 7 [cited 2025 Jan 3];10. Available from: https://www.frontiersin.org/journals/chemistry/articles/10.3389/fchem.2022.914126/full
79. Darwish MSA, Al-Harbi LM, Bakry A. Synthesis of magnetite nanoparticles coated with polyvinyl alcohol for hyperthermia application. J Therm Anal Calorim. 2022 Nov 1;147(21):11921–30.
80. Ajji Z, Maarouf M, Khattab A, Ghazal H. Synthesis of pH-responsive hydrogel based on PVP grafted with crotonic acid for controlled drug delivery. Radiation Physics and Chemistry. 2020 May 1;170:108612.
81. Ramalingam V, Varunkumar K, Ravikumar V, Rajaram R. Target delivery of doxorubicin tethered with PVP stabilized gold nanoparticles for effective treatment of lung cancer. Sci Rep. 2018 Feb 28;8(1):3815.
82. Zhu W, Zhao Y, Wu Z, Lv F, Zhang Y, Guo S. Application of UV responsive SiO_2/PVP composite hydrogels as intelligent controlled drug release patches. Polymer. 2023 Jan 3;264:125535.
83. Casares D, Escribá PV, Rosselló CA. Membrane lipid composition: Effect on membrane and organelle structure, function and compartmentalization and therapeutic avenues. Int J Mol Sci. 2019 Jan;20(9):2167.
84. Liu P, Chen G, Zhang J. A review of liposomes as a drug delivery system: Current status of approved products, regulatory environments, and future perspectives. Molecules. 2022 Jan;27(4):1372.
85. Swami R, Kumar Y, Chaudhari D, Katiyar SS, Kuche K, Katare PB, et al. pH sensitive liposomes assisted specific and improved breast cancer therapy using co-delivery of SIRT1 shRNA and docetaxel. Mater Sci Eng C. 2021 Jan 1;120:111664.

86. Salkho NM, Awad NS, Pitt WG, Husseini GA. Photo-induced drug release from polymeric micelles and liposomes: Phototriggering mechanisms in drug delivery systems. Polymers. 2022 Jan;14(7):1286.
87. Truong TT, Mondal S, Doan VHM, Tak S, Choi J, Oh H, et al. Precision-engineered metal and metal-oxide nanoparticles for biomedical imaging and healthcare applications. Adv Colloid Interface Sci. 2024 Oct 1;332:103263.
88. Lorkowski ME, Atukorale PU, Ghaghada KB, Karathanasis E. Stimuli-responsive iron oxide nanotheranostics: A versatile and powerful approach for cancer therapy. Adv Healthc Mater. 2021;10(5):2001044.
89. Pondman K, Le Gac S, Kishore U. Nanoparticle-induced immune response: Health risk versus treatment opportunity? Immunobiology. 2023 Mar 1;228(2):152317.
90. Wang X, Sun T, Zhu H, Han T, Wang J, Dai H. Roles of pH, cation valence, and ionic strength in the stability and aggregation behavior of zinc oxide nanoparticles. J Environ Manage. 2020 Aug 1;267:110656.
91. Delaney LJ, Isguven S, Eisenbrey JR, Hickok NJ, Forsberg F. Making waves: How ultrasound-targeted drug delivery is changing pharmaceutical approaches. Mater Adv. 2022 Feb 23;3(7):3023–40.
92. Kolahdouz M, Xu B, Nasiri AF, Fathollahzadeh M, Manian M, Aghababa H, et al. Carbon-related materials: Graphene and carbon nanotubes in semiconductor applications and design. Micromachines (Basel). 2022 Aug 4;13(8):1257.
93. Zhao C, Kang J, Li Y, Wang Y, Tang X, Jiang Z. Carbon-based stimuli-responsive nanomaterials: Classification and application. Cyborg Bionic Syst. 2023 Apr 11;4:0022.
94. Li L, Xing H, Zhang J, Lu Y. Functional DNA molecules enable selective and stimuli-responsive nanoparticles for biomedical applications. Acc Chem Res. 2019 Sep 17;52(9):2415–26.
95. Zarrintaj P, Jouyandeh M, Ganjali MR, Hadavand BS, Mozafari M, Sheiko SS, et al. Thermo-sensitive polymers in medicine: A review. Eur Polym J. 2019 Aug 1;117:402–23.
96. Li H, Gou R, Liao J, Wang Y, Qu R, Tang Q, et al. Recent advances in nano-targeting drug delivery systems for rheumatoid arthritis treatment. Acta Mater Medica. 2023 Jan 18;2:23–41.
97. Dixit T, Vaidya A, Ravindran S. Polymeric nanoparticles-based targeted delivery of drugs and bioactive compounds for arthritis management. Future Sci OA. 2025 Dec 31;11(1):2467591.
98. Zhang M, Hu W, Cai C, Wu Y, Li J, Dong S. Advanced application of stimuli-responsive drug delivery system for inflammatory arthritis treatment. Mater Today Bio. 2022 Mar 1;14:100223.
99. Souto EB, Blanco-Llamero C, Krambeck K, Kiran NS, Yashaswini C, Postwala H, et al. Regulatory insights into nanomedicine and gene vaccine innovation: Safety assessment, challenges, and regulatory perspectives. Acta Biomater. 2024 May 1;180:1–17.
100. Nag S, Mohanto S, Ahmed MG, Subramaniyan V. "Smart" stimuli-responsive biomaterials revolutionizing the theranostic landscape of inflammatory arthritis. Mater Today Chem. 2024 July 1;39:102178.

4 Classification and Categorization of Stimuli-Responsive Biomaterials

Umama Shahid
School of Science, Monash University Malaysia,
Darul Ehsan, Subang Jaya, Selangor, Malaysia

Sonia Dangi
Jeffrey Cheah School of Medicine and Health Sciences, Monash University Malaysia, Darul Ehsan, Subang Jaya, Selangor, Malaysia

Hock Siew Tan
School of Science, Monash University Malaysia,
Darul Ehsan, Subang Jaya, Selangor, Malaysia
Tropical Medicine and Biology Multidisciplinary platform,
Monash University Malaysia, Subang Jaya, Selangor, Malaysia

4.1 INTRODUCTION

Inflammatory diseases, such as rheumatoid arthritis (RA), inflammatory bowel disease (IBD), and psoriasis, are marked by chronic and severe inflammation caused by immune system dysregulation [1]. This instability can set off a cascade of cytokine release, recruit immune cells, and, over time, cause irreparable tissue damage and functional impairment, drastically lowering patients' quality of life. The systemic nature of inflammation in these diseases complicates treatment, as targeting one pathway often fails to address the multifaceted nature of immune dysfunction. To alleviate symptoms and manage inflammation, current treatments mostly include anti-inflammatory medications, immunosuppressants, and biologics that target specific cytokines or immune cells. However, these treatments frequently fail to achieve durable remission, owing to non-specificity and systemic distribution, which result in dose-limiting toxicities and significant side effects that impede long-term management. Corticosteroids, for example, while useful in lowering inflammation, can induce serious adverse effects such as osteoporosis, hyperglycemia, and immunosuppression if administered for an extended period. Furthermore, patients frequently develop tolerance or resistance to certain medications over time, prompting the creation of more specific, effective therapy. This lack of sustained therapeutic benefit highlights the urgent need for more targeted, personalized treatments that can more effectively modulate immune response without compromising patient safety. Given the increasing global prevalence of inflammatory illnesses, as well as the economic and social costs associated with them, there is an urgent need for novel treatments that can enhance patient outcomes while reducing treatment burdens [2].

 DOI: 10.1201/9781003560203-4

4.1.1 Role of Biomaterials in Targeted Therapies

Biomaterials have received considerable attention for their ability to overcome the limits of traditional inflammatory therapy by allowing for targeted drug delivery systems that focus directly on the affected areas. Nanoparticles, hydrogels, micelles, and liposomes can encapsulate therapeutic compounds, prevent premature degradation, and promote release at the target site, hence enhancing bioavailability and retention time. Lipid-based nanoparticles, for example, have been used to improve medication delivery in RA, with studies indicating enhanced drug accumulation in inflamed joints and less systemic toxicity [3]. Similarly, hydrogels loaded with anti-inflammatory drugs have been employed to locally release medications in IBD models, demonstrating long-term therapeutic efficacy with fewer side effects [4]. These advanced systems not only improve localized treatment but also reduce the frequency of administration, leading to better patient adherence. Advances in surface functionalization have enabled the development of biomaterials capable of recognizing molecular markers specific to inflamed tissues, such as intercellular adhesion molecule-1 (ICAM-1) and vascular cell adhesion molecule-1 (VCAM-1), which are overexpressed on endothelial cells during inflammation [5]. Drug carriers can achieve site-specific accumulation by conjugating targeting ligands to the surface of nanoparticles or liposomes, thereby increasing therapeutic efficacy and decreasing off-target effects. This precision targeting method has the potential to transform inflammatory disease therapy by allowing for lower doses, fewer systemic side effects, and better patient compliance [4].

4.1.2 Significance of Stimuli-Responsive Biomaterials in Improving Treatment Efficacy and Patient Outcomes

Stimuli-responsive biomaterials (SRBs), also known as "smart" or "intelligent" materials, are a cutting-edge class of biomaterials that respond to specific stimuli with controlled changes in their properties, making them ideal for the dynamic environments associated with inflammation [6]. As shown in Figure 4.1, SRBs can be categorized based on their response to either physiological or external stimuli, each triggering a unique material behavior tailored to the therapeutic needs of a given condition. Kost and Langer's early work on responsive drug delivery systems in 1984 revealed polymers with the ability to alter their characteristics in response to stimuli such as temperature and pH, laying the path for today's more sophisticated SRBs [7]. Modern SRBs can be programmed to respond to a variety of internal cues, including pH, enzymes, and reactive oxygen species (ROS), which are frequently dysregulated in inflammatory tissues. To achieve localized therapeutic effects while preserving healthy tissues, acidic pH-responsive polymers, for example, can release medications only in inflammatory tissues with lower pH levels. pH-sensitive nanoparticles have demonstrated preferential drug release in inflammatory joints and intestines, respectively, in models of colitis and arthritis, demonstrating the effectiveness of this mechanism. This selective drug delivery reduces the need for systemic administration, providing a more targeted and efficient treatment strategy [8]. Likewise, enzyme-responsive biomaterials provide an extra layer of specificity for targeted drug administration by breaking down in the presence of certain enzymes, such as matrix metalloproteinases (MMPs), which are overexpressed in inflamed or damaged tissues. Enzyme-sensitive hydrogels loaded with anti-inflammatory drugs in RA have shown regulated release in response to high MMP levels, lowering joint inflammation while preserving healthy tissue. Furthermore, ROS-sensitive biomaterials are especially promising for inflammation-targeted therapeutics because ROS levels are often higher in inflamed areas due to oxidative stress. Anti-inflammatory drugs loaded into ROS-responsive nanoparticles have been shown in preclinical experiments to selectively release their cargo at inflammatory sites, reducing systemic exposure and enhancing therapeutic results [9]. In addition to internal stimuli, SRBs can be programmed to respond to external stimuli such as light, ultrasound, and magnetic fields, allowing for on-demand medication delivery. For example, light-sensitive hydrogels

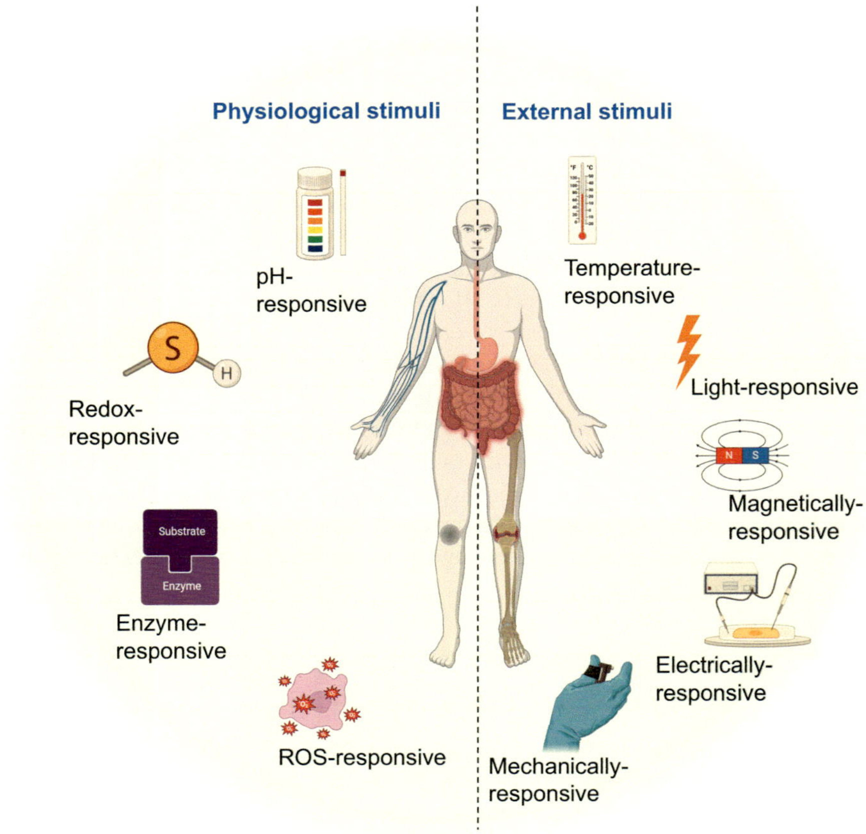

FIGURE 4.1 Classification of stimuli-responsive biomaterials (SRBs) based on their response to physiological and external stimuli. The figure categorizes SRBs into two main groups: physiological stimuli (such as pH, redox, enzyme activity, and reactive oxygen species) and external stimuli, including temperature, light, magnetic fields, electrical signals, and mechanical forces. Each class triggers a specific material response, such as drug release or structural changes, tailored to enhance therapeutic outcomes for diseases like inflammation and cancer.

have been investigated for on-site drug release in arthritis models, allowing for drug administration just when and where needed. This tunable responsiveness allows for personalized therapy based on an individual's inflammatory profile, possibly altering the treatment landscape for complicated inflammatory illnesses. Patients can benefit from lower doses, fewer side effects, and more consistent therapeutic effects by exploiting SRBs' precise and stimulus-triggered release mechanisms, hence enhancing both therapy efficacy and safety [8].

4.2 CLASSIFICATION OF STIMULI-RESPONSIVE BIOMATERIALS

SRBs are intended to respond to both physiological and environmental stimuli, providing a high level of control over drug release and therapeutic effectiveness. This precision in medication administration improves treatment outcomes, particularly for complicated illnesses such as inflammation and cancer. The major classifications of SRBs are based on their reactivity to physiological or environmental stimuli, with each category providing distinct advantages for therapeutic uses (Table 4.1).

TABLE 4.1

Classification, Mechanisms, and Applications of Stimuli-Responsive Biomaterials (SRBs). The Table Categorizes SRBs Based on Their Response to Physiological and External Stimuli, Highlighting the Underlying Mechanisms, Exemplary Materials, and Key Therapeutic Applications. A Dedicated Row on Emerging Multi-Stimuli Systems Underscores the Advancements in Integrating Multiple Triggers for Enhanced Precision and Adaptability in Complex Disease Contexts

Stimulus Type	Mechanism	Examples	Key Applications
		Physiological Stimuli	
pH-responsive [10]	Protonation or deprotonation of ionizable groups alters solubility, swelling, or degradation, leading to drug release.	Poly(acrylic acid), poly(histidine), chitosan derivatives	Drug delivery in acidic environments (tumors, inflamed tissues); oral delivery systems
Redox-responsive [33]	High glutathione (GSH) or reactive oxygen species (ROS) levels in pathological tissues reduce disulfide bonds or oxidize materials, triggering payload release.	PEG-PCL copolymers with disulfide bonds, MnO_2 nanoparticles	Targeted cancer therapy, inflammation-specific drug delivery
Enzyme-responsive [34]	Enzymes overexpressed in disease microenvironments cleave specific peptide bonds or linkages	Matrix metalloproteinase (MMP)-sensitive hydrogels, peptide-functionalized nanoparticles	Localized drug delivery in arthritis, cancer, and wound healing
ROS-responsive [35]	Oxidation of material components by high ROS levels in inflamed or tumor tissues triggers drug release	Mn_3O_4 nanozymes, thioketal-based polymers	Anti-inflammatory therapy, cancer-specific drug targeting
		External Stimuli	
Temperature-responsive [18]	Phase transitions, such as lower critical solution temperature (LCST) or upper critical solution temperature (UCST), modulate swelling, or solubility, inducing release	Poly(N-isopropylacrylamide) (PNIPAAm), PNIPAAm-PEG hydrogels	Localized hyperthermia-triggered drug delivery, cancer therapy
Light-responsive [30]	Photochemical bond cleavage or photothermal effects from light absorption release therapeutic agents	Gold nanoparticles, azobenzene-based polymers	Photodynamic therapy (PDT), spatially controlled drug release in tumors
Magnetic-responsive [36]	External magnetic fields guide nanoparticles or generate localized heat (magnetic hyperthermia) to trigger drug release	Iron oxide nanoparticles coated with PNIPAAm, magnetite nanocomposites	Tumor-targeted drug delivery, hyperthermia-based therapies
Electrical-responsive [20]	Electric fields alter conductivity, charge distribution, or material structure, leading to controlled release	Polypyrrole (PPy), Polyaniline (PANI), graphene oxide nanofibers	Neuromodulation, drug release in biosensors, and tissue regeneration
Mechanical-responsive [37]	Stress-induced changes in material properties (e.g., swelling, compression) enable release or activation	Shape memory polymers (SMPs), alginate hydrogels	Wound healing, bone regeneration, pressure-responsive drug delivery
Emerging multi-stimuli systems [38]	Integration of multiple triggers (e.g., pH + temperature, enzyme + redox) enables precise spatiotemporal control over therapeutic delivery	Thermo-pH-sensitive hydrogels, redox-enzyme hybrid systems	Personalized medicine, complex pathologies such as cancer and inflammation

4.2.1 Classification Based on Physiological Stimuli

Physiologically responsive biomaterials are designed to interact with the unique microenvironmental conditions in diseased tissues, such as altered pH, redox potential, or enzyme presence. These materials are instrumental in site-specific drug delivery, enabling targeted therapy that minimizes off-target effects.

4.2.1.1 pH-Responsive Biomaterials

pH-responsive biomaterials exploit pH changes between healthy and distressed tissues, such as tumors, inflamed regions, and cell endosomes. These locations frequently have a lower pH than typical tissues. By adding functional groups that ionize at various pH levels, these materials can modify their characteristics and induce medication release, allowing for targeted therapy at regions of inflammation or malignancy. pH-responsive biomaterials are often made up of polymers containing ionizable groups like carboxyl, amine, or imidazole. At certain pH levels, these groups can become protonated or deprotonated, affecting the material's solubility, hydrophilicity, and charge. This change in the material's properties can lead to structural transitions, such as swelling or collapsing, that result in the release of encapsulated drugs [10].

Poly(acrylic acid) (PAA) is a well-studied pH-responsive polymer. PAA's carboxyl groups ionize at pH levels above 4.5, enabling the polymer to expand and enhance medication release. At acidic pH (lower than 4.5), the carboxyl groups become protonated, resulting in polymer collapse and drug retention. This feature is especially effective for getting drugs into acidic environments like tumors or damaged tissues. For example, PAA-based hydrogels have been utilized to deliver chemotherapeutic drugs such as doxorubicin directly to cancer cells in a pH-sensitive way [11].

4.2.1.2 Redox-Responsive Biomaterials

Redox-responsive biomaterials take advantage of the differential redox potential between healthy and diseased tissues. High amounts of reducing agents such as glutathione (GSH) are frequently seen in malignant cells or areas of inflammation. These biomaterials contain disulfide linkages or other reducible bonds that can be cleaved by reducing agents, resulting in the release of encapsulated medicines or material degradation [12]. The inclusion of disulfide bonds or other reducible interactions inside the polymeric structure is the primary driving force of redox-responsive biomaterials. The disulfide bonds remain intact in normal tissues with modest concentrations of reducing agents like GSH. However, in the presence of high GSH concentrations (as observed in tumor cells or inflammatory regions), the disulfide bonds are reduced, causing the material to break down and release its pharmacological payload [12].

Polymeric nanocarriers produced from poly(ethylene glycol) (PEG)-poly(ε-caprolactone) (PCL) conjugated with disulfide linkages are a notable example. These carriers stay stable in the bloodstream, but when GSH levels rise in tumor cells, the disulfide connections break, resulting in drug release. For example, doxorubicin, a routinely used chemotherapeutic drug, can be successfully delivered to tumor sites via redox-responsive carriers while reducing systemic side effects [13].

4.2.1.3 Enzyme-Responsive Biomaterials

Enzyme-responsive biomaterials are intended to break down or release pharmaceuticals in response to the activity of certain enzymes. These materials often contain peptide sequences or chemical linkages that serve as substrates for enzymes that are overexpressed in disease states, such as MMPs in tumors or sites of inflammation [14]. The enzymatic cleavage of these sequences or bonds results in a change in material structure or the release of the encapsulated therapeutic agent. Enzyme-responsive biomaterials typically contain peptide sequences or other linkers that are particularly cleaved by overexpressed enzymes in disease environments. For example, tumor tissues frequently create MMPs, which can cleave specific peptide sequences, causing the material to deteriorate and release its therapeutic payload. This selective breakdown enables precise, localized medication distribution while minimizing systemic toxicity [15]. Peptide-functionalized nanoparticles are widely used in enzyme-controlled drug delivery systems. One such system consists of hydrogels functionalized with MMP-sensitive peptides, which break down in reaction to MMPs found in tumor environments. These hydrogels can be utilized to control the release of chemotherapy drugs such as cisplatin, which is released after enzymatic cleavage, boosting the therapeutic benefit while reducing negative effects to surrounding healthy tissue [16].

4.2.2 Classification Based on External Stimuli

External SRBs allow for precise control over therapeutic release, as they can be activated through stimuli applied outside the body. This feature enables real-time adjustment and remote regulation of drug delivery, proving particularly beneficial in applications requiring on-demand or location-specific activation.

4.2.2.1 Temperature-Responsive Biomaterials

Temperature-responsive biomaterials use temperature-induced phase transitions to alter the material's physical properties. These materials usually have a certain transition temperature, known as the lower critical solution temperature (LCST) or upper critical solution temperature (UCST), at which they experience major structural changes [17]. This thermal sensitivity can be employed to control drug release in response to localized temperature changes caused by external heat sources or fever. Temperature-responsive materials usually have a sharp phase transition around a specific temperature, known as the LCST or UCST. Below this temperature, the material often becomes hydrophilic, swells up, and thus can encapsulate drugs. When the temperature exceeds the LCST (or falls below the UCST), the material turns hydrophobic and collapses, releasing the drug. This temperature sensitivity is commonly employed in localized drug delivery systems, which use controlled heating to release drugs at specific places [17].

PNIPAAm is one of the most extensively investigated temperature-sensitive polymers. PNIPAAm goes through a phase transition at roughly 32°C (the LCST), after which the polymer turns hydrophobic and collapses, releasing the encapsulated drugs. This feature has been exploited in thermo-responsive hydrogels for targeted chemotherapy, where heat (e.g., from a localized hyperthermia treatment) causes the release of anticancer drugs such as doxorubicin at the tumor site [18].

4.2.2.2 Electrically Responsive Biomaterials

Electrical-responsive biomaterials are designed to respond to external electric fields or electrical charge changes. These materials may be triggered or modified by electrical signals, making them excellent for use in tissue engineering, brain stimulation, biosensing, and targeted medication administration [19]. Electrical impulses can control cellular behavior, such as differentiation, proliferation, and migration, as well as the release of encapsulated medicines. This makes electrically responsive biomaterials extremely useful for precisely directing biological processes. Electrical-responsive biomaterials often contain conductive polymers, nanoparticles, or charge-carrying compounds that can interact with electric fields. When an external electrical signal is supplied to certain materials, their charge distribution, ionic conductivity, and electrochemical characteristics change. This can cause structural changes such as swelling or shrinking, changes in the material's permeability, or direct electrostatic interactions with cells or biomolecules, resulting in medication release or cell activation [20].

- *Conductive polymers*: These organic polymers conduct electricity and can be activated by an electric field. They can modify their shape, charge, and ion permeability in response to electric stimuli [21].
- *Electroactive materials*: These materials, such as polypyrrole (PPy) or polyaniline (PANI), exhibit large electrochemical responses when subjected to an external electric field, allowing for controlled release or activation of encapsulated agents [22].

One example is PPy, a conductive polymer that changes volume and permeability when electrically stimulated. PPy can be employed in drug delivery systems that use an electric field to stimulate the release of medicinal drugs. For example, PPy-based nanocomposites can be utilized to transport anticancer medications to tumor areas by providing an electrical field, triggering the drug's release at the desired spot. This method has been found to improve the precision and efficiency of medication release [22]. Another example is electrospun nanofibers containing conductive elements such as graphene oxide or gold nanoparticles. In neural regeneration and muscle tissue engineering, electrical fields are employed to drive cell differentiation and improve tissue repair [23].

4.2.2.3 Magnetically Responsive Biomaterials

Magnetic-responsive biomaterials contain magnetic nanoparticles that can be controlled by an external magnetic field. These materials are especially valuable for targeted drug administration because the magnetic field may direct nanoparticles to specific regions in the body, such as tumors or infection sites. Furthermore, magnetic fields can cause localized heating (magnetic hyperthermia) to increase medication release [24]. Magnetic-responsive biomaterials contain superparamagnetic nanoparticles, such as iron oxide (Fe_3O_4) or magnetite, that react to an external magnetic field. The magnetic field allows these nanoparticles to be steered to specified sites. When subjected to an alternating magnetic field, nanoparticles create heat, causing local temperature rises and drug release from thermosensitive carriers [25]. This combination of magnetic targeting and thermally triggered release provides a highly efficient drug delivery system. Magnetic nanoparticles are frequently paired with thermoresponsive polymers to generate drug delivery systems that can be directed by an external magnet and activated by heat. Iron oxide nanoparticles coated with a temperature-sensitive polymer, such as PNIPAAm, can be used to target and treat cancers. An external magnetic field helps to concentrate nanoparticles at the tumor location, and localized heating from an alternating magnetic field can release the encapsulated drug [26].

4.2.2.4 Mechanically Responsive Biomaterials

Mechanically responsive biomaterials are designed to change properties in response to external mechanical forces such as stretching, compression, shear stress, and pressure. These materials imitate the mechanical cues required in natural biological processes, where cells and tissues react to physical stimuli such as strain or stress. Mechanically sensitive biomaterials are widely employed in applications such as wound healing, tissue engineering, medication delivery, and sensors. They enable material breakdown or medication release based on the mechanical environment, resulting in more dynamic and responsive treatment systems [27]. Mechanical-responsive biomaterials often include structural components such as elastomers, hydrogels, or nanofibers, which change their characteristics when exposed to mechanical stresses. When an external mechanical stress is applied, the material deforms (e.g., stretching, compression, or shear), affecting its physical qualities such as permeability, structure, or shape.

- *Shape memory polymers (SMPs)*: These polymers can return to a preset shape after being deformed by mechanical stress. They can be programmed to release medications or encapsulated biomolecules when activated by an external mechanical force.
- *Hydrogels and elastomers*: These materials can swell or shrink in response to mechanical strain. In drug delivery systems, mechanical stress can change the porosity or structure of the substance, triggering the release of the encapsulated drugs.
- *Nanomaterials*: Nanomaterials, such as nanofibers or nanotubes, can change mechanical characteristics when strained, allowing for targeted medication delivery or tissue regeneration.

SMPs are an excellent example of mechanically responsive materials. These polymers are designed to exist in a single shape under normal conditions but can undergo a reversible transition when subjected to mechanical stresses. For example, an SMP-based drug delivery system may be programmed to "collapse" or "open up" in response to mechanical stress (such as shear stress in blood vessels or compression at a wound site), resulting in drug release [28]. Polyurethane SMPs are one form of controlled drug delivery to tumor locations, in which the mechanical tension generated by the tumor's growth or external physical compression causes the drug to be released. Another example is hydrogel-based drug delivery devices for tissue engineering. Hydrogels derived from natural polymers like alginate or synthetic polymers like PNIPAAm are mechanically sensitive and can release medications in response to changes in pressure or deformation. Hydrogel scaffolds, for example, can release growth factors when compressed or mechanically loaded during tissue repair processes like bone regeneration [29].

4.2.2.5 Light Responsive Biomaterials

Light-responsive biomaterials use light energy to change material properties or release therapeutic chemicals. By integrating light-sensitive groups into the material, these systems can react to certain wavelengths of light, resulting in photochemical or photothermal processes that cause medication release. Light-responsive devices are particularly effective in applications requiring spatial and temporal control, such as localized tumor therapy or gene transfer [30]. Light-responsive biomaterials can undergo photochemical changes (for example, photolysis) or photothermal effects. In photochemical systems, light exposure promotes bond cleavage, rearrangement, or release of encapsulated drugs, whereas in photothermal systems, light is absorbed by the material, resulting in localized heating and drug release. Both mechanisms can be highly specific to the site of light application, offering excellent control over the release process [31]. Light-responsive biomaterials include caged compounds, which are light-sensitive groups that inhibit pharmacological activity until exposed to light. When exposed to light, the caged compound undergoes photolysis and releases the active drug. This method is commonly employed in regulated gene delivery or photodynamic therapy. In addition, gold nanoparticles that can absorb near-infrared (NIR) light are employed in photothermal therapy. When subjected to NIR light, these nanoparticles generate heat, which causes the release of encapsulated medications such as doxorubicin from the nanoparticles, hence improving localized tumor treatment [32].

4.3 DESIGN PRINCIPLES AND EMERGING TRENDS

4.3.1 Design Process for Stimuli-Responsive Biomaterials

SRBs are meticulously designed through a series of steps, including material selection, functionalization, manufacture, testing, stimulus-specific tailoring, and application-specific integration [39]. This section is a comprehensive discussion of each stage, emphasizing recent advances and uses in inflammatory conditions such as RA, IBD, and chronic wounds. Material selection is a crucial aspect of SRB design, influencing the biomaterial's biocompatibility, degradation profile, and responsiveness. The choice is based on the nature of the inflammatory condition and the appropriate treatment mechanism required. Natural polymers including chitosan, alginate, and hyaluronic acid are preferred because they are biocompatible and biodegradable. For example, chitosan is ideal for pH-responsive applications because it protonates in acidic conditions, which are typically found in inflamed tissues. Hyaluronic acid is widely utilized in rheumatology because of its ability to regenerate cartilage and modulate inflammation. However, natural materials may deteriorate too quickly in enzymatic conditions or be mechanically unstable. Chemical modifications or crosslinking with synthetic polymers are frequently used to alleviate this issue. Synthetic polymers, including PEG, PLGA, and PNIPAAm, offer controlled degradation, mechanical strength, and tunable characteristics. For example, PLGA allows for sustained drug release via hydrolytic breakdown. PNIPAAm is temperature-responsive, changing from hydrophilic to hydrophobic at body temperature, making it helpful for inflammation-induced hyperthermia applications. Hybrid materials combine the benefits of natural and synthetic polymers, resulting in systems with greater stability, mechanical characteristics, and responsiveness. PEGylated chitosan hydrogels, for example, are biocompatible as well as stable under oxidative stress. Inflammation raises ROS levels, necessitating materials that can withstand oxidative stress. Thioketal polymers are commonly employed for ROS-responsive degradation. In diseases such as RA, when joints are subjected to mechanical stress, materials must remain functioning under strain. Crosslinked hydrogels are very appropriate for these applications.

4.3.1.1 Integration of Stimulus Responsiveness

SRBs are distinguished by their ability to respond to specific stimuli, allowing for targeted therapeutic activity in response to environmental cues. Inflammatory illnesses generate a range of internal stimuli, including pH changes, ROS, and enzymes, which SRBs can use for targeted drug delivery.

- *pH-responsive systems*: Inflammation causes acidic environments (pH ~ 5.5–6.5). Polymers such as PAA or chitosan are treated with ionizable groups that swell or disintegrate in low pH settings, ensuring targeted medication release in inflamed areas. For example, anti-inflammatory medications are delivered using pH-sensitive hydrogels in cases of RA.
- *ROS-responsive systems*: Elevated ROS levels in inflamed tissues are used to cause the breakdown of thioketal links in polymers, releasing encapsulated drugs. These devices are especially useful for oxidative stress-related illnesses such as chronic wounds and arthritis.
- *Enzyme-responsive systems*: MMPs and other enzymes overexpressed in inflammation can cleave peptide linkers embedded in SRBs, allowing for site-specific material degradation and drug release. For example, MMP-sensitive nanoparticles deliver corticosteroids directly to arthritic joints.
- *Multi-stimuli systems*: To address complex inflammatory settings, multi-stimuli-responsive SRBs are engineered to respond to several inputs (e.g., pH and ROS). These systems provide more precise and reliable targeting.

4.3.1.2 Functionalization

Functionalization enhances the specificity, efficacy, and adaptability of SRBs by changing their surface or incorporating therapeutic agents.

- *Targeting ligands*: Ligands such as antibodies, peptides, and aptamers are attached to biomaterials, allowing them to bind specifically to overexpressed markers in inflammatory tissues. For example, SRBs functionalized with ICAM-1 ligands improve the targeting of endothelial cells in arthritic inflammation.
- *Drug encapsulation*: Therapeutic substances such as anti-inflammatory medicines, growth hormones, and antioxidants are encapsulated within SRBs utilizing emulsion polymerization or layer-by-layer construction. Controlled encapsulation ensures long-term medication release, minimizing the need for regular dosage.
- *Multifunctional properties*: SRBs are frequently improved with extra features. For example, antibacterial silver nanoparticles or polyphenols are used to promote wound healing, while also treating infection and inflammation. Materials functionalized with antioxidants like curcumin neutralize ROS, reducing oxidative stress in inflamed tissues.

4.3.1.3 Fabrication Techniques

Fabrication converts designed SRBs into functioning systems. Advanced approaches, such as those listed below, guarantee scalability and precision.

- *3D printing*: 3D printing enables highly customized geometries, such as porous scaffolds for cartilage regeneration. Multi-material printing allows for the integration of various responsive layers, such as a pH-sensitive core and a robust outer shell.

- *Microfluidics*: Microfluidics is frequently employed for the synthesis of SRBs at the nanoscale. It creates homogenous nanoparticles with consistent medication loading and enables high-throughput manufacture for clinical translation.
- *Self-assembly*: Self-assembly creates nanostructures without the need for external input through molecular interactions. These materials react dynamically to environmental cues such as pH and ROS, allowing for precise therapeutic administration.
- *Freeze-drying*: Freeze-drying produces porous scaffolds for tissue engineering purposes. By manipulating freezing rates, pore size, and distribution are customized to maximize drug release and cell infiltration.

4.3.1.4 Testing and Characterization

Comprehensive testing assures that SRBs are safe, effective, and responsive in physiological conditions.

- *Biocompatibility testing*: This includes various biological assays to determine the cytotoxicity, immunogenicity, and hemocompatibility of biomaterials.
- *Stimulus responsiveness*: pH-responsive materials are subjected to pH levels ranging from 5.5 to 7.4 to assess changes in swelling, degradation, or medication release. ROS-sensitive materials are evaluated for degradation rates in controlled oxidative conditions. For enzyme-responsive SRBs, materials are exposed to enzymes such as MMPs to ensure site-specific breakdown.
- *Mechanical stability*: Tensile and compressive testing ensures durability under mechanical stress, which is critical for joint applications. Dynamic mechanical analysis (DMA) determines viscoelastic characteristics to simulate the behavior of natural tissues.
- *Drug release studies*: *In vitro* drug release is assessed under simulated inflammatory circumstances using techniques such as high-performance liquid chromatography (HPLC) or UV-visible spectrophotometry. Burst release test quantifies the initial quick release, which is useful for acute inflammation. Sustained release test monitors steady medication delivery over time.
- *In vivo testing*: Animal models, such as mice with induced arthritis or colitis, are used to examine the therapeutic efficacy, systemic safety, and ability of SRBs to lower inflammatory markers.

4.3.1.5 Application Integration

Following validation, SRBs are customized to specific inflammatory conditions.

- *Localized drug delivery*: SRBs, such as pH-sensitive nanoparticles, provide tailored release at inflamed areas, reducing systemic side effects.
- *Wound healing*: Dual-responsive hydrogels (e.g., pH and ROS-responsive) adjust to the wound environment by releasing antibiotics or growth hormones in response to changing circumstances.
- *Tissue engineering*: Temperature-sensitive hydrogels serve as scaffolds for cartilage regeneration in arthritis by dynamically adjusting to inflammation-induced hyperthermia.

The comprehensive design process of SRBs, from material selection to application-specific integration [39, 40], is summarized in Figure 4.2, providing a visual overview of the key stages and their interconnections.

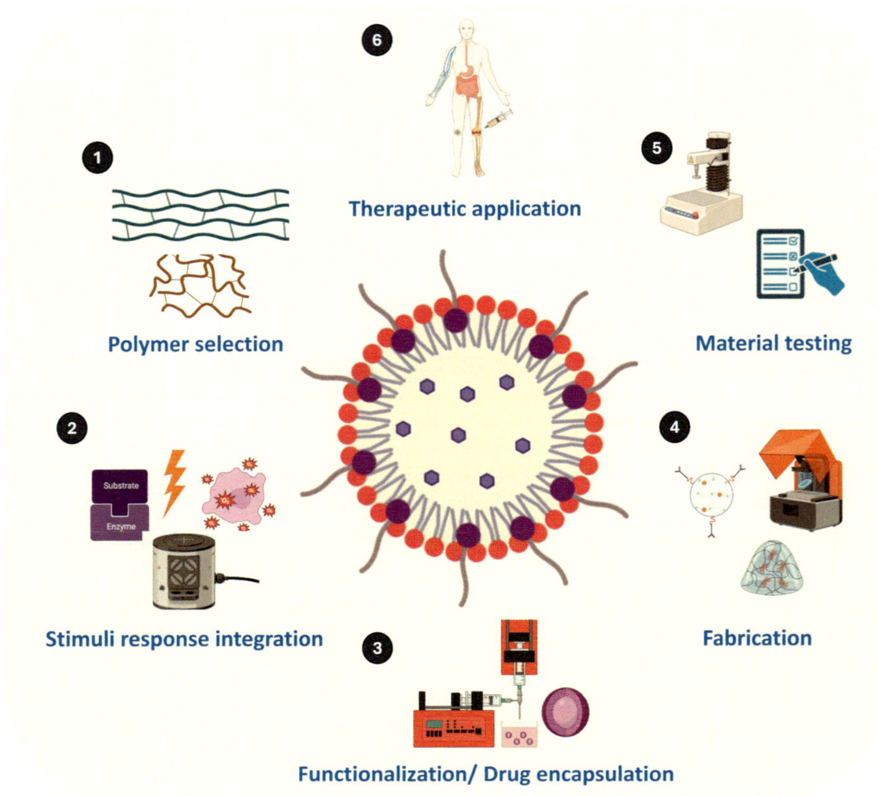

FIGURE 4.2 Step-by-step design process of stimuli-responsive biomaterials. This figure illustrates the key stages in designing stimuli-responsive biomaterials. Starting with material selection (1), appropriate polymers are chosen for biocompatibility and desired responsiveness. In stimulus-specific design (2), properties are tailored to respond to triggers like pH or temperature. Functionalization (3) adds features such as drug encapsulation or targeting ligands, followed by fabrication (4) through methods like polymerization or nanoparticle synthesis. The materials undergo testing and characterization (5) for stability and compatibility. Before application-specific integration (6) adapts them for uses like drug delivery or tissue engineering.

4.3.2 Design Considerations for Stimuli-Responsive Biomaterials

The development of SRBs requires careful consideration of various design parameters to ensure their effectiveness and compatibility with biological systems.

Stimuli selection: The choice of stimuli—whether internal (such as pH, redox potential, or enzyme presence) or external (such as temperature, light, or an electric field)—is critical to SRB efficacy. Internal stimuli rely on physiological cues from disease sites; for example, tumors frequently have an acidic environment (pH 5.5–6.5) and increased GSH levels, which can be exploited by pH- and redox-responsive biomaterials. External stimuli, on the other hand, provide exact control over the material's response and can be delivered geographically or temporally for therapeutic precision, such as initiating drug release in a specific spot using light or ultrasound. The chosen stimuli must be consistent with the disease etiology and therapy goals. External light sources, for example, are often utilized in cancer photodynamic therapy, allowing for the controlled, on-demand release of therapeutic chemicals with precise spatial control [41]. Latest research explores the incorporation of numerous stimuli-responsive parts into a single material system to improve specificity and efficiency. For example, dual-responsive devices that combine pH and enzyme triggers have a synergistic impact, releasing medicines only in the acidic, enzyme-rich tumor microenvironment [16].

Material composition: The composition and choice of polymers or hybrid materials are critical in customizing SRBs for responsiveness and biocompatibility. Polymers such as polyesters, polyacrylamides, and polyurethanes are popular because of their flexibility and ease of functionalization. These polymers are changed with certain functional groups (such as acidic or basic groups for pH responsiveness or disulfide bonds for redox sensitivity), allowing them to respond to stimuli in a controlled manner. PEG and PCL are commonly employed due to their low toxicity and good biocompatibility. Copolymerization procedures allow for the insertion of functional groups to improve responsiveness [39]. Advanced materials such as metal-organic frameworks (MOFs) and nanocomposites are increasingly being investigated for their high surface area and adjustable characteristics, enabling greater stability, targeting, and response specificity in biomedical applications [42].

Structural design: SRBs are designed across numerous scales, ranging from molecular architecture to nano- and micro-scale structures, which increases their functional adaptability and delivery potential. Nanostructures such as nanoparticles, micelles, and liposomes have several advantages, including drug encapsulation for enhanced stability, prolonged release, and targeted delivery. Hydrogels having a porous network structure, for example, can swell and release pharmaceuticals in response to a stimulus, such as pH or temperature changes, making them ideal for localized drug administration [43]. A critical part of structural design is to ensure biodegradability and non-toxicity, so that the material degrades harmlessly inside the body. Supramolecular assembly and self-assembling nanostructures are developing as design methodologies for creating dynamic, reversible materials with inherent reactivity, allowing for safe disintegration after therapy [44].

Responsive behavior: SRBs require a consistent and reversible response to stimuli to ensure reproducible performance under a wide range of physiological situations. Responsive behavior is frequently encoded into the material to allow specific drug-release mechanisms, such as diffusion, swelling, or disintegration. Temperature-responsive materials, such as PNIPAAm, undergo a phase transition around 32°C, transitioning from hydrophilic to hydrophobic, releasing encapsulated medicines when exposed to body temperature [45]. Dual or multi-responsive materials, which respond to two or more stimuli at the same time, are gaining a lot of interest. Nanoparticles that respond to both pH and temperature changes, for example, have demonstrated better specificity and therapeutic efficacy in cancer treatment [37].

Biocompatibility and toxicity: To avoid adverse immune responses or side effects during clinical translation, SRBs must be biocompatible and non-toxic. Surface changes such as PEGylation (attachment of PEG) can minimize immunogenicity, increase circulation time, and improve compatibility with biological tissues [46]. Furthermore, by integrating targeting ligands such as antibodies, peptides, or aptamers, SRBs can preferentially bind to certain cell receptors, boosting selectivity while decreasing off-target effects [44].

Scalability and manufacturing: Scalability remains an important problem as SRBs move from the experimental stage to widespread clinical application. Production processes must provide reproducibility, quality control, and cost effectiveness. Printing in 3D and microfluidics are modern manufacturing techniques that offer precise control over the geometry and composition of SRBs, allowing for batch production while retaining quality. For example, 3D-printed hydrogels and scaffolds can have regulated porosity and degradation rates, which are important in tissue engineering and regenerative medicine applications [47]. Table 4.2 further provides a concise summary of critical design parameters for SRBs, including stimulus threshold, response speed, degradability, structural robustness, and drug loading efficiency. These parameters are essential for optimizing material performance for therapeutic precision.

TABLE 4.2
Key Design Parameters and Their Functional Implications in Stimuli-Responsive Biomaterials

Physiological Stimuli	Definition	Practical Considerations	Application Impact
Stimulus threshold	The threshold level of stimulus required to trigger the response	Match threshold to physiological conditions (e.g., pH < 6 in tumors)	Enhances targeting precision and minimizes off-target effects
Response time	Time taken for the biomaterial to exhibit a functional change after stimulus	Faster responses for acute conditions (e.g., seconds for light stimuli)	Determines therapeutic efficacy and timing
Biodegradability	Capacity of the material to break down into non-toxic components after function	Use biodegradable polymers like chitosan or PLGA	Improves biocompatibility and reduces long-term risks
Structural robustness	Material's ability to maintain functionality under physiological stress	Incorporate crosslinking for hydrogels or elastomers	Ensures stability for implants and load-bearing applications
Drug-loading efficiency	Amount of therapeutic agent that can be encapsulated or conjugated effectively	Optimize material porosity or surface chemistry	Directly affects dosage and therapeutic outcome
Surface functionalization	Modification of the material surface to improve targeting or reduce immune response	Add ligands (e.g., peptides) or hydrophilic groups (PEGylation)	Enhances specificity and reduces systemic side effects
Scalability	Feasibility of producing the material on a large scale without compromising quality	Focus on simple synthesis and cost-effective methods	Accelerates clinical translation and commercialization

4.4 ADVANCES IN DYNAMIC AND MULTI-RESPONSIVE BIOMATERIALS

Traditional SRBs typically provided a single, static response to one stimulation. However, recent advancements have resulted in multi-stimuli-sensitive and adaptable biomaterials that can dynamically react to complex and changing surroundings. These developments pave the way for next-generation SRBs that promise precision control, adaptability, and high therapeutic specificity, with potential applications in personalized medicine, cancer treatment, and chronic disease management.

Multi-SRBs are intended to respond to multiple types of stimuli, such as pH, temperature, light, or enzyme activity. This capability adds another layer of control, increasing the therapeutic specificity of these compounds. For example, dual-responsive systems that respond to both pH and temperature are especially valuable in cancer therapy, where the acidic tumor microenvironment and localized hyperthermia can be used to control medication release. One such invention is pH-sensitive hydrogels, which release encapsulated pharmaceuticals in acidic conditions when heated, making them particularly effective for chemotherapy administration [38]. Similarly, triple-responsive systems have been created that respond to pH, temperature, and redox conditions. These are especially beneficial in situations involving complicated pathophysiological disorders, such as cancer or inflammation, when several biological changes can be targeted simultaneously [48]. Hydrogels are known to expand and release pharmaceuticals in response to pH and temperature changes, ensuring optimal conditions for therapeutic release in specified locations.

Adaptive biomaterials include feedback mechanisms that enable them to react dynamically to changes in their surroundings. This adaptability is especially important in chronic or progressive disorders where the pathophysiology changes with time, necessitating therapy alterations. For example, in chronic inflammatory disorders, cytokine-responsive biomaterials can modify drug release in response to varying levels of inflammatory markers, allowing for dose-dependent release in real time. A hydrogel system that releases anti-inflammatory chemicals in response to elevated cytokine levels was described, illustrating how adaptable biomaterials can accurately respond to pathogenic stimuli [49]. Self-assembling biomaterials are another example of feedback mechanisms in action, as they may adapt their structure and function in response to changes in the surrounding environment. These biomaterials undergo structural rearrangements in response to physiological stimuli, increasing their efficacy by optimizing therapeutic activity in response to disease progression. For example, self-assembling peptide hydrogels have shown promise in wound healing because their structure adjusts to tissue repair demands, encouraging cellular infiltration and regeneration at the wound site [44].

Smart drug delivery systems are at the forefront of SRB development, including a variety of stimuli and feedback loops to achieve highly targeted and controlled drug release [8]. These systems can detect and respond to real-time disease markers such as pH shifts, enzyme activity, and specific biomarkers, allowing for precise drug administration in both space and time. For example, nanoparticle-based delivery systems with embedded biosensors can only release drugs when specified biomarkers, such as cancer-associated enzymes or pH levels, surpass a predetermined threshold. This technique decreases systemic side effects while increasing therapeutic efficacy by guaranteeing that the medicine is solely released at the illness location. Furthermore, new research has produced enzyme-responsive nanoparticles that selectively release medications in response to high enzyme levels associated with specific diseases, such as MMPs in cancer. This targeted release method improves drug delivery specificity while simultaneously reducing drug exposure to healthy tissues, making it a safer and more effective therapy alternative [15]. Figure 4.3 illustrates a generalized working of SRB in therapies, highlighting how these biomaterials can localize treatment and improve outcomes in inflammatory disorders.

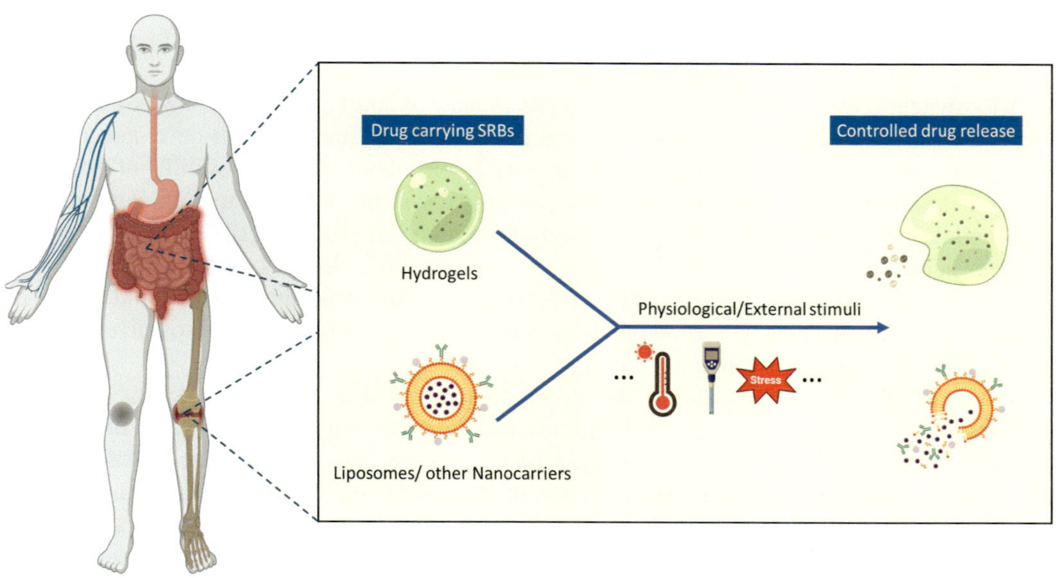

FIGURE 4.3 Illustration of stimuli-responsive biomaterials in inflammatory disorder therapy. The inflamed joints/bowel of the patient are shown, with zoomed-in views of affected sites treated with stimuli-responsive biomaterials. Hydrogels release drugs in response to local stimuli such as acidic pH or enzymes overexpressed in inflamed tissues, while nanocarriers deliver therapeutic agents triggered by reactive oxygen species or redox changes. These systems ensure precise, targeted treatment, reducing systemic side effects and improving patient outcomes.

4.4.1 Emerging Trends in Stimuli-Responsive Biomaterials Research

The future of SRBs is in continuous development of their responsiveness, adaptability, and application in real-world therapeutic conditions. As researchers investigate new stimuli and develop innovative tactics, the discipline is witnessing many significant trends. Another new trend is the use of SRBs in personalized medicine, in which biomaterials can be adapted to an individual's specific physiological and molecular profiles. By adding biomarkers or sensors into SRBs, it is feasible to create dynamic drug delivery systems that react to specific disease biomarkers or changes in an individual's condition. For example, indicators of inflammation or tumor growth can be used to trigger drug release from polymeric systems, ensuring that the patient receives the appropriate dosage at the appropriate time [50]. This method could significantly increase therapy efficacy, reduce side effects, and enable adaptive therapies in response to illness development.

Bio-inspired SRBs are gaining popularity, with materials designed to replicate natural biological processes and systems. These biomaterials are not only responsive but also biocompatible and biodegradable, which is essential for therapeutic use. DNA-based hydrogels and protein-based biomaterials have demonstrated potential due to their intrinsic biological compatibility and capacity to self-assemble in response to stimuli [51]. Bio-inspired materials offer the potential to address some of the drawbacks of synthetic polymers, including toxicity, long-term stability, and immune system recognition.

Aptamer-based SRBs are emerging as a promising technology due to their ability to specifically respond to target molecules, such as proteins, ions, and small metabolites, through conformational changes in aptamers. These materials have been incorporated into nanoparticle systems for targeted drug delivery, hydrogel matrices for controlled release, and diagnostic sensing platforms for detecting specific biomarkers. Aptamers' high specificity and adaptability make them ideal for designing SRBs that can respond to precise physiological conditions, offering advantages in minimizing side effects and enhancing therapeutic efficacy. For instance, aptamer-functionalized nanoparticles and hydrogels have been employed in cancer therapy and disease detection, responding to specific biomarkers or environmental changes such as pH and enzyme presence [52].

Riboswitches, which contain aptamer domains capable of binding to specific ligands and inducing conformational changes, represent a natural extension of aptamers in SRB development. Their ability to respond to metabolites, ions, and other small molecules opens the possibility of integrating riboswitches into biomaterials to create multi-responsive systems that react to both environmental cues and disease biomarkers [53]. By combining the aptamer functions of riboswitches with other SRB designs, it is possible to develop adaptive, dynamic drug delivery systems with enhanced specificity and therapeutic precision. This integration of riboswitches into SRBs could enable the development of materials that respond to a range of stimuli, offering a more personalized and efficient approach to disease treatment [54].

Nanotechnology is important to the development of highly precise and efficient SRBs. Nanoparticles and nanocarriers, including liposomes, micelles, and dendrimers, are increasingly being employed in stimuli-responsive drug delivery systems. These nanomaterials can be functionalized to respond to certain environmental or therapeutic circumstances, allowing for regulated medication release and increased bioavailability. For example, pH-sensitive nanoparticles can be utilized to deliver chemotherapeutic drugs directly to tumors, increasing treatment efficacy while reducing off-target effects. Recent breakthroughs in nanomedicine have also focused on using nano-sensors to monitor real-time changes in the body and provide feedback that can be utilized to dynamically adapt medication delivery systems [55]. Because of their high water content and similarity to biological tissues, hydrogels are one of the most extensively researched types of SRBs. The introduction of stimuli-responsive components into hydrogels opens up fascinating new prospects for tissue engineering and regenerative medicine. For example, pH-responsive hydrogels can be utilized to produce scaffolds for tissue regeneration, triggering medication or growth factor release in the acidic environment of wounds or tumors. The versatility of hydrogels in simulating natural tissue environments, combined with their reactivity to physiological stimuli, makes them excellent for dynamic applications that require continual adaptation to changing conditions [56].

Self-healing materials are another novel type of SRB that is meant to repair itself after damage, ensuring their functionality and longevity. These materials are especially beneficial in applications that need continuous material integrity, such as wound healing and bone regeneration. Recent research has focused on creating self-healing polymers that can respond to both environmental stimuli and mechanical stress. Materials that mend autonomously in response to physical damage or temperature changes are being investigated for use in medication delivery and tissue repair. These self-healing properties are especially crucial for the creation of long-lasting and dependable medical equipment [57].

4.5 FUTURE DIRECTIONS AND CHALLENGES

The field of SRBs has the potential to transform therapeutic techniques, particularly in drug delivery, tissue engineering, and regenerative medicine. However, bringing this technology to clinical applications presents several types of challenges and areas of improvement. Emerging trends, innovations, and barriers to SRB development are as follows:

- *Advanced technology integration*: Using cutting-edge technologies such as 3D printing, microfluidics, and nanotechnology will increase the scalability and precision of SRB production, allowing for more complex, multifunctional systems with high reproducibility. These technologies can also aid in the development of patient-specific SRBs, hence aiding personalized medicine methods in disease management [9].
- *Multi-functional systems*: Research is currently underway to produce SRBs capable of performing several functions, such as controlled drug release, tissue regeneration, and real-time biosensing. Multifunctional SRBs, for example, could release anti-inflammatory drugs while stimulating cellular growth in wound healing applications. Such breakthroughs necessitate a thorough understanding of material interactions within the body, and current research is looking into the possibilities of hybrid materials that blend synthetic and biological components to improve functionality [58].
- *Biocompatibility and immunological reaction*: Although SRBs have therapeutic benefits, biocompatibility and immunological reaction are major problems. Surface modification and biomimetic material innovations aim to increase biocompatibility and minimize immunological reactions, but more research is required to ensure the safe and long-term incorporation of SRBs in clinical settings [59].
- *Scalability and cost-effectiveness*: Producing SRBs can be exceedingly costly, particularly for complicated systems that require multi-step synthesis or accurate structural engineering. Scalable, cost-effective production methods are required to convert SRBs from laboratory to clinical application. Advances in modular assembly approaches and high-throughput manufacturing processes show promise for addressing these constraints, potentially making SRBs more accessible for medical applications [60].

4.6 CONCLUSION

The development of SRBs represents a major step ahead in overcoming the limits of traditional treatments for inflammatory disorders and other chronic diseases. These sophisticated materials adapt dynamically to physiological and environmental cues, allowing for a more targeted, controlled, and patient-specific approach to treatment. Throughout this chapter, we examined the many classes of SRBs, their mechanisms of action, design principles, and possible applications, gaining a thorough understanding of their potential to revolutionize treatment paradigms. Conventional therapies for inflammatory disorders such as RA, IBD, and chronic wounds have long been hampered by systemic toxicity, inadequate medication specificity, and resistance. While these therapies provide temporary comfort, they frequently fail to address the underlying cause of the condition and can result in adverse effects. In contrast, SRBs can respond selectively to specific disease-associated signals, such as pH shifts, higher levels of ROS, or the presence of specific enzymes, ensuring that therapeutic drugs are only released in the affected tissues. This site-specific action dramatically lowers off-target effects while increasing the therapeutic index, providing a safer and more effective alternative to standard treatments. One of SRBs' primary features is their capacity to respond to both physiological cues—such as the acidic environment and oxidative stress found in many inflammatory and malignant tissues—and external stimuli, such as light, temperature, or magnetic fields. The chapter underlined how materials that react to pH, ROS, or enzymes are especially well-suited for inflammatory illnesses, because local alterations in the microenvironment provide unique chances for targeted drug delivery. For example, pH-responsive biomaterials can use the acidic conditions in inflamed tissues, such as those present in RA or ulcerative colitis, to deliver medications directly to the site of inflammation. Similarly, ROS-responsive materials can target oxidative stress in chronic wounds or tumors, releasing payloads only when oxidative conditions cause material deterioration.

The chapter also discussed various steps involved in designing SRBs, highlighting how material selection, functionalization, and fabrication are crucial to their success. Materials are chosen based on their biocompatibility, stability, and responsiveness to intended stimuli. Natural polymers, such as chitosan or alginate, provide biocompatibility but frequently lack the mechanical strength or stability required for certain applications. In contrast, synthetic materials such as PEG, PLGA, and PNIPAAm can be adjusted for precise mechanical and degrading properties, offering the adaptability required for a wide range of therapeutic applications. Functionalizing these materials—whether by adding targeting ligands, encapsulating pharmaceuticals, or combining numerous responsive elements—increases their precision and adaptability. Moreover, the fabrication of SRBs is important to their function and clinical use. Advanced techniques like 3D printing, microfluidics, and self-assembly enable the production of complex, precise structures that are critical for achieving the desired therapeutic results. For example, 3D printing allows for the creation of scaffolds with controlled porosity for use in tissue engineering applications, whilst microfluidic devices provide exact control over the size and drug-loading capacity of nanoparticles. These advances guarantee that SRBs can be manufactured at clinically relevant scales while maintaining high levels of uniformity and performance.

Despite their enormous potential, SRBs face significant challenges before they can be broadly implemented in clinical settings. The key concerns include long-term scalability, cost-effectiveness, and biocompatibility. While laboratory-scale synthesis of SRBs has been successful, transferring these materials to industrial-scale production while keeping their functional features is a challenging task. Advanced materials, particularly those demanding sophisticated production procedures or high-purity components, might be prohibitively expensive, making them inaccessible. Furthermore, the long-term safety of SRBs, particularly in terms of potential immunological reactions or material degradation, must be extensively investigated in large-scale clinical trials to ensure their viability for chronic usage. Furthermore, regulatory approval remains a substantial hurdle. Because SRBs frequently involve new materials or unique applications, they do not necessarily comply with established regulatory systems. Obtaining regulatory approval necessitates extensive evidence on safety, efficacy, and scalability, which can cause delays in clinical application of these technologies. Looking forward, SRBs will be based on multi-stimuli-responsive systems, adaptive biomaterials, and smart technology integration. Multi-stimuli systems, which respond to several biological or environmental cues, provide more precise targeting in complex disease situations. Adaptive materials, which may modify their activity in response to oscillations in the disease environment, hold great promise for use in regenerative medicine and chronic illness management. Furthermore, including bioelectronics or machine learning into the design of SRBs has the potential to revolutionize therapy personalization by providing individualized therapeutic methods based on real-time patient data.

The SRBs have enormous potential for enhancing precision medicine, especially in the treatment of inflammatory and chronic disorders. By providing focused, adaptable, and regulated therapeutic inputs, SRBs can overcome many of the limitations associated with traditional treatments. As the field advances, the clinical translation of SRBs will be driven by the integration of new technologies, improved manufacturing processes, and a better understanding of disease biology, opening up new frontiers in healthcare and offering hope for more effective, personalized, and patient-centered therapies.

Declaration of AI and AI-Assisted Technologies

During the preparation of this work, the authors used QuillBot AI in order to paraphrase the sentences. After using this tool, the authors reviewed and edited the content as needed and take full responsibility for the content of the publication.

REFERENCES

1. Chen L, Deng H, Cui H, Fang J, Zuo Z, Deng J, et al. Inflammatory responses and inflammation-associated diseases in organs. Oncotarget 2017;9:7204. https://doi.org/10.18632/oncotarget.23208
2. McInnes IB, Gravallese EM. Immune-mediated inflammatory disease therapeutics: Past, present and future. Nat Rev Immunol 2021;21:680–6. https://doi.org/10.1038/s41577-021-00603-1
3. Chuang S-Y, Lin C-H, Huang T-H, Fang J-Y. Lipid-based nanoparticles as a potential delivery approach in the treatment of rheumatoid arthritis. Nanomaterials 2018;8:42. https://doi.org/10.3390/nano8010042
4. Yasmin F, Najeeb H, Shaikh S, Hasanain M, Naeem U, Moeed A, et al. Novel drug delivery systems for inflammatory bowel disease. World J Gastroenterol 2022;28:1922. https://doi.org/10.3748/wjg.v28.i18.1922
5. Harjunpää H, Llort Asens M, Guenther C, Fagerholm SC. Cell adhesion molecules and their roles and regulation in the immune and tumor microenvironment. Front Immunol 2019;10. https://doi.org/10.3389/fimmu.2019.01078
6. Mura S, Nicolas J, Couvreur P. Stimuli-responsive nanocarriers for drug delivery. Nat Mater 2013;12: 991–1003. https://doi.org/10.1038/nmat3776
7. Siegel RA, Langer R. Controlled release of polypeptides and other macromolecules. Pharm Res 1984;1:2–10. https://doi.org/10.1023/A:1016318423563
8. Nag S, Mohanto S, Ahmed MG, Subramaniyan V. "Smart" stimuli-responsive biomaterials revolutionizing the theranostic landscape of inflammatory arthritis. Mater Today Chem 2024;39:102178. https://doi.org/10.1016/j.mtchem.2024.102178
9. Thomas V, Bates JS, Hu J, Li L, Naleway SE. Advances in biomaterials and materials for biomedical applications. JOM 2024;76:5623–4. https://doi.org/10.1007/s11837-024-06792-z
10. Kocak G, Tuncer C, Bütün V. pH-responsive polymers. Polym Chem 2016;8:144–76. https://doi.org/10.1039/C6PY01872F
11. Tsai L-H, Yen C-H, Hsieh H-Y, Young T-H. Doxorubicin loaded PLGA nanoparticle with c/anionic polyelectrolyte decoration: Characterization, and its therapeutic potency. Polymers 2021;13:693. https://doi.org/10.3390/polym13050693
12. Quinn JF, Whittaker MR, Davis TP. Glutathione responsive polymers and their application in drug delivery systems. Polym Chem 2017;8:97–126. https://doi.org/10.1039/C6PY01365A
13. Li S, Wang Q, Duan X, Pei Z, He Z, Guo W, et al. A glutathione-responsive PEGylated nanogel with doxorubicin-conjugation for cancer therapy. J Mater Chem B 2023;11:11612–9. https://doi.org/10.1039/D3TB01731A

14. Cook AB, Palange A, Schlich M, Bellotti E, Brahmachari S, Francesco MD, et al. Matrix metalloproteinase responsive hydrogel microplates for programmed killing of invasive tumour cells. RSC Appl Polym 2023;1:19–29. https://doi.org/10.1039/D3LP00057E
15. Li M, Zhao G, Su W-K, Shuai Q. Enzyme-responsive nanoparticles for anti-tumor drug delivery. Front Chem 2020;8. https://doi.org/10.3389/fchem.2020.00647
16. Yan J, Zhang Z, Zhan X, Chen K, Pu Y, Liang Y, et al. In situ injection of dual-delivery PEG based MMP-2 sensitive hydrogels for enhanced tumor penetration and chemo-immune combination therapy. Nanoscale 2021;13:9577–89. https://doi.org/10.1039/D1NR01155C
17. Yuan Y, Raheja K, Milbrandt NB, Beilharz S, Tene S, Oshabaheebwa S, et al. Thermoresponsive polymers with LCST transition: Synthesis, characterization, and their impact on biomedical frontiers. RSC Appl Polym 2023;1:158–89. https://doi.org/10.1039/D3LP00114H
18. Jain K, Vedarajan R, Watanabe M, Ishikiriyama M, Matsumi N. Tunable LCST behavior of poly(N-isopropylacrylamide/ionic liquid) copolymers. Polym Chem 2015;6:6819–25. https://doi.org/10.1039/C5PY00998G
19. Municoy S, Álvarez Echazú MI, Antezana PE, Galdopórpora JM, Olivetti C, Mebert AM, et al. Stimuli-responsive materials for tissue engineering and drug delivery. Int J Mol Sci 2020;21:4724. https://doi.org/10.3390/ijms21134724
20. Carayon I, Gaubert A, Mousli Y, Philippe B. Electro-responsive hydrogels: Macromolecular and supramolecular approaches in the biomedical field. Biomater Sci 2020;8:5589–600. https://doi.org/10.1039/D0BM01268H
21. Kaur G, Adhikari R, Cass P, Bown M, Gunatillake P. Electrically conductive polymers and composites for biomedical applications. RSC Adv 2015;5:37553–67. https://doi.org/10.1039/C5RA01851J
22. Alkahtani ME, Elbadawi M, Chapman CAR, Green RA, Gaisford S, Orlu M, et al. Electroactive polymers for on-demand drug release. Adv Healthc Mater 2024;13:2301759. https://doi.org/10.1002/adhm.202301759
23. Heidari M, Bahrami SH, Ranjbar-Mohammadi M, Milan PB. Smart electrospun nanofibers containing PCL/gelatin/graphene oxide for application in nerve tissue engineering. Mater Sci Eng C 2019;103:109768. https://doi.org/10.1016/j.msec.2019.109768
24. Lin Y, Zhang K, Zhang R, She Z, Tan R, Fan Y, et al. Magnetic nanoparticles applied in targeted therapy and magnetic resonance imaging: Crucial preparation parameters, indispensable pre-treatments, updated research advancements and future perspectives. J Mater Chem B 2020;8:5973–91. https://doi.org/10.1039/D0TB00552E
25. Majeed MI, Lu Q, Yan W, Li Z, Hussain I, Tahir MN, et al. Highly water-soluble magnetic iron oxide (Fe_3O_4) nanoparticles for drug delivery: Enhanced in vitro therapeutic efficacy of doxorubicin and MION conjugates. J Mater Chem B 2013;1:2874–84. https://doi.org/10.1039/C3TB20322K
26. Denmark DJ, Bradley J, Mukherjee D, Alonso J, Shakespeare S, Bernal N, et al. Remote triggering of thermoresponsive PNIPAM by iron oxide nanoparticles. RSC Adv 2016;6:5641–52. https://doi.org/10.1039/C5RA21617F
27. Wang J, Kaplan JA, Colson YL, Grinstaff MW. Mechanoresponsive materials for drug delivery: Harnessing forces for controlled release. Adv Drug Deliv Rev 2016;108:68. https://doi.org/10.1016/j.addr.2016.11.001
28. Farrukh A, Nayab S. Shape memory hydrogels for biomedical applications. Gels 2024;10:270. https://doi.org/10.3390/gels10040270
29. Choi H, Choi W-S, Jeong J-O. A review of advanced hydrogel applications for tissue engineering and drug delivery systems as biomaterials. Gels 2024;10:693. https://doi.org/10.3390/gels10110693
30. Katz JS, Burdick JA. Light-responsive biomaterials: Development and applications. Macromol Biosci 2010;10:339–48. https://doi.org/10.1002/mabi.200900297
31. Xing Y, Zeng B, Yang W. Light responsive hydrogels for controlled drug delivery. Front Bioeng Biotechnol 2022;10. https://doi.org/10.3389/fbioe.2022.1075670
32. Yang N, Zhu M, Xu G, Liu N, Yu C. A near-infrared light-responsive multifunctional nanocomposite hydrogel for efficient and synergistic antibacterial wound therapy and healing promotion. J Mater Chem B 2020;8:3908–17. https://doi.org/10.1039/D0TB00361A
33. Elkassih SA, Kos P, Xiong H, Siegwart DJ. Degradable redox-responsive disulfide-based nanogel drug carriers via dithiol oxidation polymerization. Biomater Sci 2019;7:607–17. https://doi.org/10.1039/C8BM01120F
34. Mu J, Lin J, Huang P, Chen X. Development of endogenous enzyme-responsive nanomaterials for theranostics. Chem Soc Rev 2018;47:5554–73. https://doi.org/10.1039/C7CS00663B

35. Yao J, Cheng Y, Zhou M, Zhao S, Lin S, Wang X, et al. ROS scavenging Mn_3O_4 nanozymes for in vivo anti-inflammation. Chem Sci 2018;9:2927–33. https://doi.org/10.1039/C7SC05476A
36. Estelrich J, Escribano E, Queralt J, Busquets MA. Iron oxide nanoparticles for magnetically-guided and magnetically-responsive drug delivery. Int J Mol Sci 2015;16:8070–101. https://doi.org/10.3390/ijms16048070
37. Knipe JM, Peppas NA. Multi-responsive hydrogels for drug delivery and tissue engineering applications. Regen Biomater 2014;1:57–65. https://doi.org/10.1093/rb/rbu006
38. Liu Y, Ran Y, Ge Y, Raza F, Li S, Zafar H, et al. pH-sensitive peptide hydrogels as a combination drug delivery system for cancer treatment. Pharmaceutics 2022;14:652. https://doi.org/10.3390/pharmaceutics14030652
39. Tropp J, Rivnay J. Design of biodegradable and biocompatible conjugated polymers for bioelectronics. J Mater Chem C 2021;9:13543–56. https://doi.org/10.1039/D1TC03600A
40. Li M, Xia W, Khoong YM, Huang L, Huang X, Liang H, et al. Smart and versatile biomaterials for cutaneous wound healing. Biomater Res 2023;27:87. https://doi.org/10.1186/s40824-023-00426-2
41. Liao Z, Liu T, Yao Z, Hu T, Ji X, Yao B. Harnessing stimuli-responsive biomaterials for advanced biomedical applications. Exploration n.d: 20230133. https://doi.org/10.1002/EXP.20230133
42. Nguyen NTT, Nguyen TTT, Ge S, Liew RK, Nguyen DTC, Tran TV. Recent progress and challenges of MOF-based nanocomposites in bioimaging, biosensing and biocarriers for drug delivery. Nanoscale Adv 2024;6:1800–21. https://doi.org/10.1039/D3NA01075A
43. Raza A, Rasheed T, Nabeel F, Hayat U, Bilal M, Iqbal HMN. Endogenous and exogenous stimuli-responsive drug delivery systems for programmed site-specific release. Molecules 2019;24:1117. https://doi.org/10.3390/molecules24061117
44. La Manna S, Di Natale C, Onesto V, Marasco D. Self-assembling peptides: From design to biomedical applications. Int J Mol Sci 2021;22:12662. https://doi.org/10.3390/ijms222312662
45. Yang L, Fan X, Zhang J, Ju J. Preparation and characterization of thermoresponsive poly(N-isopropylacrylamide) for cell culture applications. Polymers 2020;12:389. https://doi.org/10.3390/polym12020389
46. Santhanakrishnan KR, Koilpillai J, Narayanasamy D, Santhanakrishnan K, Koilpillai J, Narayanasamy D. PEGylation in pharmaceutical development: Current status and emerging trends in macromolecular and immunotherapeutic drugs. Cureus 2024;16. https://doi.org/10.7759/cureus.66669
47. Arif ZU, Khalid MY, Tariq A, Hossain M, Umer R. 3D printing of stimuli-responsive hydrogel materials: Literature review and emerging applications. Giant 2024;17:100209. https://doi.org/10.1016/j.giant.2023.100209
48. Timin AS, Muslimov AR, Lepik KV, Saprykina NN, Sergeev VS, Afanasyev BV, et al. Triple-responsive inorganic–organic hybrid microcapsules as a biocompatible smart platform for the delivery of small molecules. J Mater Chem B 2016;4:7270–82. https://doi.org/10.1039/C6TB02289H
49. Vishwakarma A, Bhise NS, Evangelista MB, Rouwkema J, Dokmeci MR, Ghaemmaghami AM, et al. Engineering immunomodulatory biomaterials to tune the inflammatory response. Trends Biotechnol 2016;34:470–82. https://doi.org/10.1016/j.tibtech.2016.03.009
50. Mitchell MJ, Billingsley MM, Haley RM, Wechsler ME, Peppas NA, Langer R. Engineering precision nanoparticles for drug delivery. Nat Rev Drug Discov 2021;20:101–24. https://doi.org/10.1038/s41573-020-0090-8
51. Omidian H, Wilson RL, Babanejad N. Bioinspired polymers: Transformative applications in biomedicine and regenerative medicine. Life 2023;13:1673. https://doi.org/10.3390/life13081673
52. Urmi R, Banerjee P, Singh M, Singh R, Chhillar S, Sharma N, et al. Revolutionizing biomedicine: Aptamer-based nanomaterials and nanodevices for therapeutic applications. Biotechnol Rep 2024;42:e00843. https://doi.org/10.1016/j.btre.2024.e00843
53. Bowlby B. Synthetic riboswitches detect biomarker proteins. BioTechniques 2023. https://www.biotechniques.com/diagnostics-preclinical/synthetic-riboswitches-detect-biomarker-proteins/ (accessed November 19, 2024).
54. Hoang Trung Chau T, Hoang Anh Mai D, Ngoc Pham D, Thi Quynh Le H, Yeol Lee E. Developments of riboswitches and toehold switches for molecular detection—Biosensing and molecular diagnostics. Int J Mol Sci 2020;21:3192. https://doi.org/10.3390/ijms21093192
55. Liu Y, Li C, Yang X, Yang B, Fu Q. Stimuli-responsive polymer-based nanosystems for cardiovascular disease theranostics. Biomater Sci 2024;12:3805–25. https://doi.org/10.1039/D4BM00415A
56. Gupta A, Lee J, Ghosh T, Nguyen VQ, Dey A, Yoon B, et al. Polymeric hydrogels for controlled drug delivery to treat arthritis. Pharmaceutics 2022;14:540. https://doi.org/10.3390/pharmaceutics14030540

57. Quan L, Xin Y, Wu X, Ao Q. Mechanism of self-healing hydrogels and application in tissue engineering. Polymers 2022;14:2184. https://doi.org/10.3390/polym14112184
58. Multifunctional Biomaterials: Combining Material Modification Strategies for Engineering of Cell-Contacting Surfaces | ACS Applied Materials & Interfaces n.d. https://pubs.acs.org/doi/10.1021/acsami.0c01893 (accessed November 19, 2024).
59. Singh AK, Malviya R, Prajapati B, Singh S, Goyal P. Utilization of stimuli-responsive biomaterials in the formulation of cancer vaccines. J Funct Biomater 2023;14:247. https://doi.org/10.3390/jfb14050247
60. Rajvanshi J, Sogani M, Kumar A, Arora S. Biomaterials: A sustainable solution for a circular economy. Eng Proc 2023;59:133. https://doi.org/10.3390/engproc2023059133

5 Stimuli-Responsive Biomaterials for Cancer Theranostics

Kowshika Vijayan, Mohammad Suhaan Dar, and Niroj Kumar Sahu
Centre for Nanotechnology Research, Vellore Institute of Technology, Vellore, Tamil Nadu, India

5.1 INTRODUCTION

The majority of deaths globally are attributed to non-communicable diseases (NCDs), which have already become the primary cause of mortality [1]. Cancer is caused by a rapid expansion of altered cells that have evolved through natural selection [2]. Since cancer develops in a variety of organs, many contemporary definitions of the disease refer to it as a group of disorders [3]. Cancer affects many parts of body, like breast, colon, liver, skin, brain, ovary, and prostate. The procedure of treating cancer has proven to be extremely complicated [4]. Traditionally, the most widely used cancer treatments include chemotherapy, surgery, and radiation therapy. Breast cancer was the first disease to show promising outcomes from adjuvant therapy. It was also the first instance of multimodality treatment, which is now used to treat a wide variety of tumor forms [5]. The primary treatment approach for breast cancer involves surgery in most cases, although late-stage diagnosis in a subset of cases can render radical surgical interventions more complex. The goal of surgery and radiation treatment is to control the disease locally. The combination of surgical excision and radiation therapy is crucial for optimizing outcomes in breast-conserving surgery, transforming it into a safe and effective treatment option with reduced local recurrence rates [6]. The combination of loco-regional radiotherapy and chemotherapy yields a statistically significant survival advantage over chemotherapy-only approaches from two randomized trials reporting statistical results [7]. Rehabilitation for women with cancer requires managing treatment-related side effects, both during and after therapy, by addressing ongoing treatment side effects and lingering consequences of surgery, radiation, and other completed therapies, and encompasses a psychological effect, including depression, anxiety, and social isolations [8]. Because of both chemotherapy and radiation process, other organs get infected during breast cancer diagnosis. When combined, both chemotherapy and radiotherapy enhance curable rates but also elevate the major side effects like heart-related induced problem due to damage occurring in heart fibrosis. Even this combination affects bone and causes osteoporosis because of lack of calcium after the treatment. Also, it is observed that quality of ovary is affected in rats after chemotherapy treatments. Therefore, highlighting the risk caused by the treatment, it is essential to design and implement new treatment strategies to ultimately enhance patient outcomes and lifespan [9].

In contrast to conventional cancer treatments, tumor immunotherapy has made use of fully engineered nanomaterials [10], including dendrimers, polymeric nanoparticles, inorganic nanoparticles, and liposomes, to enhance the delivery of immunomodulatory agents to the tumor site, boost their bioavailability, and prevent their early degradation [11]. Many therapeutic and diagnostic agents based on nanoscale and nanostructure have been created in the past 20 years, not only for the treatment of cancer but also for its detection and prevention [12]. Some cancer treatments that make use of engineered nanomaterials include targeted cancer, photodynamic therapy (PDT), hyperthermia, and gene therapy. By

DOI: 10.1201/9781003560203-5

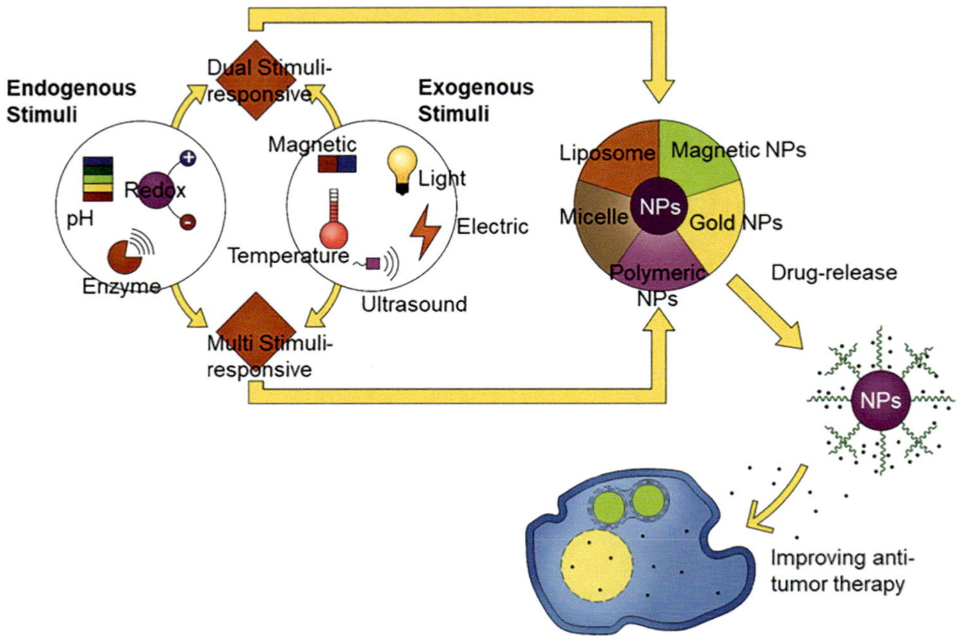

FIGURE 5.1 Graphical representation of numerous stimuli-responsive strategies. (Reprinted with permission from Ref. [13], under Creative Commons CC BY 4.0 license.)

targeting tumors (passively or actively), responding to internal or external chemical or physical stimuli, and delivering therapeutic genes to the cell nuclei, these therapies can be employed alone or in conjunction with other cancer treatments [5]. Every day, a variety of cancer-curing treatments are being developed. Meanwhile, stimuli-responsive biomaterials show positive outcomes in the treatment of cancer patients, either on their own or in combination with other therapies. There are many stimuli-responsive strategies by different biomaterials used for tumor therapy, as shown in Figure 5.1.

5.2 SIGNIFICANCE OF CANCER THERANOSTICS—GAPS AND PROSPECTS

The domain of cancer theranostics signifies a revolutionary change in oncology, integrating therapeutic and diagnostic functions to enable precision therapy. Cancer continues to be a primary cause of death globally, highlighted by its diverse characteristics and capacity to acquire resistance to standard therapies. This intricacy necessitates innovations that exceed conventional methods, frequently impeded by significant side effects, restricted therapeutic effectiveness, and insufficient tumor-specific targeting. Theranostics, which combines diagnostics and therapy on a single platform, has [10] the potential to transform cancer care by improving treatment specificity and efficacy [14]. Recent progress in nanotechnology, especially in stimuli-responsive nanomaterials, has expedited this shift, facilitating platforms that can react to specific signals—whether internal, such as redox gradients and pH, or external, such as magnetic fields, light, and temperature—to administer targeted treatment directly to the tumor microenvironment (TME).

Polymeric and inorganic nanoparticles, responsive to diverse stimuli, have demonstrated significant potential in preclinical cancer studies. The architecture of these nanomaterials facilitates meticulous regulation of drug release, triggered by TME-specific triggers. pH-responsive nanoparticles maintain stability in the bloodstream but disintegrate in the mildly acidic TME, facilitating localized release of therapeutic drugs. External stimuli-responsive therapies, like photothermal and magnetic hyperthermia (MHT), provide enhanced control by enabling on-demand activation of treatment. Light-based modalities, including PTT (photothermal therapy) and PDT, have shown efficacy in selectively targeting tumors by activating nanomaterials using near-infrared (NIR) wavelengths, resulting in localized cellular necrosis while preserving adjacent healthy tissues. Nonetheless, obstacles in light penetration restrict these therapies to accessible or superficial tumors, requiring additional advancements to expand their clinical use. The translation of these innovative platforms from preclinical research to clinical practice continues to present a significant obstacle [15–17]. Numerous stimuli-responsive nanomaterials have demonstrated substantial efficacy in preclinical models; however, their progression to clinical trials remains limited due to persistent concerns regarding biocompatibility, long-term stability, and potential systemic toxicity. In contrast, liposomal formulations have successfully transitioned into clinical use, yet the complex design of stimuli-responsive nanoparticles presents additional translational challenges. While multifunctional nanoparticles offer controlled and targeted delivery under experimental conditions, their behavior can be unpredictable within the dynamic and heterogeneous human physiological environment. Further investigations into their pharmacokinetics, chronic toxicity profiles, and biodistribution are critical to ensure safe and effective therapeutic outcomes in patients [18].

Additionally, a limited understanding of nanoparticle–TME interactions and their immunological consequences continues to hinder clinical translation. Recent studies have highlighted the role of surface modifications, such as polyzwitterionic coatings and ligand-based targeting strategies, in enhancing nanoparticle stability and tumor accumulation. For instance, transferrin-conjugated nanoparticles exploit the overexpression of transferrin receptors on cancer cells to improve targeting specificity and intracellular drug accumulation. In parallel, non-viral gene delivery systems are being developed to overcome key limitations in oncology, including endosomal entrapment and poor transfection efficiency. Notably, pH-responsive cationic polymers have shown promise in facilitating enhanced gene delivery by promoting endosomal escape, improving intracellular trafficking, and enabling robust therapeutic gene expression at the target site [19–21].

Despite the significant promise of stimuli-responsive therapeutics for non-invasive cancer treatment, there remain deficiencies in comprehending the in vivo dynamics of these materials. Photothermal and photodynamic therapies, for example, utilize targeted tumor ablation with minimal systemic damage; yet their effectiveness is sometimes constrained by issues such as light penetration and the necessity for accurate thermal regulation. Recent advancements in biodegradable nanomaterials and the integration of photodynamic treatment with immunotherapy are promising ways to improve therapeutic responses, particularly for highly resistant cancer types. The complex nature of the TME and interpatient heterogeneity present substantial challenges in attaining uniform results among varied patient populations [19–21]. Cancer theranostics has great promise for addressing the limitations of traditional medications and enabling more individualized, accurate, and minimally invasive cancer treatments. The continued research of stimuli-responsive nanoplatforms, particularly with improvements in targeting ligands, multifunctional coatings, and combination therapies, offers a promising avenue for achieving increased therapeutic specificity and patient safety despite the current constraints and difficulties. The shift from preclinical research to clinical use requires more study to improve these technologies for real-world use, guaranteeing that the therapeutic advantages seen in controlled conditions are effectively transferred to complex clinical settings [22, 23].

5.3 STIMULUS-RESPONSIVE BIOMATERIALS: VITAL FOR TARGETING CANCER

There are various forms of biomaterials used as stimuli responsive for cancer theranostics. Advanced hydrogel-based drug delivery systems (DDSs) have been developed, which can respond to multiple tumor-specific stimuli, including light, temperature, pH, and enzymatic activity, enabling precise and minimally invasive cancer treatment which can react to more than one stimulus at a time. The use of stimuli-responsive hydrogels facilitates the tailored delivery of therapeutic agents, providing targeted and efficient treatment strategies. FDA approved more than 30 types of hydrogels and in clinical practices. UGN-101 is a novel temperature-responsive polymer-based mitomycin C formulation that targets upper urothelial carcinomas. The hydrogel depot Vantas is composed of polymers (hydroxypropyl and hydroxyethyl methacrylate) that have been cross-linked using trimethylolpropane trimethacrylate. It offers treatment for advanced prostate cancer by releasing histrelin acetate into the upper arm over a 12-month period after subcutaneous application. Also, ELIGARD (Tolmar) is a gel-based product approved by FDA which delivers leuprolide acetate used in advanced prostate cancer treatments [24]. Figure 5.2 illustrates hydrogels used in enormous application, and it acts a stimuli-responsive biomaterial in cancer therapy.

A wide array of stimuli-responsive nanocarriers have been engineered based on the pathophysiological characteristics of the TME, playing a critical role in cancer imaging, diagnosis, and therapy [25]. These nanocarriers exploit biological cues—such as acidic pH,

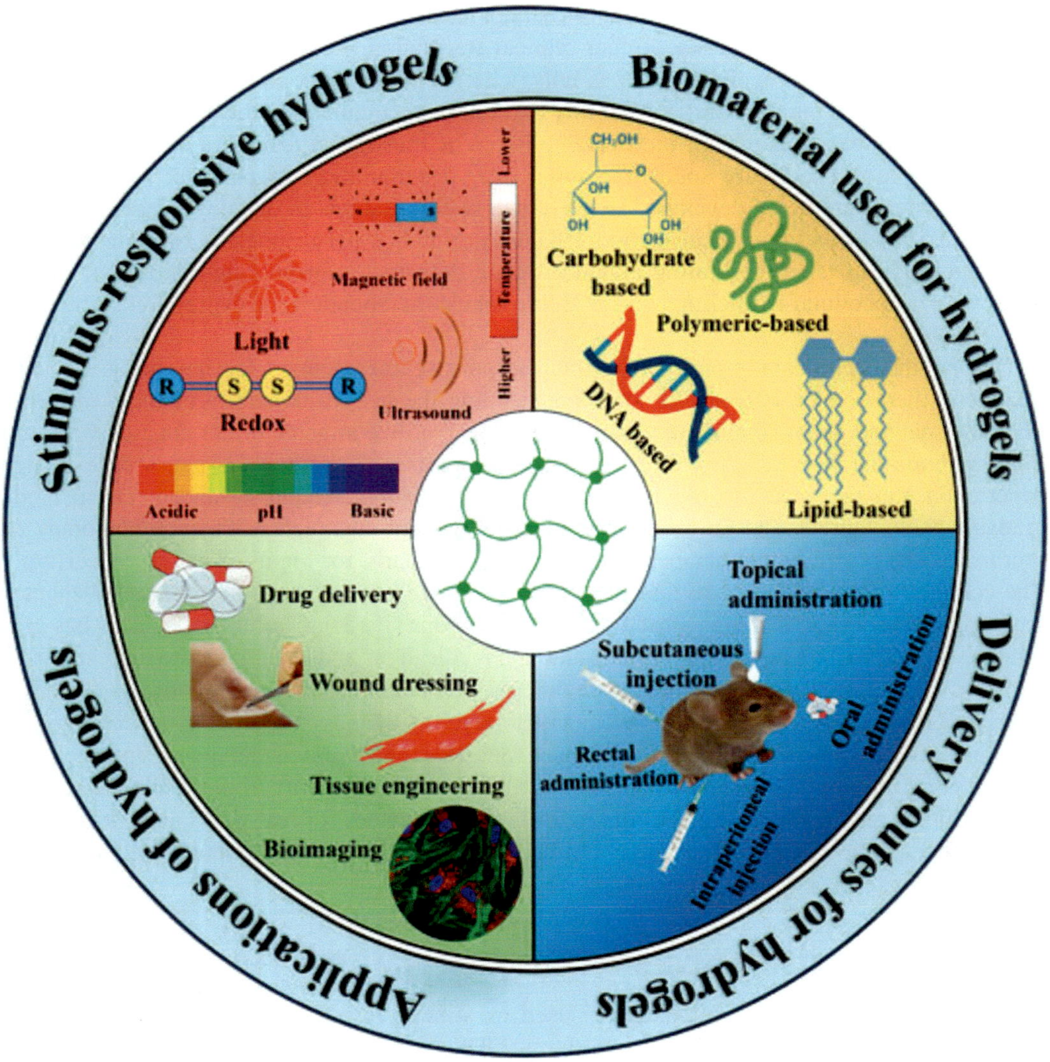

FIGURE 5.2 Hydrogel and its different field of uses. (Reprinted with permission from Ref. [24], under Creative Commons CC BY 4.0 license.)

overexpressed enzymes, and redox gradients—to achieve controlled drug release, enhance therapeutic efficacy, and minimize premature drug leakage during systemic circulation [26]. To address these challenges, Wan et al. developed a $CaCO_3$-based nanocarrier, coated with a nanoscale metal–organic framework (NMOF), enabling pH-responsive drug release within the acidic TME, while improving drug stability and preventing systemic leakage [25, 27]. Similarly, Yang et al. synthesized PNIPAM-based nanogels, which exhibited prolonged systemic circulation and demonstrated effective targeting and elimination of both cancer stem cells (CSCs) and bulk tumor cells, enhancing therapeutic selectivity and reducing recurrence [25, 28]. Fang et al. fabricated a multifunctional nanoplatform composed of hyaluronic acid–modified mesoporous silica nanoparticles (HA-MSNs), featuring a superparamagnetic Fe_3O_4 core and mesoporous SiO_2 shell. This design facilitated TME-responsive release of doxorubicin (DOX) under acidic pH conditions, thereby improving anticancer efficacy while minimizing off-target toxicity [25, 29]. Additionally, other stimuli-responsive nanocarriers, including graphene oxide (GO), MnO_2 nanoparticles, and Zr-based MOFs (Zr-MOFs), have been explored for TME-triggered drug delivery, owing to their tunable structure, high drug-loading capacity, and responsiveness to multiple tumor-associated stimuli [25]. The idea of enhancing drug delivery through conjugation to soluble macromolecules was later expanded to incorporate drug-loaded polymer nanoparticles. The conjugation of tumor particular ligands, including peptides, aptamers, and antibodies, to the surface of macromolecular and nanoparticle carriers is a strategic approach to enhance their tumor-targeting efficiency [10, 30]. Polymers such as poly(N-[2-hydroxypropyl]methacrylamide), polyethylene glycol (PEG), poly (L-glutamic acid), and styrene-maleic acid were utilized to transport anticancer treatments, including protein medications, DOX, camptothecin, and paclitaxel, to solid cancer [30]. There are still numerous biomaterials which will induce and respond to stimuli responsive which are being developed into clinical trials. Figure 5.3 shows about drug as a nanocarrier with single- or multi-responsive at tumor sites.

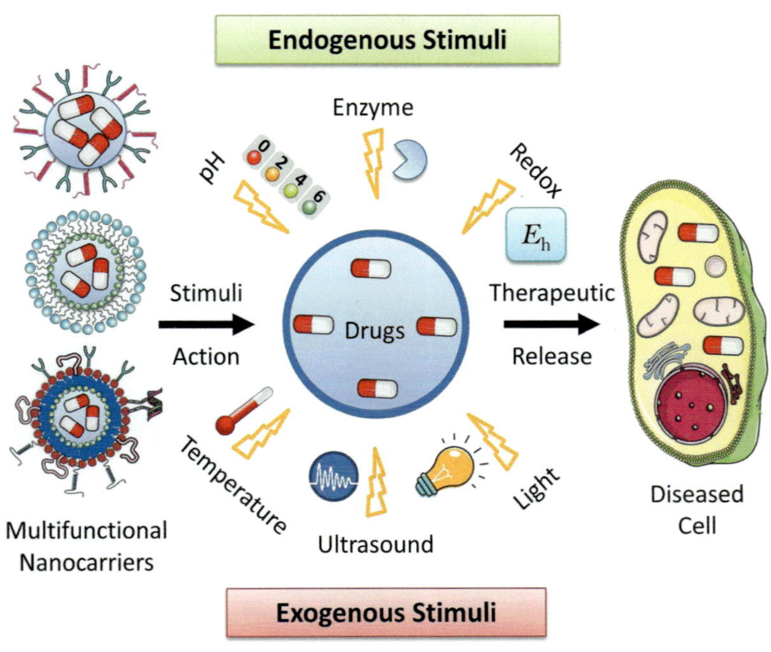

FIGURE 5.3 Representation of drug-nanocarrier response by different stimuli (Reprinted with permission from Ref. [31], under Creative Commons CC BY 4.0 license.)

5.4 SYNTHESIS, DESIGN, AND MECHANISM OF STIMULI-RESPONSE BIOMATERIALS

The development of stimuli-responsive bionanomaterials has been a major research focus over the past 20 years which are designed to exhibit molecular-level responses to specific triggers either internally or externally [32]. Certain stimuli, including changes in pH, temperature, and various external stimuli, including chemical agents, ionic strength, electrical and magnetic fields, and UV/visible light exposure, can influence the behavior of systems and cause these materials to react [32]. Internally responsive systems can be designed to respond to endogenous biological signals within the body [10], including enzymes, hypoxia, nucleic acids, ATP, glucose, pH fluctuations, and redox signals using synthetic bio-inspired elements or natural components, which is feasible across multiple length scales, from nanometers to macroscopic dimensions [33]. Physical stimulation (exogenous or external stimuli) methods used in biomedical engineering include electrical, laser, ultrasonic, and magnetic stimulation. These methods are utilized selectively according to their applicability for different purposes [14]. Figure 5.4 displays several stimuli responses for drug release at tumor areas.

5.4.1 pH-Responsive Stimuli

Because pH changes between various subcellular sites and can differ between healthy and diseased tissues, it has been used to develop stimulus-responsive systems. Cancer tissues exhibit a more acidic environment compared to normal tissues, primarily due to the increased glycolytic activity of cancer cells, which occurs under partially anaerobic conditions. Compared to healthy tissues (pH 7.4), tumors exhibit a distinct acidic environment, with pH levels ranging from 5.7 to 7.8. Furthermore, organelles with varying pH ranges include lysosomes and endosomes, which have pH values between 4.5 and 5.5. In order to release cargo in infected tissues while maintaining stability in normal tissues, numerous stimulus-responsive treatment methods have been developed having structural alterations that react to variations in pH [35].

5.4.2 Hypoxia Stimuli Responsive and Enzyme Stimuli Responsive

Compared to normal cells, cancer cells exhibit heightened oxygen requirements due to their accelerated growth and metabolism. However, tumors' irregular blood supply results in hypoxic conditions. The unique hypoxic conditions found in tumors can be exploited to design intelligent nanocarriers that selectively activate immunotherapy in response to low oxygen levels [11]. A variety of nanomaterials, including phosphodiesters, polymers, and inorganic compounds, have been utilized in the invention of enzyme-responsive DDSs, providing advantages, including improved

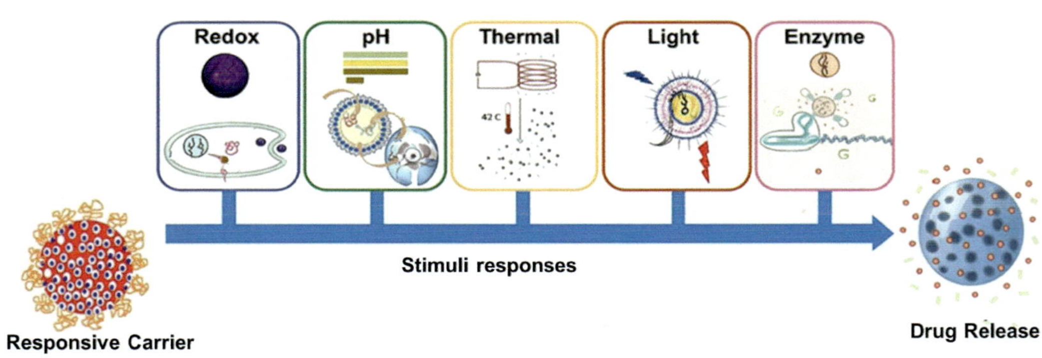

FIGURE 5.4 Various stimuli-responsive nanocarriers for drug release. (Reprinted with permission from Ref. [34], under Creative Commons CC BY 4.0 license.)

selectivity, biorecognition, sensitivity, efficiency, and catalytic efficacy. Proteases (peptidases) and phospholipases are the most employed triggering enzymes in the fabrication of enzyme-responsive DDSs [13, 36].

5.4.3 Redox Stimuli Responsive

Redox conditions can be exploited for stimulus-responsive systems, particularly (glutathione) GSH-sensitive platforms, which have garnered significant interest. These systems remain stable in healthy tissues but release payloads in diseased tissues upon detecting elevated GSH levels. ROS-responsive systems offer a targeted approach to drug release, leveraging the elevated ROS levels in inflammatory sites and diseased tissues. Notably, ROS concentrations in inflamed tissues are 10–100 times higher than in healthy tissues. ROS-responsive systems typically employ two chemical mechanisms: ROS-triggered hydrophobic-to-hydrophilic transitions and ROS-mediated structural breakdown [35].

5.4.4 Electrical-Responsive Biomaterials

Electrical-responsive biomaterials enable precise control over their biochemical and biophysical reactions through external electrical cues, altering properties like mechanical properties, redox state, hydrophobic–hydrophilic balance, and surface ligand configuration. The fabrication of electrical-responsive biomaterials typically involves the integration of electroactive components, encompassing organic polymers (polypyrrole, poly(3,4-ethylenedioxythiophene), poly(aniline)), inorganic nanomaterials (reduced GO, GO, carbon nanotubes), and novel two-dimensional materials (MXene, black phosphorus), prepared through various synthesis methods like hydrothermal synthesis, high-temperature sintering, and oxidation-reduction reactions [14].

5.4.5 Ultrasonic Responsive Biomaterials

Ultrasonic-mediated biological reactions are triggered by physical processes that occur when ultrasonic waves penetrate human tissues and interact with biological components. A number of variables affect a biomaterial's ultrasonic response characteristics, such as its shape and composition, but most significantly, its capacity to transform sound energy into forms that are more practical for applications like mechanically starting biological processes or triggering drug release. It is primarily separated into liposomes, inorganic nanoparticles, microbubbles, and nanobubbles, among others [14]. Advanced nanocarriers, including nanobubbles, calcium carbonate nanoparticles, liposomes, nanodroplets, vesicles, and nanoparticles, have been tailored for ultrasound-mediated applications and have been developed, enabling the integration of diagnostic imaging, controlled drug delivery, and cancer treatment [37].

5.4.6 Magnetic Responsive Biomaterials

Because magnetic nanoparticles (MNPs) have an inherent affinity for magnetic fields, they can be used to target tumors using magnetic-responsive nanocarriers. Additionally, these nanomaterials possess the capability to generate localized hyperthermia upon exposure to an alternating magnetic field, which can initiate medication release and tumor ablation [37]. A diverse range of magnetic nanocarriers has been engineered, including MNPs, albumin nanocapsules, polymeric micelles, magnetic nanogels, liposomes, magnetic nanocarriers, and superparamagnetic iron oxide nanoparticles (SPIONs) [38]. Magnetic sensitivity in nanocarriers is often achieved through the incorporation of magnetic materials (e.g., Fe_3O_4), other MNPs (e.g., $ZnFe_2O_4$), and also by hybrid nanomaterials (e.g., graphene/Au/Fe_3O_4), enabling both targeted therapy and magnetic resonance imaging (MRI)-based tumor imaging [37]. In addition to magnetic materials, magnetic-sensitive nanocarriers can also encapsulate various therapeutic agents, including antibodies, anticancer drugs, plasmids, contrast agents, and photosensitizers, to achieve multifunctionality and enhance multimodal therapeutic efficacy [37].

5.4.7 Light-Responsive Biomaterials

The design of light-responsive nanocarriers has emerged as a promising area of research, leveraging the versatility of light as a stimulus to enable tailored control over wavelength, intensity, and spatial distribution [39]. DDSs by light-sensitive materials exhibit wavelength-dependent responses, allowing for adjustable drug release profiles tailored to specific irradiation protocols. Light-sensitive nanocarriers, engineered for application in cancer cells and tumors, can be remotely activated using UV–Vis and NIR light irradiation, enabling precise control over targeted tumor therapy and minimizing collateral damage to normal organs. Numerous light-responsive nanocarriers have been

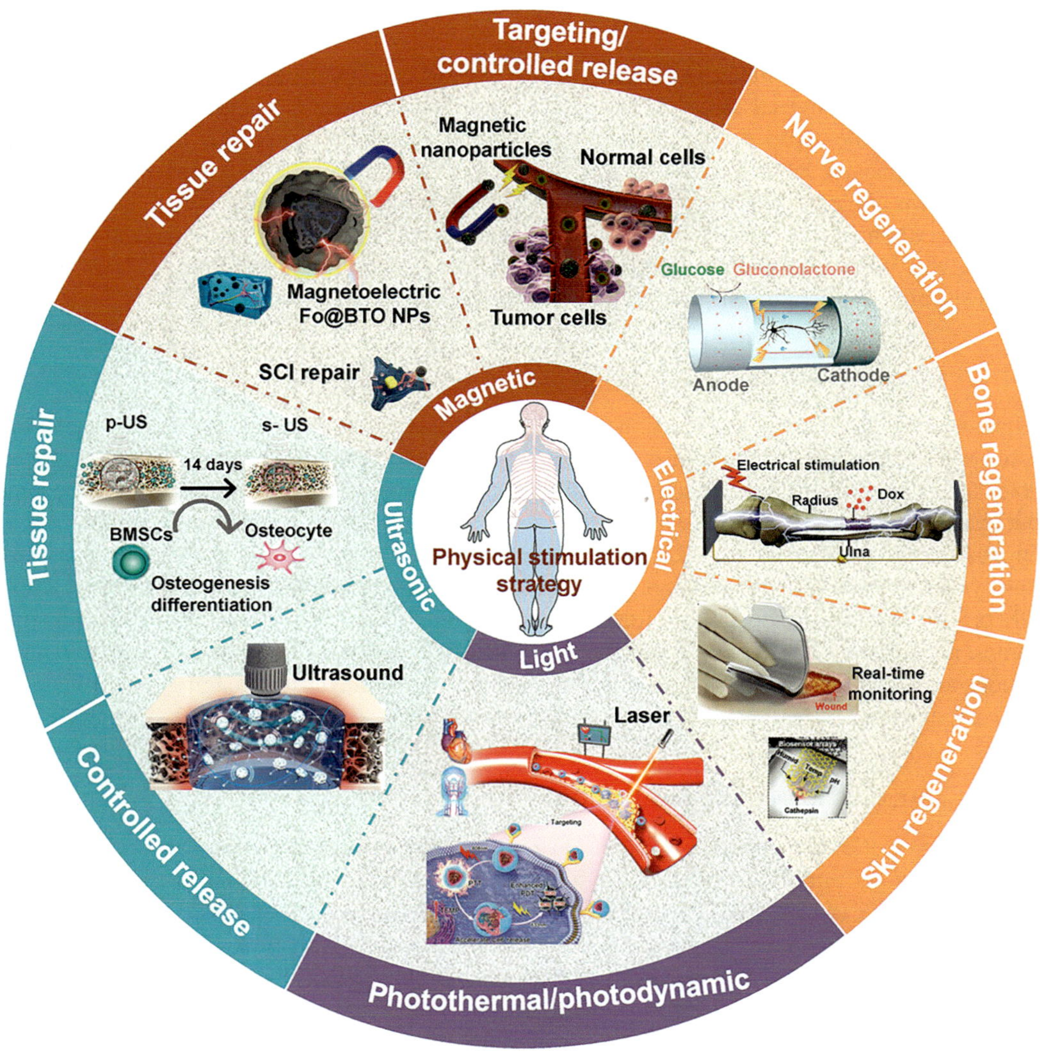

FIGURE 5.5 Several stimuli-responsive strategies with their application. (Reprinted with permission from Ref. [14], under Creative Commons CC BY 4.0 license.)

used, such as polyion complex vesicles (PICsomes), liposomes, polymersomes, polyplexes, polymeric micelles, nanoparticles, upconverting nanoparticles (UCNPs), nanorods, and nanogels. In the meantime, light-responsive materials and cargos could be used to create light-sensitive nanocarriers, such as photosensitizers [37, 39].

5.4.8 Temperature-Responsive Biomaterials

Thermo-responsive systems represent a prominent class of exogenous stimuli-responsive platforms, exhibiting considerable potential for diverse therapeutic and diagnostic applications. Nanocarriers are engineered to respond when changes in temperature occur, which deliver drugs selectively to diseased/tumor tissues, where temperatures are elevated (40–42°C), by releasing their payload upon polymer chain dehydration above the critical solution temperature. Accordingly, thermo-responsive carriers demonstrate temperature-dependent drug release, retaining the payload at normal temperatures while releasing it in the elevated temperature environment of diseased or tumor tissues [36]. As the most common thermo-responsive polymer, PNIPAM undergoes a phase transition between ambient and physiological temperatures, primarily due to entropic effects that increase with temperature. The formation of intermolecular hydrogen bonds is significant in PNIPAM systems at temperatures below the LCST (lower critical solution temperature), causing the molecular chains to stretch and turn hydrophilic; above the LCST of PNIPAM, intramolecular hydrogen bonds dominate, leading to chain collapse and hydrophobicity [37, 39]. Figure 5.5 shows physical stimulation for different biomedical applications.

5.5 THERAPEUTIC EFFECTS ON DIFFERENT CANCER TYPES

5.5.1 Breast Cancer

Breast cancer is the most frequently diagnosed and the second highest mortality rate [40], but enhanced detection and diagnostic techniques have significantly boosted survival rates [41]. To address the drawbacks of traditional surgery and chemotherapy, such as low drug efficacy, harm to healthy tissues, and an increase in side effects, new breast cancer treatments are desperately needed. In this context, the injectable hydrogel-based DDSs attracted a lot of interest [42] lately due to the promising options for regulated, localized [10], and targeted drug release to the tumor site. Injectable hydrogel offer abundant advantages over traditional systemic chemotherapy, including localized drug administration, controlled and sustained release, and improved therapeutic efficacy. All of these advancements help to lessen the adverse effects of long-term chemotherapy administered using traditional methods [43]. Oshiro-Júnior JA et al. studied the delivery of stimulus-responsive drugs in order to treat breast cancer; nanocarriers are made of materials that exhibit a dramatic shift in responses to extrinsic stimuli (for example, magnetic fields, ultrasound, light, and electric current) and intrinsic stimuli (namely enzyme, pH, and redox). DDNs have a lot of promise as novel breast cancer therapeutic options because they can enhance the pharmacological qualities of a range of medications, improving their selectivity with tumor tissue and controlling release in response to various stimuli, thereby reducing systemic harmful effects, along with some drug delivery material having theranostic effects [44]. Milad Akhlaghi et al. extracted bioactive compounds from herbs using the Soxhlet apparatus and subsequently synthesized various niosome formulations through thin film synthesis, incorporating the extracted compounds. The synthesized niosomes exhibited temperature and pH responsiveness. Analyzing cytotoxicity experiments, we discovered that nanosystems can correctly distinguish between carcinogenic and healthy cells in order to perform their harmful effects on tumor cells and avoid undesirable side effects, as well as successfully enter cells. Molecular analysis revealed that plant extracts' bioactive compounds exhibit anti-tumor properties by targeting intricate cellular pathways, including intracellular signaling and cell cycle regulation. This study shows that

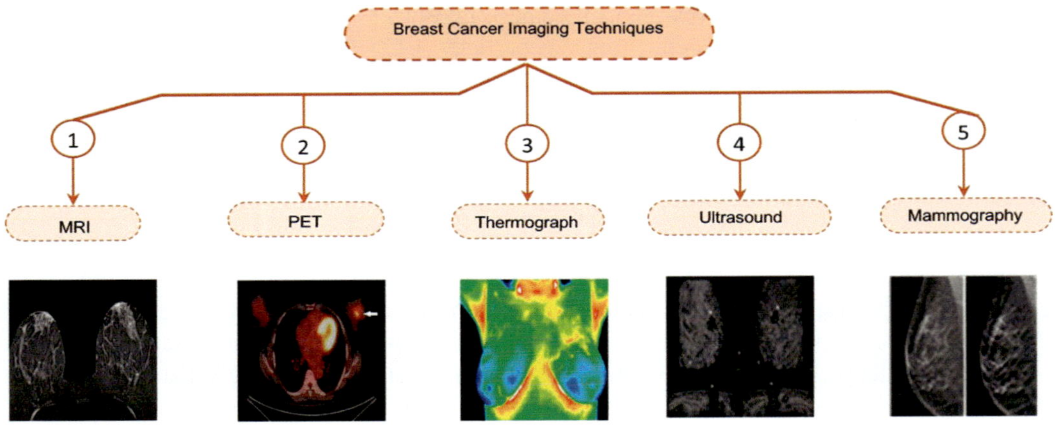

FIGURE 5.6 Various imaging techniques of breast cancer. (Reprinted with permission from Ref. [46], under Creative Commons CC BY 4.0 license.)

encapsulation boosts the anti-tumor and antibacterial properties of plant extracts [45]. Various breast cancer bioimaging techniques are shown in Figure 5.6.

5.5.2 Gastrointestinal and Liver Cancer

Gastrointestinal cancers pose a critical challenge to global health, marked by frequent occurrence, high death rates, and considerable economic and emotional burden on patients, families, and healthcare systems [47]. The majority of these tumors are detected at late stages, making treatment challenging and resulting in unfavorable outcomes [48]. Jiante Li et al. developed a novel microfluidic 3D-printed scaffold fabricated from fish gelatin and methacrylate (F-GelMA) for the targeted delivery of berberine (BBR) in postoperative gastric cancer therapy. The F-GelMA@BBR scaffold exhibited substantial in vitro cytotoxic effects against MKN-45 gastric cancer cells and remarkable in vivo anti-recurrence efficacy. The results of in vitro studies demonstrate that F-GelMA@BBR possesses potent cytotoxic activity against gastric cancer cells, while preserving the viability of non-neoplastic cells. Furthermore, in vivo studies revealed a remarkable reduction in tumor volume, with F-GelMA@BBR-treated groups exhibiting a 49.7% decrease relative to control groups. The scaffold's ordered porous structure and biocompatibility support normal cell growth, promoting tissue repair at tumor removal sites. Its potential makes it an ideal candidate for postoperative tumor treatment [49]. The stimuli-responsive hydrogel varieties, such as pH- and temperature-sensitive hydrogels, as well as their self-healing properties, have enhanced site-specific drug delivery for more targeted cancer therapy [48]. The significance of hydrogels in the clinic is further highlighted by their potential for diagnostics, circulating tumor cell isolation, and biomarker identification in gastrointestinal malignancies. As a result, hydrogels are used to diagnose and treat gastrointestinal cancers [48].

Liver cancer is a leading cancer type, with approximately 1 million incidents reported worldwide each year, placing it among the top five in global incidence [50]. One of the medications most frequently used to treat liver cancer is DOX. However, the conventional chemotherapy that uses DOX has a number of drawbacks, including a systematic release of DOX that affects both healthy and malignant tissue, resulting in the development of several side effects, poor water solubility, and multidrug resistance (MDR). Additionally, a lot of research has been done on how responsive DDSs are to various internal and external factors that affect the effectiveness of therapeutic medications. Elena Ruxandra Radu et al. synthesized and controlled DOX which is responsive to external/internal stimuli for treating liver cancer. Due to the need for several preclinical assessments of their toxicity and biocompatibility, research on stimuli-responsive DDSs for DOX is still in its early stages [51]. Based on angelica polysaccharide, Xue Liu et al. synthesized hypoxia-responsive nano-DDS for liver cancer therapy. At the liver cancer site, the drug's azobenzene (AZO) moiety responds to the hypoxic microenvironment by breaking down, resulting in enhanced drug release and accumulation at the tumor [52]. Being a hypoxia-responsive group [52], AZO breaks the main chain of the polymer through reductive cleavage in hypoxic environments, which will speed up the release of medications. Significant tumor growth inhibition was observed, highlighting the potent therapeutic effect of the hypoxia-targeted DDS [52]. Additionally, ferroptosis, a novel form of programmable death of cells, is crucial in the therapy of liver cancer and is anticipated to result in effective tumor administration [52].

5.5.3 Glioblastoma

Glioblastoma multiforme (GBM) is extremely aggressive, has a dismal prognosis, and has few available treatments. Stimuli-responsive nanocarriers for drug delivery hold tremendous promises to enhance GBM treatment approaches [53]. Carlotta Pucci et al. approached organic piezoelectric nanoparticles with drug-loaded ones which respond to ultrasound. When chemotherapy and long-term piezoelectric stimulation were combined, cell death and anti-proliferation mechanisms were activated. This anticancer nanoplatform is made up of ApoE-functionalized P(VDF-TrFE) nanoparticles loaded with nutlin-3a. These nanoparticles can be remotely activated via mechanical stimulations based on ultrasound to cause drug release while transmitting anticancer electric cues locally. Chronic piezoelectric stimulation combined with chemotherapeutic treatment activated anti-proliferation and cell apoptosis pathways, induced cell necrosis, decreased cell invasiveness, and suppressed malignant migration in drug-resistant GBM cells. Multifunctional nanomaterials (MFNs) can help overcome drug resistance in GBM with targeted, less invasive treatments [54]. Christos Tapeinos et al. created a biomimetic magnetic nano-vector based on lipids that has a prolonged release profile and a good capacity to load for the anticancer medication temozolomide. Under alternating magnetic field exposure, these nanostructures exhibited enhanced drug release, with complete release achieved through synergistic effects of low pH (4.5), 50 μm hydrogen peroxide, and magnetically induced hyperthermia. Notably, their SAR values (up to 1345 W g^{-1}) demonstrate suitability for hyperthermia applications. As the nano-vectors were triggered via alternating magnetic fields (20 mT, 750 kHz), [38] showed that these vectors exhibit slight hyperthermia (43°C) and have potent anti-tumor effects on cells (U-87 MG), which are cells with poor growth rates and high apoptosis levels. GBM may be treated using the suggested drug-loaded lipid magnetic nano-vectors, as evidenced by the synergistic combination of regulated temozolomide release and persistent hyperthermia stimulation that produced the best anticancer results [55].

5.5.4 Gynecological and Prostate Cancer

Gynecologic cancers pose a significant threat to women's health and overall quality of life. In addition to the disease burden, conventional treatment modalities—such as surgery, chemotherapy, and radiation—often carry a high risk of fertility impairment, further impacting long-term well-being. Consequently, there is an urgent need for the development of novel therapeutic strategies that are both effective and fertility-preserving for women affected by these conditions [56]. Combination treatments that combine chemotherapy and phototherapies, known as "chemophototherapy", may be more effective against cancer because they target cancer cells through a variety of mechanisms, such as thermally induced damage to the cytoskeleton and cell membrane and DNA damage. The PLGA (poly(lactic-co-glycolic)) nanoparticles were conceived and produced by Dante R. Sánchez-Ramírez et al. and contained the NIR photosensitizer indocyanine green (ICG) and chemotherapy medication carboplatin (CP). The NPs' photothermal capabilities, photodynamic ROS production, and drug release profile have all been assessed. Additionally, the SKOV-3 cells were used to test the anti-tumor effects of the nanoparticles in the in vitro model of ovarian cancer. When cells were irradiated to an 800 nm laser, an increased cytotoxic effect was seen. The evidence presented here supports the possible use of biodegradable photoresponsive nanoparticles for clinical translation, owing to their biocompatible nature, precise spatiotemporal control, and reduced likelihood of resistance development against combination regimens [57]. A DDS utilizing celastrol was created by designing, synthesizing, and assembling a tumor-targeted, ROS-sensitive nanoparticle by Weina Niu et al. The tumor cell membrane surface is the active target of nanoparticles guided by folic acid (FA) groups on their surface. Thioketal (TK) bonds in nanoparticles undergo oxidative cleavage in response to tumor-specific ROS levels, disrupting the PEG shell and facilitating celastrol release. The liberated celastrol then enhances ROS production, augmenting intracellular levels and promoting apoptosis in ovarian cancer cells [58].

Using the response of androgen PC-82 human prostate cancer xenograft as a model system, Natasha Kyprianou conducted research on the mechanisms underlying the regression of human prostatic cancer following androgen deprivation therapy. Two weeks after androgen ablation, male nude mice with PC-82 xenografts that have been castrated show a 50% tumor reduction. This retreat is caused by a series of biochemical and morphological processes that cause the androgen-dependent prostate cancer cell to stop proliferating and initiate programmed death, or apoptosis. These findings imply that, similar to healthy prostatic cells, androgen-dependent human prostate cancer cells maintain the capacity to suppress proliferation and trigger planned androgen ablation-induced cell death. Even for androgen-independent human prostatic cancer, elucidating the biochemical route that triggers this programmed death of cells should reveal new therapeutic options [59].

5.5.5 Skin Cancer

Still, there are many types of dreadful cancers occurring in the human body parts. Skin cancer has become the fifth most common type of cancer worldwide, impacting both the economic and global health [60]. The two most common localized types of skin cancer that respond well to treatment are basal cell and squamous cell carcinoma. Nevertheless, melanoma, an uncommon form of skin tumor with a high death rate, has the ability to spread and infiltrate other bodily areas. Silica-based nanomaterials offer a flexible, biocompatible, and efficient DDS with high loading capacity and targeting capabilities. Recent progress in melanoma therapy utilizing silica-based nanomaterials and hybrids is reviewed, emphasizing their adaptability and promise as DDSs for diverse molecules, including drugs, immune therapeutics, peptides, and radio-/photo-active agents [61]. Luna Gade et al. explore stimuli-responsive DDSs that focus on diseased skin, leveraging internal triggers like pH changes, reactive oxygen species (ROS), or enzyme upregulation. It emphasizes matching the delivery mechanism to the skin condition's unique pathological features [62].

5.5.6 Lung Cancer

The lung cancer (LC) is characterized by unchecked cell growth in the lung tissues, which, if ignored, may spread to other parts of body. Among the drawbacks of traditional nanocarriers are medication leakage and stability problems. Techniques like coating the NPs and using stimuli-responsive nanocarriers have been applied to get around these issues. These methods also help achieve organ-restricted delivery of drugs and enhance pre-existing features. DDSs that respond to stimuli are ones in which the medication is given or released through a stimulation. These smart nanocarriers have been used to target cancer because malignant tissues have higher enzyme levels and a distinctive pH. Additionally, several nanocarriers that contain different compounds have been developed and tested to prevent LC [63].

5.6 BIOMEDICAL IMAGING TECHNIQUES AND DIAGNOSTIC METHODS

The integration of biomedical imaging into cancer care provides unparalleled benefits, including real-time surveillance, non-destructive tissue analysis, non-invasive diagnostics, and versatility across diverse biological and pathological conditions [64]. Biomedical imaging has witnessed remarkable technological advancements, yielding innovative applications in various fields, spanning basic research to clinical practice, from cellular to organ-level investigations, through innovative techniques, including optical imaging, spectroscopy, functional imaging, as well as image-guided theranostics [65]. Advances in diagnostic imaging and targeted therapies have revolutionized radiation oncology, moving toward precision medicine, replacing traditional population-based approaches with personalized medicine. Clinicians must now navigate complex medical data to pinpoint critical parameters, enabling tailored treatment strategies that maximize cure rates [66]. Figure 5.7 represents variety of diagnosis, imaging, and treatment techniques in cancer environment of different body parts.

A variety of photophysical processes, including light absorption, scattering, and emission, are brought about by the interaction of light with biological tissues during optical imaging. These events provide essential information about cellular and tissue morphology as well as biochemistry properties. The numerous imaging and therapeutic platforms available underscore the strengths of optical technology. Absorption imaging, in particular, utilizes the varying concentrations of exogenous or endogenous chromophores in tissues to create contrast between abnormal and normal tissue which usually absorb light at the start of optical imaging [68]. The integration of imaging and physical stimuli-based therapies offers a unique opportunity for tracking and real-time monitoring, ensuring optimal dosing of external stimuli such as optical energy or X-ray radiation [69]. Thus, the idea of "theranostic" monitoring during therapy may help and enhance therapeutic approaches initiated by physical stimuli, in contrast to chemotherapy, where real-time observing of therapeutic drugs may have little clinical utility [69].

There are two distinct kinds of light-triggered treatments: PDT and PTT [69, 70]. Under light irradiation, PTT typically uses NIR absorption compounds to kill cancer cells by efficiently converting light into heat energy, which raises the tumors' local heat and causes the cancer cells to

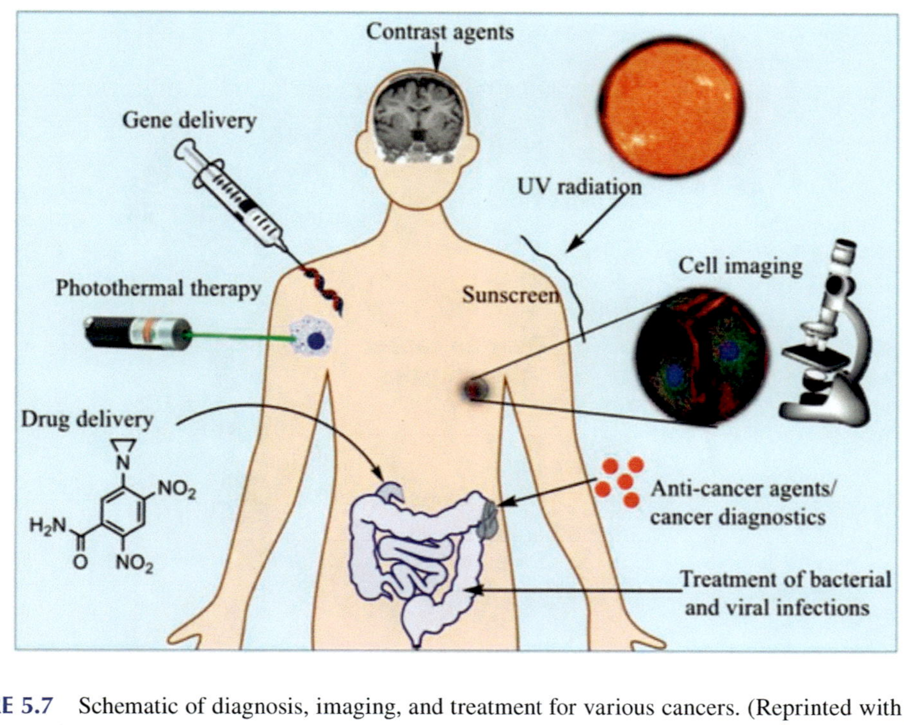

FIGURE 5.7 Schematic of diagnosis, imaging, and treatment for various cancers. (Reprinted with permission from Ref. [67], under Creative Commons CC BY 4.0 license.)

"burn". PDT, on the other hand, relies on photosensitizers that are able to convert the absorbed optical energy (light) to neighboring oxygen molecules, producing ROS or cytotoxic singlet oxygen ($^1O_2$) that harm key proteins in the vicinity and ultimately kill cancer cells [69]. An extensive range of nanoscale theranostic agents has been exploited for application in both PDT and PTT [71–73]. Along with PTT and PDT some other light-triggered responses are also widely used and incorporated in treating cancer [69]. Light-triggered drug delivery is a technique that employs photocleavable bonds to release therapeutic payloads in response to light [74].

Because of their special inherent qualities, MNPs have drawn a lot of interest for their magnetically responsive improved uses in the biomedical area, the most well-known of which is MRI. Thus, MRI is a vital medical diagnostic technology that provides soft tissue contrast and non-invasive, accurate real-time spatial resolution without the use of radiotracers or potentially hazardous ionizing radiation. When a large external MF is applied, the magnetic moment that determines the alignments of protons inside a sample causes MRI to function. When SPIONs are used in MRI, spin dephasing and a reduction in proton relaxation time result from their magnetic moment interacting with that of surrounding protons [76]. MHT has been shown to be an effective alternative or value-added treatment. MHT employs MNPs that can be put directly to the tumor, where they will encourage a controlled localized temperature increase when an external AC magnetic field is applied [77]. Ultrasound imaging is a widely employed diagnostic tool in oncology, offering comprehensive information on cancer pathology. The integration of 3D ultrasound imaging enhances diagnostic precision, allowing for detailed characterization of tumor dimensions, morphology, and spatial relationships. The addition of Doppler ultrasound and elastography enables a more comprehensive understanding of tumor pathology, including vascular patterns and tissue mechanical properties [78]. Positron emission tomography (PET) is a nuclear imaging technique that generates real-time, three-dimensional images of biological processes and functions [76]. The positron-emitting radioisotopes used in PET cancer imaging, 18F, 11C, 64Cu, 124I, 86Y, 15O, and 13N, are all produced from a cyclotron or in a generator (68Ga) [64]. To identify these photon pairs as they strike opposing detectors almost simultaneously, PET scanners are outfitted with coincidence electronics. The accompanying CT scans can be utilized for both attenuation

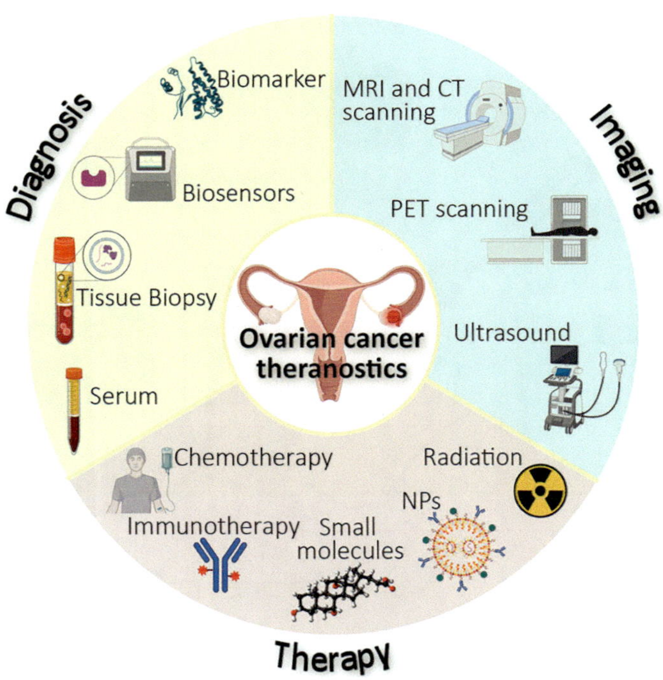

FIGURE 5.8 Outline of ovarian cancer theranostics (Reprinted with permission from Ref. [75], under Creative Commons CC BY 4.0 license.)

correction and anatomic localization, which is one benefit of hybrid PET/CT systems (23). Figure 5.8 represents imaging, diagnosis, and therapy for ovarian cancer.

5.7 MULTI-STIMULI RESPONSIVE PLATFORMS FOR CANCER MANAGEMENT

The development of multi-stimuli responsive platforms for cancer management marks a pivotal advancement in nanomedicine and targeted DDSs. These sophisticated platforms leverage various [10] endogenous (internal) and exogenous (external) stimuli to precisely control the release of therapeutic agents at specific sites within the body, particularly at diseased sites [10]. This selective approach is particularly advantageous in cancer treatment, where targeting cancer cells without affecting healthy tissue is a primary goal. By utilizing stimuli-responsive systems, researchers and clinicians can deliver drugs directly to tumor tissues, thus minimizing side effects and improving treatment efficacy. This strategy represents a departure from conventional therapies, which often rely on non-specific drug delivery and are associated with significant systemic toxicity [79–82].

Endogenous stimuli, or internal triggers, are intrinsic to the tumors' microenvironment. Tumor cells exhibit several unique characteristics compared to healthy cells, such as altered pH, higher concentrations of reducing agents like glutathione (GSH), and distinct enzymatic activity. The acidic extracellular pH of tumor tissues, a byproduct of enhanced glycolysis and lactate production in cancer cells, can be exploited in pH-responsive delivery systems [10]. These systems can be engineered to release drugs selectively in acidic environments, allowing for enhanced targeting of tumor cells. Likewise, the elevated levels of GSH in cancer cells provide an additional trigger for GSH-sensitive delivery systems. Such platforms remain inactive in normal tissues but release their payloads upon encountering the higher GSH levels found in cancer cells. Enzyme-sensitive systems also hold promise, as they can respond to the overexpression of specific enzymes, such as matrix metalloproteinases (MMPs), commonly associated with tumor progression and metastasis [83–85].

Exogenous stimuli, or external triggers, offer another layer of control and precision for these platforms. External stimuli such as light, magnetic fields, and ultrasound can activate drug release at precise locations and times, enabling real-time control over treatment [86]. For instance, light-responsive systems, particularly those responsive to NIR light, allow for the non-invasive activation of drug release, even in deeper tissues. When exposed to NIR light, these systems can produce heat or ROS, facilitating controlled drug release and photothermal or photodynamic effects [87]. Magnetic fields provide another means of external control, as MNPs can be guided and localized to tumor sites, where the magnetic field can induce hyperthermia or initiate drug release. Ultrasound, with its capacity to penetrate deep tissues, offers yet another modality, causing temporary disruptions in drug carrier structures and facilitating drug release directly at the tumor site. The precision offered by these external triggers holds great potential for personalized cancer therapy, as clinicians can adjust the intensity and duration of the stimuli to modulate drug release in real time [88].

Advancements in nanomaterials and specific chemical structures are key to the functionality of these multi-stimuli responsive platforms. Researchers have developed a range of responsive materials and chemical bonds, such as disulfide bonds, hydrazone linkages, and pH-sensitive polymers, that change or degrade in response to specific stimuli. Disulfide bonds, for example, are sensitive to reducing environments like those found within cancer cells, where high GSH levels break down the bonds, releasing the drug payload. Similarly, hydrazone linkages are pH-sensitive and can be designed to break down in the acidic TME. pH-sensitive polymers and enzyme-degradable materials further allow for controlled release, as they can swell, contract, or degrade in response to the unique biochemical conditions of tumors. These molecular and structural innovations offer high specificity and control, enabling the design of platforms that respond to multiple stimuli simultaneously, thus enhancing the precision and efficacy of cancer treatments [89, 90].

Among the recent developments, supramolecular chemistry has provided promising options for multi-stimuli responsive systems, particularly using macrocyclic compounds like pillararenes. Pillararenes can form stable host–guest complexes with drugs, allowing for stimuli-responsive release under various conditions. These molecules are highly tunable, biocompatible, and possess excellent structural stability, making them well-suited for multi-stimuli responsive applications. For instance, supramolecular nano self-assemblies using pillararenes can change to both external and internal triggers, such as light and pH [10], to deliver drugs specifically to tumor cells while avoiding healthy tissues. This versatility has led to increased interest in supramolecular systems as part of multi-stimuli responsive platforms in cancer management [91–93].

Several multi-stimuli responsive platforms have shown guaranteed results in laboratory and clinical trials, underscoring their potential for clinical translation. These platforms have been tested across various cancer varieties, such as colon, breast, and liver cancers, demonstrating improved targeting, reduced off-target effects, and enhanced therapeutic ability. Notably, the integration of imaging capabilities into these systems has advanced the field of cancer theranostics, where therapy and diagnostics are combined. Through real-time tracking of pharmacokinetics and tumor dynamics, these platforms enable clinicians to optimize treatment plans dynamically, improving therapeutic outcomes and patient care [94].

Despite their promise, multi-stimuli responsive platforms still face challenges in clinical translation, particularly related to their complexity and the need for [10] precise control over drug release timing and location. Issues such as scalability, stability, and potential immunogenicity require further investigation before these platforms can be broadly adopted in clinical practice. However, ongoing research in materials science, nanotechnology, and biomedical engineering continues to address these challenges, and with further refinement, multi-stimuli responsive platforms hold the potential to transform cancer management. Overall, multi-stimuli responsive platforms for cancer management represent a sophisticated approach that capitalizes on the unique TME and the power of external triggers to deliver therapeutic agents with unprecedented precision. By integrating a combination of stimuli-responsive strategies, these platforms offer a new level of specificity and control [10], paving the mode for safer, more efficient, and personalized cancer treatments. The ongoing development of these platforms is expected to significantly impact the field of nanomedicine, ultimately leading to improved cancer patient outcomes worldwide [95–97].

5.8 CLINICAL TRANSLATIONS AND PATENTS

Clinical applications of smart biomaterials for cancer theranostics represent a critical bridge between advanced research and real-world oncology applications. Stimuli-responsive biomaterials, which react to specific triggers like pH shifts, enzymes, temperature changes, or external stimuli (e.g., magnetic fields, light), are designed to exploit the distinctive sites of the TME. For instance, acidic pH-responsive nanoparticles remain stable in physiological pH but degrade in the acidic tumor environment, releasing therapeutic agents precisely where needed. These biomaterials enhance the specificity of cancer treatment, potentially minimizing systemic toxicity and improving therapeutic efficacy. However, translating these technologies to clinical practice involves overcoming several hurdles [22, 98]. Regulatory agencies like the FDA require extensive preclinical data demonstrating that the biomaterials are safe, biocompatible, and effective under clinically relevant conditions. This process involves assessing the pharmacokinetics, biodistribution, and immunogenicity of the stimuli-responsive agents to confirm they meet rigorous safety standards. Temperature-sensitive hydrogels and pH-responsive polymers, for example, exhibited promising efficacy in preclinical models, but further analyses are necessary to ensure they can perform consistently and safely across a broader patient population [99].

Clinical trials further validated Doxil's efficacy in treating many cancers, including ovarian cancer, breast cancer, and Kaposi's sarcoma. AmBisome is a notable advancement, comprising a liposomal version of amphotericin B. AmBisome, principally utilized for fungal infections, has a stimuli-responsive mechanism that diminishes nephrotoxicity relative to conventional formulations, highlighting the adaptability of liposomal nanocarriers in therapeutic settings. Transferrin-conjugated nanocarriers have been employed in glioblastoma therapies to exploit the upregulation of transferrin receptors in tumor cells, hence improving medication delivery and therapeutic efficacy [76]. Clinical experiments utilizing these carriers have demonstrated encouraging outcomes in enhancing targeted efficacy and reducing systemic adverse effects, as summarized in Table 5.1.

TABLE 5.1
Summary of Various Clinical Trials Indicating the Utilization of Smart Biomaterials in Various Types of Cancer

Clinical Trials	Nanoparticle/ Technology	Application	Cancer Type/ Condition	Key Findings/Significance	Last Update
NCT00984243 [101]	Hematoporphyrin	PDT	Lung cancer	PDT may replace surgery for early-stage lung cancer, reducing operations while evaluating outcomes like survival, cost, and quality of life.	2012-11-15
NCT05906407 [102]	Biomaterial	Biomarker-screening and therapy	Breast cancer	The comprehensive assessment of clinical features, genomics and further molecular markers to identify patients with early breast cancer for enrolment on marker-driven trials (COGNITION) platform identifies biomarkers for therapy-resistant breast tumors, enabling genomics-guided treatments in the COGNITION-GUIDE trial.	2024-08-26
NCT06385418 [103]	Thermosensitive hydrogel for localized drug release	Temperature-responsive hydrogel	Colorectal cancer	A thermosensitive hydrogel with 5-FU and colonic transendoscopic tubing offers a novel approach for CRC treatment, aiming to improve drug adhesion and assess its feasibility, safety, and efficacy.	2024-06-26
NCT0189589 [104]	Ferumoxytol (iron oxide)	Magnetic field-responsive	Imaging of lymph nodes and liver	Enhanced MRI clarity for cancerous lymph nodes and liver imaging.	2021-09-21
NCT00036738 [105]	Cyclosporine, dasatinib, fludarabine phosphate	Acidic pH-responsive (targeting acidic TME)	Leukemia	This phase II trial evaluates fludarabine, total-body irradiation, and donor stem cell transplants for leukemia, aiming to enhance cancer cell destruction while managing immune rejection and complications.	2020-01-29
NCT06632574 [106]	Cationic liposomes	Anti-tumor therapy	Solid tumors	Evaluation of Doxil in cancer treatment.	2024-10-09
NCT02649868 [107]	LC bead LUMI radio-opaque embolic beads	Thermal ablation	Hepatic tumors	Percutaneous trans-arterial embolization (TAE) blocks blood flow to liver tumors; researchers are testing a new material visible on imaging, sometimes combined with thermal ablation for added tumor shrinkage.	2024-07-11

Additional significant innovations encompass nanostructured lipid carriers (NLCs), examined for their capacity to transport small interfering RNA (siRNA) targeting oncogenes. These carriers have exhibited significant selectivity in gene silencing and are presently undergoing clinical tests to find their protection and efficiency. Their results have facilitated the advancement of iron oxide nanoparticles for hyperthermia-based cancer medications, utilizing Fe_3O_4 integrated into thermos-responsive hydrogels to attain localized heating, thereby eliminating tumor cells while preserving adjacent tissues. As these methodologies progress, analogous systems utilizing alternative thermos-responsive materials are being investigated for prospective clinical application [100].

The swift proliferation of stimuli-responsive biomaterials has resulted in a multitude of patents, especially for systems aimed at improving targeted specificity and therapeutic effectiveness in oncology. Patents have been granted for nanocarriers designed to release pharmaceuticals in reaction to the acidic TME. An example is a poly(L-histidine) and PEG system for DOX, which has demonstrated potential in tumor-targeted therapy by diminishing systemic exposure and enhancing intratumoral drug concentrations [108, 109]. Thermo-responsive systems including Fe_3O_4 nanoparticles have had considerable patent activity. These compounds, incorporated into biocompatible hydrogels such as GelMA, react to magnetic fields to generate hyperthermia at specific locations, thus facilitating localized treatment for solid tumors. Recent patents pertain to multifunctional and dual-responsive nanocarriers that integrate several functionalities, including imaging and therapy, into a singular platform. These theranostic nanoparticles provide concurrent treatment and monitoring, hence improving precision in cancer therapy. An exemplary instance is iron oxide nanoparticles, which function as both therapeutic agents and MRI contrast enhancers, offering significant diagnostic and therapeutic advantages. Numerous patents encompass liposomal formulations designed for controlled medication release, using pH-responsive and ultrasound-sensitive liposomes. Ultrasound-activated devices, engineered for non-invasive tumor targeting, have demonstrated potential in accessing deep-seated tumors and are currently seen as a viable option for localized cancer therapy. Iron oxide nanoparticles are crucial to patents due to their potential in diagnostic imaging and medicinal administration. These nanoparticles function as contrast agents in MRI and simultaneously carry medicines or therapeutic agents directly to tumors, providing a dual modality that is particularly advantageous in clinical applications for cancer theranostics [110, 111].

5.9 CONCLUSION

The future of stimuli-responsive biomaterials for cancer theranostics holds significant promise, with ongoing research poised to address critical challenges in cancer diagnosis and treatment. As our understanding of the TME continues to evolve, so too does the design of biomaterials that can respond to multiple triggers, providing targeted and controlled therapeutic outcomes. Future developments will likely focus on improving the responsiveness of these materials to environmental cues, enhancing their stability, and tailoring drug release to match tumor growth dynamics. Advances in nanotechnology and materials science will also play a vital role in enhancing the size, surface characteristics, and functionalization of these biomaterials, enabling better cellular uptake, prolonged circulation times, and more efficient tumor targeting. Moreover, integrating smart biomaterials with real-time molecular imaging enables non-invasive monitoring of treatment progress. The ability to visualize the location, distribution, and release of therapeutic agents in vivo will allow clinicians to adjust treatment plans dynamically, increasing the overall success rates of cancer therapies. Additionally, combining stimuli-responsive platforms with immunotherapy, gene therapy, or combination therapies will be explored to create more robust and personalized treatment regimens that maximize therapeutic efficacy while minimizing side effects. From a clinical perspective, the major hurdles in translating these innovative materials into standard practice lie in ensuring their reproducibility, scalability, and biocompatibility, as well as meeting the regulatory requirements for approval. However, with the increasing number of preclinical and clinical trials focusing on these technologies, it is likely that we will witness the emergence of stimuli-responsive biomaterials in clinical oncology soon. Furthermore, the patent landscape will continue to grow, with new intellectual property protecting novel mechanisms, formulations, and technologies that enable personalized cancer management. In conclusion, stimuli-responsive biomaterials represent a transformative step forward in cancer theranostics, offering the potential for highly targeted, personalized, and minimally invasive treatments. By responding dynamically to the unique characteristics of tumor environments, these materials can improve therapeutic outcomes, reduce side effects, and provide a more precise approach to cancer treatment. As research progresses and clinical trials advance, the future of stimuli-responsive biomaterials holds great promise in revolutionizing the way cancer is diagnosed and treated, facilitating significant advancements and patient-tailored therapies.

Declaration of AI and AI-Assisted Technologies

During the preparation of this work, the authors used QuillBot AI in order to paraphrase the sentences. After using this tool, the authors reviewed and edited the content as needed and take full responsibility for the content of the publication.

LIST OF ABBREVIATIONS

NCDs: non-communicable diseases; TME: tumor microenvironment; PTT: photothermal therapy; PDT: photodynamic therapy; NIR: near-infrared; NMOF: nano metal–organic framework; PEG: polyethylene glycol; SPIONs: superparamagnetic iron oxide nanoparticles; UCNPs: upconverting nanoparticles; LCST: lower critical solution temperature; BBR: berberine; DOX: doxorubicin; MDR: multidrug resistance; AZO: azobenzene; GBM: glioblastoma multiforme; MFNs: multifunctional nanomaterials; PLGA: (poly(lactic-co-glycolic)); ICG: indocyanine green; FA: folic acid; TK: thioketal; DDSs: drug delivery systems; LC: lung cancer; MNPs: magnetic nanoparticles; MRI: magnetic resonance imaging; MHT: magnetic hyperthermia; PET: positron emission tomography; GSH: glutathione; MMPs: matrix metalloproteinases; ROS: reactive oxygen species; NLCs: nanostructured lipid carriers; TAE: transarterial embolization.

REFERENCES

1. Bray F, Ferlay J, Soerjomataram I, Siegel RL, Torre LA, Jemal A. Global cancer statistics 2018: GLOBOCAN estimates of incidence and mortality worldwide for 36 cancers in 185 countries. CA Cancer J Clin 2018;68:394–424. https://doi.org/10.3322/CAAC.21492.
2. Ali MY, Bukhari S. (eds). Cancer Targeting Therapies: Conventional and Advanced Perspectives – 1 2024. https://www.routledge.com/Cancer-Targeting-Therapies-Conventional-and-Advanced-Perspectives/Ali-Bukhari/p/book/9781032427126?srsltid=AfmBOoohA1WL6IURJ0Yr8z9naDuTB1pGuSzasgIBma0cBnVHqgBLWHgO (accessed November 25, 2024).
3. Brown JS, Amend SR, Austin RH, Gatenby RA, Hammarlund EU, Pienta KJ. Updating the definition of cancer. Molecular Cancer Research 2023;21:1142–7. https://doi.org/10.1158/1541-7786.MCR-23-0411.
4. Debela DT, Muzazu SGY, Heraro KD, Ndalama MT, Mesele BW, Haile DC, et al. New approaches and procedures for cancer treatment: Current perspectives. SAGE Open Med 2021;9. https://doi.org/10.1177/20503121211034366.
5. Arruebo M, Vilaboa N, Sáez-Gutierrez B, Lambea J, Tres A, Valladares M, et al. Assessment of the evolution of cancer treatment therapies. Cancers (Basel) 2011;3:3279–330. https://doi.org/10.3390/cancers3033279.
6. Rutqvist LE, Rose C, Cavallin-Ståhl E. A systematic overview of radiation therapy effects in breast cancer. Acta Oncol (Madr) 2003;42:532–45. https://doi.org/10.1080/02841860310014444.
7. Bergh J, Jönsson P-E, Glimelius B, Nygren P.. A systematic overview of chemotherapy effects in breast cancer. Acta Oncol (Madr) 2001;40:253–81. https://doi.org/10.1080/02841860120784.
8. Ewertz M, Jensen AB. Late effects of breast cancer treatment and potentials for rehabilitation. Acta Oncol (Madr) 2011;50:187–93. https://doi.org/10.3109/0284186X.2010.533190.
9. Salata C, de Almeida CE, Ferreira-Machado SC, Barroso RC, Nogueira LP, Mantuano A, et al. Preliminary pre-clinical studies on the side effects of breast cancer treatment. Int J Radiat Biol 2021;97:877–87. https://doi.org/10.1080/09553002.2021.1919782.

10. Suhag D, Kaushik S, Taxak VB. Handbook of Biomaterials for Medical Applications, Volume 1 2024. https://doi.org/10.1007/978-981-97-4818-1.
11. Li XP, Hou DY, Wu JC, Zhang P, Wang YZ, Lv MY, et al. Stimuli-responsive nanomaterials for tumor immunotherapy. ACS Biomater Sci Eng 2024;10:5474–95. https://doi.org/10.1021/acsbiomaterials.4c00388.
12. Zhang L, Gu FX, Chan JM, Wang AZ, Langer RS, Farokhzad OC. Nanoparticles in medicine: Therapeutic applications and developments. Clin Pharmacol Ther 2008;83:761–9. https://doi.org/10.1038/sj.clpt.6100400.
13. Pham SH, Choi Y, Choi J. Stimuli-responsive nanomaterials for application in antitumor therapy and drug delivery. Pharmaceutics 2020;12:630. https://doi.org/10.3390/PHARMACEUTICS12070630.
14. Liao Z, Liu T, Yao Z, Hu T, Ji X, Yao B. Harnessing stimuli-responsive biomaterials for advanced biomedical applications. Exploration 2024. https://doi.org/10.1002/EXP.20230133.
15. Chu S, Shi X, Tian Y, Gao F. pH-responsive polymer nanomaterials for tumor therapy. Front Oncol 2022;12:855019. https://doi.org/10.3389/FONC.2022.855019.
16. Alsehli M. Polymeric nanocarriers as stimuli-responsive systems for targeted tumor (cancer) therapy: Recent advances in drug delivery. Saudi Pharm J 2020;28:255–65. https://doi.org/10.1016/J.JSPS.2020.01.004.
17. Chang D, Ma Y, Xu X, Xie J, Ju S. Stimuli-responsive polymeric nanoplatforms for cancer therapy. Front Bioeng Biotechnol 2021;9:707319. https://doi.org/10.3389/FBIOE.2021.707319.
18. Tenchov R, Bird R, Curtze AE, Zhou Q. Lipid nanoparticles from liposomes to mRNA vaccine delivery, a landscape of research diversity and advancement. ACS Nano 2021;15:16982–7015. https://doi.org/10.1021/acsnano.1c04996.
19. Zhang B, Huang Y, Huang Y. Advances in nanodynamic therapy for cancer treatment. Nanomaterials 2024;14:648. https://doi.org/10.3390/NANO14070648.
20. Dias D, Resina L, Ferreira FC, Sanjuan-Alberte P, Esteves T. Synthesis strategies and cancer therapy applications of PEDOT nanoparticles. Mater Adv 2024;5:7561–83. https://doi.org/10.1039/D4MA00260A.
21. Overchuk M, Weersink RA, Wilson BC, Zheng G. Photodynamic and photothermal therapies: Synergy opportunities for nanomedicine. ACS Nano 2023;17:7979–8003. https://doi.org/10.1021/acsnano.3c00891.
22. Anitha K, Chenchula S, Surendran V, Shvetank B, Ravula P, Milan R, et al. Advancing cancer theranostics through biomimetics: A comprehensive review. Heliyon 2024;10:e27692. https://doi.org/10.1016/J.HELIYON.2024.E27692.
23. Al-Thani AN, Jan AG, Abbas M, Geetha M, Sadasivuni KK. Nanoparticles in cancer theragnostic and drug delivery: A comprehensive review. Life Sci 2024;352:122899. https://doi.org/10.1016/J.LFS.2024.122899.
24. Solanki R, Bhatia D. Stimulus-responsive hydrogels for targeted cancer therapy. Gels 2024;10:440. https://doi.org/10.3390/gels10070440.
25. Fang Z, Shen Y, Gao D. Stimulus-responsive nanocarriers for targeted drug delivery. New J Chem 2021;45:4534–44. https://doi.org/10.1039/d0nj05169a.
26. Mura S, Nicolas J, Couvreur P. Stimuli-responsive nanocarriers for drug delivery. Nat Mater 2013;12:991–1003. https://doi.org/10.1038/nmat3776.
27. Wan X, Zhong H, Pan W, Li Y, Chen Y, Li N, et al. Programmed release of dihydroartemisinin for synergistic cancer therapy using a $CaCO_3$ mineralized Metal–Organic framework. Angew Chem Int Ed 2019;58:14134–9. https://doi.org/10.1002/anie.201907388.
28. Yang H, Wang Q, Li Z, Li F, Wu D, Fan M, et al. Hydrophobicity-adaptive nanogels for programmed anticancer drug delivery. Nano Lett 2018;18:7909–18. https://doi.org/10.1021/acs.nanolett.8b03828.
29. Fang Z, Li X, Xu Z, Du F, Wang W, Shi R, et al. Hyaluronic acid-modified mesoporous silica-coated superparamagnetic Fe_3O_4 nanoparticles for targeted drug delivery. Int J Nanomed 2019;14:5785–97. https://doi.org/10.2147/IJN.S213974.
30. MacEwan SR, Callahan DJ, Chilkoti A. Stimulus-responsive macromolecules and nanoparticles for cancer drug delivery. Nanomedicine 2010;5:793–806. https://doi.org/10.2217/nnm.10.50.
31. Majumder J, Minko T. Multifunctional and stimuli-responsive nanocarriers for targeted therapeutic delivery. Expert Opin Drug Deliv 2021;18:205–27. https://doi.org/10.1080/17425247.2021.1828339.
32. Shah RA, Frazar EM, Hilt JZ. Recent developments in stimuli responsive nanomaterials and their bionanotechnology applications. Curr Opin Chem Eng 2020;30:103–11. https://doi.org/10.1016/j.coche.2020.08.007.
33. Decuzzi P, Cook AB. Harnessing endogenous stimuli for responsive materials in theranostics. ACS Nano 2021;15:2068–98. https://doi.org/10.1021/acsnano.0c09115.

34. Tian M, Xin X, Wu R, Guan W, Zhou W. Advances in intelligent-responsive nanocarriers for cancer therapy. Pharmacol Res 2022;178:106184. https://doi.org/10.1016/J.PHRS.2022.106184.
35. Liu G, Lovell JF, Zhang L, Zhang Y. Stimulus-responsive nanomedicines for disease diagnosis and treatment. Int J Mol Sci 2020;21:1–44. https://doi.org/10.3390/ijms21176380.
36. Pham SH, Choi Y, Choi J. Stimuli-responsive nanomaterials for application in antitumor therapy and drug delivery. Pharmaceutics 2020;12:1–19. https://doi.org/10.3390/pharmaceutics12070630.
37. Mi P. Stimuli-responsive nanocarriers for drug delivery, tumor imaging, therapy and theranostics. Theranostics 2020;10:4557–88. https://doi.org/10.7150/thno.38069.
38. Nica V, Marino A, Pucci C, Şen Ö, Emanet M, De, Pasquale D, et al. Cell-membrane-coated and cell-penetrating peptide-conjugated trimagnetic nanoparticles for targeted magnetic hyperthermia of prostate cancer cells. ACS Appl Mater Interfaces 2023;15:30008–28. https://doi.org/10.1021/acsami.3c07248.
39. Lafuente-Gómez N, Latorre A, Milán-Rois P, Rodriguez, Diaz C, Somoza Á. Stimuli-responsive nanomaterials for cancer treatment: Boundaries, opportunities and applications. Chem Commun 2021; 57:13662–77. https://doi.org/10.1039/d1cc05056g.
40. Manzanares-Guevara LA, Licea-Claverie A, Oroz-Parra I, Bernaldez-Sarabia J, Diaz-Castillo F, Licea-Navarro AF. Smart nanoformulation based on stimuli-responsive nanogels and curcumin: Promising therapy against colon cancer. ACS Omega 2020;5:9171–84. https://doi.org/10.1021/acsomega.9b04390.
41. Libson S, Lippman M. A review of clinical aspects of breast cancer. Int Rev Psychiatry 2014;26:4–15. https://doi.org/10.3109/09540261.2013.852971.
42. Morgulchik N, Kamaly N. Meta-analysis of in vitro drug-release parameters reveals predictable and robust kinetics for redox-responsive drug-conjugated therapeutic nanogels. ACS Appl Nano Mater 2021;4:4256–68. https://doi.org/10.1021/acsanm.1c00170.
43. Xin H, Naficy S. Drug delivery based on stimuli-responsive injectable hydrogels for breast cancer therapy: A review. Gels 2022;8. https://doi.org/10.3390/gels8010045.
44. Oshiro-Júnior JA, Rodero C, Hanck-Silva G, Sato MR, Alves RC, Eloy JO, et al. Stimuli-responsive drug delivery nanocarriers in the treatment of breast cancer. Curr Med Chem 2018;27:2494–513. https://doi.org/10.2174/0929867325666181009120610.
45. Akhlaghi M, Taebpour M, Lotfabadi NN, Naghib SM, Jalili N, Farahmand L, et al. Synthesis and characterization of smart stimuli-responsive herbal drug-encapsulated nanoniosome particles for efficient treatment of breast cancer. Nanotechnol Rev 2022;11:1364–85. https://doi.org/10.1515/ntrev-2022-0080.
46. Shaban WM. Insight into breast cancer detection: New hybrid feature selection method. Neural Comput Appl 2023;35:6831–53. https://doi.org/10.1007/s00521-022-08062-y.
47. Najm A, Niculescu AG, Bolocan A, Rădulescu M, Grumezescu AM, Beuran M, et al. Chitosan and cyclodextrins—Versatile materials used to create drug delivery systems for gastrointestinal cancers. Pharmaceutics 2024;16. https://doi.org/10.3390/pharmaceutics16010043.
48. Tang M, Song J, Zhang S, Shu X, Liu S, Ashrafizadeh M, et al. Innovative theranostic hydrogels for targeted gastrointestinal cancer treatment. J Transl Med 2024;22. https://doi.org/10.1186/s12967-024-05749-9.
49. Li J, Zhu T, Jiang Y, Zhang Q, Zu Y, Shen X. Microfluidic printed 3D bioactive scaffolds for postoperative treatment of gastric cancer. Mater Today Bio 2024;24. https://doi.org/10.1016/j.mtbio.2023.100911.
50. Arciero CA, Sigurdson ER. Liver-directed therapies for patients with primary liver cancer and hepatic metastases. Curr Treat Options Oncol 2006;7:399–409. https://doi.org/10.1007/s11864-006-0008-7.
51. Radu ER, Semenescu A, Voicu SI. Recent advances in stimuli-responsive doxorubicin delivery systems for liver cancer therapy. Polymers (Basel) 2022;14. https://doi.org/10.3390/polym14235249.
52. Liu X, Wu Z, Guo C, Guo H, Su Y, Chen Q, et al. Hypoxia responsive nano-drug delivery system based on angelica polysaccharide for liver cancer therapy. Drug Deliv 2022;29:138–48. https://doi.org/10.1080/10717544.2021.2021324.
53. Ismail M, Wang Y, Li Y, Liu J, Zheng M, Zou Y. Stimuli-responsive polymeric nanocarriers accelerate on-demand drug release to combat glioblastoma. Biomacromolecules 2024. https://doi.org/10.1021/acs.biomac.4c00722.
54. Pucci C, Marino A, Şen Ö, De, Pasquale D, Bartolucci M, Iturrioz-Rodríguez N, et al. Ultrasound-responsive nutlin-loaded nanoparticles for combined chemotherapy and piezoelectric treatment of glioblastoma cells. Acta Biomater 2022;139:218–36. https://doi.org/10.1016/j.actbio.2021.04.005.
55. Tapeinos C, Marino A, Battaglini M, Migliorin S, Brescia R, Scarpellini A, et al. Stimuli-responsive lipid-based magnetic nanovectors increase apoptosis in glioblastoma cells through synergic intracellular hyperthermia and chemotherapy. Nanoscale 2019;11:72–88. https://doi.org/10.1039/c8nr05520c.

56. Lopes-Nunes J, Agonia AS, Rosado T, Gallardo E, Palmeira-de-Oliveira R, et al. Aptamer-functionalized gold nanoparticles for drug delivery to gynecological carcinoma cells. Cancers (Basel) 2021;13. https://doi.org/10.3390/cancers13164038.
57. Sánchez-Ramírez DR, Domínguez-Ríos R, Juárez J, Valdés M, Hassan N, Quintero-Ramos A, et al. Biodegradable photoresponsive nanoparticles for chemo-, photothermal- and photodynamic therapy of ovarian cancer. Mater Sci Eng C 2020;116. https://doi.org/10.1016/j.msec.2020.111196.
58. Niu W, Wang J, Wang Q, Shen J. Celastrol loaded nanoparticles with ROS-response and ROS-inducer for the treatment of ovarian cancer. Front Chem 2020;8. https://doi.org/10.3389/fchem.2020.574614.
59. Kyprianou N, English HF, Isaacs2 JT. Programmed Cell Death during Regression of PC-82 Human Prostate Cancer following Androgen Ablation1. vol. 50. 1990.
60. Zeng L, Gowda BHJ, Ahmed MG, Abourehab MAS, Chen ZS, Zhang C, et al. Advancements in nanoparticle-based treatment approaches for skin cancer therapy. Mol Cancer 2023;22. https://doi.org/10.1186/s12943-022-01708-4.
61. Trinh HT, Mohanan S, Radhakrishnan D, Tiburcius S, Yang JH, Verrills NM, et al. Silica-based nanomaterials as drug delivery tools for skin cancer (melanoma) treatment. Emergent Mater 2021;4:1067–92. https://doi.org/10.1007/s42247-021-00236-z.
62. Gade L, Boyd BJ, Malmsten M, Heinz A. Stimuli-responsive drug delivery systems for inflammatory skin conditions. Acta Biomater 2024. https://doi.org/10.1016/j.actbio.2024.08.037.
63. Dinakar YH, Karole A, Parvez S, Jain V, Mudavath SL. Organ-restricted delivery through stimuli-responsive nanocarriers for lung cancer therapy. Life Sci 2022;310. https://doi.org/10.1016/j.lfs.2022.121133.
64. Fass L. Imaging and cancer: A review. Mol Oncol 2008;2:115. https://doi.org/10.1016/J.MOLONC.2008.04.001.
65. Sun Z, Ng KH, Ramli N. Biomedical imaging research: A fast-emerging area for interdisciplinary collaboration. Biomed Imaging Interv J 2011;7:1–4. https://doi.org/10.2349/biij.7.3.e21.
66. Allen C, Her S, Jaffray DA. Radiotherapy for cancer: Present and future. Adv Drug Deliv Rev 2017;109:1–2. https://doi.org/10.1016/j.addr.2017.01.004.
67. Alromi DA, Madani SY, Seifalian A. Emerging application of magnetic nanoparticles for diagnosis and treatment of cancer. Polymers (Basel) 2021;13. https://doi.org/10.3390/polym13234146.
68. Solomon M, Liu Y, Berezin MY, Achilefu S. Optical imaging in cancer research: Basic principles, tumor detection, and therapeutic monitoring. Med Princ Pract 2011;20:397–415. https://doi.org/10.1159/000327655.
69. Chen Q, Ke H, Dai Z, Liu Z. Nanoscale theranostics for physical stimulus-responsive cancer therapies. Biomaterials 2015;73:214–30. https://doi.org/10.1016/j.biomaterials.2015.09.018.
70. Zhang Q, Zhang J, Song J, Liu Y, Ren X, Zhao Y. Protein-based nanomedicine for therapeutic benefits of cancer. ACS Nano 2021;15:8001–38. https://doi.org/10.1021/acsnano.1c00476.
71. Yang K, Zhang S, Zhang G, Sun X, Lee S-T, Liu Z. Graphene in mice: Ultrahigh in vivo tumor uptake and efficient photothermal therapy. Nano Lett 2010;10:3318–23. https://doi.org/10.1021/nl100996u.
72. Huang X, El-Sayed IH, Qian W, El-Sayed MA. Cancer cell imaging and photothermal therapy in the near-infrared region by using gold nanorods. J Am Chem Soc 2006;128:2115–20. https://doi.org/10.1021/ja057254a.
73. Dougherty TJ, Gomer CJ, Henderson BW, Jori G, Kessel D, Korbelik M, et al. Photodynamic therapy. JNCI 1998;90:889–905. https://doi.org/10.1093/jnci/90.12.889.
74. Tao Y, Chan HF, Shi B, Li M, Leong KW. Light: A magical tool for controlled drug delivery. Adv Funct Mater 2020;30. https://doi.org/10.1002/adfm.202005029.
75. Rajapaksha W, Khetan R, Johnson IRD, Blencowe A, Garg S, Albrecht H, et al. Future theranostic strategies: Emerging ovarian cancer biomarkers to bridge the gap between diagnosis and treatment. Front Drug Deliv 2024;4. https://doi.org/10.3389/fddev.2024.1339936.
76. Sheikh MM, Veeranarayanan S, Maekawa T, Kumar DS. External stimulus responsive inorganic nanomaterials for cancer theranostics. Adv Drug Deliv Rev 2019;138:18–40. https://doi.org/10.1016/j.addr.2018.10.007.
77. Graça MP, Soreto S, Gavinho S, Valente M, Salgueiro C, Nunes J, et al. Nanomaterials for Magnetic Hyperthermia. n.d.
78. Liu K, Jing B, Kang J, Han L, Chang J. Ultrasound-enabled nanomedicine for tumor theranostics. Engineering 2024. https://doi.org/10.1016/j.eng.2024.01.030.
79. Schattling P, Jochum FD, Theato P. Multi-stimuli responsive polymers – The all-in-one talents. Polym Chem 2013;5:25–36. https://doi.org/10.1039/C3PY00880K.

80. Arafat M, Sakkal M, Beiram R, AbuRuz S. Nanomedicines: Emerging platforms in smart chemotherapy treatment—A recent review. Pharmaceuticals 2024;17:315. https://doi.org/10.3390/PH17030315.
81. Ghamkhari A, Mahmoodzadeh F, Ghorbani M, Hamishehkar H. A novel gold nanorods coated by stimuli-responsive ABC triblock copolymer for chemotherapy of solid tumors. Eur Polym J 2019;115:313–24. https://doi.org/10.1016/J.EURPOLYMJ.2019.03.038.
82. Hajebi S, Chamanara M, Nasiri SS, Ghasri M, Mouraki A, Heidari R, et al. Advances in stimuli-responsive gold nanorods for drug-delivery and targeted therapy systems. Biomed Pharmacother 2024;180:117493. https://doi.org/10.1016/J.BIOPHA.2024.117493.
83. Kutoka PT, Seidu TA, Baye V, Khamis AM, Omonova CT, qizi, Wang B. Insights into tumor microenvironment (TME) and the nano approaches to suppress tumor growth. OpenNano 2022;7:100041. https://doi.org/10.1016/J.ONANO.2022.100041.
84. Zhu L, Torchilin VP. Stimulus-responsive nanopreparations for tumor targeting. Integr Biol (United Kingdom) 2013;5:96–107. https://doi.org/10.1039/C2IB20135F.
85. Lee Y, Thompson DH. Stimuli-responsive liposomes for drug delivery. Wiley Interdiscip Rev Nanomed Nanobiotechnol 2017;9. https://doi.org/10.1002/WNAN.1450.
86. Abdo GG, Zagho MM, Khalil A. Recent advances in stimuli-responsive drug release and targeting concepts using mesoporous silica nanoparticles. Emerg Mater 2020;3:407–25. https://doi.org/10.1007/S42247-020-00109-X.
87. Choudhary P, Biswas S, Kandoth N, Tayde D, Chatterjee A, Chattopadhyay S, et al. Graphene quantum dots alleviate ROS-mediated gastric damage. iScience 2022;25:104062. https://doi.org/10.1016/J.ISCI.2022.104062.
88. Liu H, Li C, Qian Y, Hu L, Fang J, Tong W, et al. Magnetic-induced graphene quantum dots for imaging-guided photothermal therapy in the second near-infrared window. Biomaterials 2020;232. https://doi.org/10.1016/J.BIOMATERIALS.2019.119700.
89. Blum AP, Kammeyer JK, Rush AM, Callmann CE, Hahn ME, Gianneschi NC. Stimuli-responsive nanomaterials for biomedical applications. J Am Chem Soc 2015;137:2140–54. https://doi.org/10.1021/ja510147n.
90. Fu X, Hosta-Rigau L, Chandrawati R, Cui J. Multi-stimuli-responsive polymer particles, films, and hydrogels for drug delivery. Chem 2018;4:2084–107. https://doi.org/10.1016/J.CHEMPR.2018.07.002.
91. kaur R, Sharma S, Rathore K. Stimuli responsive ferrocene-based supramolecular systems: New route for the design of smart devices. J Organomet Chem 2023;997:122787. https://doi.org/10.1016/J.JORGANCHEM.2023.122787.
92. Cao D, Kou Y, Liang J, Chen Z, Wang L, Meier H. A facile and efficient preparation of pillararenes and a pillarquinone. Angew Chem Int Ed 2009;48:9721–3. https://doi.org/10.1002/ANIE.200904765.
93. Zyryanov GV, Kopchuk DS, Kovalev IS, Santra S, Majee A, Ranu BC. Pillararenes as promising carriers for drug delivery. Int J Mol Sci 2023;24:5167. https://doi.org/10.3390/IJMS24065167.
94. Chehelgerdi M, Chehelgerdi M, Allela OQB, Pecho RDC, Jayasankar N, Rao DP, et al. Progressing nanotechnology to improve targeted cancer treatment: Overcoming hurdles in its clinical implementation. Mol Cancer 2023;22:169. https://doi.org/10.1186/S12943-023-01865-0.
95. Wang Z, Wang X, Xu W, Li Y, Lai R, Qiu X, et al. Translational challenges and prospective solutions in the implementation of biomimetic delivery systems. Pharmaceutics 2023;15:2623. https://doi.org/10.3390/PHARMACEUTICS15112623.
96. Lee BK, Yun YH, Park K. Smart nanoparticles for drug delivery: Boundaries and opportunities. Chem Eng Sci 2015;125:158–64. https://doi.org/10.1016/J.CES.2014.06.042.
97. Liu D, Yang F, Xiong F, Gu N. The smart drug delivery system and its clinical potential. Theranostics 2016;6:1306. https://doi.org/10.7150/THNO.14858.
98. Wei D, Sun Y, Zhu H, Fu Q. Stimuli-responsive polymer-based nanosystems for cancer theranostics. ACS Nano 2023;17:23223–61. https://doi.org/10.1021/acsnano.3c06019.
99. Chang D, Ma Y, Xu X, Xie J, Ju S. Stimuli-responsive polymeric nanoplatforms for cancer therapy. Front Bioeng Biotechnol 2021;9:707319. https://doi.org/10.3389/FBIOE.2021.707319/BIBTEX.
100. Li H, Feng Y, Luo Q, Li Z, Li X, Gan H, et al. Stimuli-activatable nanomedicine meets cancer theranostics. Theranostics 2023;13:5386–417. https://doi.org/10.7150/THNO.87854.
101. Search for: NCT00984243 | Card Results | ClinicalTrials.gov n.d. https://clinicaltrials.gov/search?cond=NCT00984243&viewType=Card (accessed January 16, 2025).
102. Search for: NCT05906407 | Card Results | ClinicalTrials.gov n.d. https://clinicaltrials.gov/search?cond=NCT05906407 (accessed January 16, 2025).
103. Search for: NCT06385418 | Card Results | ClinicalTrials.gov n.d. https://clinicaltrials.gov/search?cond=NCT06385418 (accessed January 16, 2025).

104. Search for: NCT0189589 | Card Results | ClinicalTrials.gov n.d. https://clinicaltrials.gov/search?cond=NCT0189589 (accessed January 16, 2025).
105. Search for: NCT00036738 | Card Results | ClinicalTrials.gov n.d. https://clinicaltrials.gov/search?cond=NCT00036738 (accessed January 16, 2025).
106. Search for: NCT06632574 | Card Results | ClinicalTrials.gov n.d. https://clinicaltrials.gov/search?cond=NCT06632574 (accessed January 16, 2025).
107. Search for: NCT02649868 | Card Results | ClinicalTrials.gov n.d. https://clinicaltrials.gov/search?cond=NCT02649868 (accessed January 16, 2025).
108. Khan A, Sahu NK. Hydrazone conjugated and DOX loaded PEGylated-Fe_3O_4 mesoporous magnetic nanoclusters (MNCs): Hyperthermia and in vitro chemotherapy. New J Chem 2021;45:21646–56. https://doi.org/10.1039/D1NJ03968G.
109. Wang Y, Shi W, Kuss M, Mirza S, Qi D, Krasnoslobodtsev A, et al. 3D bioprinting of breast cancer models for drug resistance study. ACS Biomater Sci Eng 2018;4:4401–11. https://doi.org/10.1021/acsbiomaterials.8b01277.
110. Xu Q, Ban X, Yang L, Chen Y, Zhang F, Wang Y, et al. MRI-visualized PTT/CDT for breast cancer ablation and distant metastasis prevention. Appl Mater Today 2024;36:102059. https://doi.org/10.1016/J.APMT.2024.102059.
111. Caspani S, Magalhães R, Araújo JP, Sousa CT. Magnetic nanomaterials as contrast agents for MRI. Materials 2020;13. https://doi.org/10.3390/MA13112586.

6 Stimuli-Responsive Biomaterials for Inflammatory Arthritis and Other Bone Disorders

Vaishali Pawar, Glynis Almeida, Divya Dubey, Sameer Patel, Sandip Sapkal, and Rohit Srivastava
Department of Biosciences and Bioengineering,
Indian Institute of Technology Bombay (IIT Bombay), Mumbai, India

6.1 INTRODUCTION TO STIMULI-RESPONSIVE BIOMATERIALS

6.1.1 Overview of Biomaterials

Biomaterials are substances which are involved in enhancing or restoring a biological function in the body, serving either a therapeutic or diagnostic purpose, without eliciting an adverse immune response. A drug delivery system is contemplated to be successful when it can deliver the desired drug at the appropriate target site, follows sustained kinetics, and does not evoke any toxic effects. Biomaterials bear testimony to these criteria and hence are considered to be ideal for drug delivery. Not much is known as to when did biomaterials come into existence but it is believed to be there since centuries. Its use dates back to the era of Second World War, wherein it provided soldiers relief from arthritic joints. However, it was in the 1970s when the term biomaterial was coined [1]. The physiochemical properties of biomaterials along with their biocompatibility and mechanical properties are of utmost importance. They are classified on the basis of their origin which could be either natural or synthetic. The examples of natural biomaterials include gelatin, heparin, hyaluronic acid, and alginate, for instance, the use of chitin-derived biomaterials for osteoarthritis (OA). But it's the synthetic biomaterials that are in higher demand as they can be easily manipulated. Vital synthetic biomaterial classes are metals, polymers, ceramics, etc. An ideal biomaterial is characterized as the one that is biocompatible, bioactive, bio-tolerant, bioresorbable, and bioinert [1]. Nanoparticles (NPs), hydrogels, and scaffolds are the forms in which biomaterials can be imparted, with properties of wettability, topography, and cross-linking capacity coming into place, thus enhancing their function [2]. Biomaterials have paved its way in several therapeutic fields from tissue engineering and organ regeneration to controlled release and regenerative medicine, thus proving to be multi-disciplinary. Its use has become evident in the prophylaxis of several detrimental diseases like cancer, AIDS, among others. Hence, biomaterials have come out as a captivating field and over the past few decades researchers have been extensively studying its interaction with the human body and their effective use in biotherapy and disease management [3].

6.1.2 Role in Inflammatory Disease Management

Inflammatory disease management is an area wherein biomaterials have been comprehensively used. Inflammation is known as a natural and vital reaction of the human body, protecting it from

DOI: 10.1201/9781003560203-6

adversities. However, a dysregulation in this inflammatory response can give rise to varied inflammatory diseases. The fascinating strategy of using biomaterials as drug carriers or incorporation of other therapeutic agents, which offer sustained release with least side effects has become quite popular [4]. They act as potent scavengers of pro-inflammatory factors or inhibit unfavourable endothelial–leucocyte interactions by blocking cell-adhesion molecules (CAM). Biomaterials can either enhance or decrease inflammation thus playing a crucial part in immune modulation and simultaneously have a hand in macrophage polarization. When embedded with signalling molecules they can regulate cell signals, morphology, and protein transport. Inter- and intra-cellular signalling can be mediated because of the degradation, stiffness, structural, and topological characteristics of biomaterials. Additionally, the biomaterial scaffolds designed can stimulate angiogenesis and promote transport of nutrients, oxygen, and waste products [2]. Early inflammation can be effectively blocked if the engineered biomaterials possess inflammatory mediator absorption, nucleic-acid binding, and reactive oxygen species (ROS)-scavenging properties. Moreover, tissue regeneration can be facilitated with the incorporation of immunomodulatory cytokines which promotes M1 to M2 macrophage transition [4].

Studies suggest that there are three major mechanisms/strategies employed by biomaterials for curbing inflammation, namely scavenging strategy, blockage strategy, and delivery strategy. An overview of the three strategies is illustrated below (Figure 6.1.) [4]. These strategies could either include passive or active targeting. Passive targeting indulges in the enhanced permeability and retention (EPR) effect, wherein a leaky vasculature delivers the drug incorporated in the biomaterial to the inflamed tissue. While, active targeting involves the binding of inflammatory compounds to biomaterial formulations and drug penetration is attained through cellular transcytosis, endocytosis, or exocytosis [4]. These biomaterial-based formulations can be made to target B-cells, T-cells, platelets, or dendritic cells to achieve better treatment efficacy. In contrast, degradation-based biomaterials have also gained momentum recently. For example, proteolytic matrix metalloproteinase (MMP)-sensitive biomaterials and biomaterials responding to myeloperoxidase can be used to deliver drugs and determine neutrophil count, respectively, in inflammatory diseases [5, 6].

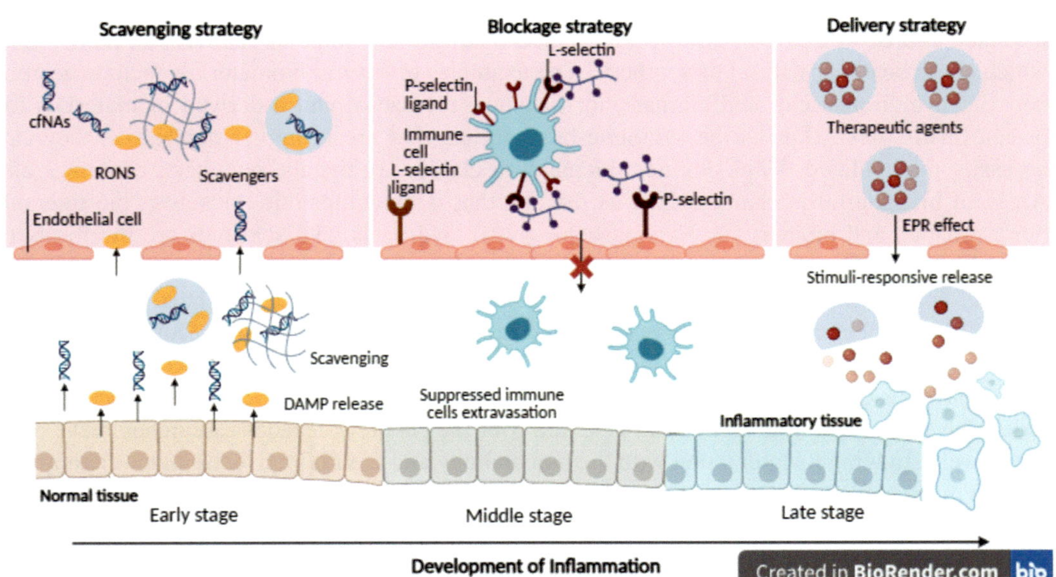

FIGURE 6.1 Biomaterial strategies for inflammation control. (Reproduced with permission from Ref. [4], Copyrights 2022, Nature.)

Hence, biomaterials well complement the existing therapies while giving the scientists an additional leeway of targeting varied pathways due to its versatility thus aiding in regulating inflammation and inflammatory-associated diseases. A biomaterial with excellent surface topography and architecture contributing to its bioactiveness and biomimicking abilities, respectively, can possess superlative functionality and prove to be a boon in disease management [2].

6.1.3 Significance of Stimuli-Responsive Systems

The unique properties of biomaterials can be further enhanced to be more personalized and tailored in order to respond to the varied conditions during the progression of an inflammatory disease, by making them stimuli-responsive. As the term suggests, stimuli-responsive biomaterials are innovative materials which can respond to internal or external stimulus like pH, temperature, light, biological signals, and many more, further undergoing reversible or irreversible modifications in their physical and chemical properties. They can monitor the inflammatory disease progression and offer targeted and controlled drug delivery. Stimuli-responsive biomaterials showcase the shape memory effect. This allows them to change their form depending on the variations in pH, light, temperature, chemical reagents, etc. They have the ability to release drugs or other molecules only when the materials encounter the right conditions for the right duration [7]. Hence, significance of stimuli-responsive materials relies on the fact that the presence of an internal/external cue is enough to elicit a response, causing a change in cross-link density, thus affecting the material's stiffness, or a change in hydrophobicity/hydrophilicity, which in turn changes the topography or swelling properties. Hence, biomaterials can respond to numerous external and internal stimuli to provide therapeutic effectiveness. They are categorized based on the type of stimulus they react to [7]. Following are few of the common stimuli-responsive biomaterials in use.

6.2 TYPES OF STIMULI-RESPONSIVE BIOMATERIALS

6.2.1 Temperature-Responsive Biomaterials

Temperature-responsive biomaterials are type of materials whose physical properties, such as solubility or phase, are altered significantly in reaction to temperature variations. Depending on the variable temperature input, they alter their conformational states. Temperature-responsive biomaterials undergo a phase transition (reversible) in response to temperature fluctuations, thereby the polymeric chains are fragmented and the hydrophobic segments form a mesh-like network, thus shrinking and squeezing out the encapsulated molecules. The two primary types of temperature-sensitive behaviours are lower critical solution temperature (LCST) and upper critical solution temperature (UCST). At LCST, the material becomes insoluble beyond a certain temperature, while at UCST, it exhibits increased solubility as temperature rises. These materials are chiefly designed to have a LCST, which essentially indicates that they shift from soluble to insoluble as the temperature rises above a predetermined threshold. This distinguishing feature makes them extremely important for numerous biomedical applications, such as tissue engineering, drug delivery, and biosensing. Temperature-responsive biomaterials help researchers accurately manipulate the release of medicinal drugs, develop tissue scaffolds, and detect biological markers by adjusting the temperature [8].

For instance, in cancer treatment, a thermo-responsive material can be placed at a tumour site and when the tumour is heated up, it causes the material to release therapeutic agents solely to that target area. In tissue engineering applications, these thermo-responsive materials serve as injectable scaffolds that are injected using a relatively simpler and less invasive technique. After their placement into the body, the said materials or scaffolds are transformed into solid-state polymers which help in creating frameworks for cell proliferation and tissue engineering [8].

6.2.2 pH-Responsive Biomaterials

pH is a characteristic feature of the microenvironment involving inflammation and encompasses different gradients. Tumour tissues typically exhibit a more acidic pH than normal tissues, allowing pH-sensitive materials to release drugs selectively in these environments. This drop in pH is attributed to the accumulation of acidic metabolites and the anaerobic conditions typical of inflamed tissues. By utilizing pH-responsive materials, researchers can exploit these pH variations to enhance treatment specificity and efficacy, especially with NPs engineered to release drugs at acidic tumour sites. In wound care, the pH-responsive nature of biomaterials can be utilized to adapt to pH shifts in the wound environment, helping to speed up healing and deliver antimicrobial agents as needed [9, 10]. The pH-responsiveness in these materials is mainly driven by the ionization of specific functional groups, which influences their electrostatic interactions, solubility, and structural stability. For example, polysaccharides containing carboxyl or amine groups react to pH changes by shifting their charge, which then affects their characteristics like swelling, gel formation, or dissolution. Their carboxyl or amine groups become protonated, which increases both the solubility and positive charge of chitosan. This adaptability makes them well-suited for applications that require a response to the environmental pH changes [11].

6.2.3 Enzyme-Responsive Biomaterials

Enzyme-responsive biomaterials are a sub-class of smart materials intended to react to peculiar enzymes in the body such as MMPs, hyaluronidases, or cathepsins to name a few, enabling controlled release, targeted drug delivery, and for diagnostic applications. These materials leverage the unique catalytic properties of enzymes, enabling site-specific activation in response to the biological environment. Enzyme-responsive biomaterials exhibit adaptability in their composition and structural design, which allows them to undergo specific chemical or physical changes in response to enzyme-catalysed reactions, thus achieving precision in biomedical applications [12]. Enzyme-responsive biomaterials typically utilize covalent or non-covalent modifications that trigger structural or chemical changes in response to enzyme presence. Common mechanisms include enzyme-catalysed cleavage, polymer degradation, and enzyme-induced solubility or phase transitions. A prominent approach involves the incorporation of enzyme-specific cleavable linkers within polymer matrices or hydrogels. These linkers break down in response to specific enzymes, releasing active agents or altering the material's physical properties. Enzyme-specific interactions ensure that biomaterial degradation or transformation occurs selectively in targeted regions, such as inflamed tissues where enzyme levels are elevated. For instance, MMPs, often found elevated in cancerous tissues, can specifically target MMP-responsive linkers within biomaterials, causing a targeted release of anticancer drugs [13].

Enzyme-responsive biomaterials can be classified on the basis of the nature of the enzyme–substrate interaction and the type of biomaterial used. Hydrogels, NPs, and micelles are frequently designed with enzyme-sensitive linkers or cross-linkers that are degraded by specific enzymes. For instance, gelatine-based hydrogels are susceptible to protease enzymes, enabling degradation and release of embedded drugs in areas of high protease activity. Additionally, polymeric NPs with peptide linkers sensitive to esterase have been shown to release encapsulated drugs upon ester bond cleavage. Design strategies often incorporate site-specific linkers or functional groups into polymer chains, which provide both structural stability and enzymatic selectivity. A typical example includes polymer systems containing peptides that are cleaved by caspase enzymes, allowing for apoptosis-specified drug delivery in cancer remedy. Hence, the targeted and controlled nature of enzyme-responsive biomaterials makes them ideal for an array of biomedical applications. In drug delivery, these materials provide site-specific activation, allowing for higher drug concentrations at diseased sites while minimizing off-target effects. Enzyme-responsive systems have also shown promise in diagnostics, where enzyme activity can be used as a biomarker to trigger signal generation, aiding in the detection of disease states [14].

6.2.4 Light-Responsive Biomaterials

Light-responsive biomaterials are a sub-set of "smart materials" that respond to external light stimuli, exhibiting a change in the physical or chemical properties involving shape, colour, conductivity, or permeability. These materials leverage specific photochromic, photothermal, and photochemical processes to trigger responses that can be precisely controlled, thus providing significant perks in biomedical engineering applications. Light-responsive biomaterials operate primarily through three mechanisms: photothermal, photochemical, and photomechanical processes. Each mechanism utilizes different molecular dynamics and reactions in response to light, depending on the wavelength and intensity [15]. The mechanisms are as follows.

6.2.4.1 Photothermal Mechanism

The photothermal mechanism relies on materials that convert absorbed light, especially in the near-infrared (NIR) region, into thermal energy. Upon exposure to light, materials like gold NPs or carbon-based materials (e.g., graphene) absorb photons, leading to localized heating. This localized heat can induce phase changes in the materials, triggering responses such as drug release, matrix degradation, or even cell death in hyperthermic therapies [16].

6.2.4.2 Photochemical Mechanism

Photochemical mechanisms involve light-induced chemical reactions, often involving a photosensitive chromophore within the biomaterial. When the chromophore absorbs specific wavelengths of light, it undergoes a chemical transformation, which could involve cleavage, polymerization, or isomerization. An example of this is the use of azobenzene-containing hydrogels, which undergo a trans-to-cis isomerization under ultraviolet (UV) light, causing reversible changes in shape or swelling of the hydrogel. Such systems have been exploited in drug delivery applications to release encapsulated therapeutics upon exposure to light [17].

6.2.4.3 Photomechanical Mechanism

Photomechanical mechanisms involve a direct conversion of light energy into mechanical energy, typically using molecular motors or materials that undergo structural changes under light. For instance, liquid-crystal elastomers (LCEs) can exhibit changes in alignment or orientation of their polymer chains upon exposure to UV or visible light, resulting in bending, stretching, or contracting movements. These mechanical responses are useful in soft robotics and dynamic cell scaffolding [18].

Therefore, the choice of wavelength, duration, and intensity is disease dependent and is subjected to the penetration depth required. Light-responsive biomaterials are widely used in delivery of drugs, tissue engineering, and biosensing. Their proficiency to provide spatially and temporally controlled responses makes them ideal for applications requiring precision and non-invasive control. These enable the controlled release of therapeutics by utilizing specific wavelengths to trigger drug release in target areas. This approach is particularly advantageous in cancer therapy, where localized drug release minimizes side effects. Moreover, in tissue engineering, light-responsive hydrogels can facilitate cell migration and scaffold remodelling by allowing controlled degradation or stiffening of the matrix. For example, hydrogels containing photodegradable linkers can be selectively degraded in response to light, allowing precise spatial control in tissue formation [19].

6.2.5 Dual and Multi-Responsive Systems

Dual and multi-responsive biomaterials represent a significant advancement in material science, offering unique properties that enable their performance to be modulated by multiple external stimuli. These materials are engineered to react to multiple variations in environmental conditions, such as pH, temperature, light, ionic strength, or mechanical forces at a given time, making them particularly suitable for drug delivery applications, tissue engineering, and environmental sensing. The adeptness to respond to two or more stimuli allows for greater control and precision in achieving desired outcomes in a wide extent of biomedical and industrial applications. The fundamental mechanism behind dual and multi-responsive biomaterials lies in the material's capability to undergo conformational or structural conversions in response to external stimuli. The responsiveness can arise from chemical bonds, polymer networks, or molecular switches incorporated into the material's design [20].

One of the most common approaches to dual or multi-responsiveness is the combination of temperature and pH sensitivity. Polymers like poly(N-isopropylacrylamide) (PNIPAM) exhibit a sharp switch in hydrophilicity as a function of temperature, transitioning from swollen to a collapsed form at a specific critical solution temperature (LCST). In contrast, pH-sensitive materials, like poly(acrylic acid) (PAA), undergo ionization changes that affect their swelling behaviour under different pH conditions. When combined in a single material, these two properties enable a system

TABLE 6.1
Types of Stimuli-Responsive Biomaterials, Examples and Applications

Type of Stimuli-Responsive Biomaterial	Examples of Biomaterials	Applications
Thermo-responsive biomaterial	Poly(N-isopropylacrylamide) (PNIPAM)	Drug delivery, tissue engineering, biosensors
	Poly(ethylene glycol) (PEG)	Drug delivery, tissue engineering, hydrogels
	Pluronic F-127	Drug delivery, gene delivery, wound healing
	Elastin-like polypeptides (ELPs)	Drug delivery, tissue engineering, actuators
	Hydroxypropyl cellulose (HPC)	Drug delivery, wound healing, tissue engineering
	Chitosan	Drug delivery, wound healing, tissue engineering
pH-responsive biomaterial	Poly(acrylic acid) (PAA)	Drug delivery (oral, targeted to tumours), hydrogels, tissue engineering
	Chitosan	Drug delivery (oral, nasal, ocular), wound healing, gene delivery
	Poly(lactic-co-glycolic acid) (PLGA)	Drug delivery (controlled release), sutures, tissue engineering
	Alginate	Drug delivery (oral, wound healing), cell encapsulation, tissue engineering
Light-responsive biomaterials	Azobenzene-containing polymers	Drug delivery (controlled release), photodynamic therapy, actuators
	Spiropyran-containing polymers	Drug delivery, sensors, switches, data storage
	Gold nanoparticles	Photothermal therapy, drug delivery, imaging
	Quantum dots	Bioimaging, sensors, drug delivery
Enzyme-responsive biomaterials	Peptide-based hydrogels (containing specific enzyme cleavage sites)	Drug delivery (controlled release), tissue engineering, biosensors
	Polymers with enzyme-cleavable linkages (e.g., ester, amide bonds)	Drug delivery (targeted release), gene delivery, biodegradable scaffolds
	Enzyme-responsive nanoparticles (e.g., liposomes, micelles)	Drug delivery (site-specific release), imaging, diagnostics
	Dextran-based hydrogels with enzyme-sensitive cross-links	Drug delivery, tissue engineering, wound healing
	Hyaluronic acid derivatives with enzyme-cleavable groups	Drug delivery, tissue engineering, ophthalmology

to respond to both temperature and pH stimulus, offering increased control in applications such as drug release systems, wherein precise regulation of delivery is necessary for therapeutic efficacy [21]. Another area of great interest involves combining light and chemical responsiveness. Photo-responsive biomaterials, typically incorporating photochromic compounds, undergo structural changes upon exposure to light, triggering various responses including swelling, degradation, or liberation of encapsulated molecules. For instance, azobenzene derivatives undergo a reversible trans–cis isomerization under UV or visible light, affecting their solubility and, consequently, their functionality. When combined with other responsive elements, such as pH or ionic strength sensitivity, these materials can exhibit complex, multi-responsive behaviour useful for controlled drug delivery or diagnostic applications [22]. Table 6.1 lists the various classes of stimuli-responsive biomaterials, examples of materials used, and its applications.

6.3 MECHANISMS OF ACTION OF STIMULI-RESPONSIVE BIOMATERIALS

6.3.1 Targeted Drug Delivery Systems

Inflammatory diseases comprehend a plethora of conditions characterized by an overactive immune response, leading to chronic inflammation that can harm tissues and impair normal physiological functions. Disorders like rheumatoid arthritis (RA), Crohn's disease, and atherosclerosis are marked by persistent inflammation that poses significant challenges for conventional treatment approaches. Traditional therapies typically utilize anti-inflammatory medications that circulate throughout the body, often resulting in undesirable side effects and insufficient targeting of the inflamed regions. In contrast, stimuli-responsive biomaterials present an innovative solution to these challenges by delivering therapeutic agents in response to particular environmental changes linked to inflammation, including variations in pH, increased temperature, heightened enzyme activity, or the occurrence of ROS. By selectively responding to these indicators, these materials facilitate localized treatment, thereby minimizing side effects and enhancing the overall efficiency of the therapy. This section delves into the mechanisms of action of stimuli-responsive biomaterials in the context of inflammatory diseases, with a focus on their potential to regulate the inflammatory response and stimulate tissue regeneration [23]. The mechanism of action employed by targeted drug delivery systems (DDS) are as follows.

6.3.1.1 pH-Responsive Mechanism

pH-responsive biomaterials exploit the acidic environmental characteristics of certain disease sites, such as tumour tissues, inflammatory sites, or intra-cellular compartments like lysosomes. In these areas, the pH is lower (often between 5.5 and 6.8 for tumours and 4.5 and 5.5 in lysosomes) compared to physiological pH (7.4). pH-responsive biomaterials are often formulated with acid-sensitive bonds or ionizable groups that become protonated in acidic conditions. This protonation changes the solubility or structure of the material, promoting the release of encapsulated drugs [9, 10].

6.3.1.2 Temperature-Responsive Mechanism

Temperature-responsive materials are engineered to undergo phase transitions at specific temperatures, often slightly above normal body temperature (~37°C). When exposed to a hyperthermic environment, as can occur in inflamed or tumour tissues, these materials undergo physical or chemical changes that lead to drug release. Typically, these materials exhibit a LCST, where they switch from a hydrophilic (soluble) to a hydrophobic (insoluble) state, resulting in aggregation or volume shrinkage that drives drug release [8].

6.3.1.3 Enzyme-Responsive Mechanism

Enzyme-responsive biomaterials cash in on the elevated levels of specific enzymes found in diseased tissues, such as proteases, lipases, or phosphatases. These enzymes cleave specific bonds within the biomaterial, initiating degradation or disassembly and allowing for the controlled release of drugs. Enzyme-responsive biomaterials are designed with peptide sequences or ester bonds tailored to be substrates for these enzymes, ensuring that the material remains stable in healthy tissues but degrades in enzyme-rich disease environments [12].

6.3.1.4 Light-Responsive Mechanism

Light-responsive biomaterials incorporate photosensitive moieties, such as azobenzene or spiropyran, which undergo structural changes or cleavage when exposed to certain wavelengths of light. Light, especially NIR light, is ideal for drug delivery due to its ability to penetrate tissue effectively. By precisely optimizing the timing and the location of light exposure, drug delivery can be confined to the target site, minimizing off-target effects [16]. Photothermal nanomaterials, like gold NPs, absorb NIR light and convert it into heat, which can either induce the breakdown of thermo-sensitive polymers or disrupt the biomaterial matrix, allowing drug release. Another example involves polymers with photocleavable linkers, where exposure to UV or NIR light triggers bond cleavage and localized drug release [16].

6.3.1.5 Magnetic Field-Responsive Mechanism

Magnetic field-responsive biomaterials contain magnetic NPs, often made from iron oxide, which can be modulated by an external magnetic field. When subjected to an alternating magnetic field, these NPs generate localized heat through magnetic hysteresis, which can disrupt the biomaterial's structure or activate temperature-sensitive mechanisms for drug release. This approach allows for the remote control of drug liberation, guiding NPs to the target site, and selectively releasing the drug. A personalized feature of this therapy is that the rate of drug release can be regulated by optimizing the direction and strength of the magnetic field [24].

6.3.1.6 Electric Field-Responsive Mechanism

Electric field-responsive biomaterials utilize conductive or dielectric properties that enable structural or conformational alterations in response to electric fields. The field can alter the physical structure of these materials, causing swelling, shrinking, or releasing charged molecules. Electric fields can also cause electrochemical reactions that disrupt the biomaterial's structure, providing a method for on-demand drug release. Conductive polymers, such as polypyrene or polyaniline, are often used in electric-responsive systems. When an electric field is applied, these polymers change their oxidation state, which can cause them to expand or contract, releasing drugs [24].

6.3.1.7 Ultrasound-Responsive Mechanism

Ultrasound-responsive biomaterials have also fascinated the research world. These biomaterials can increase drug penetration due to inertial cavitation, substantially decreasing inflammation and providing immediate pain relief. Recently, sonophoresis has become a hot topic in drug delivery aspects. Herein, the therapeutic agents encapsulated in the biomaterials have the capability to respond to ultrasound stimulation and thus are known as ultrasound-responsive biomaterials. Individualized treatment regimens are possible in relation to the progression of the disease [7].

6.3.1.8 ROS-Responsive Mechanism

ROS-responsive biomaterials respond to higher levels of hydroxy radicals ($^{\bullet}OH$), superoxide (O^{2-}) or hydrogen peroxide (H_2O_2) formed during inflammation. These ROS modify or cleave specific linkages or functional groups loaded in the biomaterials to release the encapsulated drug which could be either ROS scavengers or antioxidants [25].

6.3.2 Controlled Release in Response to Inflammatory Markers

Controlled release systems that respond to inflammatory markers represent a significant innovation in drug delivery. Such systems are designated to release therapeutic molecules in a sustained manner in response to specific stimuli linked to inflammation, providing targeted treatment with reduced side effects and enhanced efficacy. Inflammation, characterized by biochemical changes such as pH drop, enzyme production, and oxidative stress, provides a fertile ground for these systems to activate in disease-affected areas [26]. Inflammatory markers are biomolecules that are either upregulated or released in response to inflammation, indicating the presence and intensity of an inflammatory response. They play a central role in the development and progression of various diseases, including autoimmune disorders, infections, and cancer. Leveraging these markers as triggers for controlled drug release systems is a promising approach in targeted therapies, as they allow for site-specific activation of drug carriers within inflamed tissues. In inflammation, various markers are upregulated, creating a distinctive microenvironment. These markers can serve as triggers for stimuli-responsive DDS, enabling controlled drug delivery only in the presence of inflammation [12]. The following inflammatory markers act as a stimulus for controlled release.

6.3.2.1 Cytokines

Cytokines are small signalling proteins that regulate immune responses and are released by immune cells during inflammation. The key cytokines involved in inflammatory processes include the following:

- *Tumour Necrosis Factor-alpha (TNF-α)*: TNF-α is one of the primary pro-inflammatory cytokines, playing a pivotal role in the modulation of immune cells. Its levels are elevated in chronic inflammatory diseases such as inflammatory bowel disease (IBD) and RA. DDS made to respond to TNF-α can effectively target areas of inflammation by releasing anti-inflammatory agents when TNF-α is detected in high concentrations [27].
- *Interleukins (e.g., IL-1, IL-6, IL-8)*: Interleukins are produced in response to infections or injuries and promote inflammation. For instance, IL-1 and IL-6 are known to amplify inflammatory responses and are elevated in conditions such as sepsis and arthritis. Controlled-release systems that respond to interleukin levels can be designed with antibodies or aptamers that bind specifically to these cytokines, releasing therapeutic agents as a direct response to the elevated interleukin levels [27].

6.3.2.2 Reactive Oxygen Species (ROS)

Reactive oxygen species are byproducts of cellular metabolism, which are dramatically increased during inflammation due to the stimulation of immune cells like macrophages and neutrophils. ROS act as signalling molecules to further propagate the inflammatory response, but in high concentrations, they can damage tissues. ROS-responsive DDS are designed with ROS-sensitive linkers (e.g., thioketals or pro-oxidant-sensitive bonds) that degrade in the presence of elevated ROS levels, releasing the drug specifically at sites of inflammation. This is especially valuable in treating diseases characterized by oxidative stress, such as atherosclerosis, RA, and neurodegenerative disorders [28].

6.3.2.3 Matrix Metalloproteinases (MMPs)

MMPs are a group of enzymes that break down the extracellular matrix and are overexpressed in inflammatory and tumour environments. MMPs facilitate tissue remodelling and immune cell migration, crucial for the progression of inflammation. In diseases like cancer, arthritis, and cardiovascular disease, the levels of MMPs, specifically MMP-2 and MMP-9, are significantly elevated. MMP-responsive DDS often incorporate peptide sequences cleavable by these enzymes. Upon exposure to MMPs, the peptide bonds are cleaved, releasing the therapeutic payload specifically within the inflamed tissue. This strategy minimizes off-target effects, as the drug remains inactive in normal tissue where MMP levels are low [29].

6.3.2.4 Prostaglandins

Prostaglandins are lipid compounds that mediate inflammation and pain. They are synthesized by cyclooxygenase (COX) enzymes in response to inflammation and are involved in the dilation of blood vessels and the modulation of immune responses. Elevated levels of prostaglandins, such as prostaglandin E2 (PGE2), are commonly observed in conditions like arthritis and certain cancers. DDS responsive to prostaglandins are still under development, but they present potential for controlled drug release by detecting increased prostaglandin levels and responding with anti-inflammatory or pain-relieving agents [30].

6.3.2.5 C-Reactive Protein (CRP)

CRP is a protein made by the liver in response to inflammation, and it serves as a systemic marker of inflammation. Elevated levels of CRP are linked to inflammatory diseases, including cardiovascular diseases, infections, and autoimmune conditions. While CRP-responsive DDS are still in preliminary research, they hold potential for the development of treatments that respond to systemic inflammation and provide a tailored release of therapeutics [31].

6.3.2.6 Interactions with Immune Cells

The immune system responds to inflammatory markers with specific cellular interactions that activate various pathways to target infections, repair tissue, and modulate inflammation. Stimuli-responsive biomaterials interact with these immune cells to regulate inflammatory diseases [32]. Key players involving complex signalling pathways include the following.

6.3.2.7 Macrophage Activation

During infections, macrophages exhibit polarized responses (M1 for pro-inflammatory and M2 for anti-inflammatory) to eliminate pathogens and regulate inflammation. For example, studies using zebrafish models show that macrophages enhance IL-1β expression during infections, crucial for managing chronic inflammation [32].

6.3.2.8 Neutrophil Response

Neutrophils play an essential role in inflammatory responses by releasing cytokines like IL-8, which amplify the recruitment of other immunomodulatory cells to infection sites. In models of infections such as those with *Mycobacterium abscessus*, neutrophils help form protective granulomas around pathogens [32].

6.3.2.9 Cytokine Signalling

Cytokines, such as IL-1β, TNF-α and IL-6, regulate inflammatory pathways like NF-κB, pivotal for immune cell activation. For example, the NF-κB pathway is essential for recruiting leukocytes to the site of infection, promoting a balanced immune response to ensure tissue repair without excessive inflammation [32].

6.3.2.10 Inflammasomes

Inflammasomes like NLRP3 are activated by pathogens and cellular stress, inducing IL-1β production, which drives further immune cell activation and inflammation. This pathway is critical in both acute and chronic inflammation settings, underscoring the need for balance to prevent excessive immune reactions [32]. Hence, stimuli-responsive biomaterials work by varied mechanisms of action whilst curbing inflammatory diseases, from acting as targeted DDS and controlling release in response to inflammatory markers to interacting with immune cells. Several inflammatory disorders like atherosclerosis, RA, OA, IBD, central nervous system-related diseases among many others can be tackled by the introduction of stimuli-responsive biomaterials. Its application in few of the listed inflammatory diseases has been mentioned below.

6.4 BIOMATERIALS IN SPECIFIC INFLAMMATORY DISEASES

6.4.1 Rheumatoid Arthritis (RA)

RA is also known as "Inflammatory arthritis". It mainly involves the activation of various T-cells. Additionally, production of rheumatoid factor (RF) and anti-citrullinated protein antibodies (ACPA) by B-cells along with secretion of enzyme phospholipase-D (PLD) elevates inflammation and pain. Several biomarkers such as miRNA, cytokines, and enzymes are used in stimuli-responsive biomaterials for the detection and treatment of RA [7].

Literature indicates that a temperature-responsive hydrogel was formed which could counteract pain, motor impairment, and hyperalgesia associated with RA. Encapsulation efficiency of the loaded carbonic anhydrase inhibitor (CAI)—a pain-relieving molecule was around 90% and controlled released for more than 72 hours was observed. A significant reduction in inflammatory cytokines was also seen when a thermo-sensitive sodium hyaluronate and methyl cellulose (SHMC) hydrogel was formulated, incorporated with methotrexate (MTX) alginate microparticles. Similarly, a phenethyl isothiocyanate (PEITC)-loaded thermo-responsive hydrogel exhibited anti-inflammatory activity and addressed RA-associated symptoms and bone erosion issues. Further, the JAK-STAT pathway was significantly inhibited when pH-sensitive acetylated dextran NPs were encapsulated with MTX, thus lowering the severity of RA. Additionally, the macrophages were targeted through their scavenger receptors via enzyme-responsive dextran sulphate-based NPs to deliver celastrol (Cel). The NPs were modified such that it formed a dextran-sulphate-PVGLIG-Cel composite. Similar Cel-loaded NPs were engineered to be ROS-responsive as well, on modification with folic acid [7].

RA is largely found to be triggered by ROS which induces inflammation. Hence, an ultrasound-responsive 2D piezoelectric nanosheet was developed which could induce autophagy at the inflammation site, thus eliminating free radicals. Subsequently, ultrasound-based nanocomplex was developed to detect and treat RA by impeding the JAK-STAT and NF-κB pathways. Detection was facilitated by cleavage of hyaluronic acid matrix which releases aggregation-induced emission (AIE)-active chromophore and treated via release of upadacitinib. However, optimization of appropriate ultrasound parameters remains a challenge yet to be tackled. Recently, magneto-responsive biomaterials like meloxicam-loaded chitosan-magnetite nanoconjugates (MC-MNCs) were constructed for alleviation of RA symptoms and side effects and to lower the dose frequency. The release profile followed Michaelis–Menten kinetics by showing an initial burst release eventually followed by continued release. In spite of showing exemplary results, application of stimuli-responsive biomaterials for treatment of RA is accompanied with a few shortcomings. These include improper optimization of the biomaterial type, which might lead to aggregation of the formulations. Additionally, the drugs bioavailability may be affected because of the adage that inflammatory disorders constitute a high-density ECM [7]. Nonetheless, ongoing research and advancements in biomaterials will provide a much more effective solution to overcome this debilitating disease [25].

6.4.2 Osteoarthritis (OA)

OA associated with chronic low-grade inflammation is a joint disorder. The anomaly of inflammatory mediators further worsens up the situation, disturbing the balance, resulting in a joint failure. Calming down the inflammation via non-surgical remedies employs administering anti-inflammatory drugs to relieve temporary discomfort. In order to completely ward off the progression of OA, surgical interventions become a more reliable approach, which comes with its own drawbacks. Hence, biomaterials forming hydrogels, NPs, or tissue engineering scaffolds have caught the attention of researchers in recent times [2].

Hydrogel-forming biomaterials can be drug-loaded to perform cartilaginous tissue repair in a minimally invasive manner and could also stimulate the environment of ECM. A recombinant adeno-associated virus (rAAV)-loaded injectable hydrogel capable of overexpressing SOX-9 was presented to enhance cartilage repair. Another study highlights the development of a similarly administered hydrogel but this time mixed with epigallocatechin-3-gallate (EGCG) to serve a dual purpose of enhancing cartilage repair and scavenging ROS. In contrast, cleavable hydrogels loaded with BMSCs were fabricated to counter osteochondral defects. Furthermore, a composite hydrogel was formulated by combining chitosan, nanohydroxyapatite, and beta-glycerol phosphate which possessed osteogenic properties [2].

In addition to hydrogels, NP-forming biomaterials have also paved its way in OA management. Li et al. reported the downregulation of synovial inflammatory mediators by using polyethyleneimine-modified mesoporous silica nanospheres which promoted tissue self-repair. Moreover, articular cartilage ECM was prevented from being degraded by preparing folic acid and hyaluronic acid-targeted dendrimer nanocages which released carbonic acid (CO), which in turn depleted hydrogen peroxide levels hence resulting in a reduced inflammatory cytokine expression. Hydroxychloroquine-encapsulated ferritin nanocages were developed to detect the overproduction of MMP-13 and the surrounding acidic environment to release hydroxychloroquine in response. Hence, this is an example of dual-stimuli-responsive biomaterial coupling the advantages of both enzyme-responsive and pH-responsive biomaterials. Therefore, OA although incurable, the use of such biomaterials can to a great extent relieve the symptoms, suppress inflammation, promote tissue repair and regeneration, and thus keep OA in control [2]. Nevertheless, further advances in biomaterial design and synthesis can strengthen its efficiency, making it a more potent alternative not only for OA but also for several other disease treatments.

6.4.3 Inflammatory Bowel Disease (IBD)

In the management and cure of IBD, which comprises Crohn's disease and ulcerative colitis, biomaterials have shown great promise. These cutting-edge materials seek to promote tissue healing in the gastrointestinal (GI) tract, reduce inflammation, and provide targeted medicines. Biomaterials such as hydrogels and NPs are made to distribute anti-inflammatory medications straight to the gut's inflammatory areas. This focused strategy minimizes the frequency of dose, improves therapeutic efficacy, and lowers systemic adverse effects. Biocompatible scaffolds and injectable hydrogels offer a supporting matrix that can shield and encourage the healing of injured intestinal tissues. Additionally, they can be used as delivery systems for localized cell or medication therapy [33, 34]. Moreover, stem cells can be encapsulated in biomaterials to promote their viability and guide their distribution to injured tissues. IBD-affected intestinal tissues may be repaired by stem cell treatment in conjunction with biomaterial carriers. Hence, biomaterials or stimuli-responsive biomaterials provide a possible route to more individualized and successful IBD management options by combining tissue engineering, cell therapy, and drug delivery [33, 34].

6.4.4 Psoriasis

Psoriasis is a chronic inflammatory skin disease that can be treated with biomaterials, which are emerging as cutting-edge tools. Biomaterials offer a number of exciting uses by improving therapeutic efficacy and facilitating targeted medication delivery. NPs, liposomes, and hydrogels can be made to encapsulate anti-inflammatory and immunosuppressive medications, releasing them exactly at the psoriatic lesions. This targeted distribution lowers the necessary dosage and minimizes negative effects while increasing therapeutic effectiveness [35].

Bypassing the systemic circulation and reducing the effect on other body areas, biomaterial-based microneedles and patches administer medications straight via the skin. Additionally, these choices provide patients with convenient, painless administration. Scaffolds composed of biocompatible materials offer cell-based therapies, structural support, and enable the distribution of cells that alter immune responses or encourage the repair of injured skin tissue. Thus, biomaterials are creating new opportunities for more efficient and patient-centred psoriasis management by improving medication transport, facilitating cell treatments, and providing localized therapeutic choices [36].

6.4.5 Autoimmune Disorders

Through the provision of targeted therapies, the reduction of systemic effects, and the modulation of immune responses, biomaterials are revolutionizing the management of autoimmune illnesses. Localized drug distribution to certain inflammatory areas is made possible by biomaterials like hydrogels and NPs. This lowers the dosage needed and lessens the adverse effects of immunosuppressive medications used to treat autoimmune conditions including lupus and RA. Additionally, bioengineered scaffolds can help control aberrant immune responses by directly releasing cytokines or other immunomodulatory substances into afflicted tissues. By promoting tissue regeneration and regulating immunological function, these scaffolds show potential in diseases like multiple sclerosis [37]. Moreover, by encasing therapeutic cells in biocompatible materials, substances that inhibit negative immune responses can be released continuously while shielding the cells from immunological rejection. Because encapsulated cells can release insulin in reaction to glucose levels, this becomes essential for autoimmune diabetes. Therefore, biomaterials provide novel avenues for precision medicine in autoimmune diseases by combining these strategies, improving therapy effectiveness while reducing adverse effects and promoting immune system homeostasis [38].

6.5 ADVANCES IN MATERIAL DESIGN AND SYNTHESIS

6.5.1 Nanoparticles and Nanocomposites

Advances in material design and synthesis of stimuli-responsive NPs and nanocomposites have contributed significantly to the progress and efficacy of biomaterials. Nanocarrier-equipped biomaterials can pose significant advantages in addition to sustained release. It offers higher protection to drugs which are vulnerable to inactivation and at the same time prevents any prior release. While, surface modifications are one of the preliminary advancements. The importance of pH has been repeatedly highlighted when it comes to inflammation. Hence, pH-responsive NP-forming biomaterials was shaped using atom transfer radical polymerization technique and radical polymerization techniques which can self-assemble and mimic the physiological environment. To regulate macrophages, quaternized poly(β-amino ester) (QPBAE-C18) and HA-*g*-vitamin E succinate (HA-VE) NPs were engineered which were pH-responsive. Additionally, some materials are now synthesized to form higher-order assemblies such as core-shell NPs that can adapt to pH fluctuations, which enhances stability and functionality in drug delivery applications [39].

A plethora of NPs which are formed could be photo responsive, namely carbon NPs, black phosphorous-based NPs, graphene organic NPs, Au NPs, etc. Consequently, a film method was used to construct light-responsive PEG liposomes, radiolabelled with a chelator showing significant reduction in inflammation. Another study synthesized liposomes such that it contained folic acid, cyanine dye, and haemoglobin for specialized targeting, photosensitization and, to provide therapeutic effects, respectively. The NPs can be made to be magneto-responsive with the polymer coating being PVA, dextran, or PEG. These NPs respond to the external magnetic field. To overcome temperature fluctuations in the case of temperature-responsive biomaterials, an autonomous and synergetic dual drug delivery system loaded with diclofenac and kartogenin was developed. In a recent study, hermos-sensitive P (AN-co-Aam)-PEG micelles incorporated with intra-cellular adhesion molecule (ICAM-1) conjugated tofacitinib which was further developed for temperature-sensitive targeting delivery [7]. Nanozymes are another set of nanocomposites combining the properties of NPs and enzymes. They have been used to target a number of inflammatory diseases. For example, an MMP-2-responsive peptide linkage and MTX (in the hydrophobic core) were loaded into cationic PEG NPs that had the ability to scavenge cell-free DNA and provide immediate pain relief [40].

Recently, dual and multi-stimuli-responsive biomaterials are synthesized for added benefits. These respond to more than one internal or external cues [7]. Dual stimuli-responsive biomaterial was developed by Zhou F et al. comprising both enzyme-responsive and ROS-responsive strategies. Herein, rhein- and ceria oxide-loaded, thioethyl linker-based hyaluronic acid NPs were formed. Cleavage of thioethyl linker by ROS-released Ce and rhein which exhibited SOD activity to inhibit ROS and ensured therapeutic effect, respectively [41]. Hence, multi-responsive biomaterials can strike down the drawbacks of single stimulus-responsive biomaterials and thus provide better precision, specificity, and efficacy.

6.5.2 Hydrogel

Hydrogel systems are a great option especially in inflammatory disease management as they have the ability to revive the ECM microenvironment [2]. They possess innumerable properties such as sheer thinning, the ability to mimic ECM, and other physiochemical characteristics. Quite a few advances in hydrogel compositions have been observed. A study showed the use of a Schiff-based reaction to form a cross-linked PEG and chitosan hydrogel. Further advancements included the formulation of a composite hydrogel scaffold composed of sodium methacrylate and oligo polyethylene glycol fumarate (PEG-F). In order to upgrade the structure and properties of hydrogels, cross-linked hydrogels have been largely developed using cross-linking agents [42]. Moreover, UV-initiated cross-linked hydrogels which initiates cross-linking only when exposed to UV light were formed by embedding cross-linkers and photo initiators in the hydrogel biomaterial matrix which on exposure to UV forms free radicals encouraging cross-linking which in turn facilitates sustained drug release. With a similar concept, the development of near infra-red light-responsive biomaterials [7] further exhibits photocrosslinked under specific light wavelength. Enzyme-based cross-linked hydrogels are another recent technique. Fuchs S et al. formed gelatin hydrogels which cross-linked in the presence of transglutaminase enzyme. Also, an excellent biodegradable and anti-rejection, self-assembling peptide hydrogel was fabricated containing 2D nanomaterials with enzyme-like action. Furthermore, stimuli-responsive hydrogels have also undergone couple of modifications. A dual temperature and pH-responsive hydrogel was created integrating two separate polymers. Sumlar to NPs, multi-responsive biomaterials have been developed in the case of hydrogels as a single stimulus might not be sufficient enough to counter the severity of such multifaceted inflammatory diseases. Scientists are on a hunt for other distinctive stimuli apart from the ones in discussion such as ATP-responsiveness. Hence, in order to ensure optimum accuracy and maximum efficiency, research advancements in material design and synthesis of stimuli-responsive biomaterials are constant, thus revolutionizing and bringing about a paradigm shift in inflammatory disease management [7].

6.5.3 Biodegradable Polymers

In order to come up with biodegradable polymers, biomimetic designs are used for synthesizing biomaterials. This design is based on natural materials, such as peptide-based polymers, and produce degradation profiles that are both environmentally responsive and adaptable. Green Chemistry Methods utilizing low-waste procedures and renewable feedstocks to increase sustainability are also used. Further, the characteristics of polymers can be precisely regulated using methods like ring-opening and controlled radical polymerization [43].

By increasing mechanical strength and stability, nano-structuring using nanocomposites improves durability for variety of applications. Applications like tissue engineering, medication delivery, and controlled-release systems are supported by functionalized polymers. The linkages that are pH-responsive and enzyme-sensitive enable targeted degradation in particular conditions, which is helpful in the sectors of medicine. Moreover, waste can be decreased by reprocessing biodegradable polymers, such as PLA, thanks to chemical recycling and closed-loop systems. Hence, by addressing performance and cost concerns, these developments in material design and synthesis can increase the usefulness of biodegradable polymers in a variety of industries [44].

6.5.4 Smart Scaffolds

To greatly improve regenerative medicine and tissue engineering applications, advancements in the design and synthesis of smart scaffolds concentrate on developing materials that dynamically interact with cells and react to environmental stimuli. Few significant advancements include smart scaffolds that are made to react to environmental variables like temperature, pH, or certain enzymes. This supports targeted therapy by allowing regulated drug release or scaffold disintegration only in specific circumstances. Also, biofunctionalization is stimulated by growth factors, peptides, or extracellular matrix constituents. These are bioactive compounds that functionalize scaffolds, encouraging proliferation, cell adhesion, and differentiation—all of which are critical for tissue healing [45]. Additionally using bioinks in 3D printing enables accurate scaffold topologies and adaptable pore structures, which enhance diffusion and cell infiltration. Particularly in tissues like nerve and muscle, electro-conductive biomaterials used into scaffolds can encourage cell signalling and regeneration. On the other hand, adding NPs, like carbon nanotubes or hydroxyapatite, improves mechanical qualities and adds bioactivity, making them helpful for repairing bone and cartilage. Hence, these developments increase the efficacy and versatility of smart scaffolds for a series of regenerative medicine applications [45].

6.6 PRECLINICAL AND CLINICAL STUDIES

6.6.1 Overview of Preclinical Trials in Animal Models

Preclinical research in animal models has shown encouraging results, which has increased interest in the formulation of stimuli-responsive biomaterials for the healing of inflammatory illnesses in recent years. Certain physiological or pathological stimuli, such as pH shifts, oxidative stress, or temperature variations, which are frequently seen in inflammatory tissues, are what these biomaterials are made to react to. Stimuli-responsive biomaterials present a potential therapeutic method that may reduce off-target effects frequently associated with systemic anti-inflammatory medications by directly targeting inflammatory processes [46]. With the purpose of assessing the effectiveness and safety of stimuli-responsive biomaterials before clinical trials, preclinical animal models are essential. The complicated physiological circumstances that biomaterials experience in human inflammatory disorders can be simulated in vivo using animal models of inflammatory diseases. Because of their genetically manipulable nature and well-characterized immune systems, rodents—especially mice and rats—are frequently utilized in research to monitor biomaterial reactions and create specialized inflammatory situations [47].

The most commonly utilized animal models are chemically produced colitis models for IBD, high-fat diet-induced obesity models for metabolic inflammation, and collagen-induced arthritis (CIA) models for RA. The distinct inflammatory settings found in each of these models allow for the testing of the biomaterials' stimuli-responsiveness in a range of disease circumstances [48]. Following are types of stimuli-responsive biomaterials wherein animal models have been used for preclinical trails.

6.6.1.1 pH-Responsive Biomaterials

The pH-sensitive drug delivery characteristics of chitosan-based hydrogels have been extensively investigated in rodent models, demonstrating improved therapeutic efficacy in lowering local inflammation in models of colitis and arthritis. pH-sensitive nanocarriers containing anti-inflammatory medications have been shown to efficiently target arthritic joints, minimizing systemic toxicity while lowering inflammation and joint damage in animal experiments [49].

6.6.1.2 Oxidative Stress-Responsive Biomaterials

In preclinical research, oxidative stress-responsive polymers that release antioxidants or anti-inflammatory drugs only in plaques have been tested in animal models targeting atherosclerosis, demonstrating promise in lowering inflammation and plaque progression. To reduce inflammation and promote tissue healing, ROS-sensitive micelles loaded with antioxidants, for instance, have shown notable therapeutic effects in murine colitis models by specifically lowering oxidative damage in the inflamed colon [50].

6.6.1.3 Thermo-Responsive Biomaterials

These biomaterials have been examined in animal models, particularly in models of arthritis and infection-induced inflammation, where temperature-responsive hydrogels and NPs liberate therapeutic medicines when subjected to high temperatures as seen in inflammatory tissues. The use of thermo-responsive liposomes in bacterial infection models has shown promise. Liposomal formulations containing antibiotics augment therapeutic efficacy while lowering systemic exposure and related side effects by selectively releasing the drug at infection sites [51].

6.6.1.4 Multi-Stimuli-Responsive Biomaterials

As inflammation has several facets, in complex inflammatory settings, recent research in mouse models of colitis has shown the use of multi-responsive hydrogels that release anti-inflammatory medications in response to both pH and ROS levels, exhibiting better therapeutic efficacy and lesser side effects [51].

6.6.2 Clinical Translation and Trials

Preclinical studies of recent developments in stimuli-responsive biomaterials have shown promise; for instance, smart hydrogels that alter their properties in response to environmental stimuli can encapsulate anti-inflammatory agents and release them when triggered. Also, NPs engineered to release anti-inflammatory drugs at sites of inflammation have shown improved drug delivery efficiency [52]. Considering these developments, many formulations are undergoing clinical testing, making the transition from laboratory research to clinical applications. Phase I trials are performed to evaluate safety in a minimized group of human participants; Phase II trials evaluate efficacy in a larger group with the target inflammatory disease; Phase III trials involve large-scale testing compared to standard treatments; and successful trials result in submissions for regulatory approval from bodies such as the FDA. These phases comprise the research to the clinical application pathway. Only a small number of stimulus-responsive biomaterials for inflammatory illnesses are currently in advanced clinical trial stages [53].

Recent efforts have focused on creating DDS that can efficiently release therapeutic medications in response to the special conditions observed at inflammatory sites. Applications of stimuli-responsive biomaterials have shown potential in a number of inflammatory conditions, and hydrogels that react to stimuli specific to inflammation are being investigated for their capacity to release anti-inflammatory agents in a controlled manner, addressing cartilage degeneration and synovitis. Targeted NPs have been improved to deliver anti-inflammatory drugs directly to inflamed joints in RA, thereby significantly reducing cartilage destruction and joint swelling without contributing to toxic effects. Recent developments have demonstrated its use in tissue engineering and medication delivery. For example, hydrogels that mimic the extracellular matrix of the brain can release molecules drugs in accordance to environmental stimuli that help to treat brain illnesses. Furthermore, these substances are also known to promote healing in diseases such as OA and osteoporosis by modifying their characteristics to match those of the surrounding tissues, thereby improving bone regeneration [54].

Despite these developments, several restrictions prevent stimuli-responsive biomaterials from being widely used in clinical settings. One major obstacle is the complexity of the inflammatory environment; the biochemical makeup of inflammatory tissues can differ significantly between patients and even between different parts of the same tissue. This heterogeneity makes it difficult to build biomaterials that work everywhere. Furthermore, it is challenging to precisely regulate medication release rates because of competing biological molecules and material degradation rates. Moreover, there are still issues associated with biocompatibility and long-term safety, since many materials that show great biocompatibility in vitro might be harmful in vivo due to breakdown products or unexpected immune reactions. Hence, it might take a significant amount of time to navigate the regulatory environment for new biomaterials, which might in turn delay the clinical application of such promising research [55].

6.7 CHALLENGES IN CLINICAL APPLICATIONS

The most important factor for any biomaterial used in a clinical setting is biocompatibility. Stimuli-responsive materials must guarantee minimal negative effects on adjacent tissues, in addition to the efficient delivery of medications. Cytotoxicity is a major concern, as many of these materials can be harmful, especially when they break down within the body. Some polymeric nanogels, for example, may degrade and release toxic byproducts, raising concerns about their long-term safety in vivo. Immune reactions can also be triggered by introducing foreign elements. Hence, it is important to carefully develop materials to prevent systemic immunosuppression or unintended inflammatory reactions that could harm healthy tissues, even though some materials are made to positively modulate immune responses. Long-term stability is also important because erratic responses to stimuli can result in unpredictable drug release profiles, which could make the therapy unsafe [56].

There are additional challenges in producing stimuli-responsive biomaterials on a wide scale once they have been synthesized in a laboratory. It can be difficult to achieve uniformity in material quality during mass manufacturing because different synthesis conditions can result in discrepancies that impair performance. Furthermore, the cost of many sophisticated biomaterial production procedures restricts their accessibility and commercial feasibility. It is imperative to develop cost-effective techniques for mass production without sacrificing quality. In addition, incorporating new materials into well-established pharmaceutical production processes frequently necessitates extensive validation and changes, which can be expensive and time-consuming, thus further complicating the scaling-up process for mass production [57]. The clinical implementation of these novel biomaterials depends on the navigation of the regulatory environment. New materials should undergo extensive preclinical and clinical testing to meet the regulatory bodies' requirements for thorough data on their safety and effectiveness, which can greatly extend the approval process. Regulatory bodies find it challenging to evaluate the safety and effectiveness of stimuli-responsive materials regularly because of the absence of established techniques for assessing their performance. Approval delays may result from this discrepancy, as businesses may have to carry out more research to satisfy regulatory requirements. Finally, post-market surveillance is critical; continuous observation of long-term impacts is vital because regulatory frameworks need to be modified to incorporate rules designed, especially for innovative biomaterials that react dynamically to physiological changes [58].

6.8 FUTURE PERSPECTIVES AND INNOVATIONS

Biomedicine is changing due to new emerging biomaterial design technologies, especially in tissue engineering, medication delivery, and regenerative medicine. Tissues like skin and liver can be precisely constructed via 3D bioprinting, which may lead to the creation of patient-specific, transplantable tissues. Biomaterials are improved by nanotechnology with characteristics like enhanced cell adhesion and targeted medication release, which are particularly helpful in the treatment of cancer. Bioactive materials provide flexible implants and intelligent wound dressings by releasing medications in response to stimuli. Self-healing materials reduce the need for procedures and prolong implant life by imitating natural tissues. While artificial intelligence (AI) speeds up research by optimizing material compositions, decellularized scaffolds offer biocompatible frameworks for organ regeneration. Biodegradable materials decrease difficulties by disintegrating spontaneously and providing temporary support. Collectively, these developments propel safer, more individualized, and flexible medical solutions, transforming patient care in the future. By incorporating lifestyle, environmental, and genetic factors into treatment, personalized medicine customizes healthcare for each patient. One important component of pharmacogenomics is genomic medicine, which employs DNA analysis to determine illness risks and optimize medication selections based on genetic profiles. Biomarker analysis is also essential; by concentrating on tumour-specific indicators, the identification of particular proteins or gene expressions can direct targeted therapy, particularly in the treatment of cancer. Patient-derived cell models improve precision by enabling laboratory testing of therapy responses on a patient's cells. Furthermore, in order to forecast results and customize treatment regimens, AI examines vast amounts of patient data, including genetic and lifestyle information. Treatments are further improved by taking lifestyle and environmental factors into account, which address personal characteristics other than genetics. All things considered, these methods allow for extremely customized therapies, which may increase effectiveness, reduce adverse effects, and improve patient outcomes for a range of ailments.

6.9 CONCLUSION

Stimuli-responsive biomaterials possess the excellent ability to exhibit zestful variations in their properties in response to the surrounding stimulus and render theragnostic benefits, thus, emerging as a favourable approach especially for management of inflammatory diseases. In drug delivery, the ability to influence the release of therapeutics in response to multiple triggers enhances the precision of the treatment, minimizing side effects. For example, dual-responsive NPs are engineered to respond to these environmental cues, providing localized and controlled release of chemotherapeutic agents. Additionally, in tissue engineering, multi-responsive hydrogels can be used to create scaffolds that adapt to the changing microenvironment of regenerating tissues. These scaffolds can react to multiple cues, such as pH, temperature, or the existence of specific enzymes, to facilitate proliferation, differentiation, and cell adhesion. Furthermore, these materials can aid in mimicking the dynamic nature of the extracellular matrix, promoting better integration with host tissues. Moreover, multi-responsive biomaterials are also utilized in biosensing and diagnostic applications. For instance, a sensor that responds to both pH and ionic strength could provide real-time monitoring of conditions within biological systems, such as during tissue inflammation or infection. These materials can be used to detect biomarkers or changes in physiological conditions, offering valuable information for disease diagnosis and monitoring [59].

Hence, stimuli-responsive biomaterials have a potential future for the management of inflammatory disorders, but further research is needed. Research is still being conducted to improve targeting mechanisms by conjugating biomaterials with ligands specific to inflammatory indicators using active targeting strategies. Stimuli-responsive systems may also be more effective when combined with other therapeutic modalities and individualized treatment plans based on patient profiles that may optimize the therapeutic results. Nonetheless, the unique phenomenon of using stimuli-responsive biomaterials is largely leveraged to build a variety of smart technologies for addressing inflammatory diseases in future. Stimuli-responsive biomaterials have surfaced as a promising therapeutic approach for managing inflammatory diseases. These materials are designed to act in response to specific biological or environmental cues within the inflammatory microenvironment, enabling accurate control over drug delivery and biological activity, with minimal side effects. They can offer controlled release of therapeutic agents over extended periods, lessen the frequency of drug administration and enhance patient compliance. The development of stimuli-responsive biomaterials makes a potential impact on treating inflammatory diseases by providing targeted, controlled, and localized drug delivery. However, translating these systems from preclinical studies to clinical applications poses challenges related to safety, biocompatibility, scaling up for mass production, and managing regulatory approval procedures. Ongoing research is focused on optimizing these materials for enhanced therapeutic efficiency, minimal side effects, and scalability for clinical use [60]. Although stimuli-responsive biomaterials are a state-of-the-art method for treating inflammatory illnesses, their clinical implementation entails overcoming certain obstacles that require further study and advancements in research before their full potential in enhancing patient care can be realized.

Declaration of AI and AI-Assisted Technologies

During the preparation of this work, the authors used QuillBot AI in order to paraphrase the sentences. After using this tool, the authors reviewed and edited the content as needed and take full responsibility for the content of the publication.

REFERENCES

1. Biobaku-Mutingwende B. Introduction to biomaterials. Applications of 3D Printing in Biomedical Engineering 2021:1–19. https://doi.org/10.1007/978-981-33-6888-0_1
2. Mata R, Yao Y, Cao W, Ding J, Zhou T, Zhai Z, et al. The dynamic inflammatory tissue microenvironment: Signality and disease therapy by biomaterials. Research 2021;2021. https://doi.org/10.34133/2021/4189516
3. Ruterana GP, Chen J, Potin V, Tunable A-E, Si G, Photodetector V-S, et al. An overview on biomaterials and its applications in medical science. IOP Conference Series: Materials Science and Engineering 2021;1116:012178. https://doi.org/10.1088/1757-899X/1116/1/012178
4. Tu Z, Zhong Y, Hu H, Shao D, Haag R, Schirner M, et al. Design of therapeutic biomaterials to control inflammation. Nature Reviews Materials 2022;7:557–74. https://doi.org/10.1038/s41578-022-00426-z
5. Gallo J, Kamaly N, Lavdas I, Stevens E, Nguyen Q-D, Wylezinska-Arridge M, et al. CXCR4-targeted and MMP-responsive iron oxide nanoparticles for enhanced magnetic resonance imaging. Angewandte Chemie International Edition 2014;53:9550–4. https://doi.org/10.1002/ANIE.201405442
6. Guo J, Tao H, Dou Y, Li L, Xu X, Zhang Q, et al. A myeloperoxidase-responsive and biodegradable luminescent material for real-time imaging of inflammatory diseases. Materials Today 2017;20:493–500. https://doi.org/10.1016/J.MATTOD.2017.09.003
7. Nag S, Mohanto S, Ahmed MG, Subramaniyan V. "Smart" stimuli-responsive biomaterials revolutionizing the theranostic landscape of inflammatory arthritis. Materials Today Chemistry 2024;39:102178. https://doi.org/10.1016/J.MTCHEM.2024.102178
8. Li X, Su X. Multifunctional smart hydrogels: Potential in tissue engineering and cancer therapy. Journal of Materials Chemistry B 2018;6. https://doi.org/10.1039/c8tb01078a
9. Tang H, Zhao W, Yu J, Li Y, Zhao C. Recent development of pH-responsive polymers for cancer nanomedicine. Molecules 2019;24. https://doi.org/10.3390/molecules24010004
10. Chu S, Shi X, Tian Y, Gao F. pH-responsive polymer nanomaterials for tumor therapy. Frontiers in Oncology 2022;12. https://doi.org/10.3389/fonc.2022.855019
11. Keeler AJ, Salazar-Banda GR, Russell AE. Mechanistic insights into electrocatalytic reactions provided by SERS. Current Opinion in Electrochemistry 2019;17. https://doi.org/10.1016/j.coelec.2019.04.009
12. Hu Q, Katti PS, Gu Z. Enzyme-responsive nanomaterials for controlled drug delivery. Nanoscale 2014;6. https://doi.org/10.1039/c4nr04249b
13. Song Y, Li Y, Xu Q, Liu Z. Mesoporous silica nanoparticles for stimuli-responsive controlled drug delivery: Advances, challenges, and outlook. International Journal of Nanomedicine 2017;12. https://doi.org/10.2147/ijn.s117495
14. Pan Q, Fan X, Xie L, Wu D, Liu R, Gao W, et al. Nano-enabled colorectal cancer therapy. Journal of Controlled Release 2023;362. https://doi.org/10.1016/j.jconrel.2023.09.014
15. Wei H, Cui J, Lin K, Xie J, Wang X. Recent advances in smart stimuli-responsive biomaterials for bone therapeutics and regeneration. Bone Research 2022;10. https://doi.org/10.1038/s41413-021-00180-y

16. Lee HP, Gaharwar AK. Light-responsive inorganic biomaterials for biomedical applications. Advanced Science 2020;7. https://doi.org/10.1002/advs.202000863
17. Xiao L, Chen X, Yang X, Sun J, Geng J. Recent advances in polymer-based photothermal materials for biological applications. ACS Applied Polymer Materials 2020;2. https://doi.org/10.1021/acsapm.0c00711
18. Shi X, Zhang CY, Gao J, Wang Z. Recent advances in photodynamic therapy for cancer and infectious diseases. Wiley Interdisciplinary Reviews: Nanomedicine and Nanobiotechnology 2019;11. https://doi.org/10.1002/wnan.1560
19. Wang Y, Li J, Li X, Shi J, Jiang Z, Zhang CY. Graphene-based nanomaterials for cancer therapy and anti-infections. Bioactive Materials 2022;14. https://doi.org/10.1016/j.bioactmat.2022.01.045
20. Han Z, Wang P, Mao G, Yin T, Zhong D, Yiming B, et al. Dual pH-responsive hydrogel actuator for lipophilic drug delivery. ACS Applied Materials & Interfaces 2020;12:12010–7. https://doi.org/10.1021/acsami.9b21713
21. Zeng X, Wang H, Zhang Y, Xu X, Yuan X, Li J. pH-responsive hyaluronic acid nanoparticles for enhanced triple negative breast cancer therapy. International Journal of Nanomedicine 2022;17. https://doi.org/10.2147/IJN.S360500
22. Zhang X, Wang S, Cheng G, Yu P, Chang J. Light-responsive nanomaterials for cancer therapy. Engineering 2022;13. https://doi.org/10.1016/j.eng.2021.07.023
23. Municoy S, Álvarez Echazú MI, Antezana PE, Galdopórpora JM, Olivetti C, Mebert AM, et al. Stimuli-responsive materials for tissue engineering and drug delivery. International Journal of Molecular Sciences 2020;21. https://doi.org/10.3390/ijms21134724
24. Ge J, Neofytou E, Cahill TJ, Beygui RE, Zare RN. Drug release from electric-field-responsive nanoparticles. ACS Nano 2012;6. https://doi.org/10.1021/nn203430m
25. Salber J, Zoso A, Carmagnola I, Sobczak M. Enzyme-responsive hydrogels as potential drug delivery systems—State of knowledge and future prospects. International Journal of Molecular Sciences 2022;23:4421. https://doi.org/10.3390/IJMS23084421
26. Bae YH, Park K. Targeted drug delivery to tumors: Myths, reality and possibility. Journal of Controlled Release 2011;153. https://doi.org/10.1016/j.jconrel.2011.06.001
27. Gabay C. Interleukin-6 and chronic inflammation. Arthritis Research & Therapy 2006;8. https://doi.org/10.1186/ar1917
28. Prasad S, Gupta SC, Tyagi AK. Reactive oxygen species (ROS) and cancer: Role of antioxidative nutraceuticals. Cancer Letters 2017;387. https://doi.org/10.1016/j.canlet.2016.03.042
29. Overall CM, López-Otín C. Strategies for MMP inhibition in cancer: Innovations for the post-trial era. Nature Reviews Cancer 2002;2. https://doi.org/10.1038/nrc884
30. Ricciotti E, Fitzgerald GA. Prostaglandins and inflammation. Arteriosclerosis, Thrombosis, and Vascular Biology 2011;31. https://doi.org/10.1161/ATVBAHA.110.207449
31. Gabay C, Kushner I. Acute-phase proteins and other systemic responses to inflammation. New England Journal of Medicine 1999;340. https://doi.org/10.1056/nejm199902113400607
32. Leiba J, Özbilgiç R, Hernández L, Demou M, Lutfalla G, Yatime L, et al. Molecular actors of inflammation and their signaling pathways: Mechanistic insights from zebrafish. Biology (Basel) 2023;12. https://doi.org/10.3390/biology12020153
33. Radulescu DM, Neacsu IA, Grumezescu AM, Andronescu E. New insights of scaffolds based on hydrogels in tissue engineering. Polymers (Basel) 2022;14:1–30. https://doi.org/10.3390/polym14040799
34. Bertsch P, Diba M, Mooney DJ, Leeuwenburgh SCG. Self-healing injectable hydrogels for tissue regeneration. Chemical Reviews 2023;123:834–73. https://doi.org/10.1021/acs.chemrev.2c00179
35. Ferrara F, Verduci C, Laconi E, Mangione A, Dondi C, Vecchio M D, et al. Therapeutic advances in psoriasis: From biologics to emerging oral small molecules. Antibodies 2024;12(3):1–15.
36. Zhu B, Jing M, Yu Q, Ge X, Yuan F, Shi L. Treatments in psoriasis: From standard pharmacotherapy to nanotechnology therapy. Postepy Dermatol Alergol 2022;39:460–71. https://doi.org/10.5114/ada.2021.108445
37. Russo V, Khatib M, El, Prencipe G, Citeroni MR, Mauro A, Berardinelli P, et al. Scaffold-mediated immunoengineering as innovative strategy. Cells 2022;11:2266.
38. Mashayekhi K, Khazaie K, Faubion WA, Kim GB. Biomaterial-enhanced treg cell immunotherapy: A promising approach for transplant medicine and autoimmune disease treatment. Bioactive Materials 2024;37:269–98. https://doi.org/10.1016/j.bioactmat.2024.03.030
39. Xin Li J, Jiao Zhang M, Feng Shi J, Peng Wang S, Mei Zhong X, Han Wu Y, et al. pH-sensitive nano-polyelectrolyte complexes with arthritic macrophage-targeting delivery of triptolide. International Journal of Pharmaceutics 2023;632:122572. https://doi.org/10.1016/J.IJPHARM.2022.122572

40. Liu XH, Ding JY, Zhu ZH, Wu XC, Song YJ, Xu XL, et al. Recent advances in enzyme-related biomaterials for arthritis treatment. Frontiers in Chemistry 2022;10:988051. https://doi.org/10.3389/fchem.2022.988051
41. Zhou F, Li M, Chen M, Chen M, Chen X, Luo Z, et al. Redox homeostasis strategy for inflammatory macrophage reprogramming in rheumatoid arthritis based on ceria oxide nanozyme-complexed biopolymeric micelles. ACS Nano 2023;17:4358–72. https://doi.org/10.1021/acsnano.2c09127
42. Gao Y, Peng K, Mitragotri S. Covalently crosslinked hydrogels via step-growth reactions: Crosslinking chemistries, polymers, and clinical impact. Advanced Materials 2021;33:2006362. https://doi.org/10.1002/ADMA.202006362
43. Chen M, Zhong M, Johnson JA. Light-controlled radical polymerization: Mechanisms, methods, and applications. Chemical Reviews 2016;116:10167–211. https://doi.org/10.1021/acs.chemrev.5b00671
44. Wu F, Misra M, Mohanty AK. Challenges and new opportunities on barrier performance of biodegradable polymers for sustainable packaging. Progress in Polymer Science 2021;117:101395. https://doi.org/10.1016/j.progpolymsci.2021.101395
45. Saberi A, Jabbari F, Zarrintaj P, Saeb MR, Mozafari M. Electrically conductive materials: Opportunities and challenges in tissue engineering. Biomolecules. 2019;9. https://doi.org/10.3390/biom9090448
46. Tu Z, Zhong Y, Hu H, Shao D, Haag R, Schirner M, et al. Design of therapeutic biomaterials to control inflammation. Nature Reviews Materials 2022;7. https://doi.org/10.1038/s41578-022-00426-z
47. Costa-Pinto A, Santos TC, Neves NM, Reis RL. Testing natural biomaterials in animal models. Biomaterials from Nature for Advanced Devices and Therapies, 2016. https://doi.org/10.1002/9781119126218.ch30
48. Jones GW, Hill DG, Sime K, Williams AS. In vivo models for inflammatory arthritis. Methods in Molecular Biology, vol. 1725, 2018. https://doi.org/10.1007/978-1-4939-7568-6_9
49. Zhang S, Kang L, Hu S, Hu J, Fu Y, Hu Y, et al. Carboxymethyl chitosan microspheres loaded hyaluronic acid/gelatin hydrogels for controlled drug delivery and the treatment of inflammatory bowel disease. International Journal of Biological Macromolecules 2021;167. https://doi.org/10.1016/j.ijbiomac.2020.11.117
50. Petrucci G, Rizzi A, Hatem D, Tosti G, Rocca B, Pitocco D. Role of oxidative stress in the pathogenesis of atherothrombotic diseases. Antioxidants 2022;11. https://doi.org/10.3390/antiox11071408
51. Wang CPJ, Byun MJ, Kim SN, Park W, Park HH, Kim TH, et al. Biomaterials as therapeutic drug carriers for inflammatory bowel disease treatment. Journal of Controlled Release 2022;345. https://doi.org/10.1016/j.jconrel.2022.02.028
52. Lebaudy E, Fournel S, Lavalle P, Vrana NE, Gribova V. Recent advances in antiinflammatory material design. Advanced Healthcare Materials 2021;10. https://doi.org/10.1002/adhm.202001373
53. Zhang M, Hu W, Cai C, Wu Y, Li J, Dong S. Advanced application of stimuli-responsive drug delivery system for inflammatory arthritis treatment. Materials Today Bio 2022;14. https://doi.org/10.1016/j.mtbio.2022.100223
54. Serna JA, Rueda-gensini L, Céspedes-valenzuela DN, Cifuentes J, Cruz JC, Muñoz-camargo C. Recent advances on stimuli-responsive hydrogels based on tissue-derived ECMs and their components: Towards improving functionality for tissue engineering and controlled drug delivery. Polymers (Basel) 2021;13. https://doi.org/10.3390/polym13193263
55. Bernard M, Jubeli E, Pungente MD, Yagoubi N. Biocompatibility of polymer-based biomaterials and medical devices-regulations, *in vitro* screening and risk-management. Biomaterials Science 2018;6:2025–53. https://doi.org/10.1039/c8bm00518d
56. Ozturk S, Ayanoğlu FB, Parmaksiz M, Elçin AE, Elçin YM. Chapter 11: Clinical and Surgical Aspects of Medical Materials' Biocompatibility. Handbook of Biomaterials Biocompatibility; 2020, p. 219–50. https://doi.org/10.1016/B978-0-08-102967-1.00012-8
57. Chandra P, Yoo JJ, Lee SJ. Biomaterials in Regenerative Medicine: Challenges in Technology Transfer from Science to Process Development. Translational Regenerative Medicine, Elsevier Inc.; 2015, p. 151–67. https://doi.org/10.1016/B978-0-12-410396-2.00013-X
58. Song X, Tang Z, Liu W, Chen K, Liang J, Yuan B, et al. Biomaterials and regulatory science. Journal of Materials Science and Technology 2022;128:221–7. https://doi.org/10.1016/j.jmst.2022.04.018
59. Wang J, Wei L, Luo G, Li Z, Zhao C, Zhang H, et al. Synergistic effect of well-defined dual site boosting oxygen reduction reaction. Electronic Supplementary Information (ESI) for Energy & Environmental Science 2018;11:3375–9.
60. Zhou Y, Li Q, Wu Y, Li X, Zhou Y, Wang Z. Molecularly stimuli-responsive self-assembled peptide nanoparticles for targeted imaging and therapy. ACS Nano 2023;17. https://doi.org/10.1021/acsnano.3c01452

7 Stimuli-Responsive Biomaterials for Neuroinflammatory and Neurological Disorders

Swagath Valsan
Department of Bio-Medical Sciences,
School of Bio Sciences and Technology (SBST),
Vellore Institute of Technology (VIT), Vellore, India

Ravi Sudesh
Department of Biosciences,
School of Bio Sciences and Technology (SBST),
Vellore Institute of Technology (VIT), Vellore, India

Faraz Ahmad
Department of Biotechnology,
School of Bio Sciences and Technology (SBST),
Vellore Institute of Technology (VIT), Vellore, India

7.1 INTRODUCTION

Millions of people worldwide suffer from neuroinflammatory and neurological illnesses, which represent a substantial global health burden. In fact, neurological disorders rank as most prevalent cause of disability, and the second commonest factor associated with mortality among humans [1]. Incidences of neurological disease-related deaths and disabilities have exponentially increased worldwide over the last few decades, and additional increases are anticipated because of enhanced life expectancy and aged population expansion. Rapid changes in demographics and increased prevalence of risk factors, including obesity, cardiovascular ailments, and psychological stress, have aggravated the situation globally, making the burden of neurological diseases unbearable.

Neuropathological states of Alzheimer's disease (AD), Parkinson's disease (PD), multiple sclerosis (MS), and traumatic brain injury (TBI) are characterized by complex pathophysiologies involving oxidative stress, neuronal damage and dysfunction, and neuroinflammation. In particular, recent studies have underscored the crucial role of neuroinflammation as both a mediator and a consequence of these disorders, contributing to disease progression and exacerbating neurological damage [2]. Consequently, effective therapeutic strategies that target inflammation and promote neuronal repair are urgently needed. In this context, stimuli-responsive biomaterials have appeared as an encouraging class of agencies for the treatment of neuroinflammatory and neurological disorders. These advanced biomaterials are fabricated to specifically respond to pathophysiological cues, such as temperature, pH, oxidative species, or the presence of certain enzymes or ions, which are often dysregulated in diseased states. By modulating local environments in a controlled manner, stimuli-responsive biomaterials can provide targeted and personalized treatment options that enhance therapeutic efficacy while

DOI: 10.1201/9781003560203-7

limiting adverse side effects [3]. Stimuli-responsive systems offer significant advantages in the regulation of neuroinflammation in multiple neuropathological states by enabling the spatial and temporal control of drug release, cell targeting, and tissue regeneration. For example, pH-sensitive hydrogels [4] can deliver anti-inflammatory agents or neuroprotective drugs specifically to inflamed brain regions in conditions like MS or AD. Likewise, temperature-responsive polymers [5, 6] have shown promise in facilitating the controlled release of therapeutic proteins or gene-therapy vectors in response to the elevated temperatures characteristic of neuroinflammatory sites.

This chapter aims to provide an overview of recent advancements in the development and application of stimuli-responsive biomaterials for the amelioration of aberrantly activated neuroinflammatory pathways in neurological disorders. Various categories of stimuli-responsive systems, including pH-sensitive polymers, thermoresponsive materials, and redox-sensitive nanomaterials are explored, highlighting their design principles, mechanisms of action, and recent *in vivo* and clinical developments. Moreover, the challenges and future directions for integrating these innovative biomaterials into clinical practice for the therapy of neurological diseases are also discussed, with a focus on improving therapeutic outcomes and overcoming current limitations.

7.2 SIGNIFICANCE OF NEUROINFLAMMATORY AND NEUROLOGICAL DISORDERS—GAPS AND PROSPECTS

Neuroinflammatory and neurological disorders represent a diverse group of conditions that profoundly impact the quality of life of millions of people globally. This group of disorders, which includes AD, PD, MS, TBI, and stroke, are associated with progressive neuronal dysfunction, degeneration, and chronic inflammation in the central nervous system (CNS). While the pathogenesis of neurodegenerative disorders involves protein conformational changes and aggregation, and the consequent synaptic and neuronal toxicity are the main causes of these neurological conditions [7–9], neuroinflammation, the aberrant stimulation of immune cells and excessive presence of pro-inflammatory mediators within the CNS, plays a crucial role in the pathogeneses of these diseases [10–12]. Macrophages, cytokines, the complement system, and pattern recognition receptors are important participants in this inflammation. Aging, trauma, dementia, high blood pressure, stroke, depression, diabetes, medications, and toxins are some of the factors that mediate overactivation of neuroinflammatory pathways. Neuroinflammation is actually a defensive pathophysiological reaction that shields the brain from both internal and external insults; however, excessive and prolonged release of inflammatory mediators is detrimental and results in neurodegenerative outcomes [13]. Typically, pro-inflammatory caspase, a sensor protein, and an adapter protein make up cytosolic molecular factories, also known as inflammasomes. Among the most studied inflammasome is nucleotide-binding oligomerization domain leucine-rich repeat and pyrin domain-containing protein 3 (NLRP3), which is identified as a key contributor to neurodegenerative illnesses [14]. Inflammatory mediators including prostaglandins and pro-inflammatory cytokines are produced by CNS cells and excite glial cells, attract immune cells, and trigger chemokines and adhesion molecules. Neuroinflammation is caused by the overproduction of pro-inflammatory cytokines [15]. Neurodegenerative illnesses can result from glial cells' overproduction of cytokines, which are essential for neurogenesis. Intercellular communication relying on secreted cytokines, chemokines, and other mediators stimulate microglia, which take part in innate immune responses [16]. Upon pathogen penetration, damaged cells release chemical signals such as adenosine triphosphate (ATP), which acts as a chemoattractant for microglia and raises the quantity of purine nucleotides [17]. Abnormal nervous system development, neurodegenerative diseases, or neuronal dysfunction resulting in massive morphofunctional alterations in neurons rely on inherited genetic variants. Environmental variables may cause inflammatory events linked to neurological diseases like AD, as well as genetic and epigenetic alterations [18]. As a result, molecular, signaling, and metabolic processes within the CNS are heavily altered in neurodegenerative diseases. These show up as aberrant protein aggregation, oxidative damage, and inflammation, which are caused by an increase in free radical generation. Furthermore, because of the increased activity of enzymes, neurotransmitters may be depleted, broken down, or not produced enough in the synaptic cleft. Additional conditions include mitochondrial malfunction, neuronal excitation toxicity, and blood–brain barrier (BBB) damage [19].

A significant challenge in the therapy of neuroinflammatory and neurological disorders is the lack of specificity in targeting the underlying inflammatory processes without affecting healthy brain tissue. Traditional pharmacological treatments, such as nonsteroidal anti-inflammatory drugs (NSAIDs) or corticosteroids, often fail to address the root causes of neuroinflammation and may cause adverse effects, including immune suppression and systemic toxicity. In addition, many of these treatments cannot cross the BBB efficiently, rendering them less effective in treating neurological disorders [20]. Another key challenge is the heterogeneity of neuroinflammatory conditions. Disorders like AD, PD, and MS differ not only in their underlying etiology but also in the types of inflammatory responses they provoke. The presence of distinct immune cell populations, such as microglia and astrocytes, which exhibit differential activation states across these diseases, complicates the development of universal therapies [21]. The chronic nature of neuroinflammation, often coupled with neuronal damage, necessitates therapies that can mitigate inflammation while promoting tissue regeneration and neuroprotection. Moreover, current diagnostic tools for neuroinflammatory and neurological disorders primarily rely on symptomatic assessment and neuroimaging, which may fail to detect subtle, early-stage neuroinflammation. There is a growing need for biomarkers that can more accurately detect and monitor neuroinflammatory processes, for example, in conditions such as early-stage AD or in the acute phase of stroke. Moreover, despite encouraging advancements in the understanding of the underlying molecular mechanisms, effective therapeutic strategies remain limited, majorly due to the complexity of the neuroinflammatory system and the BBB, which restricts the efficient delivery of most drugs [22].

The advent of stimuli-responsive biomaterials offers promising new prospects for addressing the above gaps for an effective treatment strategy against neuroinflammatory and neurological disorders. These materials may be engineered to dynamically and specifically respond to changes in temperature, pH, ionic strength, or enzymatic activity, all of which are often altered during neuroinflammatory processes [23]. For instance, inflammation is typically associated with changes in the local pH and increased oxidative stress, both of which can serve as triggers for the spatiotemporally controlled release of therapeutic agents using pH-sensitive hydrogels or redox-responsive nanomaterials [24]. Such materials can deliver anti-inflammatory or neuroprotective drugs specifically to inflamed brain sites, thereby limiting the risk of adverse systemic side effects. Moreover, neuroinflammation in diseases such as AD or PD is often localized in specific brain regions, making stimuli-responsive systems potent candidates for targeted drug delivery [25]. For example, thermoresponsive hydrogels can release their payloads when encountered with mild hyperthermia, a characteristic feature of inflammation in the brain, allowing for a spatiotemporally regulated release of therapeutic agents at the site of injury or disease [6]. Additionally, the ability to incorporate biomolecules such as cytokines, growth factors, or RNA-based therapies into these materials opens new avenues for not only controlling inflammation but also promoting tissue repair and regeneration [26]. Furthermore, nanomaterials—particularly those capable of crossing the BBB—represent an exciting prospect for overcoming a significant challenge in the therapy of neurological disorders [27]. Bioengineering of appropriate nanoparticles may allow response to specific biomolecular signatures associated with neuroinflammation, such as the presence of certain enzymes or receptors expressed by activated microglia and astrocytes [28]. By functionalizing these nanoparticles with ligands that target these cell types, it is possible to attain high specificity and selectivity in the delivery of therapeutic agents to areas of active inflammation, enhancing both efficacy and safety. Additionally, the multi-modal therapeutic approach that integrates stimuli-responsive biomaterials with other advanced technologies, such as gene editing (e.g., CRISPR/Cas9), nanorobots, or optogenetics, could further improve the precision and efficacy of treatments for neurological diseases [29]. For instance, gene therapies could be delivered directly to targeted neurons or glial cells using stimuli-responsive nanocarriers, enabling the direct modulation of gene expression involved in inflammation and neuroprotection.

7.3 IDEAL STIMULI-RESPONSIVE MATERIALS FOR NEUROINFLAMMATORY AND NEUROLOGICAL DISORDER MANAGEMENT

The fabrication and appropriate usage of ideal stimuli-responsive biomaterials for the treatment of neuroinflammatory and neurological disorders requires an intricate balance between target specificity, therapeutic efficacy, biocompatibility, and controlled responsiveness to specific environmental cues (Figure 7.1). These materials must not only respond to disease-specific stimuli (e.g., changes in pH, temperature, oxidative stress, or enzymatic activity) but also provide precise, localized delivery of ameliorative agents to mitigate neuroinflammation, promote neuroprotection, and stimulate tissue repair in the CNS [30]. In this section, we outline the key characteristics of ideal stimuli-responsive biomaterials, discuss the materials that meet these criteria, and explore their potential in the management of neuroinflammatory conditions. For stimuli-responsive materials (SRM) to be effective in the management of neurological disorders, they must possess several critical characteristics:

- *Targeted response to pathological stimuli*: SRM should be capable of specifically responding to the unique environmental cues associated with neuroinflammation and neurodegeneration [31]. For instance, inflammation often leads to changes in pH, oxidative stress, or the overexpression of certain enzymes or receptors, all of which may be harnessed to serve as triggers for the appropriate spatiotemporal release of therapeutic agents.
- *Biocompatibility and safety*: Given the delicate nature of brain tissue and the high risk of side effects, SRM must be biocompatible and biodegradable. They should not provoke an immune response or toxicity even during the long run. Materials that degrade into non-toxic byproducts are particularly advantageous [32].
- *Efficient BBB penetration*: A primary hurdle in treating neurological disorders is the presence of BBB, which restricts the delivery of most therapeutics to the brain. Ideal stimuli-responsive formulations must either cross the BBB effectively or be delivered via non-invasive techniques that bypass it, such as focused ultrasound (FUS) [33].
- *Controlled release and sustained delivery*: Neurotherapeutic stimuli-responsive material should not only allow the release of their bioactive payloads in response to the desired

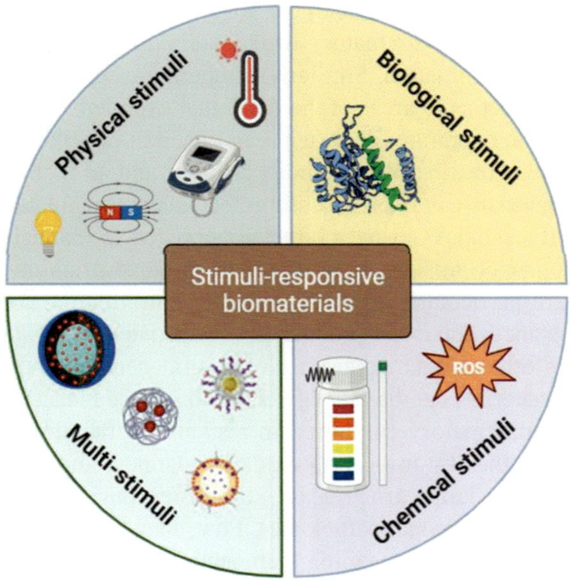

FIGURE 7.1 Properties of an ideal stimuli-responsive biomaterial for diagnosis and therapy of neuroinflammatory pathologies.

stimulus but also do so in a spatiotemporally regulated manner, ensuring sustained release at inflamed sites over time. This is particularly important for chronic conditions like AD and PD, for which long-term treatment is often necessary [34].

- *Ease of fabrication and scalability*: Last, for the SRM to transition from the laboratory to clinical applications, they must be easy to fabricate, reproducible, and scalable for large-scale production, all while maintaining their effectiveness.

7.4 STIMULUS-RESPONSIVE BIOMATERIALS: VITAL FOR TARGETING NEUROINFLAMMATORY AND NEUROLOGICAL DISORDERS

Stimulus-responsive biomaterials, also known as "smart" materials, represent a potentially transformative approach in the therapy of pathologies associated with neuroinflammation. These materials have an ability to elicit appropriate responses to changes in pH, temperature, light, magnetic fields, particular ions/metabolites, or specific enzymes, all of which are often dysregulated in the context of neuronal diseases. The unique ability of these materials to respond to localized pathological stimuli offers significant benefits over conventional therapeutic systems, particularly in the treatment of complex and heterogeneous conditions like neuroinflammation and neurodegeneration. SRM respond to variations in environmental factors including light, temperature, magnetic fields, or electricity [35]. SRM can alter their structure, chemical makeup, or mechanical properties in reaction to these stimuli. Pathological characteristics of brain disease usually include vascular dysfunction, inflammation, oxidative stress, elevated expression of matrix metalloproteinases (MMPs), and neuronal loss or death in damaged tissues [36].

Neuroinflammation, a key pathological feature of many CNS diseases such as AD, PD, and MS, is associated with aberrant activation of immune cells (e.g., microglia and astrocytes), enhanced secretion of pro-inflammatory mediators, and disruption of the BBB. These neuroinflammatory responses not only exacerbate neuronal damage but also create an ideal environment for the application of stimuli-responsive biomaterials that can target specific pathological cues, including pro-inflammatory signals. For instance, pH-responsive hydrogels are particularly useful in neuroinflammatory environments where the local pH may be lowered due to the accumulation of acidic metabolites produced by activated immune cells. Upon sensing the acidic pH characteristic of inflamed tissue, these hydrogels can undergo a conformational change, releasing encapsulated therapeutic agents such as anti-inflammatory drugs, antioxidants, or neuroprotective molecules specifically at the site of inflammation. Similarly, temperature-sensitive polymers can be for the delivery of bioactive therapeutics to areas of the brain that experience localized hyperthermia due to inflammation. Elevated temperatures are often seen in conditions like TBI or stroke, where ischemic damage leads to the activation of heat shock proteins and an increase in local temperature. Thermoresponsive biomaterials can release neuroprotectants in a regulated manner upon reaching a specific temperature threshold, offering a targeted approach to manage inflammation and promote healing [37]. Another promising class of stimuli-responsive biomaterials is redox-sensitive nanomaterials, which are particularly advantageous for neuroinflammatory diseases that involve oxidative stress. For instance, enhanced production of reactive oxygen species (ROS) and oxidative neuronal damage is often a defining feature of neurodegenerative diseases like AD and PD [38]. Redox-responsive materials can be bioengineered to release bioactive neuroprotectants, such as antioxidants or anti-inflammatory cytokines, in response to the elevated levels of ROS found in inflamed brain regions, thereby mitigating oxidative damage and restoring homeostasis [39]. Because of their ability of regulating drug release, stimuli-responsive biomaterials offer significant advantages for the therapy of neuronal pathologies. First, they allow for fine-tuning spatiotemporal release of their bioactive payload, meaning therapeutic agents are released only in presence of specific disease-associated cues at the site of inflammation or injury [40]. This reduces the risk of adverse side effects in non-target tissues/areas, particularly in the highly sensitive brain. Second, these materials can be engineered for specific cellular targeting, using ligands or antibodies that recognize disease-specific markers on the surface of immune cells or neurons [41]. This enables highly selective drug delivery to degenerating cells, improving therapeutic outcomes. Moreover, the biodegradability of many SRM ensures that they do not accumulate in the body, further enhancing their safety profile [42]. Interestingly, upon fulfillment of their desired functions, these materials can also be engineered to degenerate into non-toxic byproducts, which may abolish the requirement of often invasive removal procedures.

AD, PD, MS, stroke, and other neurological illnesses have been linked to prolonged activation of reactive astrocytes and microglia [43]. Accumulation of pathogenic proteins like α-synuclein and amyloid-β (Aβ) in PD and AD, respectively, can increase the reactivity of microglia [44, 45]. Many therapeutic medications and biomolecules that may be helpful in treating these illnesses are blocked from being delivered by the BBB/blood cerebrospinal fluid barrier (BCSB) or to the complex regions in the brain. In order to modify neuroinflammation, biomaterials can offer a way to go around the BB or BSC barriers and deliver medications to the site of illness or damage. Biomaterial strategies for regulating neuroinflammation and neurological disorders include the use of coatings to extend the longevity of implantable neural probes [46, 47], nanoparticles that can penetrate BB/BSC barriers [48–50], hydrogels to allow for the controlled administration of immunomodulatory therapeutics [51, 52], and scaffolds implanted to foster an environment supporting neural regeneration and growth [53, 54]. Below we summarize some of the pertinent researches which have focused on stimuli-responsive biomaterials for the therapy of different classes of neuronal pathologies.

Hydrogels containing growth factors or mesenchymal stromal cells (MSCs) can boost their anti-inflammatory properties and endorse brain regeneration. Injectable thermos-responsive hydrogel consisting of materials such as hyaluronic acid, chitosan, and hydroxyethyl cellulose become hard at body temperature and liquid at less than 25°C. Injection of human umbilical cord-derived MSCs into rodents with TBI have been shown to stimulate MSC retention, survival and proliferation, boosting neuron survival, and learning and memory by stimulating signaling through brain-derived neurotrophic factor (BDNF) [55]. Light-induced crosslinking of hydrogel-based nanoparticles composed of imidazole-modified gelatin methacrylate and functionalized with polydopamine and stromal cell-derived factor-1 loaded with human amniotic mesenchymal stem cells (hAMSCs) were shown to induce repair of cryogenically damaged rat brains by promoting hAMSC migration to damage site for neuronal development [56]. Similarly, implantation of 3D bioprinted neural stem cells (NSCs) fabrications restored neuronal functional deficits induced by TBI in adult zebrafish [57]. Relying on the aberrantly expressed enzymes in damaged brain tissues as baits, hydrogels functionalized with peptides recognizing MMP9 were created for limiting neuronal damage in a TBI model. MMP9-mediated cleavage of PLGL tetrapeptide linker allowed these hydrogels to release neuroprotective peptides at the hippocampal injury sites and stimulate neurogenesis [58]. Similarly, a poly(ethylene) glycol-bis-(acryloyloxy acetate) hydrogel formulation was shown to reduce the levels of pro-inflammatory cytokines and mitigate motor dysfunctions in a rat model of TBI [59]. An injectable ROS and enzyme-responsive hydrogel constructed using poly(propylene sulfide)120 (PPS120) and triglycerol monostearate (TM), and functionalized with curcumin was fabricated to improve drug delivery and release for potential applications in brain damage [60]. Iron overload increases the creation of ROS, which exacerbates neurodegeneration [61]. Functionalization with an iron chelator, deferoxamine mesylate allowed a 3-aminophenylboronic acid-grafted hyaluronic acid and polyvinyl alcohol (PVA) hydrogel construct aided the improvements in motor functions, and learning, and memory skills by reducing iron overload and oxidative stress in brain-injured rats [62].

pH-sensitive biomaterials are another class of therapeutic agents which are being envisioned as significant therapeutic tools. Various tissues and subcellular compartments within the human body have varying pH values; the cytosol has a pH of 7.4, endosomes have a pH of 5.5–6.0, and lysosomes have a pH of 4.5–5.5. Targeting specific regions, releasing medicinal substances with low toxicity, and reacting to certain pH triggers are all features of specialized nanocarriers. Because of this, pH-responsive nanoparticles are an intriguing medication delivery strategy. The flash nanoprecipitation technique was used to develop a multipurpose pH-responsive nanoplatform that targets ROS. The systems of nanocarriers demonstrated lower cytotoxicity in cells and good stability. Hydrophilic, high molecular weight species have been encapsulated with good loading efficiency using the flash nanoprecipitation technique [63].

Thermoresponsive nanoplatforms are being researched for AD treatment because of their substantial latent heat of fusion and because of their ability to undergo reversible temperature-dependent solid–liquid transition. The sustained release of biodegradable dendritic nanoparticles containing nerve growth factor and composed of poly(L-lactic acid), poly(L-lysine), and poly(N-isopropylacrylamide) was assessed on PC12 neuron cells. At temperatures over 37°C, these nanoparticles demonstrated 6–13 times more cellular absorption than at 25°C. Their capacity to transfer neuroprotective peptides and proteins across the BBB in AD models is evidenced by the fact that they elicit sustained nerve growth factor release and stimulate neurite outgrowth and synaptogenesis [64]. Thermoresponsive nanoplatforms are appropriate for managing medication release because of their significant latent heat of fusion and reversible solid–liquid transition over a limited temperature range. After being extensively employed in cancer treatment, these nanoplatforms are currently being researched for AD treatment. The ability of sustained release of nerve growth factor in response to temperature changes of biodegradable thermoresponsive dendritic nanoparticles has been successfully evaluated in PC12 cells. The cellular absorption of these nanoparticles was significantly greater at temperatures in the range of 37°C, compared to lower temperatures of 25°C. A non-invasive and successful method for dissolving Aβ peptides and fibrils in AD is hyperthermia, or local heat generating. A more modern method of causing hyperthermia is near-infrared (NIR) laser irradiation, which can cause localized hyperthermia with sufficient intensities and great spatial precision. A novel multifunctionalized nanosystem for photothermal therapy of AD was created using graphene oxide functionalized with Aβ fibril staining dye, thioflavin-S (ThS). Relying on graphene's strong NIR optical absorption characteristics, this nanosystem was able to successfully target Aβ fibrils, shielding neurons from the latter's toxicity in NIR-exposed mice [65]. Similarly, polyoxometalate (POM) nanoplatform which responded to NIR stimulation was developed and found to demonstrate high antioxidant functions, in addition to photothermal-responsive ability to suppress Aβ oligomerization and fibrillization. As ROS scavengers, POMs help prevent the aggregation of Aβ monomers. Mesoporous silicon nanoparticles, a thermoresponsive copolymer called poly(N-isopropylacrylamide-co-acrylamide), and a copolymer including POM comprised the nanoplatform under investigation [66].

A new non-invasive drug delivery nanoplatform which was electrically responsive was created by combining graphene mesoporous silica (GSN) and polypyrrole nanohybrids, and functionalized with a metal chelator clioquinol. Neurite outgrowth is stimulated, cellular ROS are decreased, and Aβ de-aggregation is facilitated by the platform. The low conductivity of mesoporous silica nanoparticles (MSN) led to their replacement with GSN. When the polypyrrole–GSN nanohybrids are electrically stimulated, clioquinol is produced in a regulated manner, enabling it to chelate Cu^{2+} and disassemble Aβ plaques. The interfacial characteristics of the nanoplatform were characterized using electrochemical impedance spectroscopy. This is the first study to combine pharmaceutical and non-pharmacological therapy methods for AD into a single system [64].

A popular thermo-ablative technique for administering medications in pathological models of Parkinson's, Alzheimer's, and brain malignancies is FUS. In AD transgenic animal models, it has been demonstrated to breach the BBB without the use of drugs, lowering amyloid load, preventing memory deficits, and improving synaptic plasticity [65, 66]. Injectable microbubbles combined with magnetic resonance guided focused ultrasound (MRgFUS) is a related, largely non-invasive technique that has great spatial and temporal specificity for breaching the BBB [67, 68]. As a clinical pilot study, this method was applied to allow permeability across BBB in patients who were diagnosed as amyloid-positive. Verifying the procedure's viability and safety as well as assessing its potential clinical and therapeutic benefits for AD were the main goals. Because of its excellent specificity and accuracy for opening the BBB and its ability to image the target area in real time, the study demonstrated the viability and safety of this non-invasive method. With or without a treatment for BBB opening alone, this method may assist target the disease in its early stages and may be employed as a potential therapeutic strategy against AD [69]. One potential target for anti-AD therapy is mitigation of metal dysregulation. Metal chelators, including as derivatives of 8-hydroxyquinoline and chloroquine, are used to prevent the production of ROS and metal ion-induced Aβ aggregation. Nevertheless, their incapacity to penetrate the BBB and engage with metal ions restricts their application in traditional delivery systems. Targeted medication delivery with ROS-responsive nanoparticles is being used to release therapeutic metal chelators at disease sites in order to get around these restrictions. In order to prevent the development of Aβ fibrils and serve as capping agents for MSNs, anionic gold nanoparticles were modified using β-D-glucose. This responsive nanoplatform demonstrated strong BBB permeability and good compatibility while reducing Cu^{2+}–$A\beta_{40}$ complex-induced oxidative stress-mediated cell death. Receptor for advanced glycation end-products (RAGE) was discovered to be upregulated on neurons, microglia, and the BBB in AD. Effective neuroprotection and enhanced oxidative stress were demonstrated by targeting this receptor using a polymeric micelle that contained curcumin, ROS-responsive polymer ((polyethylene glycol)-LysB), and a peptide that targets the RAGE receptor [70].

The combination of the antidepressant medication genipin with hydroxypropyl-β-cyclodextrin and P407/P188/PEG8000 constructs shows that thermoresponsive gels can efficiently transport medications to brain tissue. In mouse brains, these hydrogels released genipin in a sustained manner, enhancing its antidepressant effects [71]. Another instance featured icariin-integrated hydrogel for its sustained release following intranasal administration and encapsulated in alginate nanogels. This resulted in quick antidepressant effects in rat and mouse models [72]. Another method delivers the antidepressant olanzapine (Olz) by combining hydrogels with nanoparticles to make amino borane-based nanoconstructs. These were delivered into the brain via nasal administration after being enclosed in a P407/P188 hydrogel. Interestingly, Olz was only released when NP broke down due to elevated ROS levels in the brain [73]. Hydrogels made of carboxymethyl chitosan and oxidized starch nanoparticles considerably decreased schizophrenia-like symptoms in rats treated with PAOPA, a D2 allosteric modulator via the nose-to-brain route of administration, significantly enhancing the bioavailability, compared to the intraperitoneal route [74]. To improve the administration oxcarbazepine, a potential anti-seizure agent in poloxamer P407 and sodium carboxymethyl cellulose hydrogel, chitosan nanoparticles were used. When administered intranasally, this mixture demonstrated enhanced antiepileptic and anti-inflammatory properties [75].

7.5 THERAPEUTIC EFFECTS ON DIFFERENT NEUROINFLAMMATORY AND NEUROLOGICAL DISORDERS

Multiple studies have indicated the multi-modal therapeutic potential of stimuli-responsive biomaterials in different neuropathologies. In recent years, a variety of constructs have been devised which have been shown to be responsive toward a plethora of external and internal stimuli for the manifestation of their complete ameliorative effects (Figure 7.2). Below, we discuss the major categories of stimuli-responsive and their relevance for mitigation of neuroinflammatory and neurological conditions.

7.5.1 pH-Responsive Systems

pH-responsive biomaterials are among the most commonly studied stimuli-responsive systems for the targeted delivery of bioactive therapeutics in neuroinflammatory and neurological diseases. These materials exploit the localized acidic microenvironments that are characteristic of inflammation and injury. In conditions like MS and AD, areas of demyelination or amyloid plaque deposition create a distinct acidic pH that can be exploited for stimuli-induced drug release. pH-sensitive hydrogels, such as those composed of poly(2-dimethylamino)ethyl methacrylate (PDMAEMA) or

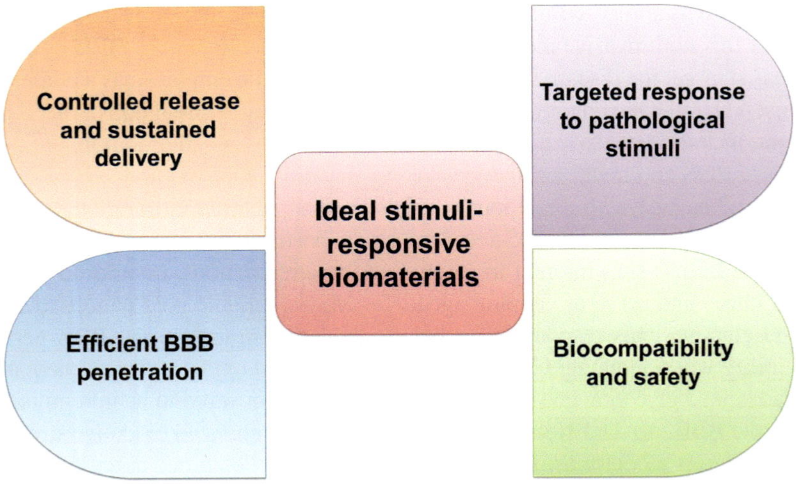

FIGURE 7.2 The various categories of stimuli-responsive biomaterials for the amelioration of neuroinflammation in brain pathologies.

polymeric micelles, undergo conformational changes when exposed to acidic environments which induces release of encapsulated bioactive payloads [76]. These hydrogels can be functionalized with anti-inflammatory drugs, antioxidants, and neuroprotective agents to precisely target inflamed brain regions. Moreover, pH-responsive materials have the advantage of minimizing systemic side effects, as they can be fabricated to release bioactive constituents only in the acidic microenvironment of inflamed tissues, enhancing therapeutic efficiency while reducing toxicity to healthy brain tissue. Indeed, the acidic microenvironment created by inflammation provides a unique prospect to design pH-sensitive polymers for localized drug delivery in neuroinflammatory diseases [77]. Many of these materials typically consist of weak acids or bases that ionize at specific pH values. For instance, pH-sensitive polymeric micelles and nanogels may be employed for targeted delivery of anti-inflammatory agents, such as corticosteroids, to areas of the brain affected by neuroinflammation. The low pH in the diseased or injured regions triggers the release of the bioactive payload, while minimizing systemic toxicity. These materials are particularly effective in conditions like MS, where localized acidity occurs due to demyelination and immune cell infiltration. In the brain parenchyma, 3D6 antibody fragments (3D6-Fab) effectively prevent Aβ aggregation. They create negatively charged citraconylated-Fab when they react with citraconic anhydride. A dual pH/redox-sensitive nanomicelle is formed by crosslinked poly-polymers of cationic disulfides. The major amino group in citraconylated-Fab reverses the Fab's charge to improve its antigen-binding capacity when it reaches an endocytic acidic pH [78].

In ischemic stroke, the blocked blood vessels may further affect the brain tissue or ischemic region to become acidic, called as acidosis. To address this, pH-sensitive micro-DDSs can be used for ischemic stroke therapy. A polyionic complex was created using anionic PAA and cationic poly(ethylene glycol)-b-poly [4-(2, 2, 6, 6-tetramylpiperidine-1-oxy) amino methyl styrene] (PEG-B-PMNT). The nanoparticles showed significant thrombolysis activity at pH 6.2 but retained its structure at pH 7.4. The nanoparticles also increased t-PA's half-life from 8.2 minutes to 71.2 minutes. In a cerebral ischemia mouse model, t-PA@iRNP injection decreased infarct volume and diminished neuronal impairments. pH-sensitive PEG-conjugated nanogels containing urokinase accelerated clot dissolution, lowered neurotoxicity and apoptosis, preserved the BBB integrity, and reduced neurological impairments [79]. A Ca^{2+}/NT nanocomplex coated with branched polyethyleneimine was also used as a pH-responsive construct for the release of ATP. Intranasal administration of this nanoconstructs was found to be beneficial in dramatically decreasing the infarct volume and mitigating neuronal deficits associated with middle cerebral artery occlusion (MCAO) [80]. A pH-sensitive nanoparticle laden with the anti-inflammatory and antioxidant medication succinobucol successfully assisted in lowering the infarct volume of cerebral ischemia rats by targeting cerebral ischemic lesions, as demonstrated by fluorescence labeling and MRI imaging [81]. A pH-responsive platform was constructed using hydroxypropyl methyl cellulose and carbopol for the controlled nose-to-brain delivery of paliperidone, an anti-schizophrenia drug [82].

7.5.2 ROS-Responsive Systems

ROS are produced in a variety of typical biological conditions and are important for many processes, such as learning and memory, synaptic plasticity, and the immune system's defense against infections [83]. Excess ROS can cause oxidative stress; certain neurodegenerative diseases, like AD and PD, have been linked to deficits in cognitive function due to elevated ROS levels. Cells create several antioxidant enzymes that inhibit the production of ROS. Redox-responsive biomaterials exploit the differences in oxidative stress between healthy and inflamed tissues [84]. In neurodegenerative diseases like AD and PD, elevated levels of ROS and increased oxidative stress may serve as inducers for the release of neuroprotectants from redox-sensitive nanoparticles. For example, polymeric nanoparticles conjugated with thiol groups undergo cleavage in the presence of oxidative species, enabling spatiotemporal regulation of the delivery of encapsulated anti-inflammatory drugs or neuroprotective agents directly at the site of oxidative damage. These materials hold promise in reducing neuroinflammation and protecting neurons from further degeneration. Redox-responsive materials, particularly those based on disulfide bonds or thiol groups, can be designed to deliver therapeutic agents including anti-inflammatory drugs, when exposed to elevated levels of ROS. These materials are highly selective, responding only to the oxidative environment in inflamed or injured brain regions. These systems have shown significant promise in preclinical models, demonstrating their ability to reduce neuroinflammation and protect neurons from further degeneration [85]. By responding directly to the disease-associated oxidative environment, redox-responsive materials can minimize drug loss and improve therapeutic outcomes.

ROS-responsive drug carriers can be engineered to release the bioactive payload in a selective and sustained manner in response to elevated ROS levels. These loaded molecules have the ability to either affect the neuropathology-related pathways or reduce inflammation by scavenging ROS or downregulating inflammatory pathways. Among these compounds are anti-inflammatory and antioxidant medications like dexamethasone, ibuprofen, indomethacin, and epigallocatechin gallate, as well as medications that are particular to neurological disorders like resveratrol and simvastatin. A study used polypropylene sulfide nanoparticles to reduce inflammation after electrode-brain implantation in a rat model. A polyethylene oxide coating was applied to immobilize the nanoparticles on a flexible microelectrode. Over nine days, the loaded antioxidant released, resulting in smoother integration of neural tissue with the nanoparticle-coated electrodes [86]. Simvastatin, which increases the synthesis of BDNF and thereby mitigates spatial learning deficits, and lethal-7b (let7b) antisense oligonucleotide, a promoter of NSC differentiation, were combined using a ROS unit with a diselenide link particle. Simvastatin-functionalized nanoparticles which encapsulated let-7b and superparamagnetic iron oxide nanocubes were found to significantly improved memory and BDNF production in mice with AD [87].

Boronic esters, similar to thioketal bonds, undergo oxidation, making them suitable for burst drug release in response to inflammation. This specific type of chemistry has been successfully implemented in the treatment of stroke which is associated with high levels of ROS. Thus, researchers bioengineered dextran nanoformulations modified with boronic esters to encapsulate NR2B9C, a neuroprotective agent with a potent ability to target degenerating neurons at injury sites. The particles efficiently delivered NR2B9C across BBB in a rat model of cerebral ischemia with minimal toxic side effects [88]. Poly[(2-acryloyl)ethyl(p-boronic acid benzyl) dimethylammonium bromide] (B-PDEAEA) constructs with a cationic lipid cover may be employed for DNA-based therapeutics in pathologies associated with neuroinflammation. Cationic lipid covering on these formulations aid in achieving effective gene transfections in the intended cells. Similar bi-layered particles have been successfully employed for the expression of tumor suicide genes in an *in vivo* cancer model, overcoming barriers like lysosomal trapping and serum instability [89]. Last, gold nanofabrication capped with mesoporous silica have been employed for H_2O_2-sensitive release of clioquinol, a metal chelator [90]. Employment of this ROS-responsive delivery system was reported to robustly mitigate Cu^{2+}-induced Aβ aggregation, consequently increasing cell survival and reducing ROS-mediated apoptosis.

7.5.3 Enzyme-Responsive Systems

Enzyme-responsive biomaterials have been developed to recognize and respond to specific enzymes that are overexpressed during neuroinflammation, such as MMPs or cathepsins. These enzymes play critical roles in the breakdown of the BBB and the extracellular matrix in neuroinflammatory conditions. By designing biomaterials that degrade or release their therapeutic payloads in the presence of these enzymes, it may be possible to accomplish localized drug delivery that is both selective and efficient. Enzyme-responsive systems can be particularly useful in treating conditions like stroke, where the disruption of the BBB and subsequent neuroinflammation require targeted intervention [91]. The activation of specific enzymes is another hallmark of neuroinflammation and neurological disorders. Enzymes such as cathepsins and MMPs are upregulated in conditions like stroke and neurodegenerative diseases, where they contribute to tissue degradation and inflammation. Enzyme-sensitive materials can be engineered to degrade or release drugs upon encountering these specific enzymes. Enzyme-responsive hydrogels and nanocarriers can be functionalized with peptide sequences that are cleaved by overexpressed enzymes in inflamed brain regions. This approach enables the localized delivery of neuroprotective agents or anti-inflammatory drugs with high specificity, reducing the need for systemic treatment and enhancing therapeutic efficacy. Transferrin is one of the preferred targets for allowing penetration of drug-loaded nanosystems. Thus, transferrin functionalized liposomal constructs have been evidenced to deliver neuroprotectant and improve AD-related pathology in mice [92]. In addition to transferrin, penetration may also enhance the BBB penetrating capabilities of liposomes to deliver apolipoprotein E2 (apoE2) expressing plasmid for the treatment of AD [93]. Lactoferrin, similarly can be used to target BBB for delivering neurotherapeutics, such as acetylcholinesterase inhibitor huperzine A [94]. Angiopep, a high-affinity ligand for BBB component, low-density lipoprotein receptor-related protein-1, has also been used to functionalize nanocarriers for the delivery of siRNAs to injured sites in the CNS [95]. Last, an enzyme-responsive helical micromotor has been recently constructed for delivering NSCs in a magnetic field-dependent manner in order to restore neural networks in *Xenopus laevis* [96].

7.5.4 Temperature-Responsive Systems

Thermoresponsive materials are another promising class of stimuli-responsive systems. Localized temperature changes in the brain often occur in response to neuroinflammatory processes. Elevated temperatures can result from ischemia, injury, or inflammation, providing a natural cue for the release of therapeutic agents. Poly (N-isopropylacrylamide) (pNIPAAm) has been one of the most prominent materials of choice for the fabrication of thermoresponsive hydrogels and micelles due to its reversible temperature-dependent gel-to-sol transition. Hence, these temperature-sensitive hydrogels can be designed to reversibly change their physical properties in response to a range of temperature fluctuations. Most extensively researched thermoresponsive hydrogels often include various hydrophobic methyl, ethyl, and propyl groups which can alter their physical and structural characteristics in response to temperature changes [97]. Both synthetic and natural polymers can be exploited for the creation of thermoresponsive hydrogels. Polysaccharides (e.g., cellulose, chitosan, and xyloglucan) and proteins (e.g., gelatin) are examples of natural polymers. Among the synthetic polymers are dimethylamine (ethyl methacrylate), poly(N-isopropylacrylamide) (pNIPAAm), poly(ethylene oxide)–poly(propylene oxide)–poly(ethylene oxide) (PEO–PPO–PEO), and poly(organophosphoronitrile) [98].

In the context of neurological disorders, where localized tissue damage often leads to changes in temperature, thermoresponsive hydrogels have been shown to be efficient in targeted and regulated release of therapeutic biomolecules. These biomaterials have been shown to release drugs, growth factors, and even gene-therapeutic agents in response to temperatures changes associated with neuroinflammatory processes, such as those seen in neurodegenerative conditions and TBI. Additionally, thermoresponsive nanoparticles have been shown to cross the BBB and respond to temperature shifts, making them suitable candidates for the therapy of neurodegenerative diseases [99]. Thermoresponsive hydrogels have extensive application in cell encapsulation and medication release. Thermoresponsive hydrogels composed of natural polymer chitosan, due to their mucoadhesive properties, have been suggested for intranasal administration of neuroprotectants in models of AD and PD [100]. For instance, ibuprofen has delivered by thermosensitive chitosan hydrogels using the nose-to-brain route [101]. The formulation was optimized for intranasal administration with no harmful effects on nasal epithelial cells with the use of chitosan at a molecular weight of 110–150 kDa, and with a sol-to-gel conversion 2.9 times quicker than clearance by the mucociliary system [102]. Chitosan-based thermosensitive hydrogels composed of hydroxyethyl cellulose-collagen-β-phosphoglycerate have been tested for delivery of bone marrow-derived MSCs to aid neuronal repair in spinal cord injury (SCI) models [103]. Similarly, temperature-dependent release of antioxidant ferulic acid was carried out using chitosan-gelatin-β-phosphoglycerate hydrogels and showed robust anti-inflammatory and cell-protective actions in N2A cells exposed to H_2O_2 [104].

Hydrogels composed of another natural polymer collagen have been suggested as suitable platforms for the temperature-responsive release of neurotrophic and growth factors, potentially providing neuroprotection in brain and SCIs as well as neurodegenerative conditions. Indeed, collagen hydrogels incorporating a crosslinker, genipin were used for the delivery of growth factors which could regulate astrocyte-mediated recovery of neurons [105]. Similarly, collagen hydrogels were used as carriers for the delivery of neurotrophin-3 in an experimental model of SCI and elicited robust anti-inflammatory effects and neuroprotection [106]. Collagen hydrogel has also been tested for regulated delivery of glial-derived neurotrophic factor (GDNF) for functional upliftment of dopaminergic neurons as a therapeutic approach for PD [107]. GDNF-collagen hydrogel greatly increased striatal re-innervation and dopaminergic neuron survival, which in turn greatly increased functional recovery. Research also suggests that hydrogels may provide a supporting matrix for transplanted cells, increasing cell survival. Thus, MSCs were encapsulated in thermoresponsive collagen-genipin constructs for their subsequent release in order to aid neuronal survival and recovery [105]. Last, thermoresponsive 3D bioprinted nanoconstructs composed of water-soluble and biodegradable polyurethane polymers have been used for encapsulation of NSCs for neuronal repair in a zebrafish model of TBI [54].

Apart from the natural polymers, hydrogels composed of synthetic versions have also been tested as delivery agents for neurotherapeutics in recent years. Anti-tumorigenic agent, paclitaxel has been shown to be delivered to glioma sites in rats using temperature-responsive system composed of poly(1,3-bis(carboxyphenoxy)propane)-co-sebacic acid (PCPP-SA) and temozolomide, an alkylating agent [108]. Temperature-responsive hydrogels composed of synthetic polymers have also been used to deliver milk fat globule–epidermal growth factor 8 to control neuroinflammatory responses in SCI [109]. pNIPAAm-based hydrogels, for example, exhibit a reversible phase transition at specific temperatures, enabling the release of encapsulated drugs only when the local temperature reaches a critical threshold [110]. This feature is particularly useful in post-injury or post-stroke and oncological settings, where hyperthermic conditions promote inflammation and cell death. Indeed, pNIPAAm-based thermoresponsive hydrogels have been successfully used for controlled release of neurotrophins, BDNF, and neurotrophin-3 to aid recovery processes of axonal regeneration in SCI [111, 112]. pNIPAAm-based temperature-responsive constructs have also been employed to supply nasal olfactory ecto-mesenchymal stem cells to injured neurons and reduce neuroinflammatory processes associated with SCI [113]. pNIPAAm–keratin hydrogels may act as delivery agents for iron chelator, deferoxamine mesylate for reducing oxidative damage and inflammation in the therapy of conditions such as intracerebral hemorrhage [114]. Doxorubicin has been shown to be efficiently delivered by temperature-responsive gelation polymer and consequently enhance anti-tumorigenic pathways under *in vitro* and *in vivo* conditions [115].

7.5.5 Photo-Responsive Systems

Light-responsive materials react to light through photocleavable crosslinkers or photosensitive molecules like azobenzene, spiropyran, or dithienylethene. The chemical characteristics of these molecules, including hydrophobicity and crosslinking patterns, change when illumination alters the molecular conformation, configuration, or isomerization status of the photo-responsive moiety. Photo-stimulation can precisely and remotely regulate the target zone without being intrusive or causing injury to cells, so it is a potential technique for biological applications. Photo-responsive hydrogels have constituents which elicit dynamic changes in crosslinking patterns upon photothermal cues, such as visible, NIR, and UV light [116]. These moieties absorb light of specific wavelengths and transform them into chemical signals by means of the processes of cleavage, dimerization, and isomerization, which results in structural or property changes like swelling, shrinking, or crosslinking [117]. In addition to the more commonly employed pH, temperature, and redox-responsive systems, light-responsive materials are gaining attention for their ability to offer non-invasive control over drug delivery. These materials are especially useful in deep brain delivery and in situations where localized treatment is required, allowing spatial and temporal precision in the treatment of neurological diseases [118].

Several groups have designed efficient light-responsive systems for the delivery of neuromodulators, such as neurotransmitters [119], neuropeptides [120, 121], and opioid receptor modulators [122, 123]. DNA nanoconstructs functionalized with light-responsive components have also been employed for the release of neurotransmitter glutamate [124], and for neurosteroid dehydroepiandrosterone [125]. Light-responsive zeolitic imidazolate-based upconversion nanoparticle carrying nitric oxide donor, S-nitrosocysteine has been evidenced to repress gliosis and neuroinflammation and promote repair processes in SCI models [126]. Dopamine receptor agonist SKF-81297 has also been demonstrated to be released in a light-dependent manner from azobenzene–phosphatidylcholine nanofabrication [127]. Rwei and co-workers proposed the employment of NIR light-sensitive nanoplatforms capable of controlled release of tetrodotoxin for local anesthesia-mediated pain relief [128]. Similarly, light-responsive liposomes attached with gold nanorods have been shown to effectively deliver tetrodotoxin and dexmedetomidine for anesthetic effects in rat footpad [129]. NIR illumination has also been used as an initiator for the controlled release of Kv7.4 voltage-gated potassium channel agonist fasudil from light-responsive nanosystems in order to modulate ventral tegmental dopaminergic neuronal activity patterns [130]. Modulators of calcium signaling such as inositol triphosphate have also been effectively delivered to neuronal cells using light-responsive systems [131]; and this approach has been extended to living mice [132]. Last, photo-responsive gold-based nanofabrications have been shown to inhibit Aβ fibrillization [133] and may be considered for anti-AD therapy in future.

7.5.6 Ultrasound and Magnetic Field-Responsive Systems

Ultrasound is a safer, non-invasive kind of brain stimulation than intrusive methods like deep brain stimulation and spinal cord stimulation. Additionally, compared to non-invasive techniques like transcranial electrostimulation and transcranial magnetic stimulation, FUS provides more spatial precision and the capacity to efficiently target deeper brain structures (a clinical penetration of several cm). Sonoporation-mediated targeting of BBB in recent years has been as a potent technique for aiding targeting drug release for the therapy of neurological disorders [134]. For instance, ultrasound-responsive nanoconstructs were successfully employed for targeted localized delivery of GABA receptor agonist, muscimol in rat motor cortices and found to result in the intended neuromodulatory effects [135]. Propofol has also been administered using FUS/ultrasound-responsive system-based technology in epileptic rats without any significant damage to the BBB and resulted in drastic reduction in seizure intensity [136]. Wang and co-workers have also shown the utility of ultrasound-responsive nanoemulsions in delivering propofol to the targeted brain sites [137]. In another study, pentobarbital was shown to release from nanodroplets under FUS for local anesthesia in motor cortices of rat brains, all while maintaining the integrity of the BBB [138]. Ultrasound-responsive release of another anesthetic, tetrodotoxin was successfully demonstrated using liposomes containing protoporphyrin IX which produces ROS when stimulated by ultrasound for the precisely regulated release of the neurotoxin for localized anesthesia [139].

Magnetic fields are thought to be one of the best external physical stimuli for precisely activating drug release since they don't require direct contact with the subject's body and give a real-time response. Magnetic nanoparticles, which have the ability to transform magnetic fields into signals that biological receptors can perceive, are essential to techniques which rely on changes in magnetic field for controlled release of payload. Magnetothermal-responsive systems which release encapsulated drugs by generating heat upon changes induced in magnetic fields are particularly generating a lot of interests among researchers. For instance, a transient receptor potential vanilloid 1 (TRPV1) channel agonist, allyl isothiocyanate bound by a temperature-sensitive 4,4′-azobis(4-cyanovaleric acid) linker was shown to be effectively released from iron oxide magnetic nanoparticles upon presentation of magnetothermal stimuli [140]. A similar approach was used by Rao and colleagues who fabricated magnetic field-responsive iron oxide nanoliposomes containing payloads which were released after heat was locally generated in the nanoconstructs, while maintaining the overall temperature of the bulk medium. They tested the technique for delivery of SKF-38393, an agonist of dopamine receptor D1 (DRD1) in mice brain, specifically causing alterations in neuronal signaling in the nucleus accumbens, thereby modulating social interactions [141]. Magnetothermal-controlled release of dopamine, and the consequent enhancement of striatal neuronal activity, was also demonstrated using magnetic nanoparticles functionalized with thermo-labile poly [oligo(ethylene glycol) methyl ether methacrylate] coating [142]. Magnetic field-stimulated delivery of a potential anti-PD agent, levodopa has been successfully accomplished using alginate–xanthan gum hydrogels [143]. Similarly, resveratrol, a potential anti-AD therapeutic has been brain delivered via intranasal administration using superparamagnetic iron oxide nanofabrication in mice. Results from this study indicated robust improvements in cognitive functions, mitigation of pro-inflammatory mediators and suppression of AD markers [144]. Magnetic hyperthermia mediated spatiotemporally controlled release of chemotherapeutic temozolomide was shown to improve multiple outcomes, including those related to neuroinflammation in an *in vivo* model of glioblastoma [145].

7.6 BIOMEDICAL IMAGING TECHNIQUES AND DIAGNOSTIC METHODS

Diagnostic methods based upon neurochemical assessments provide critical information regarding altered morpho-functional aspects of neurons in different brain pathophysiological states. Engineering of smart electrochemical nanosensors which are highly sensitive for the various neurochemicals are handy tools in this regard. Additionally, nanoelectrode with switchable surface properties may be advantageous for better controlling of the assay. Surface properties which allow appropriate recognition of external stimuli will enhance correct targeting of these nanoformulations, thereby improving the selectivity as well as sensitivity. Recently, there have been several successful attempts of developing stimuli-responsive neurochemical sensors. For instance, Ding and co-workers developed a graphene electrode for determination of sugars in an enantio-selective manner which could detect even 1 nM concentrations of D-glucose [146]. Phenylboronic acid-based electrochemical stimuli-responsive biosensor, with poly(N-isopropylacrylamide) as a switcher was successfully employed for the detection of sialic acid in mice brain at a detection limit of 0.4 pM [147]. Phenylboronic acid- and poly(N-isopropylacrylamide)-based multi-stimuli-responsive hydrogel with $[Ru(bpy)_3]^{2+}$ redox centers has also been created to recognize fructose and produce output as changes in the electrical signals [148]. Another multi-stimuli-responsive enzyme-based microgel has been fabricated to detect glucose in the physiological concentration ranges in a temperature-sensitive manner [149]. A similar temperature-regulated electrochemical biosensor composed of poly(N-isopropylacrylamide)-b-poly(2-acrylamidoethyl benzoate)/graphene oxide and functionalized with hemoglobin was fabricated for the detection of H_2O_2 [150]. Stimuli-responsive gels which swell in presence of target metabolites and thereby cause changes in the electrical conductance of their constituent semiconductors have been devised against glucose [151] and calcium ions [152].

Nanochannels, which allow ion-specific transport for output signals, are another class of smart stimuli-responsive biosensors which have been exploited for electrochemical quantitation of biomarkers. For instance, a polyethylene terephthalate nanochannel with phenyl guanidine as the identifier has been fabricated to monitor the levels of phosphorylated tyrosine [153]. A biomimetic ATP-responsive nanochannel has also been devised based upon the properties of ATP-gated cellular ion channels [154], which may serve as a potent indicator of ATP levels and metabolic states in living systems. Indeed, polyimidazolium-based micropipettes have been proposed to aid cerebral ATP measurements in concentration ranges of 5–100 nM [155]. In conclusion, smart stimuli-responsive micro- and nanoconstructs have created immense possibilities; the possibility of measuring critical metabolites and biomarkers in biological fluids, such as cerebrospinal fluid, which has even been extended to brain tissues in living organisms. A dual electrochemical and florescence-sensitive quantum dot fabrication has been proposed to identify ApoE4 allele in human blood samples for possible identification of AD cases [156].

Neural probes, which interact with CNS components to either stimulate or record electrical activities, can be integrated into biomaterials to help integrate implants for the CNS. This has boosted the treatment of neuropathologies, improved our understanding of neural connectivity, and made it possible to construct neuro-prosthetics. BBB is compromised when probes are usually placed straight into parenchymal tissue, which can cause tissue injury, local glia activation, and a foreign body reaction. For implanted probes to remain reliable over the long term, glial responsiveness to the implant and regulatory neuroinflammatory signals are essential [157]. There are two considerations for deciding the materials to use to make brain probes and their coatings. These are satisfied by materials that promote cell and protein adhesion can be utilized to encourage the development of neurons that are close to the probes to enhance neural signal detection, and biomaterials which reduce neuroinflammatory reactions and prevent harm to the probes. Both strategies seek to limit neuroinflammatory processes and the development of glial scars and increase the sustained operation of the neural probes. Graphene's beneficial electrical conductivity, chemical inertness, and mechanical flexibility make it an attractive material for creating brain probes [158]. It promotes the development of NSCs, axonal sprouting, and neural adhesion [159]. Graphene works better than other materials at electrode interfaces because it causes less glial scarring and neuronal retraction. Indeed, graphene has been envisioned as a suitable probe material for monitoring neuronal activity for extended periods of time [44]. However, there are questions regarding appropriateness of graphene for *in vivo* applications due to its vulnerability to phagocyte-released peroxidase-mediated oxidation. To avoid possible device failure and particle bioaccumulation, methods for shielding brain probes' graphene covering layer from deterioration are essential [160]. Regarding SRM, hyaluronic acid, a major component of the parenchymal extracellular matrix of the CNS, is a particularly interesting target for neural probe coatings [161]. When hyaluronic acid thin films are combined with the cationic polymers such as poly-L-lysine, there is increased adherence of these constructs with neurons through electrostatic interactions with the cell membrane with a negative charge. Electrodes inside the brain have been coated with this thin film mixture [162]. A study found that a hyaluronic acid/poly-L-lysine coating on graphene monolayers enhanced adhesion of neurons, thereby aiding their outgrowth. The coating adhered to the monolayer without significantly affecting its crystalline quality, demonstrating its potential for neural probe integration, indicating that this coating could potentially enhance neural probe integration [163]. Hydrogels are cytocompatible and have variable mechanical characteristics which can potentially be modified by functionalization with cell-adhesive peptides or stimuli-responsive crosslinkers, making them robust materials for coating neural probes. Due to its resistance to cell and protein attachment, PEG hydrogels are frequently utilized to prevent the immune system from detecting implants [164].

Among the mediators of neuroprotection and recovery in injuries, implantable scaffolds are excellent systems. As there can be a substantial loss of functional tissue as a result of CNS pathologies such as TBI, SCI, and stroke neural regeneration may be aided by implantable scaffolds which can guide cell migration, fill holes, and offer mechanical support. Particularly, for spinal cord damage, these scaffolds are very alluring as they allow delivery of stem cells which can proliferate and assist injured neuronal cells to regenerate. A variety of techniques, such as templated molds, tissue decellularization, additive manufacturing, microfluidic devices, and cryogenic procedures, like freeze-drying, are used to generate implantable scaffolds [165]. Supporting neural networks, these scaffolds can be fibrous, multichannel, or microporous in structure. Controlled porosity and orientation for cellular alignment can be produced using additive manufacturing. Direct implantation of exosomes, cells, nanoparticles, and proteins is made possible by bioprinting viscoelastic hydrogels. The mechanical strength and adjustable porosities of scaffolds are improved by freeze-drying polymers. Hydrogels and hydrophobic polymers such as fibrin, polylactic acid (PLGA), and PCL can be used to create them. Axonal regeneration, synapse forms, and functional recovery are all frequently facilitated by implantable scaffolds [166]. Through SCIs, anisotropic channels promote axon extension and cell migration. In order to treat SCIs, aligned collagen scaffolds are utilized to encourage the neuronal differentiation and neurite outgrowth of fetal brain and spinal cord NSCs of human origin. The promise for treating SCI was demonstrated by the fact that spinal cord-derived NSCs outperformed those derived from the brain in controlling neuroinflammation and encouraging neuronal regeneration. Synthetic polymers can be used to create implantable scaffolds that can modulate inflammation by adjusting the degradation rate and products of PLGA. This is because the PLGA degradation is associated with an acidic and inflamed microenvironment. Indeed, changing the degeneration rate of and byproducts obtained upon PLGA degradation can influence inflammatory responses [167]. Neuroprotective bioactives and neurotrophic and growth factors can also be released in a sustained manner using implantable scaffolds (Figure 7.3); for example, a collagen/heparin scaffold encapsulating vascular endothelial growth factor (VEGF) that was freeze-dried has been utilized to treat TBI in rat models [168]. The scaffold alleviated edema, decreased lesion size, enhanced neuronal survival, and encouraged angiogenesis. Additionally, it markedly reduced levels of pro-inflammatory cytokines, IL-1b and IL-6. A multicomponent gelatin scaffold encapsulating polydopamine-containing nanoconstructs which also delivered GDNF to treat SCI is one example of a combination strategy involving different biomaterials that has been recently investigated [169]. By reducing neuronal apoptosis and neuroinflammation, GDNF released from the polydopamine nano delivery systems enhanced axonal regeneration and neuronal survival. The scaffold confirmed the effectiveness of combinatorial treatment approaches for controlling aberrantly active neuroinflammatory pathways, and supplying neurotrophic sustenance at the same time in order to allow robust neuronal and synaptic recovery.

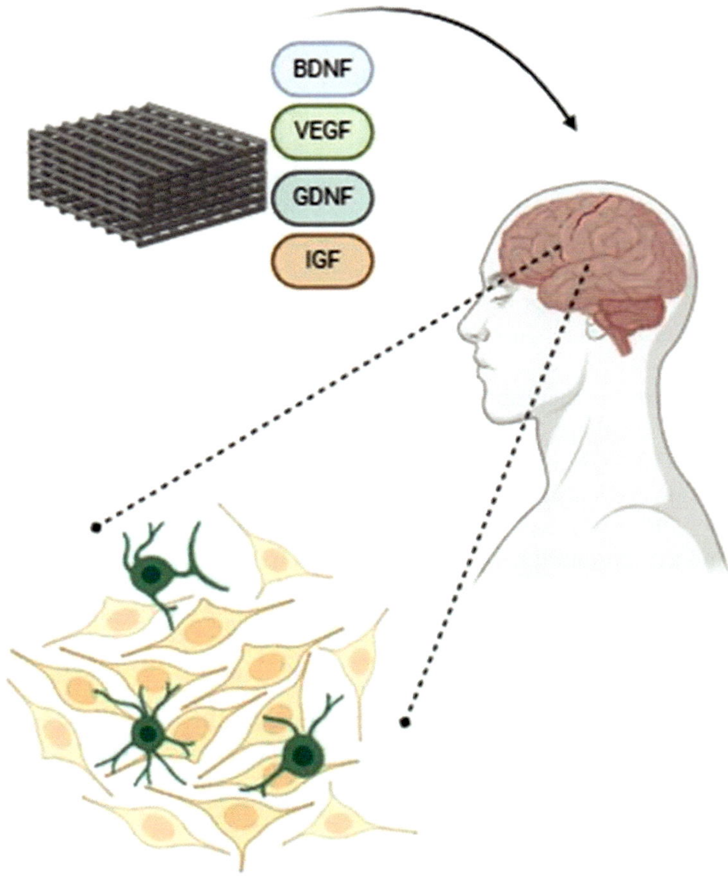

FIGURE 7.3 Implantable scaffolds as delivery systems for growth factors limiting neurodegeneration and aiding regeneration.

7.7 MULTI-STIMULI-RESPONSIVE PLATFORMS FOR NEUROINFLAMMATORY AND NEUROLOGICAL DISORDERS

Multi-stimuli reactive materials react to three or more stimuli and are less studied but essentially intriguing. Several primary studies of various responsive materials have shed light on the external factors that must be adjusted in order to include three or more responsive elements in a single responsive material [34]. The specifications for the molecular design of a system that must react to three or more stimuli are undoubtedly more intricate. Even more specific responses to three or more stimuli at the same time are possible with these systems. Materials with promising properties for biological applications should result from a better grasp of the design principles. Due to their capacity to react to two or more stimuli in the microenvironments of CNS pathologies, multiply responsive nanocarriers have garnered increased interest [173]. For improving treatment efficacy, the medication release profile from this nanofabrication can be accurately controlled under intricate disease states.

Based on MSNs and other materials, a wide range of nanocarriers that respond to dual and multiple stimuli, such as pH-temperature, pH-voltage, pH-specific metabolites, pH-specific enzymes, dual enzyme, and pH-temperature-metabolites/enzyme, may be designed to transport medicinal agents to alleviate neuroinflammatory conditions. For example, Don et al. use a dual stimuli-responsive fucoidan–chitosan-based nanocarriers, which respond to P-selectin and acidic microenvironment, for the delivery of curcumin, a potent anti-neuroinflammatory agent [170]. Thermo and pH-responsive nanocarriers have been proposed as delivery agents for tumoricidal agents for the therapy of gliomas [171]. Similarly, dual stimuli-responsive nanocarriers loaded with chemotherapeutic docetaxel, and functionalized with pH-responsive angiopep-2 moiety and histidine for glioma cell targeting, have shown promising results [172]. Further, using the knowledge of the primary features of metastasis, elevated MMP2 levels and decreased extracellular pH, dual microenvironment responsive nanocarrier may be considered for brain delivery of therapeutics for glioma treatment. In this regard, Huang and colleagues have created a cell-penetrating peptide which requires activation by simultaneous presence of increased MMP2 enzyme levels and decreased pH. This nanocarrier can target angiogenesis pathways as well as activate death of glioma cells by co-delivering shRNA against VEGF and doxorubicin [173]. Vinpocetine, a therapeutic used for cerebrovascular ailments, was shown to be released in a regulated manner by employing temperature and pH-responsive carbopol–HPMC–alginate hydrogels [174].

Reversible addition-fragmentation chain transfer (RAFT) polymerization chemistry was used to fabricate a boronic acid block copolymer with N-isopropylacrylamide (NIPAm) with a self-assembly property in response to changes in pH, temperature, and sugar concentrations [175]. At temperatures higher than the pNIPAAm block's lower critical solution temperature (LCST) of 32°C, the PAPBA-b-pNIPAAm block copolymers dehydrate and organize as micelles. The PAPBA component is polyanionic at basic and neutral pH but turns to hydrophobic in acidic medium. The polymer's hydrophilicity is also increased when boronate esters are formed in the presence of diols. PAPBA-b-pNIPAAm's multi-responsive nature was illustrated by the reversible aggregation and disintegration in response to changes in pH, temperature, and glucose concentration. Each block's dehydration was further investigated using NMR spectroscopy in conjunction with temperature and pH changes. Dextran nanofabrication functionalized with phenylboronic acid have been used as pH- and ROS-responsive delivery systems for naproxen, a NSAID [176], and could be tried for controlling pathological neuroinflammatory conditions.

A dual temperature and pH-responsive hydrogel carrier has been proposed as a delivery agent for timosaponin BII, a potential anti-AD drug. *In vivo* experiments showed that intranasal administration of this construct prevented aberrant activation of neuroinflammatory mediators, and concomitantly stimulated behavioral attributes of memory in animal model of AD [177]. Another multi-stimuli-responsive material which relies on magnetic and pH signals has been tested for the delivery of siRNA against beta-site amyloid precursor protein cleaving enzyme 1 (BACE-1) for the therapy of AD [178]. Bruun and co-workers designed a multi-stimuli-responsive lipid nanoplatform for the brain delivery of siRNA. Functionalization with angiopep permitted entry of the nanocarriers across BBB, while recognition sequences for MMPs allowed targeted delivery to tumor microenvironment. Further, cleavage of the sequence resulted in the release of glutamic acid residues which changed the lipid nanoplatform charge to positive, allowing release of the siRNA payload [95].

7.8 CLINICAL TRANSLATIONS AND PATENTS

The patent landscape for stimuli-responsive biomaterials in the field of neurological disorders has been rapidly evolving, reflecting the growing interest in their therapeutic potential. Many patents have been filed on novel designs of stimuli-responsive biomaterials, including those based on nanomaterials, hydrogels, and polymeric carriers with dual or multi-stimuli responsiveness (Table 7.1). These patents cover various aspects of drug delivery systems that can address neuroinflammation and neurodegeneration by targeting specific biomarkers or responding to changes in the microenvironment of neurological tissues. One key aspect of innovation in the patent landscape is the bioengineering of nanocarriers with the ability to deliver multiple therapeutic bioactives in response to different stimuli. For example, patent applications have

TABLE 7.1

Summary of Some of the Stimuli-Responsive Systems Patented as Therapeutic Tools for Delivery of Therapeutics and/or Cellular Regeneration

Country of Approval	Year	Name	Patent No.	Institution	Inventor	Description
WIPO (PCT)	2001	Magnetically responsive microspheres	WO2001078087A2	Luminex Corporation	Donald J. Chandler and Michael A. Herren	Construction of hybrid fluorescent or luminescent magnetic nanoparticle-based microspheres constructed; reactive surface biomoieties can be used as baits for attachment to biologically active molecules, allowing selective separations and analytical assays to be performed
WIPO (PCT)	2001	Magnetically responsive microparticles	WO1996037313A1		James J. Sutor	Fabrication of magnetite-based magnetically responsive constructs with the ability to be coated for precise functionalization
USA	2008	Photo-responsive hydrogels	US20080044472A1	Arizona Technology Enterprises LLC and Arizona State University	Antonio Garcia, Rohit Rosario, John Gust, Mark Hayes, Manuel Marquez, Zhibing Hu, and Tong Cai	Photo-responsive spiropyran-based hydrogel precursors, whose properties can be changed by exposure to light, pH, and temperature, can be used for targeted delivery of pharmaceutical bioactives
Japan	2012	Temperature-responsive composite polymer	JP2012232961A	Osaka University and Osaka Prefecture University	Chie Kojima	Temperature-responsive composite polymer functionalized with a XPGXG peptide moiety, which undergoes phase transition between hydrophilic and hydrophobic states, capable of carrying pharmaceutical payloads and delivering them in a temperature-sensitive manner
USA	2016	Nanoparticles with pH triggered drug release	US20180318230A1	Brigham and Women's Hospital Inc. and Massachusetts Institute of Technology	Sunandini Chopra, Rohit Karnik, Amy Wang, Omid C. Farokhzad, and Xue-Qing Zhang	Nanoconstruct comprising of a pH-responsive polymer, can act as a system for delivery of bioactive payload that releases it in a pH-sensitive manner
USA	2016	Temperature-responsive substrate for cell culture	US9279102B2	Tokyo Women's Medical University	Masamichi Nakayama and Teruo Okano	Temperature-responsive surface composed of water-insoluble polymer and temperature-sensitive segments for cell culture propagation capable of efficiently culturing cells, adherent cells can be removed by changing the temperature

USA	2018	Library of pH-responsive polymers and nanoprobes	US20170143852A1	University of Texas	Jinming Gao, Gang Huang, Tian Zhao, Xinpeng MA, Yiguang Wang, Yang Li, and Baran D. Sumer	Micellar nanoprobes composed of hydrophobic and hydrophilic segments which are sensitive to pH, resulting in altered fluorescence signal in presence of a particular pH value, efficient for imaging of cellular or extracellular environment and delivering a drug in a pH-dependent manner
USA	2018	Methods, devices, and systems for on-demand ultrasound-triggered drug delivery	US20130041311A1	Columbia University, Children's Medical Center Corp, and Massachusetts Institute of Technology	Daniel S. Kohane, Hila Epstein-Barash, and Mark A. Borden	Implantable or injectable microbubble-containing drug delivery nanosystems for ultrasound-triggered targeted and localized release of encapsulated bioactives
USA	2018	Enzyme-responsive nanocapsules for protein delivery	US9993440B2	University of California	Yunfeng Lu, Tatiana Segura, Suwei Zhu, and Jing Wen	Enzyme-responsive polymer shell for the delivery of polypeptides in the specific vicinity of the microenvironment expressing the particular enzymes which degrade the polymer shell, consequentially allowing delivery of one or polypeptide payloads, polymer shell disintegration relies on the peptide-based interconnections which are cleaved by environmental conditions, such as presence of a particular protease
USA	2020	pH-responsive mucoadhesive polymeric-encapsulated microorganisms	US10548844B2	Massachusetts Institute of Technology	Aaron C. Anselmo, Robert S. Langer, and Ana Jaklenec	Bioengineering of microbes for targeted enteric delivery of therapeutics within gastrointestinal sites in a pH-dependent and sustained manner may be used for altering resident microbial population
Europe	2020	Tumor imaging using photon-emitting phosphors having therapeutic properties	EP3134122B1	Immunolight LLC, and Duke University, and North Carolina State University	Harold Walder, Frederic A. Bourke, Zakaryae Fathi, Wayne F. Beyer, Mark W. Dewhirst, Mark Oldham, Justus Adamson, and Michael Nolan	Combinatorial constructs with the ability to deliver therapeutics in a photo-sensitive manner and phosphors capable of emitting light in the visible or UV range for imaging of the disease sites
USA	2020	Photo-responsive protein hydrogels	US10647755B2	Hong Kong University of Science and Technology	Fei Sun and Ri Wang	Hydrogels capable of releasing therapeutic bioactives in a light-dependent manner; applications extend to cell encapsulation and culturing

(Continued)

TABLE 7.1 (*Continued*)
Summary of Some of the Stimuli-Responsive Systems Patented as Therapeutic Tools for Delivery of Therapeutics and/or Cellular Regeneration

Country of Approval	Year	Name	Patent No.	Institution	Inventor	Description
USA	2021	Ultrasound-responsive devices and systems	US20160296203A1	Columbia University, Children's Medical Center Corp., and Massachusetts Institute of Technology	Elisa E. Konofagou, Jean Provost, Jianwen Luo, Stanley J. Okrasinski, Stéphane Thiébaut, and Vu Thanh-Hieu Nguyen	Bioengineered ultrasound-sensitive scaffolds and materials for the localized and targeted delivery of bioactives provide mechanical stimulation to cells and increase perfusion of fluids in the microenvironment
USA	2022	Enzyme-responsive shape memory polymers	US20190301064A1	Syracuse University	James Henderson, Patrick T. Mather, and Shelby Buffington	Enzyme-responsive shape memory polymers formed by crosslinking with ester bonds that are sensitive to the presence of specific enzymes, such as Amano lipase PS; the presence of a thermoplastic elastomer component allows enzyme-responsive contraction or expansion upon changes in the elastomeric phase of the scaffold
Europe	2022	Functionalized linkers in responsive biomaterials	EP4412600A1	University of Cincinnati	John Robert Martin, Karina Ann Bruce, Dylan Widder Marques, and Alan Joseph Fullenkamp	Incorporation of labile linkers (keto, thiol, or thioketal) into stimuli-responsive biomaterial
China	2023	ROS-responsive hyperbranched poly(beta-amino ester) nanofabrications	CN115449072A	Suzhou University	Yin Lichen and Wu Qinghua	Construction of an ROS-responsive hyperbranched nano-core which can be encapsulated in fusion membrane derived from platelet or microglial cells; nano-composite can be used for the delivery of nucleic acid-based therapies drug to target cells at inflamed sites, particularly for the treatment of conditions like cerebral ischemia
USA	2010	Temperature and pH-responsive poly(amidoamine) oligomer hydrogels	US8383153	Sungkyunkwan University, and Foundation for Corporate Collaboration	Doo Sung Lee, Bong Sup Kim, and Minh Khanh Nguyen	Fabrication of a dual responsive (temperature and pH) nanoplatform for the delivery of therapeutic agents

USA	2002	pH-responsive hydrogel-based delivery system	US7066904B2	Boston Scientific Scimed Inc.	Arthur Rosenthal, James J. Barry, and Ronald Sahatjian	Hydrogel capable of being delivered at target sites by catheters, which deliver encapsulated therapeutics in a pathological environment (such as pH or ionic strength changes) which controls the swelling and contraction properties of the polymer
Europe	1992	Polyurethane hydrogels for iontophoretic drug delivery	EP0524718A1	Sicor Inc.	Soonkap Hahn	Iontophoretic (electric current dependent) dermal delivery of therapeutics using polyurethane hydrogel matrices
USA	2010	Swellable hydrogel plugs for drug delivery	US8409606B2	Incept LLC	Amarpreet S. Sawhney, Peter Jarrett, Michael Bassett, and Charles Blizzard	Swellable hydrogels for delivery of therapeutics to the eye, capable of swelling in presence of physiological water molecules in the ocular environment to release drugs
WIPO (PCT)	1998	pH-responsive hydrogel gels for oral protein delivery	WO1998043615A1	Purdue Research Foundation and Hoshi University	Nicholas A. Peppas, Anthony M. Lowman, Tsuneji Nagai, and Mariko Morishita	pH-responsive hydrogels encapsulating proteins (e.g., insulin) which protect the cargo from the stomach acids, but elicit swelling-induced protein release when exposed to higher pH conditions of the small intestines

been filed for ROS- and pH-sensitive nanoparticles designed to target amyloid plaques in AD, enabling the dual release of anti-inflammatory and neuroprotective agents upon encountering the characteristic oxidative and acidic microenvironment of Alzheimer's-affected tissues. These multifunctional systems are designed to release drugs in a highly localized and regulated manner, providing therapeutic efficacy while curtailing adverse side effects [179]. In addition to nanoparticles, patent filings for stimuli-responsive hydrogels have gained attention as a therapeutic strategy against SCIs, stroke, and brain trauma. These systems often involve enzyme-sensitive, temperature-responsive, or light-sensitive materials that can be injected or implanted at the site of injury, where they undergo a controlled release upon encountering the stimuli from the local tissue environment [180]. Despite the progress in stimuli-responsive biomaterial-based therapeutic approaches (Table 7.2), several challenges remain that must be addressed before widespread clinical adoption:

a. *Regulatory hurdles*: The FDA and other regulatory bodies have stringent requirements for neurological drug delivery systems, especially regarding the safety and lasting stability of new biomaterials. *In vivo* toxicity studies and long-term safety evaluations are crucial before clinical approval can be granted.
b. *Scalability*: While small-scale production of stimuli-responsive biomaterials has been demonstrated in laboratories, scaling up these systems for clinical use requires significant investment in manufacturing processes that can guarantee consistency, purity, and quality control.
c. *Personalization of treatment*: As the pathophysiology of neurological diseases is often patient-specific, developing personalized stimuli-responsive systems that respond to the unique biomarker profiles of individual patients is an area of active research.

Looking forward, multifunctional and multi-stimuli-responsive biomaterials are likely to play increasingly significant roles in the clinical management of neuroinflammatory and neurological disorders. Future developments will likely focus on:

a. Optimizing BBB penetration and enhancing targeted brain delivery of therapeutic bioactives.
b. Personalized medicine approaches that tailor the treatment to individual patients' disease profiles.
c. Multi-modal therapies that combine stimuli-responsive systems with other treatments, such as gene therapy, immunotherapy, or neuroprotective agents.
d. The development of clinically viable platforms that can be easily manufactured and scaled for widespread use in clinical settings.
e. As these systems move closer to clinical application, it is anticipated that the patent landscape will continue to evolve, with further innovation in the design and application of SRM for neurological diseases.

7.9 CONCLUSION

The advent of stimuli-responsive biomaterials has introduced significant avenues for therapeutic advancements against neuroinflammation associated with CNS disorders. As our understanding of the molecular mechanisms driving these conditions deepens, the role of these smart materials in providing targeted, dynamic, and controlled therapeutic interventions becomes ever more promising. While the application of stimuli-responsive systems in neurobiology is still in its infancy, several future directions stand poised to enhance their clinical viability and effectiveness. One of the most exciting directions for stimuli-responsive biomaterials is their integration into personalized medicine. The ability to design materials that respond to specific pathophysiological

TABLE 7.2
Summary of Clinical Trials for the Evaluation of the Therapeutic Potential of Stimuli-Responsive Systems in Different Pathologies

Title	Year of Initiation	Condition or Disease	Clinical Trial ID	Investigators	Institute	Summary	Status/Last Known Status	Phase
Evaluation of the cell detachment ratio on pH-responsive chitosan as a prognostic factor in lung cancer	2019	Lung cancer	NCT04218188	Tai-Horng Young	National Taiwan University Hospital	Chitosan-based pH-responsive biomaterials for culturing patient-derived tumor cell in order to evaluate the cellular detachment ratio and expression of surface markers measures of predicting patient survival	Recruiting	–
Photoactivated composite biomaterial for soft tissue restoration in rodents and in humans	2011	Soft tissue injury	IRB #143574 Health Canada	Alexander T Hillel, and Jennifer H Elisseeff	Johns Hopkins University	PEG-hyaluronic acid-based injectable composites which are photo-crosslinked transdermal light exposure; useful for soft tissue replacement and reconstruction in abdominal tissues, for example	Unknown	–
Temperature-sensitive liposomal doxorubicin and hyperthermia in treating women With locally recurrent breast cancer	2006	Breast cancer	NCT00346229	Kimberly L. Blackwell	Duke University	High temperature-responsive liposomal delivery of chemotherapeutic doxorubicin, combined with localized hyperthermic signal for causing death of cancer cells	Terminated	Phase 1
Monitoring local tissue oxygen changes using the Wireless Lumee Oxygen Platform in correlation to transcutaneous oxygen pressure (TcPO2)	2020	Peripheral artery disease	NCT04514861	Kerstin Rebrin	Profusa, Inc.	Lumee Oxygen is the soft injectable oxygen-responsive hydrogel component of the Wireless Lumee Oxygen Platform and allows determination of subcutaneous oxygen levels	Unknown	Not applicable
Magnetic nanoparticles system in acute coronary syndrome	2014	Acute coronary syndrome	NCT02226523	Yen-Wen Wu	Far Eastern Memorial Hospital	Magnetic field-activated nanoplatforms functionalized with bioprobes such as antibodies for rapid assay of biomolecules like cardiac tissue-expressed enzymes, troponins, and myoglobulin; the technique was called "immunomagnetic reduction (IMR)"	Completed	Not applicable

(Continued)

TABLE 7.2 (*Continued*)
Summary of Clinical Trials for the Evaluation of the Therapeutic Potential of Stimuli-Responsive Systems in Different Pathologies

Title	Year of Initiation	Condition or Disease	Clinical Trial ID	Investigators	Institute	Summary	Status/Last Known Status	Phase
Plasmonic photothermal and stem cell therapy of atherosclerosis versus stenting	2010	Atherosclerosis, coronary artery disease	NCT01436123	Alexander Kharlamov	Ural State Medical University	Au-nanoconstructs with silica–iron oxide shells encapsulated in stem cells which release the cargo upon targeted localized exposure to high-energy plasmonic photothermic (NIR) which causes a burning or melting effect disintegrating the carrier stem cells	Terminated	Phase I
Plasmonic nanophotothermal therapy of atherosclerosis	2007	Cardiovascular diseases	NCT01270139	Alexander Kharlamov	De Haar Research Task Force	Silica–Au–Fe nanoconstructs delivered via bioengineered arterial patches capable of providing microbubbles or stem cell-based therapy for the functional restoration of vessel walls	Completed	Not applicable
Phase II study of combined temozolomide and SGT-53 for treatment of recurrent glioblastoma	2014	Glioblastoma	NCT02340156	John deGroot	SynerGene Therapeutics, Inc.	SGT-53, cationic liposomal construct capable of delivering p53 cDNA to tumor cells; ability of the delivery system to cross BBB conferred by functionalization with anti-transferrin receptor antibody	Terminated	Phase II
Targeted silica nanoparticles for real-time image-guided intraoperative mapping of nodal metastases	2014	Head and neck cancer	NCT02106598	Hilda Stambuk	Memorial Sloan Kettering Cancer Center	NIR fluorophore and radiolabeled silica nanocarriers for real-time imaging lymph node metastasis	Active	Phase I, II
Anti-EGFR-immunoliposomes loaded with doxorubicin in patients with advanced triple negative EGFR positive breast cancer	2016	Breast cancer	NCT02833766	Ralph Winterhalder	Swiss Group for Clinical Cancer Research	EGFR-responsive nanoconstructs for the targeted delivery of doxorubicin	Terminated	Phase II

A Study to Evaluate the Safety, Tolerability and Immunogenicity of EGFR(V)-EDV-Dox in Subjects With Recurrent Glioblastoma Multiforme (GBM)	2016	Glioblastoma multiforme	NCT02766699	Jennifer MacDiarmid, Himanshu Brahmbhatt, Gary L Gallia, and Stuart A Grossman	Engeneic Pty Limited	EGFR-responsive biomimetic mini-cell derived from bacterial cells capable of delivering doxorubicin for chemotherapeutic purposes	Unknown	Phase I
Ultrasound-based blood–brain barrier opening and albumin-bound paclitaxel and carboplatin for recurrent glioblastoma	2020	Glioblastoma	NCT04528680	Adam M Sonabend	Northwestern University	FUS-responsive brain delivery of chemotherapeutics, paclitaxel, and carboplatin	Recruiting	Phase I, II

cues related to altered states of temperature, pH, and ionic concentration, and presence of specific enzymes/metabolites may hold potential for precise and patient-specific treatment strategies under clinical settings. Future developments in bioinformatics and molecular diagnostics may allow for the creation of individualized biomaterial systems that can tailor therapeutic release profiles specifically taking into account the individual's unique pathogenic features, genetic background, and therapeutic needs. This is crucial as many neuroinflammatory and neurological disorders, such as AD, PD, and MS, are multifaceted and require multifactorial therapeutic approaches. Stimuli-responsive biomaterials that combine drug delivery, neuroprotection, and regenerative capabilities in a single system could be game-changers. For example, multifunctional nanomaterials that respond to both inflammatory mediators and oxidative stress could simultaneously alleviate symptoms and promote tissue repair, offering a more holistic approach to treatment. Stimuli-responsive biomaterials may also serve as ideal platforms for combination therapies. By integrating with gene therapy, cell-based therapies, or immunomodulatory approaches, these materials could offer synergistic effects that enhance the overall therapeutic outcome. For instance, incorporating CRISPR/Cas9 gene-editing tools within a smart material matrix could allow for the in-situ correction of genetic defects in neurodegenerative diseases, while the material itself regulates the release of both gene-editing tools and neuroprotective agents.

The application of stimuli-responsive biomaterials in the therapy of neuroinflammatory and neurological disorders holds enormous potential, but several key challenges must be addressed. First, scalability and manufacturing processes for these materials remain a concern. While many stimuli-responsive systems have been demonstrated in preclinical studies, translating these materials into large-scale, cost-effective production for clinical use is a complex task. Furthermore, the enduring bioavailability, biocompatibility, and safety of these systems need to be rigorously evaluated under clinical settings. Moreover, a more comprehensive understanding of the brain's immune environment across various neurological diseases is crucial to designing highly specific stimuli-responsive biomaterials. Personalized medicine approaches that take into account the heterogeneity of the immune response in individual patients will be essential for optimizing treatment regimens. The invention of advanced *in vivo* imaging tools and techniques and real-time diagnostic tools will likely play significant roles in monitoring the progress of treatment and evaluating the effectiveness of stimuli-responsive therapies.

Moreover, a more comprehensive understanding of the brain's immune environment across various neurological diseases is crucial to designing highly specific stimuli-responsive biomaterials. Personalized medicine approaches that take into account the heterogeneity of the immune response in individual patients will be essential for optimizing treatment regimens. The development of real-time diagnostic tools is expected to streamline monitoring the progress of treatment and evaluating the effectiveness of stimuli-responsive therapies. While short-term applications of stimuli-responsive biomaterials have shown promise in preclinical models, the long-term bioavailability, biocompatibility, stability, and biodegradability of these materials remain critical concerns. Future development of advanced responsive biomaterials with improved resistance to degradation and optimized interaction with neural tissue will be essential to establish their long-term efficacy and safety. Furthermore, exploring non-invasive or minimally invasive methods of monitoring the material's performance *in vivo* will be crucial for assessing therapeutic outcomes over extended periods. A significant note of mention here is the regulatory and ethical considerations associated with the clinical employment of diagnostic and therapeutic stimuli-responsive biomaterials. As stimuli-responsive biomaterials progress from preclinical to clinical stages, rigorous attention must be paid to the regulatory frameworks and ethical considerations surrounding their use. The potential for materials to be manipulated externally or respond to various endogenous triggers necessitates careful evaluation of their long-term safety profiles. Additionally, ethical questions regarding patient consent, the complexity of material design, and the potential societal implications of advanced neurotherapeutic technologies must be addressed proactively.

In conclusion, stimuli-responsive biomaterials may represent a transformative approach in the treatment of neuroinflammatory and neurological disorders, offering unprecedented opportunities for targeted, controlled, and dynamic therapeutic interventions. Their capacity to appropriately respond to specific environmental cues holds immense potential in improving both the effectiveness and safety of treatments for a range of conditions, from acute neuroinflammation to chronic neurodegeneration. Although significant challenges remain in terms of optimizing material properties, ensuring long-term safety, and translating findings from bench to bedside, on-going advancements in materials science, neurobiology, and nanotechnology are rapidly bridging these gaps. Ultimately, integration of stimuli-responsive systems into clinical practice has the potential to revolutionize the management of CNS pathologies, beneficially altering patient disease outcomes and overall quality of life. As research continues to evolve, these materials are expected to become a cornerstone of next-generation neurotherapeutics, making personalized, responsive treatments a reality for those suffering from debilitating neurological conditions.

Declaration of AI and AI-Assisted Technologies

During the preparation of this work, the authors used QuillBot AI in order to paraphrase the sentences. After using this tool, the authors reviewed and edited the content as needed and take full responsibility for the content of the publication.

LIST OF ABBREVIATIONS

AD: Alzheimer's disease; apoE: apolipoprotein E; BACE-1: beta-site amyloid precursor protein cleaving enzyme 1; BBB: blood–brain barrier; BCSB: blood cerebrospinal fluid barrier; BDNF: brain-derived neurotrophic factor; CNS: central nervous system; B-PDEAEA: poly[(2-acryloyl) ethyl(p-boronic acid benzyl) dimethylammonium bromide]; DRD1: dopamine receptor D1; FUS: focused ultrasound; GDNF: glial-derived neurotrophic factor; GSN: graphene mesoporous silica; hAMSC: human amniotic mesenchymal stem cells; let7b: lethal-7b; MCAO: middle cerebral artery occlusion; MMP: matrix metalloproteinase; MRgFUS: magnetic resonance guided focused ultrasound; MS: multiple sclerosis; MSC: mesenchymal stromal cells; MSN: mesoporous silica nanoparticles; NIPAm: N-isopropylacrylamide; NLRP3: nucleotide-binding oligomerization domain leucine-rich repeat and pyrin domain-containing protein 3; NSAID: nonsteroidal anti-inflammatory drug; NSC: neural stem cells; Olz: olanzapine; PCPP-SA: poly(1,3-bis(carboxyphenoxy) propane)-co-sebacic acid; PD: Parkinson's disease; PDMAEMA: poly(2-dimethylamino) ethyl methacrylate; PEG: poly(ethylene) glycol; PEG-B-PMNT: poly(ethylene glycol)-b-poly [4-(2, 2, 6, 6-tetramylpiperidine-1-oxy) amino methyl styrene]; PEO–PPO–PEO: poly(ethylene oxide)–poly(propylene oxide)–poly(ethylene oxide); PLGA: polylactic acid, pNIPAAm: poly(N-isopropylacrylamide); POMs: polyoxometalates; PPS120: poly(propylene sulfide)120; PVA: polyvinyl alcohol; RAFT: reversible addition-fragmentation chain transfer; RAGE: receptor for advanced glycation end-products; ROS: reactive oxygen species; SCI: spinal cord injury; TBI: traumatic brain injury; ThS: thioflavin-S; TM: triglycerol monostearate; TRPV1: transient receptor potential vanilloid 1; VEGF: vascular endothelial growth factor.

REFERENCES

1. Feigin VL, Vos T, Nichols E, Owolabi MO, Carroll WM, Dichgans M, et al. The global burden of neurological disorders: Translating evidence into policy. Lancet Neurol 2020;19:255–65. https://doi.org/10.1016/S1474-4422(19)30411-9.
2. Mishra A, Bandopadhyay R, Singh PK, Mishra PS, Sharma N, Khurana N. Neuroinflammation in neurological disorders: Pharmacotherapeutic targets from bench to bedside. Metab Brain Dis 2021;36:1591–626. https://doi.org/10.1007/s11011-021-00806-4.

3. Zheng R, Yu C, Yao D, Cai M, Zhang L, Ye F, et al. Engineering stimuli-responsive materials for precision medicine. Small 2024:e2406439. https://doi.org/10.1002/smll.202406439.
4. Rizwan M, Yahya R, Hassan A, Yar M, Azzahari A, Selvanathan V, et al. pH sensitive hydrogels in drug delivery: Brief history, properties, swelling, and release mechanism, material selection and applications. Polymers (Basel) 2017;9:137. https://doi.org/10.3390/polym9040137.
5. Nag S, Mohanto S, Ahmed MG, Subramaniyan V. "Smart" stimuli-responsive biomaterials revolutionizing the theranostic landscape of inflammatory arthritis. Mater Today Chem 2024;39:102178. https://doi.org/10.1016/j.mtchem.2024.102178.
6. Karimi M, Sahandi Zangabad P, Ghasemi A, Amiri M, Bahrami M, Malekzad H, et al. Temperature-responsive smart nanocarriers for delivery of therapeutic agents: Applications and recent advances. ACS Appl Mater Interfaces 2016;8:21107–33. https://doi.org/10.1021/acsami.6b00371.
7. Ahmad F, Liu P. Synaptosome as a tool in Alzheimer's disease research. Brain Res 2020;1746:147009. https://doi.org/10.1016/j.brainres.2020.147009.
8. Sami N, Rahman S, Kumar V, Zaidi S, Islam A, Ali S, et al. Protein aggregation, misfolding and consequential human neurodegenerative diseases. Int J Neurosci 2017;127:1047–57. https://doi.org/10.1080/00207454.2017.1286339.
9. Soto C, Pritzkow S. Protein misfolding, aggregation, and conformational strains in neurodegenerative diseases. Nat Neurosci 2018;21:1332–40. https://doi.org/10.1038/s41593-018-0235-9.
10. Ciccocioppo F, Bologna G, Ercolino E, Pierdomenico L, Simeone P, Lanuti P, et al. Neurodegenerative diseases as proteinopathies-driven immune disorders. Neural Regen Res 2020;15:850. https://doi.org/10.4103/1673-5374.268971.
11. Schain M, Kreisl WC. Neuroinflammation in neurodegenerative disorders—A review. Curr Neurol Neurosci Rep 2017;17:25. https://doi.org/10.1007/s11910-017-0733-2.
12. Liu Z, Cheng X, Zhong S, Zhang X, Liu C, Liu F, et al. Peripheral and central nervous system immune response crosstalk in amyotrophic lateral sclerosis. Front Neurosci 2020;14:575. https://doi.org/10.3389/fnins.2020.00575.
13. Shastri A, Bonifati DM, Kishore U. Innate immunity and neuroinflammation. Mediators Inflamm 2013;2013:1–19. https://doi.org/10.1155/2013/342931.
14. Piancone F, La Rosa F, Marventano I, Saresella M, Clerici M. The role of the inflammasome in neurodegenerative diseases. Molecules 2021;26:953. https://doi.org/10.3390/molecules26040953.
15. Veerhuis R, Nielsen HM, Tenner AJ. Complement in the brain. Mol Immunol 2011;48:1592–603. https://doi.org/10.1016/j.molimm.2011.04.003.
16. Monif M, Burnstock G, Williams DA. Microglia: Proliferation and activation driven by the P2X7 receptor. Int J Biochem Cell Biol 2010;42:1753–6. https://doi.org/10.1016/j.biocel.2010.06.021.
17. Franke H, Verkhratsky A, Burnstock G, Illes P. Pathophysiology of astroglial purinergic signalling. Purinergic Signal 2012;8:629–57. https://doi.org/10.1007/s11302-012-9300-0.
18. Sharma VK, Mehta V, Singh TG. Alzheimer's disorder: Epigenetic connection and associated risk factors. Curr Neuropharmacol 2020;18:740–53. https://doi.org/10.2174/1570159X18666200128125641.
19. Rasool M, Malik A, Qureshi MS, Manan A, Pushparaj PN, Asif M, et al. Recent updates in the treatment of neurodegenerative disorders using natural compounds. Evid-Based Complement Alternat Med 2014;2014:321. https://doi.org/10.1155/2014/979730.
20. Jarrott B, Williams SJ. Chronic brain inflammation: The neurochemical basis for drugs to reduce inflammation. Neurochem Res 2016;41:523–33. https://doi.org/10.1007/s11064-015-1661-7.
21. Muzio L, Viotti A, Martino G. Microglia in neuroinflammation and neurodegeneration: From understanding to therapy. Front Neurosci 2021;15:742065. https://doi.org/10.3389/fnins.2021.742065.
22. Bors LA, Erdő F. Overcoming the blood–brain barrier. Challenges and tricks for CNS drug delivery. Sci Pharm 2019;87:6. https://doi.org/10.3390/scipharm87010006.
23. Agrawal M, Dayaramani R. Stimuli-Responsive Polymers for Brain Delivery. Application of Nanocarriers in Brain Delivery of Therapeutics, Singapore: Springer Nature Singapore; 2024, p. 263–83. https://doi.org/10.1007/978-981-97-2859-6_10.
24. Deng Z, Liu S. Inflammation-responsive delivery systems for the treatment of chronic inflammatory diseases. Drug Deliv Transl Res 2021;11:1475–97. https://doi.org/10.1007/s13346-021-00977-8.
25. Mozafari N, Ashrafi H, Azadi A. Targeted drug delivery systems to control neuroinflammation in central nervous system disorders. J Drug Deliv Sci Technol 2021;66:102802. https://doi.org/10.1016/j.jddst.2021.102802.
26. Han X, Alu A, Liu H, Shi Y, Wei X, Cai L, et al. Biomaterial-assisted biotherapy: A brief review of biomaterials used in drug delivery, vaccine development, gene therapy, and stem cell therapy. Bioact Mater 2022;17:29–48. https://doi.org/10.1016/j.bioactmat.2022.01.011.

27. Kumar M, Sharma P, Maheshwari R, Tekade M, Shrivastava SK, Tekade RK. Beyond the Blood–Brain Barrier. Nanotechnology-Based Targeted Drug Delivery Systems for Brain Tumors, Elsevier; 2018, p. 397–437. https://doi.org/10.1016/B978-0-12-812218-1.00015-4.
28. Hanif S, Muhammad P, Chesworth R, Rehman FU, Qian R, Zheng M, et al. Nanomedicine-based immunotherapy for central nervous system disorders. Acta Pharmacol Sin 2020;41:936–53. https://doi.org/10.1038/s41401-020-0429-z.
29. Kumar R, Aadil KR, Mondal K, Mishra YK, Oupicky D, Ramakrishna S, et al. Neurodegenerative disorders management: State-of-art and prospects of nano-biotechnology. Crit Rev Biotechnol 2022;42:1180–212. https://doi.org/10.1080/07388551.2021.1993126.
30. Dai X, Li W, Xie D, Liu B, Gong L, Han H. Stimuli-responsive nano drug delivery systems for the treatment of neurological diseases. Small 2025;21:2410030. https://doi.org/10.1002/smll.202410030.
31. Eleftheriadou D, Kesidou D, Moura F, Felli E, Song W. Redox-responsive nanobiomaterials-based therapeutics for neurodegenerative diseases. Small 2020;16:e1907308. https://doi.org/10.1002/smll.201907308.
32. Mura S, Nicolas J, Couvreur P. Stimuli-responsive nanocarriers for drug delivery. Nat Mater 2013;12:991–1003. https://doi.org/10.1038/nmat3776.
33. Lochhead JJ, Thorne RG. Intranasal delivery of biologics to the central nervous system. Adv Drug Deliv Rev 2012;64:614–28. https://doi.org/10.1016/j.addr.2011.11.002.
34. Li J, Mooney DJ. Designing hydrogels for controlled drug delivery. Nat Rev Mater 2016;1:16071. https://doi.org/10.1038/natrevmats.2016.71.
35. Rivera-Tarazona LK, Campbell ZT, Ware TH. Stimuli-responsive engineered living materials. Soft Matter 2021;17:785–809. https://doi.org/10.1039/D0SM01905D.
36. Ghosh S, Ghosh S, Sharma H, Bhaskar R, Han SS, Sinha JK. Harnessing the power of biological macromolecules in hydrogels for controlled drug release in the central nervous system: A review. Int J Biol Macromol 2024;254:127708. https://doi.org/10.1016/j.ijbiomac.2023.127708.
37. Kim Y-J, Matsunaga YT. Thermo-responsive polymers and their application as smart biomaterials. J Mater Chem B 2017;5:4307–21. https://doi.org/10.1039/C7TB00157F.
38. Singh A, Kukreti R, Saso L, Kukreti S. Oxidative stress: A key modulator in neurodegenerative diseases. Molecules 2019;24:1583. https://doi.org/10.3390/molecules24081583.
39. Liu J, Han X, Zhang T, Tian K, Li Z, Luo F. Reactive oxygen species (ROS) scavenging biomaterials for anti-inflammatory diseases: From mechanism to therapy. J Hematol Oncol 2023;16:116. https://doi.org/10.1186/s13045-023-01512-7.
40. Das SS, Bharadwaj P, Bilal M, Barani M, Rahdar A, Taboada P, et al. Stimuli-responsive polymeric nanocarriers for drug delivery, imaging, and theragnosis. Polymers (Basel) 2020;12:1397. https://doi.org/10.3390/polym12061397.
41. Chowdhury A, Kunjiappan S, Panneerselvam T, Somasundaram B, Bhattacharjee C. Nanotechnology and nanocarrier-based approaches on treatment of degenerative diseases. Int Nano Lett 2017;7:91–122. https://doi.org/10.1007/s40089-017-0208-0.
42. Ahmadi S, Rabiee N, Bagherzadeh M, Elmi F, Fatahi Y, Farjadian F, et al. Stimulus-responsive sequential release systems for drug and gene delivery. Nano Today 2020;34:100914. https://doi.org/10.1016/j.nantod.2020.100914.
43. Hickman S, Izzy S, Sen P, Morsett L, El Khoury J. Microglia in neurodegeneration. Nat Neurosci 2018;21:1359–69. https://doi.org/10.1038/s41593-018-0242-x.
44. Su X, Maguire-Zeiss KA, Giuliano R, Prifti L, Venkatesh K, Federoff HJ. Synuclein activates microglia in a model of Parkinson's disease. Neurobiol Aging 2008;29:1690–701. https://doi.org/10.1016/j.neurobiolaging.2007.04.006.
45. Heurtaux T, Michelucci A, Losciuto S, Gallotti C, Felten P, Dorban G, et al. Microglial activation depends on beta-amyloid conformation: Role of the formylpeptide receptor 2. J Neurochem 2010;114:576–86. https://doi.org/10.1111/j.1471-4159.2010.06783.x.
46. Cui Y, Zhang F, Chen G, Yao L, Zhang N, Liu Z, et al. A stretchable and transparent electrode based on PEGylated silk fibroin for in vivo dual-modal neural-vascular activity probing. Adv Mater 2021;33:e2100221. https://doi.org/10.1002/adma.202100221.
47. Bourrier A, Shkorbatova P, Bonizzato M, Rey E, Barraud Q, Courtine G, et al. Monolayer graphene coating of intracortical probes for long-lasting neural activity monitoring. Adv Healthc Mater 2019;8:e1801331. https://doi.org/10.1002/adhm.201801331.
48. Cho H, Kambhampati SP, Lai MJ, Zhou L, Lee G, Xie Y, et al. Dendrimer-triamcinolone acetonide reduces neuroinflammation, pathological angiogenesis, and neuroretinal dysfunction in ischemic retinopathy. Adv Ther (Weinh) 2021;4:2000181. https://doi.org/10.1002/adtp.202000181.

49. Hollinger KR, Sharma A, Tallon C, Lovell L, Thomas AG, Zhu X, et al. Dendrimer-2PMPA selectively blocks upregulated microglial GCPII activity and improves cognition in a mouse model of multiple sclerosis. Nanotheranostics 2022;6:126–42. https://doi.org/10.7150/ntno.63158.
50. Zhang F, Zhang Z, Alt J, Kambhampati SP, Sharma A, Singh S, et al. Dendrimer-enabled targeted delivery attenuates glutamate excitotoxicity and improves motor function in a rabbit model of cerebral palsy. J Cont Release 2023;358:27–42. https://doi.org/10.1016/j.jconrel.2023.04.017.
51. Zhang D, Ren Y, He Y, Chang R, Guo S, Ma S, et al. In situ forming and biocompatible hyaluronic acid hydrogel with reactive oxygen species-scavenging activity to improve traumatic brain injury repair by suppressing oxidative stress and neuroinflammation. Mater Today Bio 2022;15:100278. https://doi.org/10.1016/j.mtbio.2022.100278.
52. Albashari A, He Y, Zhang Y, Ali J, Lin F, Zheng Z, et al. Thermosensitive bFGF-modified hydrogel with dental pulp stem cells on neuroinflammation of spinal cord injury. ACS Omega 2020;5:16064–75. https://doi.org/10.1021/acsomega.0c01379.
53. Liu X, Zhang G, Wei P, Hao L, Zhong L, Zhong K, et al. 3D-printed collagen/silk fibroin/secretome derived from bFGF-pretreated HUCMSCs scaffolds enhanced therapeutic ability in canines traumatic brain injury model. Front Bioeng Biotechnol 2022;10:995099. https://doi.org/10.3389/fbioe.2022.995099.
54. Liu X, Zhang J, Cheng X, Liu P, Feng Q, Wang S, et al. Integrated printed BDNF-stimulated HUCMSCs-derived exosomes/collagen/chitosan biological scaffolds with 3D printing technology promoted the remodelling of neural networks after traumatic brain injury. Regen Biomater 2023;10:rbac085. https://doi.org/10.1093/rb/rbac085.
55. Yao M, Chen Y, Zhang J, Gao F, Ma S, Guan F. Chitosan-based thermosensitive composite hydrogel enhances the therapeutic efficacy of human umbilical cord MSC in TBI rat model. Mater Today Chem 2019;14:100192. https://doi.org/10.1016/j.mtchem.2019.08.011.
56. Zheng Y, Wu G, Chen L, Zhang Y, Luo Y, Zheng Y, et al. Neuro-regenerative imidazole-functionalized GelMA hydrogel loaded with hAMSC and SDF-1α promote stem cell differentiation and repair focal brain injury. Bioact Mater 2021;6:627–37. https://doi.org/10.1016/j.bioactmat.2020.08.026.
57. Hsieh F-Y, Lin H-H, Hsu S. 3D bioprinting of neural stem cell-laden thermoresponsive biodegradable polyurethane hydrogel and potential in central nervous system repair. Biomaterials 2015;71:48–57. https://doi.org/10.1016/j.biomaterials.2015.08.028.
58. Adak A, Das G, Khan J, Mukherjee N, Gupta V, Mallesh R, et al. Extracellular matrix (ECM)-mimicking neuroprotective injectable sulfo-functionalized peptide hydrogel for repairing brain injury. ACS Biomater Sci Eng 2020;6:2287–96. https://doi.org/10.1021/acsbiomaterials.9b01829.
59. Jeong DU, Bae S, Macks C, Whitaker J, Lynn M, Webb K, et al. Hydrogel-mediated local delivery of dexamethasone reduces neuroinflammation after traumatic brain injury. Biomed Mater 2021;16:035002. https://doi.org/10.1088/1748-605X/abc7f1.
60. Qian F, Han Y, Han Z, Zhang D, Zhang L, Zhao G, et al. In Situ implantable, post-trauma microenvironment-responsive, ROS Depletion Hydrogels for the treatment of Traumatic brain injury. Biomaterials 2021;270:120675. https://doi.org/10.1016/j.biomaterials.2021.120675.
61. Tang L, Wang L, Yang X, Feng Y, Li Y, Feng W. Poly(N-isopropylacrylamide)-based smart hydrogels: Design, properties and applications. Prog Mater Sci 2021;115:100702. https://doi.org/10.1016/j.pmatsci.2020.100702.
62. Qiu Y, Zeng Y, Zhang C, Lv X, Ling Y, Si Y, et al. A ROS-responsive loaded desferoxamine (DFO) hydrogel system for traumatic brain injury therapy. Biomed Mater 2024;19:025016. https://doi.org/10.1088/1748-605X/ad1dfd.
63. Tang C, Amin D, Messersmith PB, Anthony JE, Prud'homme RK. Polymer directed self-assembly of pH-responsive antioxidant nanoparticles. Langmuir 2015;31:3612–20. https://doi.org/10.1021/acs.langmuir.5b00213.
64. Kim YS, Gulfam M, Lowe TL. Thermoresponsive-co-biodegradable linear–dendritic nanoparticles for sustained release of nerve growth factor to promote neurite outgrowth. Mol Pharm 2018;15:1467–75. https://doi.org/10.1021/acs.molpharmaceut.7b01044.
65. Li M, Yang X, Ren J, Qu K, Qu X. Using graphene oxide high near-infrared absorbance for photothermal treatment of Alzheimer's disease. Adv Mater 2012;24:1722–8. https://doi.org/10.1002/adma.201104864.
66. Gopalan D, Pandey A, Udupa N, Mutalik S. Receptor specific, stimuli responsive and subcellular targeted approaches for effective therapy of Alzheimer: Role of surface engineered nanocarriers. J Contr Release 2020;319:183–200. https://doi.org/10.1016/j.jconrel.2019.12.034.
67. Wu L, Wang J, Gao N, Ren J, Zhao A, Qu X. Electrically pulsatile responsive drug delivery platform for treatment of Alzheimer's disease. Nano Res 2015;8:2400–14. https://doi.org/10.1007/s12274-015-0750-x.

68. Jordão JF, Thévenot E, Markham-Coultes K, Scarcelli T, Weng Y-Q, Xhima K, et al. Amyloid-β plaque reduction, endogenous antibody delivery and glial activation by brain-targeted, transcranial focused ultrasound. Exp Neurol 2013;248:16–29. https://doi.org/10.1016/j.expneurol.2013.05.008.
69. Burgess A, Nhan T, Moffatt C, Klibanov AL, Hynynen K. Analysis of focused ultrasound-induced blood–brain barrier permeability in a mouse model of Alzheimer's disease using two-photon microscopy. J Contr Release 2014;192:243–8. https://doi.org/10.1016/j.jconrel.2014.07.051.
70. Jordão JF, Ayala-Grosso CA, Markham K, Huang Y, Chopra R, McLaurin J, et al. Antibodies targeted to the brain with image-guided focused ultrasound reduces amyloid-β plaque load in the TgCRND8 mouse model of Alzheimer's disease. PLoS One 2010;5:e10549. https://doi.org/10.1371/journal.pone.0010549.
71. Nisbet RM, Van der Jeugd A, Leinenga G, Evans HT, Janowicz PW, Götz J. Combined effects of scanning ultrasound and a tau-specific single chain antibody in a tau transgenic mouse model. Brain 2017;140:1220–30. https://doi.org/10.1093/brain/awx052.
72. Lipsman N, Meng Y, Bethune AJ, Huang Y, Lam B, Masellis M, et al. Blood–brain barrier opening in Alzheimer's disease using MR-guided focused ultrasound. Nat Commun 2018;9:2336. https://doi.org/10.1038/s41467-018-04529-6.
73. Lu Y, Guo Z, Zhang Y, Li C, Zhang Y, Guo Q, et al. Microenvironment remodeling micelles for Alzheimer's disease therapy by early modulation of activated microglia. Adv Sci 2019;6:1801586. https://doi.org/10.1002/advs.201801586.
74. Qi X-J, Xu D, Tian M-L, Zhou J-F, Wang Q-S, Cui Y-L. Thermosensitive hydrogel designed for improving the antidepressant activities of genipin via intranasal delivery. Mater Des 2021;206:109816. https://doi.org/10.1016/j.matdes.2021.109816.
75. Xu D, Lu Y-R, Kou N, Hu M-J, Wang Q-S, Cui Y-L. Intranasal delivery of icariin via a nanogel-thermoresponsive hydrogel compound system to improve its antidepressant-like activity. Int J Pharm 2020;586:119550. https://doi.org/10.1016/j.ijpharm.2020.119550.
76. Liu L, Liu M, Xiu J, Zhang B, Hu H, Qiao M, et al. Stimuli-responsive nanoparticles delivered by a nasal-brain pathway alleviate depression-like behavior through extensively scavenging ROS. Acta Biomater 2023;171:451–65. https://doi.org/10.1016/j.actbio.2023.09.038.
77. Majcher MJ, Babar A, Lofts A, Leung A, Li X, Abu-Hijleh F, et al. In situ-gelling starch nanoparticle (SNP)/O-carboxymethyl chitosan (CMCh) nanoparticle network hydrogels for the intranasal delivery of an antipsychotic peptide. J Contr Release 2021;330:738–52. https://doi.org/10.1016/j.jconrel.2020.12.050.
78. Abou-Taleb BA, El-Ganainy SO. Thermoresponsive gel-loaded oxcarbazepine nanosystems for nose-to-brain delivery: Enhanced antiepileptic activity in rats. Pharm Res 2023;40:1835–52. https://doi.org/10.1007/s11095-023-03552-7.
79. Madhu CR, Patel BH. pH-sensitive polymers with their important applications (a review). Curr Phys Chem 2024;14:93–115. https://doi.org/10.2174/0118779468296209240427102827.
80. Gomte SS, Agnihotri TG, Khopade S, Jain A. Exploring the potential of pH-sensitive polymers in targeted drug delivery. J Biomater Sci Polym Ed 2024;35:228–68. https://doi.org/10.1080/09205063.2023.2279792.
81. Xie J, Gonzalez-Carter D, Tockary TA, Nakamura N, Xue Y, Nakakido M, et al. Dual-sensitive nanomicelles enhancing systemic delivery of therapeutically active antibodies specifically into the brain. ACS Nano 2020;14:6729–42. https://doi.org/10.1021/acsnano.9b09991.
82. Cui W, Liu R, Jin H, Lv P, Sun Y, Men X, et al. pH gradient difference around ischemic brain tissue can serve as a trigger for delivering polyethylene glycol-conjugated urokinase nanogels. J Contr Release 2016;225:53–63. https://doi.org/10.1016/j.jconrel.2016.01.028.
83. Choi YS, Cho DY, Lee H-K, Cho J-K, Lee DH, Bae YH, et al. Enhanced cell survival of pH-sensitive bioenergetic nucleotide nanoparticles in energy/oxygen-depleted cells and their intranasal delivery for reduced brain infarction. Acta Biomater 2016;41:147–60. https://doi.org/10.1016/j.actbio.2016.05.037.
84. He W, Mei Q, Li J, Zhai Y, Chen Y, Wang R, et al. Preferential targeting cerebral ischemic lesions with cancer cell-inspired nanovehicle for ischemic stroke treatment. Nano Lett 2021;21:3033–43. https://doi.org/10.1021/acs.nanolett.1c00231.
85. Sherje AP, Londhe V. Development and evaluation of pH-responsive cyclodextrin-based in situ gel of paliperidone for intranasal delivery. AAPS PharmSciTech 2018;19:384–94. https://doi.org/10.1208/s12249-017-0844-8.
86. Beckhauser TF, Francis-Oliveira J, De Pasquale R. Reactive oxygen species: Physiological and physiopathological effects on synaptic plasticity. J Exp Neurosci 2016;10:23–48. https://doi.org/10.4137/JEN.S39887.

87. Tyagi N, Gambhir K, Kumar S, Gangenahalli G, Verma YK. Interplay of reactive oxygen species (ROS) and tissue engineering: A review on clinical aspects of ROS-responsive biomaterials. J Mater Sci 2021;56:16790–823. https://doi.org/10.1007/s10853-021-06338-7.
88. Liu J, Li Y, Chen S, Lin Y, Lai H, Chen B, et al. Biomedical application of reactive oxygen species – Responsive nanocarriers in cancer, inflammation, and neurodegenerative diseases. Front Chem 2020;8:00838. https://doi.org/10.3389/fchem.2020.00838.
89. Mercanzini A, Reddy ST, Velluto D, Colin P, Maillard A, Bensadoun J-C, et al. Controlled release nanoparticle-embedded coatings reduce the tissue reaction to neuroprostheses. J Contr Release 2010;145:196–202. https://doi.org/10.1016/j.jconrel.2010.04.025.
90. Li Y, Li Y, Ji W, Lu Z, Liu L, Shi Y, et al. Positively charged polyprodrug amphiphiles with enhanced drug loading and reactive oxygen species-responsive release ability for traceable synergistic therapy. J Am Chem Soc 2018;140:4164–71. https://doi.org/10.1021/jacs.8b01641.
91. Lv W, Xu J, Wang X, Li X, Xu Q, Xin H. Bioengineered boronic ester modified dextran polymer nanoparticles as reactive oxygen species responsive nanocarrier for ischemic stroke treatment. ACS Nano 2018;12:5417–26. https://doi.org/10.1021/acsnano.8b00477.
92. Xiang J, Liu X, Zhou Z, Zhu D, Zhou Q, Piao Y, et al. Reactive oxygen species (ROS)-responsive charge-switchable nanocarriers for gene therapy of metastatic cancer. ACS Appl Mater Interfaces 2018;10:43352–62. https://doi.org/10.1021/acsami.8b13291.
93. Yang L, Yin T, Liu Y, Sun J, Zhou Y, Liu J. Gold nanoparticle-capped mesoporous silica-based H_2O_2-responsive controlled release system for Alzheimer's disease treatment. Acta Biomater 2016;46:177–90. https://doi.org/10.1016/j.actbio.2016.09.010.
94. Dou Y, Li C, Li L, Guo J, Zhang J. Bioresponsive drug delivery systems for the treatment of inflammatory diseases. J Contr Release 2020;327:641–66. https://doi.org/10.1016/j.jconrel.2020.09.008.
95. Kong L, Li X, Ni Y, Xiao H, Yao Y, Wang Y, et al. Transferrin-modified osthole PEGylated liposomes travel the blood–brain barrier and mitigate Alzheimer's disease-related pathology in APP/PS-1 mice. Int J Nanomedicine 2020;15:2841–58. https://doi.org/10.2147/IJN.S239608.
96. dos Santos Rodrigues B, Kanekiyo T, Singh J. ApoE-2 brain-targeted gene therapy through transferrin and penetratin tagged liposomal nanoparticles. Pharm Res 2019;36:161. https://doi.org/10.1007/s11095-019-2691-7.
97. Jiang Y, Liu C, Zhai W, Zhuang N, Han T, Ding Z. The optimization design of lactoferrin loaded HupA nanoemulsion for targeted drug transport via intranasal route. Int J Nanomedicine 2019;14:9217–34. https://doi.org/10.2147/IJN.S214657.
98. Bruun J, Larsen TB, Jølck RI, Eliasen R, Holm R, Gjetting T, et al. Investigation of enzyme-sensitive lipid nanoparticles for delivery of siRNA to blood-brain barrier and glioma cells. Int J Nanomedicine 2015;10:5995–6008. https://doi.org/10.2147/IJN.S87334.
99. Liu S, Chen B, Feng Y, Gao C, Du D, Jiang T, et al. Helical hydrogel micromotors for delivery of neural stem cells and restoration of neural connectivity. Chem Eng J 2024;479:147745. https://doi.org/10.1016/j.cej.2023.147745.
100. Ávila-Salas F, Durán-Lara EF. An overview of injectable thermo-responsive hydrogels and advances in their biomedical applications. Curr Med Chem 2020;27:5773–89. https://doi.org/10.2174/0929867325666190603110045.
101. Klouda L. Thermoresponsive hydrogels in biomedical applications. Eur J Pharm Biopharm 2015;97:338–49. https://doi.org/10.1016/j.ejpb.2015.05.017.
102. Bellotti E, Schilling AL, Little SR, Decuzzi P. Injectable thermoresponsive hydrogels as drug delivery system for the treatment of central nervous system disorders: A review. J Contr Release 2021;329:16–35. https://doi.org/10.1016/j.jconrel.2020.11.049.
103. Perkušić M, Nižić Nodilo L, Ugrina I, Špoljarić D, Jakobušić Brala C, Pepić I, et al. Chitosan-based thermogelling system for nose-to-brain donepezil delivery: Optimising formulation properties and nasal deposition profile. Pharmaceutics 2023;15:1660. https://doi.org/10.3390/pharmaceutics15061660.
104. Gholizadeh H, Cheng S, Pozzoli M, Messerotti E, Traini D, Young P, et al. Smart thermosensitive chitosan hydrogel for nasal delivery of ibuprofen to treat neurological disorders. Expert Opin Drug Deliv 2019;16:453–66. https://doi.org/10.1080/17425247.2019.1597051.
105. Mohebbi S, Nezhad MN, Zarrintaj P, Jafari SH, Gholizadeh SS, Saeb MR, et al. Chitosan in biomedical engineering: A critical review. Curr Stem Cell Res Ther 2019;14:93–116. https://doi.org/10.2174/1574888X13666180912142028.
106. Zhang J, Cheng T, Chen Y, Gao F, Guan F, Yao M. A chitosan-based thermosensitive scaffold loaded with bone marrow-derived mesenchymal stem cells promotes motor function recovery in spinal cord injured mice. Biomed Mater 2020;15:035020. https://doi.org/10.1088/1748-605X/ab785f.

107. Dong G-C, Kuan C-Y, Subramaniam S, Zhao J-Y, Sivasubramaniam S, Chang H-Y, et al. A potent inhibition of oxidative stress induced gene expression in neural cells by sustained ferulic acid release from chitosan based hydrogel. Mater Sci Eng: C 2015;49:691–9. https://doi.org/10.1016/j.msec.2015.01.030.
108. Macaya D, Ng KK, Spector M. Injectable collagen – Genipin gel for the treatment of spinal cord injury: In vitro studies. Adv Funct Mater 2011;21:4788–97. https://doi.org/10.1002/adfm.201101720.
109. Breen BA, Kraskiewicz H, Ronan R, Kshiragar A, Patar A, Sargeant T, et al. Therapeutic effect of neurotrophin-3 treatment in an injectable collagen scaffold following rat spinal cord hemisection injury. ACS Biomater Sci Eng 2017;3:1287–95. https://doi.org/10.1021/acsbiomaterials.6b00167.
110. Moriarty N, Pandit A, Dowd E. Encapsulation of primary dopaminergic neurons in a GDNF-loaded collagen hydrogel increases their survival, re-innervation and function after intra-striatal transplantation. Sci Rep 2017;7:16033. https://doi.org/10.1038/s41598-017-15970-w.
111. Vellimana AK, Recinos VR, Hwang L, Fowers KD, Li KW, Zhang Y, et al. Combination of paclitaxel thermal gel depot with temozolomide and radiotherapy significantly prolongs survival in an experimental rodent glioma model. J Neurooncol 2013;111:229–36. https://doi.org/10.1007/s11060-012-1014-1.
112. Gong Z, Wang C, Ni L, Ying L, Shu J, Wang J, et al. An injectable recombinant human milk fat globule–epidermal growth factor 8–loaded copolymer system for spinal cord injury reduces inflammation through NF-κB and neuronal cell death. Cytotherapy 2020;22:193–203. https://doi.org/10.1016/j.jcyt.2020.01.016.
113. Shaibie NA, Ramli NA, Mohammad Faizal NDF, Srichana T, Mohd Amin MCI. Poly(N-isopropylacrylamide)-based polymers: Recent overview for the development of temperature-responsive drug delivery and biomedical applications. Macromol Chem Phys 2023;224:2300157. https://doi.org/10.1002/macp.202300157.
114. Comolli N, Neuhuber B, Fischer I, Lowman A. In vitro analysis of PNIPAAm–PEG, a novel, injectable scaffold for spinal cord repair. Acta Biomater 2009;5:1046–55. https://doi.org/10.1016/j.actbio.2008.10.008.
115. Conova L, Vernengo J, Jin Y, Himes BT, Neuhuber B, Fischer I, et al. A pilot study of poly(N-isopropylacrylamide)-g-polyethylene glycol and poly(N-isopropylacrylamide)-g-methylcellulose branched copolymers as injectable scaffolds for local delivery of neurotrophins and cellular transplants into the injured spinal cord. J Neurosurg Spine 2011;15:594–604. https://doi.org/10.3171/2011.7.SPINE11194.
116. Bonnet M, Trimaille T, Brezun J-M, Feron F, Gigmes D, Marqueste T, et al. Motor and sensitive recovery after injection of a physically cross-linked PNIPAAm-g-PEG hydrogel in rat hemisectioned spinal cord. Mater Sci Eng: C 2020;107:110354. https://doi.org/10.1016/j.msec.2019.110354.
117. Zhu Q, Gong Y, Guo T, Deng J, Ji J, Wang B, et al. Thermo-sensitive keratin hydrogel against iron-induced brain injury after experimental intracerebral hemorrhage. Int J Pharm 2019;566:342–51. https://doi.org/10.1016/j.ijpharm.2019.05.076.
118. Arai T, Joki T, Akiyama M, Agawa M, Mori Y, Yoshioka H, et al. Novel drug delivery system using thermoreversible gelation polymer for malignant glioma. J Neurooncol 2006;77:9–15. https://doi.org/10.1007/s11060-005-9001-4.
119. Ji W, Wu Q, Han X, Zhang W, Wei W, Chen L, et al. Photosensitive hydrogels: From structure, mechanisms, design to bioapplications. Sci China Life Sci 2020;63:1813–28. https://doi.org/10.1007/s11427-019-1710-8.
120. Li L, Scheiger JM, Levkin PA. Design and applications of photoresponsive hydrogels. Adv Mater 2019;31:1807333. https://doi.org/10.1002/adma.201807333.
121. Shi J, Tan C, Ge X, Qin Z, Xiong H. Recent advances in stimuli-responsive controlled release systems for neuromodulation. J Mater Chem B 2024;12:5769–86. https://doi.org/10.1039/D4TB00720D.
122. Nakano T, Mackay SM, Wui Tan E, Dani KM, Wickens J. Interfacing with neural activity via femtosecond laser stimulation of drug-encapsulating liposomal nanostructures. eNeuro 2016;3(6): ENEURO.0107-16.2016. https://doi.org/10.1523/ENEURO.0107-16.2016.
123. Banghart MR, Sabatini BL. Photoactivatable neuropeptides for spatiotemporally precise delivery of opioids in neural tissue. Neuron 2012;73:249–59. https://doi.org/10.1016/j.neuron.2011.11.016.
124. Layden AE, Ma X, Johnson CA, He XJ, Buczynski SA, Banghart MR. A biomimetic C-terminal extension strategy for photocaging amidated neuropeptides. J Am Chem Soc 2023;145:19611–21. https://doi.org/10.1021/jacs.3c03913.
125. Ma X, Johnson DA, He XJ, Layden AE, McClain SP, Yung JC, et al. In vivo photopharmacology with a caged mu opioid receptor agonist drives rapid changes in behavior. Nat Methods 2023;20:682–5. https://doi.org/10.1038/s41592-023-01819-w.

126. McClain SP, Ma X, Johnson DA, Johnson CA, Layden AE, Yung JC, et al. In vivo photopharmacology with light-activated opioid drugs. Neuron 2023;111:3926–40.e10. https://doi.org/10.1016/j.neuron.2023.09.017.
127. Kohman RE, Cha SS, Man H-Y, Han X. Light-triggered release of bioactive molecules from DNA nanostructures. Nano Lett 2016;16:2781–5. https://doi.org/10.1021/acs.nanolett.6b00530.
128. Veetil AT, Chakraborty K, Xiao K, Minter MR, Sisodia SS, Krishnan Y. Cell-targetable DNA nanocapsules for spatiotemporal release of caged bioactive small molecules. Nat Nanotechnol 2017;12:1183–9. https://doi.org/10.1038/nnano.2017.159.
129. Jiang Y, Fu P, Liu Y, Wang C, Zhao P, Chu X, et al. Near-infrared light-triggered NO release for spinal cord injury repair. Sci Adv 2020;6:eabc3513. https://doi.org/10.1126/sciadv.abc3513.
130. Xiong H, Alberto KA, Youn J, Taura J, Morstein J, Li X, et al. Optical control of neuronal activities with photoswitchable nanovesicles. Nano Res 2023;16:1033–41. https://doi.org/10.1007/s12274-022-4853-x.
131. Rwei AY, Wang BY, Ji T, Zhan C, Kohane DS. Enhanced triggering of local anesthetic particles by photosensitization and photothermal effect using a common wavelength. Nano Lett 2017;17:7138–45. https://doi.org/10.1021/acs.nanolett.7b04176.
132. Zhan C, Wang W, Santamaria C, Wang B, Rwei A, Timko BP, et al. Ultrasensitive phototriggered local anesthesia. Nano Lett 2017;17:660–5. https://doi.org/10.1021/acs.nanolett.6b03588.
133. Li B, Wang Y, Gao D, Ren S, Li L, Li N, et al. Photothermal modulation of depression-related ion channel function through conjugated polymer nanoparticles. Adv Funct Mater 2021;31:2010757. https://doi.org/10.1002/adfm.202010757.
134. Li X, Che Z, Mazhar K, Price TJ, Qin Z. Ultrafast near-infrared light-triggered intracellular uncaging to probe cell signaling. Adv Funct Mater 2017;27:1605778. https://doi.org/10.1002/adfm.201605778.
135. Xiong H, Li X, Kang P, Perish J, Neuhaus F, Ploski JE, et al. Near-infrared light triggered-release in deep brain regions using ultra-photosensitive nanovesicles. Angew Chem Int Ed 2020;59:8608–15. https://doi.org/10.1002/anie.201915296.
136. Abidi SMS, Dar AI, Acharya A. Multifunctional gold nanoparticle-conjugated cellulose nanoonions alleviate Aβ42 fibrillation-induced toxicity via regulation of oxidative stress and ion homeostasis. Biomacromolecules 2021;22:2419–35. https://doi.org/10.1021/acs.biomac.1c00228.
137. Patel PB, Latt S, Ravi K, Razavi M. Clinical applications of micro/nanobubble technology in neurological diseases. Biomimetics 2024;9:645. https://doi.org/10.3390/biomimetics9100645.
138. Ozdas MS, Shah AS, Johnson PM, Patel N, Marks M, Yasar TB, et al. Non-invasive molecularly-specific millimeter-resolution manipulation of brain circuits by ultrasound-mediated aggregation and uncaging of drug carriers. Nat Commun 2020;11:4929. https://doi.org/10.1038/s41467-020-18059-7.
139. Airan RD, Meyer RA, Ellens NPK, Rhodes KR, Farahani K, Pomper MG, et al. Noninvasive targeted transcranial neuromodulation via focused ultrasound gated drug release from nanoemulsions. Nano Lett 2017;17:652–9. https://doi.org/10.1021/acs.nanolett.6b03517.
140. Wang JB, Aryal M, Zhong Q, Vyas DB, Airan RD. Noninvasive ultrasonic drug uncaging maps whole-brain functional networks. Neuron 2018;100:728–738.e7. https://doi.org/10.1016/j.neuron.2018.10.042.
141. Lea-Banks H, O'Reilly MA, Hamani C, Hynynen K. Localized anesthesia of a specific brain region using ultrasound-responsive barbiturate nanodroplets. Theranostics 2020;10:2849–58. https://doi.org/10.7150/thno.41566.
142. Rwei AY, Paris JL, Wang B, Wang W, Axon CD, Vallet-Regí M, et al. Ultrasound-triggered local anaesthesia. Nat Biomed Eng 2017;1:644–53. https://doi.org/10.1038/s41551-017-0117-6.
143. Romero G, Christiansen MG, Stocche Barbosa L, Garcia F, Anikeeva P. Localized excitation of neural activity via rapid magnetothermal drug release. Adv Funct Mater 2016;26:6471–8. https://doi.org/10.1002/adfm.201602189.
144. Rao S, Chen R, LaRocca AA, Christiansen MG, Senko AW, Shi CH, et al. Remotely controlled chemomagnetic modulation of targeted neural circuits. Nat Nanotechnol 2019;14:967–73. https://doi.org/10.1038/s41565-019-0521-z.
145. Guntnur RT, Muzzio N, Gomez A, Macias S, Galindo A, Ponce A, et al. On-demand chemomagnetic modulation of striatal neurons facilitated by hybrid magnetic nanoparticles. Adv Funct Mater 2022;32:2204732. https://doi.org/10.1002/adfm.202204732.
146. Kondaveeti S, Semeano ATS, Cornejo DR, Ulrich H, Petri DFS. Magnetic hydrogels for levodopa release and cell stimulation triggered by external magnetic field. Colloids Surf B Biointerfaces 2018;167:415–24. https://doi.org/10.1016/j.colsurfb.2018.04.040.
147. Abbas H, Refai H, El Sayed N, Rashed LA, Mousa MR, Zewail M. Superparamagnetic iron oxide loaded chitosan coated bilosomes for magnetic nose to brain targeting of resveratrol. Int J Pharm 2021;610:121244. https://doi.org/10.1016/j.ijpharm.2021.121244.

148. Beola L, Iturrioz-Rodríguez N, Pucci C, Bertorelli R, Ciofani G. Drug-loaded lipid magnetic nanoparticles for combined local hyperthermia and chemotherapy against glioblastoma multiforme. ACS Nano 2023;17:18441–55. https://doi.org/10.1021/acsnano.3c06085.
149. Ding S, Cao S, Zhu A, Shi G. Wettability switching of electrode for signal amplification: Conversion of conformational change of stimuli-responsive polymer into enhanced electrochemical chiral analysis. Anal Chem 2016;88:12219–26. https://doi.org/10.1021/acs.analchem.6b03278.
150. Ding S, Cao S, Liu Y, Lian Y, Zhu A, Shi G. Rational design of a stimuli-responsive polymer electrode interface coupled with in vivo microdialysis for measurement of sialic acid in live mouse brain in Alzheimer's disease. ACS Sens 2017;2:394–400. https://doi.org/10.1021/acssensors.6b00772.
151. Li H, Voci S, Ravaine V, Sojic N. Tuning electrochemiluminescence in multistimuli responsive hydrogel films. J Phys Chem Lett 2018;9:340–5. https://doi.org/10.1021/acs.jpclett.7b03119.
152. Marcisz K, Kaniewska K, Mackiewicz M, Nowinska A, Romanski J, Stojek Z, et al. Electroactive, mediating and thermosensitive microgel useful for covalent entrapment of enzymes and formation of sensing layer in biosensors. Electroanalysis 2018;30:2853–60. https://doi.org/10.1002/elan.201800459.
153. Zhou Y, Cao J, Zhao J, Xie Y, Fei J, Cai Y. Temperature-responsive amperometric H_2O_2 biosensor using a composite film consisting of poly(N-isopropylacrylamide)-b-poly (2-acrylamidoethyl benzoate), graphene oxide and hemoglobin. Microchimica Acta 2016;183:2501–8. https://doi.org/10.1007/s00604-016-1893-5.
154. Fujita H, Yamagishi K, Zhou W, Tahara Y, Huang SY, Hashimoto M, et al. Design and fabrication of a flexible glucose sensing platform toward rapid battery-free detection of hyperglycaemia. J Mater Chem C Mater 2021;9:7336–44. https://doi.org/10.1039/D1TC00667C.
155. Matsumoto A, Endo T, Yoshida R, Miyahara Y. Electrical visualization of chemo-mechanical signal transduction using a smart gel-modified gate field effect transistor. Chem Commun 2009:5609–11. https://doi.org/10.1039/b911689c.
156. Li M, Xiong Y, Lu W, Wang X, Liu Y, Na B, et al. Functional nanochannels for sensing tyrosine phosphorylation. J Am Chem Soc 2020;142:16324–33. https://doi.org/10.1021/jacs.0c06510.
157. Liu Q, Ding S, Gao R, Shi G, Zhu A. A highly selective ATP-responsive biomimetic nanochannel based on smart copolymer. Anal Chim Acta 2021;1188:339167. https://doi.org/10.1016/j.aca.2021.339167.
158. Zhang K, He X, Liu Y, Yu P, Fei J, Mao L. Highly selective cerebral ATP assay based on micrometer scale ion current rectification at polyimidazolium-modified micropipettes. Anal Chem 2017;89:6794–9. https://doi.org/10.1021/acs.analchem.7b01218.
159. Mars A, Hamami M, Bechnak L, Patra D, Raouafi N. Curcumin-graphene quantum dots for dual mode sensing platform: Electrochemical and fluorescence detection of APO*e4*, responsible of Alzheimer's disease. Anal Chim Acta 2018;1036:141–6. https://doi.org/10.1016/j.aca.2018.06.075.
160. Sharafkhani N, Kouzani AZ, Adams SD, Long JM, Lissorgues G, Rousseau L, et al. Neural tissue-microelectrode interaction: Brain micromotion, electrical impedance, and flexible microelectrode insertion. J Neurosci Methods 2022;365:109388. https://doi.org/10.1016/j.jneumeth.2021.109388.
161. Pampaloni NP, Lottner M, Giugliano M, Matruglio A, D'Amico F, Prato M, et al. Single-layer graphene modulates neuronal communication and augments membrane ion currents. Nat Nanotechnol 2018;13:755–64. https://doi.org/10.1038/s41565-018-0163-6.
162. Wang S-X, Lu Y-B, Wang X-X, Wang Y, Song Y-J, Wang X, et al. Graphene and graphene-based materials in axonal repair of spinal cord injury. Neural Regen Res 2022;17:2117. https://doi.org/10.4103/1673-5374.335822.
163. Fabbri R, Saracino E, Treossi E, Zamboni R, Palermo V, Benfenati V. Graphene glial-interfaces: challenges and perspectives. Nanoscale 2021;13:4390–407. https://doi.org/10.1039/D0NR07824G.
164. Djoudi A, Molina-Peña R, Ferreira N, Ottonelli I, Tosi G, Garcion E, et al. Hyaluronic acid scaffolds for loco-regional therapy in nervous system related disorders. Int J Mol Sci 2022;23:12174. https://doi.org/10.3390/ijms232012174.
165. Galindo AN, Frey Rubio DA, Hettiaratchi MH. Biomaterial strategies for regulating the neuroinflammatory response. Mater Adv 2024;5:4025–54. https://doi.org/10.1039/D3MA00736G.
166. Faussner A, Deininger MM, Weber C, Steffens S. Direct addition of poly-lysine or poly-ethylenimine to the medium: A simple alternative to plate pre-coating. PLoS One 2022;17:e0260173. https://doi.org/10.1371/journal.pone.0260173.
167. Hume PS, Bowman CN, Anseth KS. Functionalized PEG hydrogels through reactive dip-coating for the formation of immunoactive barriers. Biomaterials 2011;32:6204–12. https://doi.org/10.1016/j.biomaterials.2011.04.049.
168. Meghri NW, Donius AE, Riblett BW, Martin EJ, Clyne AM, Wegst UGK. Directionally solidified biopolymer scaffolds: Mechanical properties and endothelial cell responses. JOM 2010;62:71–75. https://doi.org/10.1007/s11837-010-0112-9.

169. Sousa JPM, Stratakis E, Mano J, Marques PAAP. Anisotropic 3D scaffolds for spinal cord guided repair: Current concepts. Biomater Adv 2023;148:213353. https://doi.org/10.1016/j.bioadv.2023.213353.
170. Du B, Yin H, Chen Y, Lin W, Wang Y, Zhao D, et al. A waterborne polyurethane 3D scaffold containing PLGA with a controllable degradation rate and an anti-inflammatory effect for potential applications in neural tissue repair. J Mater Chem B 2020;8:4434–46. https://doi.org/10.1039/D0TB00656D.
171. Zhang J, Liu X, Ma K, Chen M, Xu H, Niu X, et al. Collagen/heparin scaffold combined with vascular endothelial growth factor promotes the repair of neurological function in rats with traumatic brain injury. Biomater Sci 2021;9:745–64. https://doi.org/10.1039/C9BM01446B.
172. Ma J, Li J, Wang X, Li M, Teng W, Tao Z, et al. GDNF-loaded polydopamine nanoparticles-based anisotropic scaffolds promote spinal cord repair by modulating inhibitory microenvironment. Adv Healthc Mater 2023;12:2202377. https://doi.org/10.1002/adhm.202202377.
173. Zhou J, Patel TR, Sirianni RW, Strohbehn G, Zheng M-Q, Duong N, et al. Highly penetrative, drug-loaded nanocarriers improve treatment of glioblastoma. Proc Nat Acad Sci 2013;110:11751–6.
174. Don T-M, Chang W-J, Jheng P-R, Huang Y-C, Chuang E-Y. Curcumin-laden dual-targeting fucoidan/chitosan nanocarriers for inhibiting brain inflammation via intranasal delivery. Int J Biol Macromol 2021;181:835–46. https://doi.org/10.1016/j.ijbiomac.2021.04.045.
175. King JL, Maturavongsadit P, Hingtgen SD, Benhabbour SR. Injectable pH thermo-responsive hydrogel scaffold for tumoricidal neural stem cell therapy for glioblastoma multiforme. Pharmaceutics 2022;14:2243. https://doi.org/10.3390/pharmaceutics14102243.
176. Martins C, Araújo M, Malfanti A, Pacheco C, Smith SJ, Ucakar B, et al. Stimuli-responsive multifunctional nanomedicine for enhanced glioblastoma chemotherapy augments multistage blood-to-brain trafficking and tumor targeting. Small 2023;19:2300029. https://doi.org/10.1002/smll.202300029.
177. Huang S, Shao K, Liu Y, Kuang Y, Li J, An S, et al. Tumor-targeting and microenvironment-responsive smart nanoparticles for combination therapy of antiangiogenesis and apoptosis. ACS Nano 2013;7:2860–71. https://doi.org/10.1021/nn400548g.
178. Nafee N, Ameen AER, Abdallah OY. Patient-friendly, olfactory-targeted, stimuli-responsive hydrogels for cerebral degenerative disorders ensured >400% brain targeting efficiency in rats. AAPS PharmSciTech 2021;22:6. https://doi.org/10.1208/s12249-020-01872-0.
179. Mitchell MJ, Jain RK, Langer R. Engineering and physical sciences in oncology: Challenges and opportunities. Nat Rev Cancer 2017;17:659–75. https://doi.org/10.1038/nrc.2017.83.
180. Vigata M, Meinert C, Hutmacher DW, Bock N. Hydrogels as drug delivery systems: A review of current characterization and evaluation techniques. Pharmaceutics 2020;12. https://doi.org/10.3390/pharmaceutics12121188.

8 Stimuli-Responsive Biomaterials for Diabetes and Obesity Management

Shrestha Dutta, Diganta Chaudhury, and Soumya Deep Phadikar
Department of Pharmaceutical Science and Engineering,
Indian Institute of Technology (IIT-ISM), Dhanbad, Jharkhand, India

Chandrawali Goyal
School of Life Sciences, Central University of Gujarat,
Gandhinagar, Gujarat, India

Souhrid Sarkar
School of Cancer Sciences, Department of Medical,
Veterinary and Life Sciences,
University of Glasgow, Glasgow, United Kingdom

Chinnaperumal Kamaraj
Interdisciplinary Institute of Indian System of Medicine,
Directorate of Research, SRM Institute of Science and Technology,
Kattankulathur, Tamil Nadu, India

8.1 INTRODUCTION

In contrast to conventional biomaterials, smart stimuli-responsive biomaterials react to external and internal cues that stimulate or activate them [1]. As a result, researchers have been focusing more on these innovative biomaterials in recent years. Various materials, including polymers, liposomes, micelles, dendrimers, carbon-based nanomaterials, nanogels, and metallic nanoparticles (NPs), are increasingly used to develop smart systems due to their ability to respond to a wide range of endogenous stimuli (such as redox potential, pH, and enzyme presence) and exogenous stimuli (such as ultrasound, temperature, light, electric, and magnetic fields). These materials, which can react to changes in their internal or external environments, are referred to as stimuli-responsive or stimuli-reactive materials. When exposed to specific signals from their internal or external environments, these materials undergo activated changes. They are easy to fabricate, biocompatible, and highly adaptable, offering varying degrees of responsiveness to different biomaterials, making them ideal for personalized therapy and future diagnostic applications. Additionally, these materials exhibit detectable or measurable changes at the nano- or microscale, such as molecular bond reorganization, morphological alterations, or molecular movement, which in turn lead to macroscopic changes in properties like shape, color, and function [2]. Stimuli-sensitive materials can be designed by altering their chemical, mechanical, electrical, biological, optical, or other properties, taking advantage of their versatile functional groups and molecular backbones. These materials can also be engineered in various forms, such as bulk, thin films, NPs or microparticles, and composites [3]. Clinical applications of first-generation stimuli-responsive materials have primarily

DOI: 10.1201/9781003560203-8

focused on developing pharmacological carriers for drug delivery. These materials enhance the effectiveness, half-life, circulation, and bioavailability of medications. To advance to next-generation stimuli-responsive materials, researchers have developed multifunctional platforms designed for environmental responsiveness, controlled release, and targeted molecular or cellular delivery [4]. Diabetes is characterized by elevated blood glucose levels. By 2030, the number of people living with diabetes mellitus is expected to exceed 552 million, making it one of the most prevalent and deadly diseases worldwide. Despite significant advances in research and treatment, insulin remains the primary medication used to regulate blood glucose levels and extend the lives of diabetic patients. The traditional method of insulin delivery involves regular subcutaneous injections, which can lead to several adverse effects, including discomfort, infection, local tissue damage, and also damage in nerve. There is a great need to develop self-regulating insulin delivery systems capable of automatically adjusting insulin doses in response to fluctuations in blood glucose levels. In this context, researchers are increasingly focused on stimuli-responsive systems due to their potential for improved efficacy and reduced side effects. Stimuli-responsive polymers, in particular, can alter their physical and chemical properties when exposed to external environmental changes, often referred to as stimuli. While recent advancements have led to the discovery of various thermal, electrochemical, and redox-responsive polymeric systems, most stimuli-responsive insulin delivery systems still primarily rely on changes in pH and/or glucose concentration. These systems are designed to facilitate rapid insulin release by undergoing quick structural changes or responding to fluctuations in pH, temperature, glucose levels, and other environmental factors [5].

Obesity has become a major global public health issue, contributing to a rise in comorbidities, such as fatty liver disease, cardiovascular disease, and type 2 diabetes mellitus (T2DM). The primary approach to managing obesity and its associated health problems is pharmacotherapy, often combined with lifestyle changes or surgery. However, most anti-obesity medications face challenges related to potential side effects, target selectivity, and bioavailability. Currently, only a few drugs, such as liraglutide, and orlistat, are approved for the clinical treatment of obesity. As a result, there is a pressing need for alternative therapeutic approaches. In light of recent advancements in understanding the pathophysiology of obesity, as well as the growing integration of materials science, chemistry, biotechnology, and pharmacy, innovative treatment strategies are increasingly advancing through preclinical and clinical research [6]. Chitosan, a natural polymer composed of glucosamine and N-acetylglucosamine copolymers, has been shown to possess anti-obesity properties and can be used as a dietary supplement to reduce cholesterol levels. Initially, it was thought that chitosan's anti-obesity effects were primarily due to its fat-binding ability, which prevents the intestinal absorption of dietary lipids. However, recent studies suggest that its anti-obesity action may be linked to a more complex endocrine mechanism, potentially involving the regulation of adipokines such as serum leptin and C-reactive protein (CRP). As mentioned earlier, adipocytes release the hormone leptin. When body fat increases or energy levels are high, serum leptin levels rise, signaling the hypothalamus in the brain to reduce food intake. However, despite elevated leptin production, leptin resistance can occur when the brain and leptin receptors become insensitive to the hormone, preventing the brain from detecting the signals from adipocytes [7].

Poly(lactide-co-glycolide) (PLG) is a synthetic biodegradable polymer widely used in drug delivery and tissue engineering. It can be processed into various forms, such as hydrogels, scaffolds, and NPs [8]. Studies have shown that PLG scaffolds, when implanted into the epididymal fat pad, integrate well with the surrounding tissue, demonstrating excellent biocompatibility [9]. The PLG scaffold has been shown to protect mice from diet-induced obesity and glucose intolerance, as indicated by the unexpectedly high expression of glucose transporter protein 1 (GLUT1), insulin-like growth factor I (IGF-I), and the glucose transporter proteins GLUT1 and GLUT4, which are involved in wound healing and regulation of blood glucose levels. This resulted in enhanced glucose uptake in the epididymal fat pad and reduced blood glucose levels in mice, even when the scaffold was implanted without any drug loading [10]. PLG scaffolds show great promise as a platform for treating advanced metabolic disorders, and their therapeutic potential can be further enhanced through cellular or pharmacological applications. In another study, a nanogold shell was functionalized with hyaluronic acid to improve its stability and biosafety. Furthermore, the surface of the particles was coated with an adipocyte-targeting peptide (ATP), which specifically binds to prohibition on the surface of adipocytes. This chapter deals with how the stimuli-responsive biomaterials are used to manage diabetes and obesity.

8.2 CROSSTALK BETWEEN DIABETES AND OBESITY

Obesity-associated diabetes mellitus, a chronic metabolic affliction accounting for 90% of all diabetic patients, has been affecting humanity extremely badly and escalating the risk of developing other serious disorders. It is observed that 0.4 billion people globally have diabetes, whose major cause is obesity. Currently, innumerable synthetic drugs like alogliptin and rosiglitazone are being used to get through diabetes, but they have certain complications, restrictions with severe side effects, and toxicity issues. Recently, the frequency of plant-derived phytochemicals as advantageous substitutes against diabesity is increasing progressively due to their unparalleled benefit of producing less side effects and toxicity. Of these phytochemicals, dietary polyphenols have been accepted as potent agents against the dual sword. These polyphenols target certain genes and molecular pathways through dual mechanisms such as adiponectin upregulation, cannabinoid receptor antagonism, free fatty acid oxidation, ghrelin antagonism, glucocorticoid inhibition, sodium–glucose cotransporter inhibition, oxidative stress and inflammation inhibition which sequentially help to combat both diabetes and obesity (Figure 8.1).

8.2.1 Genetic and Environmental Aspects

Genetics clearly plays an important role in conferring the risk for the development of metabolic diseases. Variant genes determine the individual susceptibility toward known risk factors and may explain why only a fraction of obese individuals develop T2DM whereas the majority of diabetics are obese. In recent genome-wide association studies (GWAS), numerous variant genes were identified that predispose to diabetes or obesity [11]. However, due to the relatively small contribution of the individual single nuclear polymorphisms (SNPs) to the overall disease risk, the predictive value of the gene variants is relatively small, and the pathophysiological relevance of many of these SNPs remains to be clarified. When combined, the genes identified so-far by GWAS explain only 15%–20% of the heritable variance of metabolic diseases [12, 13]. An example of contradictory results of GWAS versus functional in vivo data represents the fat mass and obesity-associated (FTO) gene. In different GWAS, SNPs located in the first intron of the FTO gene were associated with an altered body mass index (BMI) [14], whereas FTO knockout mice develop postnatal growth retardation and exhibit a reduced body length. In contrast, no association of FTO was detected for height in humans [15]. Although new in vivo data exist that reflect the human pathophysiology more

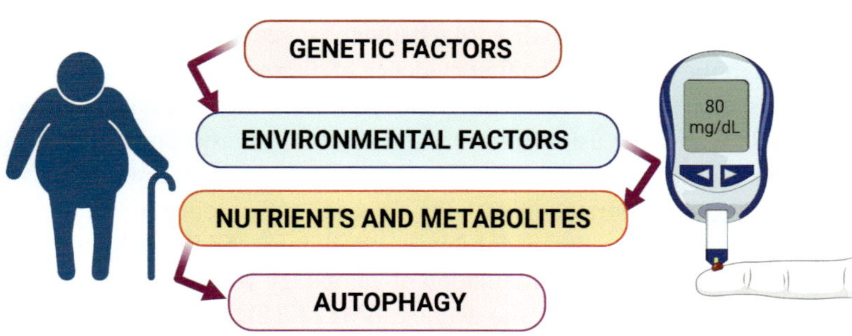

FIGURE 8.1 Summarizes major factors of crosstalk between diabetes and obesity.

precisely, the discrepancies of the GWAS and functional approaches remain apparent [16]. Thus, even though many studies have confirmed FTO and TCF7L2 as two major genes implicated in obesity and diabetes in humans, respectively, GWAS have provided only limited mechanistic insights into the pathophysiology of these diseases. Novel approaches combining classical familial linkage analysis methods with whole-genome sequencing (WGS) are currently emerging as an important and powerful analysis method, especially since rare variants, which are not well-interrogated by GWAS, could be responsible for a substantial proportion of complex human diseases [17].

Polygenic mouse models have proven to be important tools to investigate molecular mechanisms that link obesity and T2DM. Despite novel advancements in the sequencing technology, the most successful strategy to identify and characterize new risk alleles is represented by a positional cloning approach [12, 18]. This approach capitalizes on a combination of breeding of multiple recombinant congenic mouse lines and of expression profiling of critical genomic regions that confer the phenotype. Using this approach, nine gene variants were identified as candidates for type 2 diabetes (T2D) and/or obesity during the last years. Sorcs1 encodes for a protein of largely unknown function that binds to a transcription factor responsible for islet vascularization [13]. Lisch-like factor was described to be responsible for reducing β-cell mass and β-cell replication rates [13]. Zfp69, a zinc-finger transcription factor, was described as causal gene for the diabetogenic Nidd1 quantitative trait locus (QTL) derived from the lean SJL (Swiss Jim Lambert) mouse strain and responsible for the distribution of lipids between different organs. Although immune system, ectopic fat, and macro/micronutrients all contribute in part to the susceptibility for diabetes in the obese state, most of the underlying molecular mechanisms are still poorly understood. The identification of susceptibility genes mediating the progression of T2D is crucial to prevent the massive epidemics of the disease. Future research will be focused not only on gene–gene interactions but also on the interplay of genetic and environmental risk factors [15, 16].

8.2.2 Autophagy

Autophagy, an evolutionarily conserved process, plays a crucial role in maintaining cellular homeostasis. Its dysfunction has been implicated in the development of various metabolic diseases, including obesity, T2D, and metabolic dysfunction-associated steatotic liver disease (MASLD). In obesity, evidence suggests that autophagy is upregulated during the early stages of autophagosome formation, possibly as a response to proinflammatory conditions in adipose tissue (AT). Similarly, autophagosome formation appears to be elevated under hyperglycemic or insulin-resistant conditions in T2D patients, potentially serving as a compensatory mechanism to remove damaged organelles and proteins [19].

However, prolonged hyperglycemia and impaired insulin signaling may disrupt autophagic flux, leading to the accumulation of dysfunctional cellular components and contributing to β-cell dysfunction. In MASLD, studies indicate that autophagy inhibition may play a role in disease progression. Despite these findings, it remains challenging to determine whether autophagy is consistently enhanced or suppressed in these metabolic conditions, as autophagy marker levels vary depending on the metabolism of specific organs, tissues, experimental conditions, and disease duration. These variations make it difficult to discern whether changes in autophagic activity are a cause or consequence of metabolic diseases. The first evidence of altered autophagy in obese patients was reported in 2010 by Öst et al., who observed an increased number of autophagosomes in adipocytes from obese individuals with T2D using transmission electron microscopy (TEM). This increase coincided with elevated levels and turnover of the autophagy marker microtubule-associated protein 1 light chain 3 (LC3), demonstrated in both the presence and absence of the autophagy inducer rapamycin and the lysosomal degradation inhibitor chloroquine. Additionally, reduced mTORC1 activity supported these findings. The upregulation of autophagy was also linked to the fragmentation of large lipid droplets. In this study, the average BMI of T2D patients was approximately 40 (obesity class II/III), although overweight individuals (BMI $\geq$ 27) were also included. Control subjects without T2D were overweight on average [20]. Similarly, Kovsan et al. demonstrated increased

TABLE 8.1
Tabular Representation of Various Stimuli-Responsive Biomaterials and Their Mechanism of Actions

Stimuli	Mechanism/Response	Applications
Temperature (e.g., RFA, microwave hyperthermia, HIFU)	Phase transition in polymers (e.g., sol–gel transformation, swelling/deswelling). Hydrophilic to hydrophobic transitions (e.g., PNIPAM).	Localized drug delivery, thermo-sensitive hydrogels, tissue engineering, diabetes/obesity management.
Increased body temperature (e.g., exercise)	Controlled release of therapeutic agents like insulin, metformin, GLP-1 receptor agonists, or appetite suppressants.	Diabetes and obesity management; targeted, sustained drug release.
Hybrid stimuli (thermal + glucose or pH)	Enhanced specificity and biomimicry for hyperglycemia management.	Advanced glucose-monitoring systems, multi-agent drug delivery.
Temperature-sensitive scaffolds	Controlled delivery of pancreatic islet cells, brown adipose tissue, or growth factors.	Regenerative medicine for tissue repair and pancreatic tissue regeneration.
Injectable hydrogels	Encapsulation and controlled release of growth factors or drugs (e.g., EGF with doxycycline in chitosan nanoparticles).	Diabetic wound healing, inflammation reduction, collagen synthesis, and epithelial regeneration.
Thermo-sensitive nano vectors	Enhanced Permeability and Retention (EPR) effect; chemo- and radiotherapy sensitivity.	Cancer treatments, controlled drug delivery, regenerative medicine.
Wearable devices (e.g., wristbands)	Continuous glucose monitoring and temperature-triggered drug release.	Personalized diabetes and obesity control; non-invasive monitoring and therapy.

autophagophore formation in AT from obese patients, independent of glycemic status. This effect was particularly pronounced in omental fat compared to subcutaneous fat, as shown by mRNA and protein expression levels (Table 8.1). The upregulation of autophagy correlated positively with obesity severity, visceral fat distribution, and adipocyte hypertrophy [21]. Subsequent studies have consistently reported increased autophagy marker levels in AT from individuals with obesity and obesity-related T2D compared to lean controls without T2D [22, 23]. Positive correlations between the expression of autophagy-related genes and glucometabolic status [24], as well as elevated transcript levels of autophagy genes in AT from individuals with obesity and T2D compared to those with normal glycemia, have also been noted. Notably, autophagosome formation appears more pronounced in visceral AT than in subcutaneous AT. In individuals without T2D, LC3 was not detected in subcutaneous or visceral AT samples. Furthermore, a study revealed that an initially increased number of autophagosomes in the subcutaneous AT of obese patients, with or without T2D, was undetectable one year after undergoing bariatric surgery. It has been proposed that heightened autophagy in AT of individuals with obesity may help modulate obesity-induced AT inflammation. This hypothesis is supported by findings that autophagy inhibition significantly increases the transcriptional expression of proinflammatory cytokines in obese human and murine AT samples [25].

8.3 STIMULI-RESPONSIVE MATERIALS

8.3.1 Physical Stimuli

8.3.1.1 Light Responsive

Light-sensitive biomaterials have become a frontier in the advancement of treatment options for diabetes and obesity [26]. These biomaterials are often referred to as "smart" materials. They are engineered to respond to light in a regulated and predictable manner. This enables control over their physical characteristics [27]. This special characteristic provides opportunities for developing non-invasive therapies that can be controlled spatially and temporally. These therapies include targeted drug delivery methods and the activation of signaling pathways to alter behavior [26]. The potential of biomaterials to transform treatment strategies for common metabolic disorders is substantial and it can enhance patient outcomes and overall quality of life significantly.

The way these materials react to light is due to the inclusion of molecules known as chromophores in their inherent structures [27]. When exposed to specific light wavelengths, these chromophores undergo changes in their structure or conformation leading to a chain of reactions that produce the intended therapeutic outcome [28]. This precise management of the materials properties enables drug delivery triggering cellular responses and adjusting tissue functions effectively. Light responsive biomaterial seems like an attractive therapeutic choice, for addressing challenging metabolic conditions such as diabetes and obesity that call for treatment approaches.

Light-sensitive biomaterials exert their influence through a process known as photoisomerization [29]. In this process the atoms within a molecule undergo rearrangement upon absorption resulting in a change in its isomeric structure. An example is the conversion between cis and trans isomers of azobenzene derivatives which occurs with variations, in light wavelengths exposure. The modification in composition can greatly impact the characteristics of the biomaterial like its water-repelling nature or charge and solubility levels are altered accordingly. This could result in the regulated release of medication or modifications in how the substance engages with cells. For example, a hydrogel embedding an azobenzene derivative could be crafted to dispense insulin upon exposure to UV light, as a way to possibly facilitate insulin delivery when needed.

Another key process involves photocleavage which utilizes light to disrupt chemical bonds in a molecule [27]. This method enables controlled release of substances, from a biomaterial or modification of its characteristics. For instance, by integrating sensitive connectors into polymer structures, drugs or bioactive compounds can be liberated when exposed to a certain light wavelength. This approach has been utilized in creating sensitive medications that stay dormant until they are triggered by light at a specific location; they are needed to reduce unintended effects and enhance treatment effectiveness.

Apart from these alterations at the molecular level, light exposure can also bring about significant changes in the characteristics of materials due to photothermal effects [27]. Some materials like gold NPs have light absorption abilities and can produce heat when illuminated by light rays resulting in local temperature rises. This heat generation effect from exposure to light can be utilized to activate the release of drugs from temperature-sensitive carriers or induce the death of cells, in specific tissues. For example, a hydrogel-containing particles of gold can release trapped medicines when exposed to near-infrared (NIR) light offering a way to administer drugs in a controlled manner without invasive procedures. The use of sensitive biomaterial in controlling diabetes shows great potential because it allows for the creation of insulin delivery systems that can be triggered as needed. The conventional method of insulin treatment involves injections that can be bothersome and do not always replicate the body's natural insulin release rhythms. Light-sensitive biomaterial presents a possible remedy by enabling on-demand insulin administration when exposed to signals. For instance, a small needle patch, with a responsive gel could be utilized for delivering insulin through the skin. When light hits the hydrogel substance, it contains insulin which works to reduce the levels of glucose in the blood [27].

Light-sensitive biomaterials have the potential to do more than administer insulin; they can also be utilized to distribute other beneficial substances for managing diabetes effectively such as glucagon-like peptide-1 (GLP-1), a hormone that boosts insulin production and has displayed encouraging outcomes in addressing T2D. Light-responsive NPs can be engineered to release this hormone systematically, a method that might offer a viable substitute for conventional GLP-1-based injections. In the field of managing obesity issues in individuals' health conditions using methods involving light-responsive biomaterials is quite a promising approach for delivering drugs and other treatments in a controlled manner. The idea of controlling the release of appetite-suppressing medications using light shows potential. Light-sensitive hydrogels containing these drugs can be placed under the skin to allow for controlled drug delivery via exposure, to light stimuli. This can actually provide a non-invasive technique to manage obesity by controlling appetite and at the same time reducing food intake. Using photothermal therapy, several people are exploring a new way to reduce fat deposits in the body by harnessing light to activate photosensitizers that produce reactive oxygen species (ROS) capable of specifically targeting and eliminating cells. This technique displays promise in addressing health issues linked to obesity, such as non-alcoholic fatty liver disease (NAFLD), as it can selectively eliminate excess fat cells while preserving the well-being of neighboring tissues.

Despite the capabilities of light-reactive biomaterials for managing diabetes and obesity-related issues, there are still obstacles to overcome in their advancement and practical implementation in clinical settings. A key hurdle is the depth to which light can penetrate tissues, especially with shorter wavelengths. This constraint makes these materials mostly suitable for surface-level tissues or necessitates methods to enable light delivery to deeper tissue layers. Scientists are actively investigating ways to address this challenge by looking into the utilization of NIR light with tissue penetration capabilities and the creation of up-conversion NPs capable of converting NIR light, into higher energy wavelengths.

One concern is the risk of phototoxicity when exposed to UV light arising from certain photoactive molecules producing ROS that could harm normal tissues. The key is to choose molecules wisely and fine-tune the amount of light to reduce the chances of phototoxicity occurring. Creating materials that are both biocompatible and stable under the influence of light poses its own set of challenges in terms of design and synthesis complexity. These materials must maintain stability in environments while being non-toxic and capable of reacting to light stimuli in a reliable and controllable way. Researchers are therefore exploring different strategies to modify and optimize the synthesis of these materials—including but not limited to the use of biocompatible polymers, surface modifications and nanotechnology.

8.3.1.2 Thermo-Responsive

Advanced smart materials, thermo-responsive biomaterials possess reversible physical and chemical transformations upon changes in temperature, thus their application in biomedical fields, especially in diabetes and obesity management. These are primarily polymer-based matrices: poly(N-isopropylacrylamide) (PNIPAM), chondroitin sulfate (CS), and derivatives of Pluronic that benefit from phase transitions triggered by temperature to ultimately result in localized and controlled therapies. The mechanism of action entails external thermal stimuli by means of radiofrequency ablation (RFA), microwave hyperthermia, or high-intensity-focused ultrasound (HIFU). Through these stimuli, a temperature gradient between the lesion site and normal tissue can be created, resulting in phase transitions in the polymers, which in turn triggers changes in physical properties such as sol–gel transformation, swelling, or deswelling. PNIPAM, for example, transitions at its lower critical solution temperature (LCST) of ~32°C. Below this temperature, it is hydrophilic and traps drugs while above that temperature, it becomes hydrophobic and releases therapeutic agents in a controlled manner. Analogous temperature-dependent sol–gel transitions occur in chitosan, that is suitable for injectable hydrogels for applications in wound healing or tissue engineering applications, and micelles or gels form from Pluronic polymers with heating, acceptable for drug delivery or thermo-sensitive coatings. These can mimic the natural physiological processes of biological systems and their controlling steps, such as insulin secretion, to release therapeutic agents like insulin, metformin, or GLP-1 receptor agonists in a targeted and sustained fashion. For obesity management, thermo-responsive systems can encapsulate appetite suppressants or fat metabolism modulators, which might be released in response to increased body temperature as in physical exercise. Multi-agent systems could further enhance treatment by delivering multiple drugs simultaneously, targeting both diabetes and obesity pathways.

In regenerative medicine, thermo-responsive scaffolds promote the repair of tissues through controlled delivery of pancreatic islet cells or brown AT. Hybrid systems in which thermal responsiveness is combined with other stimuli like glucose or pH make them more accurate and biomimetic, providing highly advanced hyperglycemia management solutions. These polymers also allow the implantation of minimally invasive glucose-monitoring systems that respond to temperature fluctuations that are coupled with glucose levels. To summarize, there is innovative work in localized drug delivery and regenerative medicine by finely tuned temperature-sensitive mechanisms without systemic side effects across thermo-responsive polymers. One innovative application is the development of a thermo-responsive injectable hydrogel for diabetic wound healing, which is one of the most severe complications affecting morbidity and mortality in diabetic patients [30]. It contains Epidermal Growth Factor, known to be critical during all phases of wound healing, conjugated with doxycycline, a non-antibiotic anti-inflammatory and antibacterial agent. In this formulation, the challenge of epidermal growth factor's (EGF) lower stability was confronted by encapsulating it within chitosan NPs through an ionic gelation process. Optimized for size at 203 nm, zeta potential at +28.5 mV, and entrapment efficiency at 83.43%, these NPs were later on encapsulated into hydrogels along with the protease inhibitor. These hydrogels exhibited good biocompatibility and injectability in addition to showing thermo-response for sustained, controlled release.

In vitro experiments demonstrated strong antibacterial activity and enhanced cell migration. Further, in vivo experiments in diabetic rat models showed important reductions in inflammation, increasing collagen synthesis, and better epithelial regeneration, which progressed through all stages of wound healing: proliferation, remodeling, and maturation. These findings hold great promise for the use of thermo-responsive biomaterials in the treatment of diabetic complications—the suppression of inflammation with tissue regeneration, an innovative new therapeutic approach in chronic wound care in diabetes. The most significant benefits of thermo-responsive polymers include their ability to improve the so-called Enhanced Permeability and Retention (EPR) effect and sensitivity to chemo- and radiotherapy and, therefore, are perfect for targeted treatments. Another benefit is the relatively straightforward synthesis and versatility in various therapeutic areas, such as nano vectors for controlled drug delivery, hydrogels, and scaffolds that support cell growth [30]. However, these polymers suffer from drawbacks such as potential off-target delivery and minimal differences or variations in internal body temperatures, making their precision challenging. Furthermore, the NPs introduced within these systems need to be stable enough to ensure performance uniformity and therapeutic effect. Thermo-responsive biomaterials offer controlled drug release triggered by temperature changes, making them ideal for treatments like diabetes and obesity. They are biocompatible, allowing long-term use without immune reactions, and can be injected minimally invasively, improving patient compliance. However, their effectiveness can be compromised if body temperature falls outside the optimal range for activation, leading to poor drug release. Additionally, some thermo-sensitive hydrogels have poor mechanical stability, limiting their use in dynamic environments. Developing these systems is also complex and costly, raising manufacturing challenges (Table 8.1). Thermo-sensitive biomaterials have enormous potential for moving forward the drug delivery and therapeutic treatments of disease states like diabetes or obesity. In the future, research directions would apparently be geared to smart drug delivery systems that respond to natural physiological temperature changes. Devices would thus be engineered for the controlled release of insulin or other agents against diabetes at individual real-time fluctuations in physiological conditions. This should have direct benefit to enhance the precision and efficacy of therapy. Another very great expansion is that of the use of thermo-sensitive biomaterials in regenerative medicine, more so as a tissue engineer for the repair and regeneration of damaged pancreatic tissues by diabetes. Controlled delivery of growth factors or stem cells via these materials will significantly improve outcomes. Innovations will also lead the way to integrate thermo-sensitive biomaterials in wearable devices, such as wristbands, to monitor blood glucose continuously. Such devices could then be designed to release medications due to temperature changes, creating an easy and efficient means for diabetes and obesity control. These developments together point to a revolutionary change that could be brought by thermo-sensitive biomaterials to personalized healthcare and regenerative medicine.

8.3.1.3 Magneto Responsive

Magneto-responsive biomaterials are a class of smart materials with novel properties conferred by magnetic nanoparticles (MNPs). Material properties open up a brand-new perspective for the treatment and management of diabetes and obesity. These biomaterials, sensitive to external magnetic field solicitations, will achieve both targeted therapeutic delivery and bioactive stimulation, and thus metabolic regulation. In most of these systems, MNP inclusion-iron oxide (Fe_3O_4), cobalt, or nickel-interacts with magnetic stimuli to ensure precision in the physical, chemical, or mechanical transformation in therapeutic intervention. It is with these capabilities in site-specific delivery and modulation of therapeutic agents that make magneto-responsive biomaterials very promising for reducing the global burden of diabetes and obesity.

The underlying mechanism of magneto-responsive biomaterials is based on the manipulation of MNPs through external magnetic fields. Magnetic targeting allows such NPs to be directed to specific anatomical sites, hence allowing therapy with minimum systemic side effects. In addition, an alternating magnetic field may cause heating through magnetic hyperthermia, which can also be used for triggering drug release or modulating biological processes. Examples are magnetic fields that, in diabetes treatment, may promote insulin delivery or the stimulation of regeneration in pancreatic tissue [31]. Magnetic hyperthermia, which may cause localized heating, either to disrupt AT directly or to stimulate the release of appetite-suppressing drugs, could potentially be used for weight loss in obesity management. One notable application of magneto-responsive biomaterials is in glucose-responsive insulin delivery systems. These systems have glucose-sensitive enzymes, like glucose oxidase (GOx), which work in synergy with MNPs embedded within hydrogels or polymer matrices. In response to increased blood glucose levels, enzymatic activity causes a change in the local environment, which initiates a magnetic response and promotes insulin release. The release kinetics can be further enhanced by the application of an external magnetic field, hence offering a dual control mechanism that may mimic physiological glucose regulation. This approach minimizes the risk of hypoglycemia and improves the precision of diabetes management.

Besides drug delivery, magneto-responsive biomaterials hold immense promise in tissue engineering and regenerative medicine applied to diabetes. The magnetically responsive scaffolds could be designed to support pancreatic islet regeneration and be loaded with growth factors and stem cells. Magnetic fields applied to such systems provoke cell proliferation, differentiation, and migration, hence creating an environment that can allow tissue repair. It was determined that magnetic stimulation of stem cells in these scaffolds improves insulin production and, thus, has the potential to be a curative approach for type 1 diabetes. Because of these factors, magneto-responsive biomaterials are an excellent strategy for managing obesity, in which there is excess accumulation of fat and appetite dysregulation. Appetite-reducing drugs like leptin or GLP-1 receptor agonists can be encapsulated within polymeric matrices using magnetic NPs. Controlled drug release is triggered by externally applied magnetic fields at targeted sites, such as the gastrointestinal tract or hypothalamus, leading to a decrease in hunger and increase in satiety [31, 32]. This local delivery thus assures effectiveness while keeping systemic exposure and side effects as minimal as possible.

Other innovative applications in obesity management by magnetic hyperthermia are the magnetic induction of lipolysis or apoptosis in AT. The localized heating of MNPs, by the alternating magnetic fields, breaks down fat cells without damage to surrounding healthy tissues. This minimally invasive approach might be combined with physical exercise or dietary intervention to improve weight-loss therapies. Moreover, magneto-responsive implants have been developed to control the long-term release of anti-obesity medications. Such devices can be remotely turned on and off, thus enabling personalized adaptive treatment regimens. The development of hybrid magneto-sensitive systems, which incorporate several stimuli, such as pH, glucose, or temperature into magnetic sensitivity, represents significant progress in biomaterials development. For example, magneto-glucose-responsive hydrogels combine magnetic NPs with GOx. The resulting system will react appropriately to changes in blood glucose level and to external magnetic fields applied. This double responsiveness provides exact control of insulin release. It improves glycemic controls and reduces the burden from frequent monitoring for patients. Similarly, combining magnetic properties with thermo-responsive ones makes the treatment of obesity effective by ensuring the drug releases only under certain physiological conditions.

Despite the great potential of magneto-responsive biomaterials, there are also some challenges, for instance, ensuring that MNPs are biocompatible and stable in the body to avoid long-term toxicity or immune reactions. Full exploitation of such materials often necessitates specialized equipment capable of providing controlled magnetic field generation—a factor that probably reduces access to technology and scalability. Manufacturing complexity due to increasing levels of functionality by multi-stimuli-responsiveness further extends the barrier against the possibility of widespread usage. In any case, the future of magneto-responsive biomaterials is bright, and active research is being done to further develop their precision, biocompatibility, and multifunctionality. Wearable magneto-responsive systems are also being explored for non-invasive solutions for real-time glucose monitoring and drug delivery. For instance, insulin or appetite suppressants might be released from wristbands embedded with magneto-responsive reservoirs upon user-specific magnetic triggers [33]. At the same time, developments in tissue engineering allow the creation of magnetically responsive scaffolds to promote regeneration of the pancreatic and ATs as a completely new way of treating diabetes and obesity. Magneto-responsive biomaterials represent the state of the art in smart therapeutic technologies owing to the dynamic and patient-centered methodologies they can offer in diabetes and obesity management. The capabilities that are enabled to realize precise, localized, and controlled therapy go a long way toward assuring new treatment paradigms for improved outcomes and enhancement in the quality of life of patients globally. Continued research into the current set of challenges places these materials as a promise to become a crucial component in the future of personalized medicine.

8.3.1.4 Electroresponsive

Electroresponsive (ER) biomaterials are recognized as a class of smart materials capable of modifying their mechanical, physical, or chemical properties in response to external electric fields [31]. This adaptability enables its applications across various biomedical domains, particularly in developing advanced drug delivery systems and bioelectronic devices, and is noted for combining electrical responsiveness with biocompatibility, making them highly suitable in precision medicine for conditions such as obesity and diabetes [32, 33]. These ER biomaterials present a promising platform for on-demand therapeutic delivery, leveraging electrical stimulation to trigger drug release precisely at target sites [34, 35]. Unlike conventional systems, which rely on passive release, these materials allow for dynamic modulation of treatment in response to patient-specific physiological requirements, thereby enhancing therapeutic effectiveness while minimizing adverse effects [35, 36]. The functionality of ER biomaterials primarily relies on their interaction with applied electric fields which influences their structure and behavior. Common conductive materials such as conjugated polymers, carbon-based nanostructures, and metallic NPs are often incorporated to facilitate electron mobility and enable electrochemical reactions. Under electrical stimulation, conformational or chemical changes are induced within the biomaterial matrix which triggers the controlled release of encapsulated drugs or bioactive agents [37]. For example, polypyrrole (PPy), polyaniline (PANI), and poly(3,4-ethylenedioxythiophene) (PEDOT) are sensitive to the electric field, and reversible oxidation-reduction reactions occur within the polymer matrix. Volumetric shifts of redox leading to material swelling enable controlled release of pharmacological agents. Similarly, thiolated biomaterials are engineered to break selectively through disulfide bonds that form when electrical stimulation is applied, modulating material swelling so drugs can diffuse. Carbon-based materials, such as graphene, impart conductivity and mechanical stability, further enabling stimulus-responsive behavior to be effective [37].

In a study by [38], poly vinylidene fluoride (PVDF) films were and have been demonstrated as intestinal implants for the treatment of obesity and diabetes. These films, characterized by a high β-crystalline phase and enhanced mechanical strength, showed significant weight and glycemic control improvements, thus elucidates electroactive implants as a potential replacement to bariatric surgery with no invasive procedures. However, [39] suggested a thiol–yne polyethylene glycol

(PEG) click-hydrogel, functionalized with PEDOT NPs, as an ER platform for insulin delivery. With electrochemical stimulation of the hydrogel system, sustained, yet controlled, insulin release can be achieved. PEDOT–PEG interactions further exhibited a capability for sustained in vitro release of insulin, suggesting that it has the potential for bioelectronic applications. And in another study by [40], thiolated silk fibroin (TSF) microneedles improved with graphene for conductive enhancement have been studied to understand their delivery capabilities for insulin. Electrical stimulation was shown to break the disulfide bonds within TSF which caused swelling of the microneedles and eventually helped well with the delivery of insulin. It is reversible and thus dynamically controlled drug delivery. Researchers conducted in vivo studies in type 1 diabetic mice have shown effective glucose regulation within safe limits over extended durations, highlighting the potential for integrating such systems with glucose-monitoring technologies.

The benefits of ER biomaterials are numerous which makes them an attractive choice for modern medical treatments. A key advantage is their drug delivery capability that can administer medications with accuracy either continuously or in pulses based on specific medical requirements. This feature helps reduce exposure to drugs and potential side effects while guarantee that the medications reach their intended destinations, in the right amounts. Moreover, these substances are extremely adaptable and may be modified to react to triggers such as electric fields alterations in pH levels and changes in temperature expanding their range of uses. Their ability to work well with device shapes also improves their effectiveness in developing therapeutic systems. Another key benefit is their capacity to decrease reactions, a factor especially, in long-term treatments, where recurring doses may result in issues. In the realm of metabolic conditions such as obesity and diabetes, these substances provide a chance for treatments that are less intrusive or minimally invasive which may help ease the traditional treatments, like surgery or frequent injections. The ER biomaterials offer several benefits; however, several literatures further reported the challenges of ER biomaterials to overcome. The primary concern is expensive nature of materials and manufacturing processes. Moreover, materials like graphene may encounter challenges in compatibility with the body, which restrict their range of applications. Another issue of importance is ensuring the durability of these materials when subject to repeated signals as any degradation could jeopardize their effectiveness and safety. Additionally relying on power sources introduces complexities.

The significant potential exists for the field of ER biomaterials to transform the treatment of obesity and diabetes. In future emerging advancements in material science, such as hybrid composites and nanoscale architectures, are likely to enhance conductivity, biocompatibility, and mechanical properties. Wireless and implantable devices represent an exciting direction, offering remote-controlled, patient-specific therapies. For instance, closed-loop systems that combine glucose sensors with ER insulin delivery platforms could revolutionize diabetes management. Moreover, advancements in energy-harvesting technologies are anticipated to reduce dependency on external power sources, facilitating fully autonomous systems. As research progresses, addressing challenges related to scalability, regulatory compliance, and long-term safety will be essential. Collaborative efforts between material scientists, bioengineers, and clinicians will drive the translation of these technologies from laboratory settings to clinical applications, ultimately advancing therapeutic outcomes for patients with metabolic disorders.

8.3.1.5 Ultrasound Responsive

Ultrasound-sensitive materials are becoming increasingly popular in the field of medicine because of their capacity to react to ultrasound signals in a very precise way [41]. This unique responsiveness enables the management of drug release timing and location and the triggering of healing substances while influencing biological functions—qualities that make these materials highly suitable for various drug delivery methods and tissue repair and regeneration purposes. The process of ultrasound-triggered drug release hinges on the interaction between thermal and nonthermal impacts [42]. Thermal effects stem from transforming energy into warmth and may result in heightened drug dispersion and improved cell permeability as well, as potential disruption of the cell membrane to aid in the absorption and internal distribution of medicinal substances. This method is especially important for delivering medications that target cells internally or those that benefit from improved absorption. Conversely, the non-heating effects are mostly linked to cavitation. A process that includes the creation, oscillation, and bursting of bubbles, within the biological material or nearby tissues [43]. This cavitation procedure produces shock waves and shear stress therefore advancing drug discharge, sonoporation, and increased vascular permeability. Sonoporation involves creating pores, in cell membranes, using ultrasound technology to aid in the delivery of large molecules or genetic material that would normally face challenges crossing the cell membrane.

Various ultrasound-sensitive biomaterial options have been created for purposes with distinct features and benefits of their own unique nature in mind. One example is microbubbles which have attracted interest for their strong response to ultrasound and capacity to transport substantial loads. This makes them appropriate for applications such as drug delivery and ultrasound imaging [44]. Their capability to vibrate and collapse when exposed to ultrasound enables the controlled discharge of enclosed medications or therapeutic substances. Nano-sized bubbles present benefits in delivering drugs due to their smaller size and better ability to gather in specific tissues. This is especially advantageous in cancer treatment as it aids in penetration and retention within the tumor environment. The reduced size of these nanobubbles enables them to exit blood vessels and reach deeper into tissues to enhance the presence of healing substances locally. When tiny liquid particles made of chemicals are exposed to ultrasound waves in the body, they can change into gas bubbles as a way to release drugs and improve imaging techniques. This transformation ability offers a method for releasing medications when needed. The droplets stay unchanged in the bloodstream until ultrasound is used at the specific area, for treatment. Micelles formed by combining amphiphilic block copolymers have the flexibility to hold and release both water- and oil-soluble medications efficiently. This property makes them appealing choices for delivering drugs through ultrasound stimulation [44]. By accommodating a variety of drugs in one carrier structure using ultrasound micelles widens the scope of treatment options available for patients.

Stimuli-responsive hydrogels have become popular for their ability to act as drug delivery systems that can react to different stimuli like ultrasound. These hydrogels can be customized to alter their chemical characteristics when exposed to ultrasound waves for controlled drug release purposes. This makes them ideal, for delivering drugs and therapeutic proteins effectively. The use of ultrasound biomaterials goes way beyond traditional drug delivery methods. Focal ultrasound combined with microbubbles or nanodroplets has demonstrated promise in temporarily opening the blood–brain barrier—a significant challenge that restricts the delivery of medications to the brain. This non-invasive method presents an avenue, for addressing different neurological conditions by aiding in the movement of drugs through the blood–brain barrier. Moreover, drug delivery systems that respond to ultrasound have shown effectiveness in treating diseases by targeting the delivery of agents to bacteria and other pathogens like biofilms can increase their efficiency. In drug delivery science, ultrasound technology at lower frequencies has the potential to improve the skin permeability. This allows for the transfer of therapeutic substances through the skin, without requiring injections or other invasive techniques [45]. This method is especially beneficial for individuals who need to take medication or face challenges with conventional drug delivery techniques.

Even though there have been advancements in creating and using biomaterial that responds to ultrasound waves, there are still a number of obstacles yet to overcome. Enhancing the effectiveness of these biomaterials relies heavily on increasing the capacity for drug loading to improve their outcomes. It's important to find the balance in ultrasound intensity since using high levels can harm healthy tissues and low levels may not activate the desired drug release or therapeutic benefits effectively. Tailoring ultrasound stimulation to applications and maximizing therapeutic outcomes while minimizing potential adverse effects involves optimizing parameters, like frequency, intensity, and pulse duration [44].

The global burden of diabetes continues to rise, with current pharmacological treatments primarily focused on glycemic control rather than disease reversal. Given this limitation, the regulation of glucose homeostasis remains the cornerstone of diabetes management. In this context, the exploration of non-invasive therapeutic strategies has garnered growing interest. One such emerging approach is the use of low-intensity-focused ultrasound (LIFU) for modulating physiological processes, including glucose metabolism. A recent study investigated the potential of ultrasonic stimulation as a non-pharmacological method to lower blood glucose levels and improve glucose tolerance. The research employed a custom-built, smartphone-controlled ultrasonic stimulation system, designed to deliver targeted therapy to specific acupoints. The acupoint CV12, located midway between the xiphoid process and the umbilicus, was selected for its traditional association with gastrointestinal and metabolic regulation. To simulate T2D, Sprague-Dawley rats were subjected to a high-fat diet (HFD) followed by intraperitoneal injection of streptozotocin (STZ), a protocol known to induce insulin resistance and hyperglycemia. The ultrasonic stimulation was applied at a frequency of 1 MHz, a pulse repetition frequency of 15 Hz, a duty cycle of 10%, and a sonication duration of 30 minutes per treatment session. Remarkably, a single session of ultrasonic stimulation led to an acute and statistically significant reduction in blood glucose levels by 11.5% ± 3.6% within just 5 minutes of treatment ($p < 0.001$). This rapid glycemic response suggested a potential neuromodulatory mechanism triggered by mechanical stimulation of the targeted tissue. Further assessments, conducted after intermittent treatments on days 1, 3, and 5 of the first week, revealed sustained improvements in glucose tolerance. By the sixth week, treated animals displayed a significantly smaller area under the glucose tolerance curve compared to untreated diabetic controls ($p < 0.05$). To elucidate the underlying mechanisms, hematological analyses were performed. The results indicated a significant increase in circulating β-endorphin levels (58% ± 71.9%, $p < 0.05$), a neuropeptide associated with pain modulation and metabolic regulation. While insulin levels also rose by 56% ± 88.2%, this change did not reach statistical significance ($p = 0.15$), possibly due to variability in individual responses or sample size limitations. These findings highlight the potential of low-intensity ultrasound as a non-invasive and portable modality for modulating glucose homeostasis. The observed enhancement in glucose tolerance and acute hypoglycemic response supports its future application as an adjunctive therapy alongside conventional diabetic medications. As the field of ultrasonic neuromodulation continues to evolve, such studies pave the way for the development of wearable, app-integrated systems for real-time metabolic regulation.

In the realm of ultrasound biomaterial research, it is crucial to tackle these hurdles and broaden their possibilities ahead. The key lies in crafting materials that are eco-friendly and harmonious with the body to guarantee the lasting well-being and effectiveness of such biomaterial creations [45]. It is paramount to optimize drug loading capabilities and attain control over release mechanisms, for enhanced treatment results and reduced adverse effects. It is essential to conduct preclinical and clinical research to fully assess the long-term safety and effectiveness of these biomaterials in different applications. This will help pave the way for their use, in clinical settings [1]. Biomaterials that respond to ultrasound show potential to transform different areas of healthcare. By tackling existing obstacles and pushing boundaries through innovation, these advanced materials have the ability to revolutionize the management of illnesses, enhance patient results, and influence the trajectory of healthcare moving forward.

8.3.1.6 Mechanical Responsive

Mechano-responsive biomaterials represent a very young family of smart materials engineered to sense environmental mechanical stimuli. In contrast to a passive interface of the traditional biomaterial, mechano-active biomaterials assume an active response toward fluctuations in mechanical forces, including tensile strain, compressive strain, and shear strains. Since biomaterials are sensitive to mechanical stress, they are generally used for special purposes in repairing and regenerating tissues. The basic principle of mechano-responsive biomaterials works on the concept of identifying and responding to the mechanical forces applied to tissues during movements or stresses [46].

Biomaterials are engineered for their structure or properties to be altered upon such mechanical forces applied. For instance, these can be physicochemical changes, like swelling, shrinking, or reshaping due to strain. These changes enable the materials to be active in their effect on the tissue microenvironmental functions, thus supporting regeneration and repair of tissues. To understand the interplay between genetic background and metabolic response to dietary challenges is crucial in unraveling the complexity of obesity and T2D. In a comparative study exploring the effects of HFD on metabolic health, multiple inbred mouse strains were subjected to either a low-fat diet or an HFD for a period of eight weeks. The objective was to characterize differences in whole-body energy metabolism, body composition, and molecular markers related to mitochondrial function, inflammation, oxidative stress, and lipid handling. Among the strains tested—C57BL/6 (BL6), 129X1, DBA/2, FVB/N, and BALB/c—most displayed varying degrees of susceptibility to HFD-induced obesity, glucose intolerance, and insulin resistance. These phenotypes align with commonly reported outcomes in rodent models of diet-induced metabolic dysfunction. However, a notable exception emerged in the form of BALB/c mice, which demonstrated a relative resistance to these deleterious effects. Despite HFD exposure, BALB/c mice maintained more favorable glucose homeostasis and insulin sensitivity profiles compared to their counterparts. This metabolic resilience prompted further investigation into potential underlying mechanisms. However, comprehensive assessments revealed no significant differences in mitochondrial metabolism or oxidative stress markers in liver and muscle tissues that could account for this protection. Similarly, levels of inflammation within AT—a known contributor to insulin resistance—did not distinguish BALB/c mice from the more susceptible strains. The key to their metabolic advantage appeared to lie in hepatic lipid handling. Unlike the other strains, BALB/c mice did not accumulate excessive hepatic lipids, including triacylglycerols and diacylglycerols, which are strongly implicated in insulin resistance. Importantly, this absence of lipid accumulation was not attributable to reduced lipogenesis or increased lipid oxidation. Instead, the data suggest a more nuanced mechanism: BALB/c mice exhibited lower fatty acid uptake in the liver, potentially reducing the substrate burden for ectopic lipid deposition. This observation underscores the significance of tissue-specific lipid fluxes in determining metabolic outcomes and highlights the BALB/c strain as a genetically determined model of resistance to HFD-induced hepatic steatosis and systemic insulin resistance. These findings emphasize the importance of genetic background in metabolic studies and suggest that interventions targeting fatty acid uptake may offer therapeutic potential in the management of diet-induced metabolic disorders.

They can be employed to actively control drug or cell delivery inside a tissue that will respond to the mechanical conditions of the tissue, thereby delivering therapeutic agents at the right place and time. It is also possible to reconstruct or retain the original mechanical properties of tissues while maintaining a favorable healing environment. Biomaterials hence allow tissue remodeling as well as provide accelerated healing within muscular, osseous, and vascular tissues, responding to mechanical cues [46]. Such materials, especially those for musculoskeletal and cardiovascular tissues, have been quite promising because the mechanical forces play a critical role in normal functions and repair. Despite the major challenges in developing these materials, there are advancements in the field of regenerative medicine that bring new hopes for improving tissue repair and regeneration. Jariwala et al. demonstrated the promising use of piezoelectric poly(vinylidene fluoride-trifluoroethylene) nanofibers as a mechano-responsive drug release system [47]. The nanofibers have a high surface area-to-volume ratio and some piezoelectric properties, which allow for controlled, demand-driven drug release under the influence of mechanical stimuli. The negative zeta potential enables electrostatic loading with cationic drugs, which is released in response to a change in surface potential when exposed to mechanical forces, such as pressure or shockwaves. Drug release kinetics may be tailored by modification of the fiber diameter, affecting piezoelectric properties, and the quantity of release can also be controlled by modulating the mechanical stimulus. Both in vitro and ex vivo models verified the efficacy of the platform. This study shows the potential for piezoelectric P(VDF-TrFE) nanofibers in highly sensitive, controlled drug delivery for applications in personalized medicine and targeted therapies.

Strain-sensitive biomaterials can be very useful in wide applications where there is a dynamic environment, and the ability to adapt and react to changes in physiological conditions enhances performance. They improve health monitoring because their properties change with strain, giving an instantaneous glimpse into the body's functions. For example, if the scaffolds can be prepared from materials sensitive to strain, the matching with tissue and its mechanical properties would further improve integration and functionality in tissue engineering. Biomaterials will also allow for the potential controlled release of drugs when therapeutic agents are released due to specific mechanical stimuli whereby therapeutic treatments may appear more precise and efficient, especially in chronic conditions such as diabetes and obesity. Also, its biocompatibility minimizes the adverse reactions when implanted, especially for long-term medical devices like stents and implants. But these have their own limitations. The manufacturing process for strain-sensitive biomaterials is highly complex and technology-intensive, making them costly with longer production times. Finding the right balance between strength, flexibility, and responsiveness is particularly challenging. Furthermore, some of these strain-sensitive materials lack enough mechanical strength to be used as load-bearing devices in cases such as bone or cartilage regeneration and degrade with time. Another major concern is degradation due to sustained mechanical stress, which might precipitate functional failure. So, long-term behavior of these materials in the body is an important issue for their successful use in clinical applications.

Mechanosensitive biomaterials signify a promising route in tissue engineering and regenerative medicine. They may be used to create a new avenue toward active adaptation to mechanical stimuli in the body. Traditionally, conventional biomaterials are known to react passively to mechanical forces. Mechano-active biomaterials, on the other hand, exhibit active responses toward the local mechanical environment. Their functional performance is, therefore, constantly mediated by such forces. This characteristic places them in an advantageous position regarding enhanced repair and regeneration of tissues, mainly musculoskeletal and cardiovascular tissues. Nonetheless, there are many challenges still in the development and application of mechano-active biomaterials. The conceptual understanding of such materials at a theoretical level in tissue repair modeling is still an area that needs exploration. Advanced simulation approaches can be applied to fine-tune the principles under which such materials operate and to determine their eventual integration into tissue engineering strategies. Although a lot of efforts have been paid toward coupling the mechanical cues with biochemical approaches for enhancing the regenerative potential of the presented materials, this field of study is still at its nascent stages. Other approaches have been reported; however, most of them have been at the basic levels, like efforts toward constructing mechano-active systems that could better harness these biomaterials for the control of enzyme-assisted biocatalysis. Another area of research to be critical in design and fabrication for mechano-active materials. The current methods are still not accessible or realistic enough toward universal usage. Along these lines, there is a need for more efficient strategies for creation of such advanced biomaterials. Despite such challenges, biologically active biomaterials give much promise for advanced tissue repair and regeneration. Exciting opportunities for personalized and more effective therapeutic approaches exist with these new materials. The continued research and innovation may address some of the challenges put forward in this chapter and, consequently, introduce these new materials into clinical practice. This progress further increases their potential to revolutionize healthcare by giving patients who require regenerative treatments more satisfactory results (Table 8.2).

8.3.2 Chemical Stimuli

8.3.2.1 Moisture Responsive

Moisture-sensitive biomaterials are lately developed materials that respond dynamically to environmental humidity, thus being truly very suitable for such applications as drug delivery, wound healing, and tissue engineering. These make use of hydrophilic polymers, which respond drastically with regard to physical state or structure when exposed to moisture. Upon contact with humidity,

TABLE 8.2
Strain-Responsive Biomaterials Depicting the Type of Stimuli, Mechanism of Response and Applications

Stimuli	Mechanism/Response	Applications
Tensile, compressive, and shear strain	Alters properties like swelling, shrinking, reshaping, or physicochemical changes when mechanical forces are applied.	Alters properties like swelling, shrinking, reshaping, or physicochemical changes when mechanical forces are applied.
Mechanical stress	Drug release through piezoelectric properties of biomaterials, responding to surface potential changes caused by strain or shockwaves.	Controlled drug delivery for personalized medicine and chronic conditions like diabetes and obesity.
Dynamic strain	Adapts material properties (strength, flexibility) to match tissue mechanical environments, improving integration and functionality.	Tissue engineering, especially scaffolds for musculoskeletal and vascular tissue regeneration.
Piezoelectric properties	Adapts material properties (strength, flexibility) to match tissue mechanical environments, improving integration and functionality.	Targeted therapies with enhanced precision, especially using piezoelectric materials like P(VDF-TrFE).
Sustained mechanical stress	Potential degradation and loss of mechanical strength over time, challenging their use in load-bearing application.	Long-term implants and medical devices like stents.
Mechanical cues	Coupled with biochemical processes for enzyme-assisted biocatalysis or tissue remodeling.	Advanced tissue engineering strategies for enhanced repair and regenerative outcomes.

such water-absorbing polymers may swell or alter their mechanical properties, such as permeability and elasticity. These swelling facilitate the controlled release of encapsulated drugs or bioactive substances, tailoring therapeutic delivery to the conditions of the surrounding environment. The mechanism relies on adsorption of water molecules onto the surface and diffusion through the polymer matrix before desorption within its inner structure. Such changes cause relaxation of polymer chains and thus result in enhanced release of buried drug molecules. Furthermore, the rate of water absorption and drug delivery may be controlled by changing the molecular weight or cross-linking density of the polymers. Moisture-sensitive biomaterials thus provide a smart approach for developing adaptive therapeutic systems optimized according to physiological demands.

Moisture-responsive materials represent an innovative class of smart materials that have the ability to evolve their properties or their shape based on changes in environmental humidity. Moisture-responsiveness has gained much attention—particularly within the umbrella of 4D printing—due to dynamic and responsive conditions [48]. Applications range from agriculture and food safety to biomedical engineering and far beyond, when including moisture-responsive materials within 4D printing. A study done [49] highlighted the chemical modification of cellulose with stearoyl moieties that includes cellulosic stearoyl esters (CSEs) of different degrees of substitution (DSs). Interestingly, the CSE films at a low DS of 0.3, called CSE0.3, were discovered to have a moisture-sensitive property that could not be seen with higher DSs of 1.3 or 3 of CSE1.3 and CSE3 films. This reversible folding and unfolding of the CSE0.3 films can be attributed to the adsorption and desorption of the water molecules on their surface. The bending performance of the films was improved further by spray-coating CSE3 NPs onto the CSE0.3 films, the latter exhibiting changes in bending movements over shorter timescales and sustained shape transitions over water. Bilayer films, comprising a CSE0.3 layer sandwiched between a CSE3 layer, exhibited both moisture- and temperature-dependent responses. The thickness of the CSE0.3 films proved easily accessible for adjusting the extent of bending, thus allowing movement to start from the thinner side due to changes in mechanical resistance. This type of work emphasizes the potentiality for the flexible use of cellulose-derived materials to create moisture-sensitive smart systems with adjustable, multifunctional properties.

The notable advantage of moisture-responsive materials is related to optimizing processes in which environmental control plays a crucial role. For example, there are agricultural applications in the creation of adaptive plant supports that react to changes in humidity variations for optimal greenhouse plant care. This not only builds up plants but also provides better agricultural practices. Similarly, moisture-sensitive seals for grain silos might prevent moisture ingress and thereby ensure the safety of stored grains against spoilage and promote food security [12]. Controlled release of drugs or bioactive agents through moisture-sensitive mechanisms in biomedical applications provides targeted and efficient therapeutic delivery systems with reduced side effects and improved patient outcome. A drawback remains for moisture-responsive materials despite their promise; namely, the large initial investment required to produce these materials does not yet support commercial-scale applications. Their production costs are still relatively high, although efforts to scale up their manufacturing processes to permit large industrial use have been extremely difficult. In addition, their sustainability and long-term behavior under repeated humid fluctuations will require more deeply contemplated research and optimization (Table 8.3).

Even though these are drawbacks, the ability of the moisture-responsive materials to provide precision and adaptability in dynamic environments can be potentially very far-reaching in realizing transformative potential within these materials. Furthermore, their sustainability and long-term behavior under repeated humid fluctuations will need more deeply contemplated research and optimization. While these represent drawbacks, the ability of moisture-responsive materials to provide precision and adaptability in dynamic environments can be very far-reaching in realizing transformative potential within such materials. Continued advancements in material science

TABLE 8.3
Moisture-Responsive Biomaterials, Its Mechanism of Response and Its Applications

Stimuli	Mechanism/Response	Applications
Environmental humidity	Polymers swell or alter their mechanical properties (permeability, elasticity) in response to water adsorption and diffusion.	Controlled drug delivery, wound healing, and tissue engineering.
Adsorption/desorption	Relaxation of polymer chains causes release of encapsulated drugs or bioactive substances.	Adaptive therapeutic delivery systems optimized for specific physiological demands.
Humidity variations	Cellulose-based materials show reversible shape transitions (e.g., bending or unfolding) upon exposure to moisture.	Smart systems for 4D printing, agricultural plant supports, and moisture-sensitive seals for grain silos.
Molecular weight or cross-linking density	Tailor rate of water absorption and drug delivery, enhancing adaptability and precision.	Moisture-sensitive drug formulations for antidiabetic therapies, improving bioavailability and patient outcomes.
Repeated humid fluctuations	Changes in material sustainability and functionality over time, requiring optimization for long-term behavior.	Personalized medicine and dietary supplements targeting diabetes and obesity by modulating hydration levels for appetite regulation and weight management.
Combined moisture and temperature sensitivity	Bilayer films with moisture and temperature responses enable enhanced movement and shape changes in dynamic environments.	Changes in material sustainability and functionality over time, requiring optimization for long-term behavior.

and engineering will cause such materials to transform industries through more sustainable efficient systems that are intelligent. Despite these current limitations, these promising applications can bring moisture-responsive materials to the forefront for future innovations and developments.

The future of moisture-sensitive biomaterials appears incredibly bright for managing diabetes and obesity challenges and broad biomedical applications. They will revolutionize drug formulations in stabilizing the more sensitive antidiabetic drugs, enabling shelf stability and maximally improving bioavailability. Patients will thus be able to realize consistent therapeutic benefits with lower and more effective dosages. Moisture-sensitive biomaterials also have promising applications in personalized medicine. Ultimately, this may be tailored for even more sensitivity to the average moisture levels or specific physiological conditions of a particular individual. An example would be the optimization of drug delivery for diabetes and obesity treatments to be therefore more targeted and effective. To add to this, in a world that is experiencing continuously increasing levels of obesity, there is increasingly more pressure for novel approaches like moisture-sensitive dietary supplements or drugs that could modulate hydration levels, which would have a biological effect on appetite regulation, provide enhanced satiety, and lead to better weight management overall. All in all, these recent developments suggest that moisture-sensitive biomaterials might be set on a pathway for revolutionizing healthcare by offering smart, responsive answers to complex healthcare needs.

8.3.2.2 Redox Responsive

Redox-responsive biomaterials technology is the chemistry of redox as most substances undergo an oxidation-reduction process which is the movement and transfer of electrons, and this happens in cellular metabolic pathways. Inside the body, oxidative stress which is excessive generation of ROS and reactive nitrogen species (RNS) is usually associated with chronic diseases. Redox-responsive types of materials avail themselves with some functional moieties which are affected by and responsive to these oxidative stresses. When such biomaterials faced with any ROS or microenvironment change such as the perturbed redox state in its vicinity, alterations in redox, they chemically react, for instance, by breaking some bond in a substrate that is sensitive to ROS or by changing shape, and hereby, activate therapy. Such activities may include the release of the drug from the depot, destruct of the polymer drug depot, or change of the biological material structural properties [50]. Redox-responsive biomaterials essentially provide a cascading series of events. A redox reaction is the initiation event, where the functional groups of the material come into contact with oxidative or reductive agents present in the microenvironment to initiate a conformational or structural alteration such as pore formation and degradation of the biomaterial that changes its behavior [51–53]. For instance, disulfide-cross-linked hydrogels swell responsive to the redox environment through thiol–disulfide exchange and reverse from a gel to a sol state that frees up the encapsulated bioactive molecules [52]. Similarly, materials with ROS-cleavable linkers such as thioketals experience degradation when placed in an oxidative environment that leads to precision cargo release at the site of activity [54]. These mechanisms are especially useful for targeting tissues with heightened oxidative stress, such as in the inflamed AT of obesity or hyperglycemic environments of diabetes.

There are some promising novel applications studied for redox-sensitive biomaterials [55] studied glucose biosensing with the use of manganese dioxide nanosheets toward diabetes management. These MnO_2 nanosheets combined with upconversion nanoparticles (UCNPs) quench fluorescence under physiological conditions, but the fluorescence was recovered in response to the presence of H_2O_2 produced through glucose oxidation catalyzed by GOx. This fluorescence recovery allowed sensitive and fast glucose detection in human serum, representing an interesting avenue for non-invasive glucose monitoring. Another study by [56] developed photoluminescence system with application in the concurrent sensing of H_2O_2 and glucose using $NaYF_4^+/Er_3^+$ UCNPs. Examples in this group displayed very high sensitivity and specificity without interference from other biomolecules through systems like this but have limitations such as interference from nonspecific biomolecules and system complexity, however, to be ready for practical applications much work needed to be done. Besides diagnostics, redox-sensitive hydrogels have also been found to be highly promising for therapeutic applications [57], genetically engineered collagen-like protein hydrogels which have been designed for the treatment of diabetic wounds, which undergone gel–sol transitions in response to oxidative stress and allowed the release of therapeutic agents and increased cellular migration at the wound site. That is, these materials not only assisted in healing by reducing oxidative damage and facilitated tissue regeneration but also reduced complications that occur with diabetes like chronic ulcers. Despite such promising prospects, the scalability and long-term stability remained concerning factors for these hydrogels that requires further research to optimize their utility in clinical settings. The advantages of redox-responsive biomaterials are multifaceted. Dynamic responsiveness to endogenous signals offers high specificity with minimum chances of off-target effects. In addition, adaptability in design for concurrent drug delivery, diagnostic monitoring, and therapeutic feedback makes the multifunctional platforms highly relevant for complex systems such as diabetes and obesity, where co-occurring conditions usually require complex treatment regimens. Additionally, the biocompatibility and biodegradability of many redox-responsive systems enhance their appeal for clinical use, as they minimize the risk of adverse immune reactions and environmental persistence. However, these materials have their limitations too. The complexity of the designs they require can pose significant manufacturing challenges. Moreover, interindividual differences in redox environment stemming from diet, genetics, and the state of disease play a potential role in altering how redox-responsive biomaterials behave. Thereby, personalized approaches to use become inevitable. The stability and reliability of these materials in vivo, especially the long-term exposure to fluctuating redox conditions, remain an active area of study. Controlled release of therapeutics enhances the efficacy of drugs and limits systemic side effects, which is critical for chronic disease management. Looking forward, further integration of redox-responsive biomaterials with digital health technologies offers new promise for personalized medicine. The ability to monitor redox states in real time through wearable devices may allow dynamic adjustment of therapy and optimize treatment efficacy while reduce side effects. Other targeting strategies using biomarkers specific to oxidative stress in diabetes and obesity may also improve the accuracy of these materials. For example, the ligands targeted could be peptides or antibodies that would bind to Ox-LDL in obesity or advanced glycation end-products (AGEs) in diabetes to make the localization of therapeutic actions even more specific. There could also be multifunctional systems responsive to pH, temperature, and mechanical forces in addition to redox changes that would allow these materials to be used in a wide variety of therapeutic scenarios.

8.3.3 Combination of Multiple Stimuli/Dual or Hybrid Stimuli

There has been the development of several hybrid systems that have begun to integrate multiple-stimuli-responsive elements to provide better specificity and functionality. This in turn allows for more widespread applications in drug delivery systems, tissue engineering, or biosensing. Dual-stimuli-responsive peptides and proteins have inherent biocompatibility and structural flexibility giving them significant advantages over other commonly used materials. One very frequently used system is a combination of temperature and pH responsive biomaterials. Elastin-like polypeptides (ELPs), for example, are temperature-sensitive materials. They undergo a phase change at the LCST depending on the amino acid sequence as well as chain length. If we add acidic or basic residues to ELPs we can essentially make them sensitive to pH as well, thus allowing them to alter their structure in acidic environments. This dual responsiveness is actually perfect for drug delivery systems in case of cancers, where tumors have warmer and more acidic conditions [5].

A combination of enzyme- and pH-sensitive systems have also been observed to be highly effective, especially in case of cancer treatments. Several tumors are also known to produce high levels of matrix metalloproteinases (MMPs). This makes them useful for enzyme-sensitive biomaterials. This method of combining MMP sensitivity with pH sensitivity helps improve targeting as well as ensuring that the drugs are released only when they are necessary. They are also used for delivering drugs in case of diabetes treatment for increased precision. NPs that can respond to both enzymatic activity and acidic pH environments are programmed to release GLP-1 analogs which in turn helps regulate blood sugar without causing hypoglycemia [58]. These systems ensure selective activation in only the desirable targets/conditions, thus improving drug availability and reducing side effects. These systems can be utilized for personalized treatment for diabetes. pH- and glucose-responsive biomaterials are also widely used in closed-loop insulin delivery systems. These systems are designed to mimic pancreatic beta cells and their release of insulin in response to high blood sugar. GOx is crucial in many of these designs since it is responsible for converting glucose to gluconic acid and lowering the local pH. This change in pH causes hydrogels/NPs to swell and release insulin. Systems that combine GOx with the enzyme catalase can also stabilize the response by breaking down hydrogen peroxide byproducts that are formed. Temperature- and glucose-responsive systems are also being explored for their therapeutic potential. Thermo-responsive polymers, like PNIPAM, are known to change their solubility with change in temperature, while glucose-binding molecules regulate drug release. Insulin can therefore be designed to be released only when blood sugar is high and external heat is applied, thus creating the possibility of wearable transdermal devices. Microneedle-array patches with glucose-sensitive vesicles also offer continuous glucose monitoring and effective insulin delivery.

For the treatment of obesity, scientists are developing multi-stimuli systems that can help control hormones related to appetite and energy balance. Light- and temperature-sensitive hydrogels are being developed for on-demand release of hunger-suppressing hormones. NIR light triggers gold nanoparticle-based systems to generate heat, causing structural changes that in turn release therapeutic agents. Since the method is non-invasive and highly effective, it provides precise control over drug delivery while the same time reducing patient discomfort and the need for frequent dosing. Redox-sensitive carriers containing sulfide bonds break down in reducing environment. This can allow for targeted drug release inside diseased cells. Additional investigation using computational modeling can help optimize glucose- and enzyme-responsive biomaterial systems by refining reaction speeds and improving their predictability inside the body. Researchers are focused on preventing hypoglycemia through balanced insulin release. This paves the way for developing future systems that can deliver both insulin and glucagon as and when needed [59].

8.4 CHALLENGES AND FUTURE PERSPECTIVES

Stimuli-responsive biomaterials, which respond to internal, external, or environmental cues, have emerged as promising solutions for managing chronic conditions, enabling controlled and precise drug delivery. Physical stimuli-responsive biomaterials are especially useful for drug delivery that is sensitive to environmental changes within the body. For instance, thermo-responsive hydrogels release therapeutic agents such as insulin or anti-obesity drugs according to the body's temperature fluctuations to provide tailored treatment. ER materials can allow for on-demand drug delivery that is controlled by electrical signals to optimize treatment for individual patients. Similarly, ultrasound-responsive materials can non-invasively target specific tissues, such as delivering drugs to AT in obesity or the pancreas in diabetes. Strain-responsive materials, which respond to mechanical cues, are promising for tissue regeneration, aiding in diabetic wound healing or restore obesity-related tissue damage.

Chemical stimuli-responsive biomaterials have additional benefits. Moisture-responsive materials can release bioactive agents in response to changes in humidity, allowing for controlled drug delivery. pH-responsive materials can release drugs at specific body sites, like the gastrointestinal tract, optimizing therapeutic efficacy while minimizing systemic side effects. Redox-responsive materials react to oxidative stress, common in diseases like diabetes and obesity, thus targeting the delivery of therapeutic agents to tissues with heightened oxidative stress, improving precision and reducing off-target effects.

Even though the clinical application of these biomaterials shows significant potential, their development is still accompanied by several challenges. One key challenge is the complexity and high cost of manufacturing, thus limiting their accessibility for routine clinical use. Additionally, scalability remains a significant barrier. Long-term stability is another concern, as materials like thermo-responsive hydrogels may degrade over temperature changes, and ER systems may lose functionality upon repeated cycles. Ensuring biocompatibility is crucial, as materials need to be safe without causing any adverse reactions. ER systems, for instance, must provide safe electrical stimulation, while strain-responsive materials should maintain mechanical strength for load-bearing applications. Physiological variability also poses challenges, especially for pH-responsive materials, as the pH environment varies across body compartments, affecting material performance. Similarly, moisture-responsive materials need to be very finely tuned to respond to fluctuating humidity levels, which affects drug release profiles. Overcoming these challenges requires ongoing research and optimization to ensure reliability and sustainability.

Despite all these challenges, stimuli-responsive biomaterials hold great potential for improving the management of chronic disorders. The ability to control drug release based on environmental stimuli allows for personalized treatment, which is crucial for chronic conditions requiring long-term care. Moreover, non-invasive drug delivery can improve patient compliance by reducing the need for injections. These materials further support tissue regeneration and repair and thus offer hopes for better healing outcomes in conditions like diabetic wounds or obesity-related complications. Additionally, integration of stimuli-responsive biomaterials with technologies such as 4D printing and wearable devices may further enhance their potential. 4D printing could create devices that dynamically respond to changes in moisture, pH, or mechanical stress, offering customizable solutions for drug delivery and tissue regeneration. Wearable devices could monitor physiological conditions in real time, enabling dynamic adjustments to drug delivery and optimizing treatment. These innovations will likely drive advancements in the biomedical application of stimuli-responsive biomaterials.

8.5 CONCLUSION

Stimuli-responsive biomaterials represent a transformative frontier in the development of advanced therapeutic systems for managing complex metabolic disorders such as diabetes and obesity. These smart materials possess the unique capability to interact with biological systems through precise responses to specific internal (e.g., pH, enzymes, glucose levels) or external (e.g., temperature, light, ultrasound) stimuli. Their dynamic and tunable properties allow for controlled and site-specific drug release, modulation of cellular behavior, and mimicry of physiological functions—offering a level of precision and adaptability far beyond that of traditional biomaterials.

In the context of diabetes, the urgent need for self-regulating insulin delivery systems that can respond to fluctuating glucose levels has driven the innovation of glucose-responsive platforms. These systems utilize molecular mechanisms such as enzymatic oxidation and reversible binding to regulate insulin release in real time, closely emulating the natural function of pancreatic β-cells. Such responsive delivery systems not only enhance therapeutic efficacy but also reduce systemic side effects and improve patient adherence by minimizing the burden of frequent injections and glycemic variability. Similarly, in obesity management, stimuli-responsive materials show promise in delivering appetite-suppressing drugs and metabolic regulators in a controlled fashion. The use of polymers like chitosan and synthetic scaffolds such as PLG demonstrates how materials can influence metabolic pathways, adipokine signaling, and glucose uptake, even in the absence of pharmacological agents. Innovations such as adipocyte-targeted NPs and hormone-regulating scaffolds highlight the potential for personalized and minimally invasive therapeutic interventions. The integration of materials science, biotechnology, and medicine has enabled the engineering of responsive systems that are not only biocompatible and biodegradable but also multifunctional and scalable for clinical translation. As research progresses, future directions should focus on enhancing the specificity, responsiveness, and safety profiles of these biomaterials while exploring synergistic approaches involving cellular therapy, genetic modulation, and microenvironmental engineering. In summary, stimuli-responsive biomaterials hold considerable potential to revolutionize the therapeutic landscape of metabolic diseases. By offering intelligent, adaptive, and patient-centric solutions, these materials are poised to play a pivotal role in the next generation of drug delivery systems and regenerative medicine strategies aimed at combating diabetes and obesity.

Declaration of AI and AI-Assisted Technologies

During the preparation of this work, the authors used QuillBot AI in order to paraphrase the sentences. After using this tool, the authors reviewed and edited the content as needed and take full responsibility for the content of the publication.

REFERENCES

1. Wei H, Cui J, Lin K, Xie J, Wang X. Recent advances in smart stimuli-responsive biomaterials for bone therapeutics and regeneration. Bone Research. 2022;10(1):17.
2. McCall AL, Farhy LS. Treating type 1 diabetes: from strategies for insulin delivery to dual hormonal control. Minerva Endocrinologica. 2013;38(2):145.
3. Sarmento B, Martins S, Ferreira D, Souto EB. Oral insulin delivery by means of solid lipid nanoparticles. International Journal of Nanomedicine. 2007;2(4):743–9.
4. Chiang JL, Kirkman MS, Laffel LM, Peters AL. Type 1 diabetes through the life span: a position statement of the American Diabetes Association. Diabetes Care. 2014;37(7):2034.
5. Li J, Duan H, Liu Y, Wang L, Zhou X. Biomaterial-based therapeutic strategies for obesity and its comorbidities. Pharmaceutics. 2022;14(7):1445.
6. Lewis JS, Allen RP. An introduction to biomaterial-based strategies for curbing autoimmunity. Experimental Biology and Medicine. 2016;241(10):1107–15.
7. Myers MG, Leibel RL, Seeley RJ, Schwartz MW. Obesity and leptin resistance: distinguishing cause from effect. Trends in Endocrinology & Metabolism. 2010;21(11):643–51.
8. Gao Y, Ji H, Peng L, Gao X, Jiang S. Development of PLGA-PEG-PLGA hydrogel delivery system for enhanced immunoreaction and efficacy of Newcastle disease virus DNA vaccine. Molecules. 2020;25(11):2505.
9. Żywicka B, Krucińska I, Garcarek J, Szymonowicz M, Komisarczyk A, Rybak ZJM. Biological properties of low-toxic PLGA and PLGA/PHB fibrous nanocomposite scaffolds for osseous tissue regeneration. Evaluation of Potential Bioactivity. Molecules. 2017;22(11):1852.
10. Hendley MA, Murphy KP, Isely C, Struckman HL, Annamalai P, Gower RM. The host response to poly(lactide-co-glycolide) scaffolds protects mice from diet induced obesity and glucose intolerance. Biomaterials. 2019;217:119281.
11. McCarthy MI, Zeggini E. Genome-wide association studies in type 2 diabetes. Current Diabetes Reports. 2009;9:164–71.
12. DIAbetes Genetics Replication And Meta-analysis (DIAGRAM) Consortium. Large-scale association analysis provides insights into the genetic architecture and pathophysiology of type 2 diabetes. Nature Genetics. 2012;44(9):981–90.
13. So HC, Gui AH, Cherny SS, Sham PC. Evaluating the heritability explained by known susceptibility variants: a survey of ten complex diseases. Genetic Epidemiology. 2011;35(5):310–7.
14. Frayling TM, Timpson NJ, Weedon MN, Zeggini E, Freathy RM, Lindgren CM, et al. A common variant in the FTO gene is associated with body mass index and predisposes to childhood and adult obesity. Science. 2007;316(5826):889–94.
15. Fischer J, Koch L, Emmerling C, Vierkotten J, Peters T, Brüning JC, et al. Inactivation of the Fto gene protects from obesity. Nature. 2009;458(7240):894–8.
16. Hakanen M, Raitakari OT, Lehtimaki T, Peltonen N, Pahkala K, Sillanmaki L, et al. FTO genotype is associated with body mass index after the age of seven years but not with energy intake or leisure-time physical activity. The Journal of Clinical Endocrinology & Metabolism. 2009;94(4):1281–7.
17. Church C, Lee S, Bagg EA, McTaggart JS, Deacon R, Gerken T, et al. A mouse model for the metabolic effects of the human fat mass and obesity associated FTO gene. PLoS Genetics. 2009;5(8):e1000599.

18. Stančáková A, Laakso M. Genetics of metabolic syndrome. Reviews in Endocrine and Metabolic Disorders. 2014;15:243–52.
19. Jakubek P, Pakula B, Rossmeisl M, Pinton P, Rimessi A, Wieckowski MR, et al. Autophagy alterations in obesity, type 2 diabetes, and metabolic dysfunction-associated steatotic liver disease: the evidence from human studies. Internal and Emergency Medicine. 2024;19(5):1473–91.
20. Öst A, Svensson K, Ruishalme I, Brännmark C, Franck N, Krook H, et al. Attenuated mTOR signaling and enhanced autophagy in adipocytes from obese patients with type 2 diabetes. Molecular Medicine. 2010;16:235–46.
21. Kovsan J, Blüher M, Tarnovscki T, Klöting N, Kirshtein B, Madar L, et al. Altered autophagy in human adipose tissues in obesity. The Journal of Clinical Endocrinology & Metabolism. 2011;96(2):E268–77.
22. Nuñez C, Rodrigues V, Gomes F, De Moura R, Victorio S, Bombassaro B, et al. Defective regulation of adipose tissue autophagy in obesity. International Journal of Obesity. 2013;37(11):1473–80.
23. Kosacka J, Kern M, Klöting N, Paeschke S, Rudich A, Haim Y, et al. Autophagy in adipose tissue of patients with obesity and type 2 diabetes. Molecular and Cellular Endocrinology. 2015;409:21–32.
24. Xu Q, Mariman EC, Roumans NJ, Vink RG, Goossens GH, Blaak EE, et al. Adipose tissue autophagy related gene expression is associated with glucometabolic status in human obesity. Adipocyte. 2018;7(1):12–9.
25. Jansen H, Van Essen P, Koenen T, Joosten L, Netea M, Tack C, et al. Autophagy activity is up-regulated in adipose tissue of obese individuals and modulates proinflammatory cytokine expression. Endocrinology. 2012;153(12):5866–74.
26. Liao Z, Liu T, Yao Z, Hu T, Ji X, Yao B. Harnessing stimuli-responsive biomaterials for advanced biomedical applications. Exploration. 2024;5(1): 20230133.
27. Lee HP, Gaharwar AK. Light-responsive inorganic biomaterials for biomedical applications. Advanced Science. 2020;7(17):2000863.
28. Khizar S, Zine N, Errachid A, Elaissari A. Introduction to stimuli-responsive materials and their biomedical applications. Journal of Materials Chemistry B 2023;12:6993–6995.
29. Municoy S, Alvarez Echazu MI, Antezana PE, Galdopórpora JM, Olivetti C, Mebert AM, et al. Stimuli-responsive materials for tissue engineering and drug delivery. International Journal of Molecular Sciences. 2020;21(13):4724.
30. Tallapaneni V, Mude L, Pamu D, Palanimuthu VR, Magham SV, Karri VVSR, et al. Growth factor loaded thermo-responsive injectable hydrogel for enhancing diabetic wound healing. Gels. 2022; 9(1):27.
31. Dong X, Li B, Peng Q, Tian T. Editorial: Preparation, properties and applications of electro-responsive smart materials. Frontiers in Materials. 2022;9:943315.
32. Famm K. Drug discovery: a jump-start for electroceuticals. Nature. 2013;496(7445):159–61.
33. Greenway F, Zheng J. Electrical stimulation as treatment for obesity and diabetes. Journal of Diabetes Science and Technology. 2007;1(2):251–9.
34. Murdan S. Electro-responsive drug delivery from hydrogels. Journal of Controlled Release. 2003;92(1–2):1–17.
35. Xie C, Li P, Han L, Wang Z, Zhou T, Deng W, et al. Electroresponsive and cell-affinitive polydopamine/polypyrrole composite microcapsules with a dual-function of on-demand drug delivery and cell stimulation for electrical therapy. Nature. 2017;9(3):e358-e.
36. Ashton MD, Hardy JG. Progress in active ingredient formulations. Johnson Matthey Technology Review. 2019;63(3):211–25.
37. Magaz A, Ashton MD, Hathout RM, Li X, Hardy JG, Blaker JJ. Electroresponsive silk-based biohybrid composites for electrochemically controlled growth factor delivery. Pharmaceutics. 2020;12(8):742.
38. Chang H-M, Zhan W-P, Tsai H-C, Yang M-R. Poly(vinylidene fluoride) intestinal sleeve implants for the treatment of obesity and type 2 diabetes. Polymers. 2022;14(11):2178.
39. Muñoz-Galán H, Enshaei H, Silva JC, Esteves T, Ferreira FC, Casanovas J, et al. Electroresponsive Thiol–Yne click-hydrogels for insulin smart delivery: tackling sustained release and leakage control. ACS Applied Polymer Materials. 2024;6(14):8093–104.
40. Qi Z, Tao X, Tan G, Tian B, Zhang L, Kundu SC, et al. Electro-responsive silk fibroin microneedles for controlled release of insulin. International Journal of Biological Macromolecules. 2023;242:124684.
41. Athanassiadis AG, Ma Z, Moreno-Gomez N, Melde K, Choi E, Goyal R, et al. Ultrasound-responsive systems as components for smart materials. Chemical Reviews. 2021;122(5):5165–208.
42. Yeingst TJ, Arrizabalaga JH, Hayes DJ. Ultrasound-induced drug release from stimuli-responsive hydrogels. Gels. 2022;8(9):554.
43. Tu L, Liao Z, Luo Z, Wu YL, Herrmann A, Huo S, editors. Ultrasound-controlled drug release and drug activation for cancer therapy. Exploration. 2021;1(3):20210023.

44. Cai L, Xu J, Yang Z, Tong R, Dong Z, Wang C, et al. Engineered biomaterials for cancer immunotherapy. MedComm. 2020;1(1):35–46.
45. Wei W, Cardes F, Hierlemann A, Modena MM. 3D in vitro blood-brain-barrier model for investigating barrier insults. Advanced Science. 2023;10(11):2205752.
46. Lin X, Bai Y, Zhou H, Yang L. Mechano-active biomaterials for tissue repair and regeneration. Journal of Materials Science & Technology. 2020;59:227–33.
47. Jariwala T, Ico G, Tai Y, Park H, Myung NV, Nam J. Mechano-responsive piezoelectric nanofiber as an on-demand drug delivery vehicle. ACS Applied Bio Materials. 2021;4(4):3706–15.
48. Al Nahari B, Zarbane K, Beidouri Z. The use of moisture-responsive materials in 4D printing. Journal of Achievements of Materials and Manufacturing Engineering. 2023;119(1).
49. Zhang K, Geissler A, Standhardt M, Mehlhase S, Gallei M, Chen L, et al. Moisture-responsive films of cellulose stearoyl esters showing reversible shape transitions. Nature. 2015;5(1):1–13.
50. Song C-C, Du F-S, Li Z-C. Oxidation-responsive polymers for biomedical applications. Journal of Materials Chemistry B. 2014;2(22):3413–26.
51. Gaddimath S, Payamalle S, Channabasavana Hundi Puttaningaiah KP, Hur J. Recent advances in pH and redox responsive polymer nanocomposites for cancer therapy. Journal of Composites Science. 2024;8(1):28.
52. Lu H, Yuan L, Yu X, Wu C, He D, Deng J, et al. Recent advances of on-demand dissolution of hydrogel dressings. Burns & Trauma. 2018;29(6):35.
53. Uskoković V. Supplementation of polymeric reservoirs with redox-responsive metallic nanoparticles as a new concept for the smart delivery of insulin in diabetes. Materials. 2023;16(2):786.
54. Rinaldi A, Caraffi R, Grazioli MV, Oddone N, Giardino L, Tosi G, et al. Applications of the ROS-responsive thioketal linker for the production of smart nanomedicines. Polymers. 2022;14(4):687.
55. Yuan J, Cen Y, Kong X-J, Wu S, Liu C-L, Yu R-Q, et al. MnO_2-nanosheet-modified upconversion nanosystem for sensitive turn-on fluorescence detection of H_2O_2 and glucose in blood. ACS Applied Materials & Interfaces. 2015;7(19):10548–55.
56. Liu J, Lu L, Li A, Tang J, Wang S, Xu S, et al. Simultaneous detection of hydrogen peroxide and glucose in human serum with upconversion luminescence. Biosensors and Bioelectronics. 2015;68:204–9.
57. Jia S, Wang J, Wang X, Liu X, Li S, Li Y, et al. Genetically encoded in situ gelation redox-responsive collagen-like protein hydrogel for accelerating diabetic wound healing. Biomaterials Science. 2023; 11(24):7748–58.
58. Li Y, Yang G, Gerstweiler L, Thang SH, Zhao CX. Design of stimuli-responsive peptides and proteins. Advanced Functional Materials. 2023;33(7):2210387.
59. Yu J, Zhang Y, Bomba H, Gu ZJ. Stimuli-responsive delivery of therapeutics for diabetes treatment. Bioengineering & Translational Medicine. 2016;1(3):323–37.

9 Stimuli-Responsive Biomaterials for Cardiovascular and Cerebrovascular Disorders (CCVDs)

Rajnish Srivastava, Naveen Singh, and Ankita Thakur
Chitkara School of Pharmacy, Chitkara University, Baddi, Himachal Pradesh, India

Amit Kumar Srivastava
Department of Biosciences and Bioengineering, Indian Institute of Technology, Roorkee, Uttarakhand, India

9.1 INTRODUCTION

9.1.1 Overview of Stimuli-Responsive Biomaterials

Biomaterials that respond to specific internal or external triggers are termed "stimuli-responsive" biomaterials or "smart" biomaterials and are generally considered advanced materials with the ability to change their physicochemical properties in response to specific stimuli. For complex diseases like cardiovascular and cerebrovascular disorders (CCVDs), conventional therapies often feel frustrated and cannot get to the target well. Biomaterials developed with the ability to respond to stimuli, such as pH, temperature, reactive oxygen species (ROS), or external inputs (light, ultrasound, and magnetic fields), can be developed to release therapeutic agents only at the site of disease, in a selective manner. These materials are versatile, and their applications include investigations in targeted drug delivery, tissue engineering, and regenerative medicine. Nanoparticle-based systems can be designed to respond to biochemical signals in atherosclerotic lesions, ischemic heart tissue, or inflamed cerebrovascular sites by releasing encapsulated agents such as anti-inflammatory drugs, genes, or peptides. Another prominent category of responsive biomaterials, hydrogels are engineered for controlled degradation and release and are set to respond to enzymatic activity or oxidative stress in damaged cardiac tissues to facilitate myocardial regeneration [1]. In the last few years, by bringing stimuli-responsive biomaterials to bioengineered tissues, we continue to expand our knowledge on refining their selectivity, biocompatibility, and efficacy to maximize therapeutic outcomes and minimize adverse effects. Stimuli-responsive biomaterials have transformative potential for CCVDs, as these early-stage therapeutic interventions provide a means for the treatment of CCVDs using precision medicine.

9.1.2 Importance in Cerebral and Cardiovascular Disorders

There is a huge importance for stimuli-responsive biomaterials to manage cerebral and cardiovascular disorders owing to their ability to adapt to specific pathological cues and generate fine therapeutic responses. CCVDs, including ischemic heart disease and stroke, are among the top causes of mortality worldwide. Due to short therapeutic windows and adverse effects such as hemorrhagic

DOI: 10.1201/9781003560203-9

transformation, the application of conventional treatments, such as thrombolytic therapies, is often restricted. To overcome these limitations, in response, stimuli-responsive biomaterials have been developed as a potential strategy to achieve rational and controllable therapeutic impact. Diseased tissues can be detected and respond to specific environmental changes in pH, ROS, enzyme activity, or external stimuli such as magnetic fields and light, and these "smart" biomaterials can release therapeutic agents or modify their structural properties precisely where and when needed. This is particularly important in CCVDs, where restoring blood flow and minimizing damage to brain or heart tissue are priorities. Using such responsive systems allows for increased therapeutic efficacy, decreased risk of off-target effects, and increased patient outcomes [2, 3].

9.1.3 Need for Stimuli-Responsive Biomaterials for CCVDs

Medical treatment of cerebral and cardiovascular disorders is unique because of the dynamic nature of these disorders and the limited effectiveness of traditional therapies in targeting diseased sites. Such biomaterials based on stimuli-responsive materials are a promising solution given that they can be engineered to release therapeutic agents in response to the internal cues present in the body, such as pH variations, oxidative stress, and enzyme activity, which are most commonly occurring at the disease site. This target approach may help control drug release, which in turn improves the therapeutic effects on the disease site with minimal impact on healthy tissues. In addition, pH-sensitive formulations are beneficial because of the acidic state of ischemic brain tissues or atherosclerotic-modified plaques, and antioxidant formulations are useful due to the oxidative stress accompanying these diseases. This selectivity enhances considerable ability to fine-tune the delivery and timing of drug release to respond to complex disease disorders of the cerebral and cardiovascular systems. The ability to incorporate such specific activating cues in stimuli-sensitive materials opens the way for innovation in treatment instruments that model the ever-changing biochemical milieu of these diseases [4]. The objectives of this chapter are to highlight and expand upon various cutting-edge stimuli-responsive biomaterials in hydrogels and nanoparticle applications for critical CCVDs. New developments in biomaterials for theranostics such as stimuli-responsive biomaterials are reviewed together with confidence in the betterment of CCVD patients.

9.2 CARDIOVASCULAR AND CEREBROVASCULAR DISORDERS (CCVDs) – GAPS AND PROSPECTS

Vascular diseases are conditions that affect the vascular system or blood vessels, arteries, and veins, which can lead to various conditions, including ischemic stroke (IS), carotid artery disease, pulmonary embolism, myocardial ischemia, and peripheral artery disease. These diseases affect the brain and heart and can cause increased mortality and morbidity rates around the world, including individuals in the cerebrovascular and cardiovascular diseases (CCVDs) categories [1]. Over the years, CCVDs have remained to be the leading causes of death worldwide according to the global burden of disease report. CCVDs are estimated to have caused 20.5 million deaths in 2021, which is almost one-third of total deaths all over the world. The United Nations has identified non-communicable diseases (NCDs), including CCVDs, as a foremost global health issue and has presented enormous strategies to lessen the effects of the disease in all parts of the world [5]. CCVDs have been recognized globally, with their risk factors including high-sugar and high-fat diets, smoking, obesity, no exercise, alcohol consumption, hypertension (HTN), diabetes, and hyperlipidemia. In fact, the majority of CCVDs can be prevented if people embrace healthier diets and engage in physical activities [6]. In general, the synthetic drugs and natural products that have been used for the treatment of several CCVDs are known to have drawbacks such as side effects, low selectivity, lesser bioavailability, and tolerance [7]. Though there have been some improvements in the management of CCVDs, there is still so much to be achieved. Diagnostic impairment at early stages, therapies that lack individualization, and problems with medicine administration hinder modern approaches [8]. The incomplete understanding of and inability to diagnose CCVD in its early stages or accurately in low-resource environments remains one of the biggest deficits in the disease's current management. The management of chronic disorders depends a lot on early identification to enhance early management to prevent severe stages. However, the instruments used in efficient screening, including imaging, blood biomarkers, and genetic testing, may be costly and demand special equipment. Low-income countries have less access to diagnostic and certain kinds of treatment, which are important factors in explaining mortality differences between the developed and the developing world [9].

CCVDs are also known to be determined by genetic factors, environmental factors, and lifestyle factors that vary significantly from one individual to another. Conventional method on the other hand takes an organized approach from one patient to another without considering that everybody may not respond to treatment in the same way, depending on disease etiology, metabolism, or response to therapy [10]. Though molecular and cellular pathology also implements the concept of personalized treatment depending on the patient's biological characteristics, the concept holds special promise as treatment could be targeted at specific pathways. However, this approach is still principally investigational and not widely practiced, mainly due to reasons such as high cost, absence of broadly established biomarkers for patient selection, and relatively low implementation in clinical practice [11]. Drug delivery in CCVDs is a major concern because the cardiovascular and cerebrovascular systems are integrated structures with multi-faceted functions. The systemic application of therapeutic agents is limited to low concentrations of the drug within the target tissues since traditional drug delivery systems are ineffective in providing optimal concentrations of the active agent. For instance, in treating cerebrovascular disorders, the blood–brain barrier (BBB) poses a major challenge, because it prevents the release of most therapeutic agents to the brain. Similarly, delivering drugs precisely to damaged heart tissue without affecting healthy tissues is challenging due to the dynamic and high-flow nature of the cardiovascular system [7, 12]. To address certain issues, including physiological barriers, off-target effects, low efficiency of drugs, and potentially undesirable side effects, different stimuli-sensitive biomaterials drug delivery systems have been developed [13]. Several "smart" strategies have been proposed to overcome the limitations of modern treatments in medicine and enhance the therapeutic effect. These strategies concern using biomaterials that can sense the biochemical changes in the diseased microenvironment and act in a prescribed manner. These "smart" biomaterials or stimuli-responsive materials may change one or several of their physicochemical characteristics or structures in response to stimuli. The inclusion of the various internal stimuli from the physiological microenvironment, including pH, redox potential, temperature, enzyme, and mechanical force, or some available, easily manipulated external stimuli such as light, ultrasound, electric, or magnetic, has resulted in highly controlled smart systems [14]. Stimuli-responsive biomaterials may help fill these gaps by enhancing the first-line treatment, targeting delivery, and personalizing treatments. However, current studies related to biomaterials also focus on issues such as accessibility, cost, and the ability to integrate with existing therapeutic procedures [13].

9.3 STIMULI-RESPONSIVE BIOMATERIALS FOR CEREBRAL DISORDERS

Cerebral disorders like stroke, neurodegenerative diseases such as Alzheimer's or Parkinson's, and traumatic brain injuries (TBIs) are chronic diseases with limited treatment options. These diseases are difficult to treat due to the BBB, which acts as a barrier by being selectively permeable. To overcome these barriers, stimuli-responsive biomaterials have been developed to deliver therapeutic agents more effectively to the brain (Figure 9.1). These biomaterials act as a specific response to specific internal or external stimuli, which makes it possible to achieve targeted drug delivery, controlled drug release, and interaction with the specific microenvironment of the brain [15].

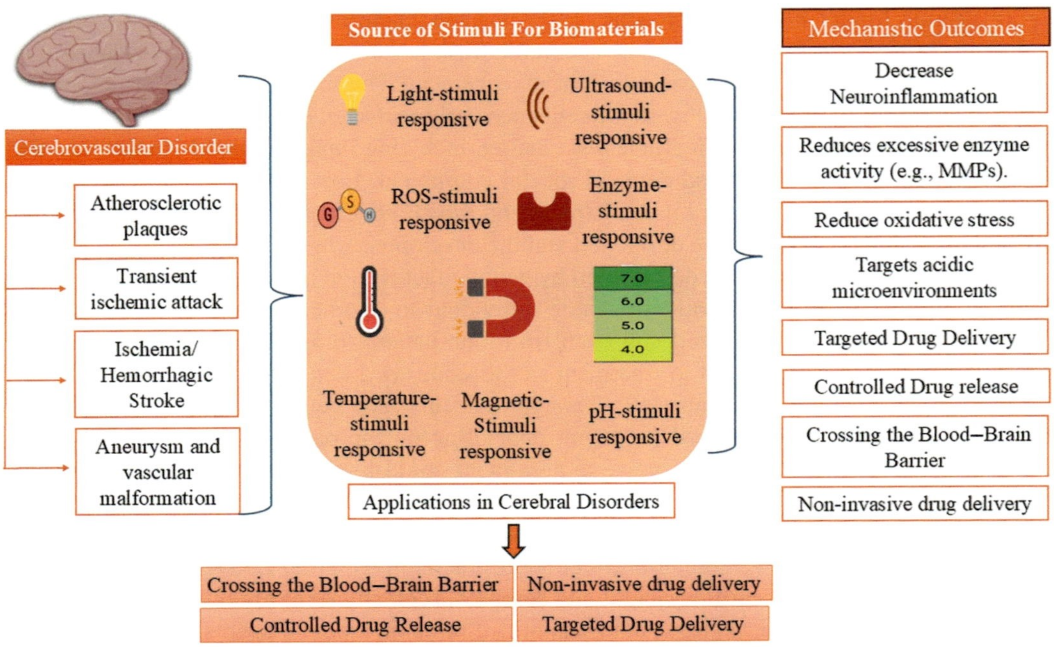

FIGURE 9.1 Role and application of stimuli-responsive biomaterials in cerebrovascular disorders.

9.3.1 Pathophysiology of Cerebral Disorders

Cerebrovascular disease is a medical condition that affects the blood vessels of the brain and cerebral circulation. Cerebrovascular disease can develop from various congenital or idiopathic causes (e.g., cerebral autosomal dominant arteriopathy, amyloid angiopathy, and fistulas). However, the most common cause is the formation of atherosclerotic plaques. These plaques, which consist of, among others, cholesterol, fats, calcium, and foam cells, accumulate in the blood vessels, resulting in the formation of clots or thrombi, subsequently leading to transient ischemic attack (TIA) and IS. Besides stroke and TIA, vascular malformations and aneurysms are two more conditions that affect the cerebrovascular unit. It comprises a variety of separate pathologies with various epidemiological and therapeutic characteristics, including stroke, TIA, aneurysm, and vascular malformation. Owing to its ability to alter blood vessel structure, high blood pressure (BP) or HTN has been considered a crucial contributing factor for developing or worsening cerebrovascular disorders. Notably, most of the diseases mentioned above share common characteristics (e.g., inflammation, hypoxia, oxidative stress, acidosis, and others) that are used as targets for developing stimuli-responsive biomaterials [16]. These biomaterials can "read" the microenvironmental alterations in the diseased tissue and respond in predetermined ways, helping mitigate, inhibit, and sometimes reverse the disease's symptoms [13]. The pathophysiology of cerebral disorders, particularly strokes, is primarily characterized by a disruption in blood flow to the brain, which leads to a cascade of damaging cellular and molecular events. Strokes are classified into two main types: ischemic and hemorrhagic, each with distinct mechanisms of injury. It is the most common form, accounting for about 85% of all stroke cases. It occurs when there is an insufficient supply of blood and oxygen to the brain. This can be caused by two main types of occlusions: thrombosis and embolism. In thrombosis, blood vessels narrow due to the buildup of atherosclerotic plaques, which eventually leads to clot formation and a blockage in the flow of blood. On the other hand, embolic strokes occur when an embolus (a clot or fat deposit) travels to the brain, obstructing blood flow and reducing oxygen delivery. This results in severe stress and untimely cell death (necrosis). Necrosis in brain tissue is followed by disruption of the plasma membrane, organelle swelling, and the leakage of cellular contents into the extracellular space, leading to further damage [17]. Other pathological events that have been implicated in the development of IS include inflammation, energy failure, increased calcium levels within the cell, acidosis, oxidative stress, excitotoxicity, and activation of glial cells. The disruption of the BBB and infiltration of leukocytes are also critical in increasing neuronal damage [18]. Hemorrhagic stroke, occurring in 10–15% of all strokes, results from bleeding in the brain. This type of stroke is often more deadly and is classified into two types: intracerebral hemorrhage (ICH) and subarachnoid hemorrhage (SAH). In ICH, there is bleeding into the parenchyma of the brain, thereby resulting in infarction through blood vessel rupture. Major causes of ICH include HTN, disruption of blood vessels, and complications relating to the use of anticoagulants or thrombolytic agents. SAH results from bleeding within the subarachnoid space caused by a head injury or a burst cerebral aneurysm. Blood clotting represents toxic effects in the vascular system and provokes a worsening of brain tissue condition and intracranial pressure. These two types of hemorrhagic stroke caused severe ventricular and cellular injury, making the later rehabilitation even more challenging [19]. In both ischemic and hemorrhagic strokes, the interruption of the balanced cerebral blood flow (CBF) leads to a variety of pathological processes such as inflammation, oxidative stress, and glial activation. All these processes lead to neuronal death and loss of function, which is the main characteristic feature of stroke-induced brain damage [18, 19]. The pathophysiology of cerebral injury following TBI unfolds in a two-stage cascade of cellular and metabolic disruptions. In the initial stage, direct tissue damage causes impaired CBF and metabolism, creating an "ischemia-like" state. This leads to anaerobic glycolysis, resulting in lactic acid accumulation, acidosis, increased membrane permeability, and subsequent edema formation. As anaerobic metabolism is insufficient to maintain cellular energy levels, ATP stores deplete, causing failure of energy-dependent ion pumps and exacerbating cellular dysfunction. In the second stage, terminal membrane depolarization occurs, accompanied by excessive release of excitatory neurotransmitters like glutamate and aspartate. This activates receptors such as NMDA (N-methyl-D-aspartate), AMPA (α-amino-3-hydroxy-5-methyl-4-isoxazolpropionate), and voltage-dependent Ca^{2+} and Na^{+} channels. The influx of calcium and sodium ions triggers catabolic intracellular processes, activating enzymes like lipid peroxidases, proteases, and phospholipases, which elevate the intracellular levels of free fatty acids and free radicals, leading to cellular damage. Additionally, the activation of caspases and endonucleases causes DNA fragmentation and inhibits DNA repair mechanisms. Together, these events result in the degradation of cellular and vascular membranes, ultimately leading to necrosis or programmed cell death (apoptosis), which contributes to the progressive damage seen in TBI [20] (Figure 9.1).

9.3.2 Types of Stimuli-Responsive Biomaterials in Cerebral Disorders

9.3.2.1 pH-Responsive Biomaterials

pH-sensitive materials are attractive drug delivery appliances because they can respond to minor pH changes at the tumor site, especially in cerebral conditions that have a more acidic environment than normal tissue. This pH difference allows the development of materials that transport medications to specific body sites, enhancing treatment results and decreasing side effects. Active polymers like carboxylic acid or amine are used to make these materials. These groups can be protonated and deprotonated by pH changes to affect the material's structure. Some of these materials contain acid-sensitive linkers like acetals or hydrazones that release the medication in the tumor tissues' acidic environment [21]. As an example, alginate, a biodegradable anionic copolymer with low toxicity, could be administered orally. Acidic environments cause polymer carboxylic acid groups to become –COOH and generate hydrogen bonding, which prevents swelling and limits drug release. Composite materials have been designed to improve the hydrogel's mechanical strength and prevent burst discharge. When calcium hydrogen phosphate is combined with alginate, hydrogen bonding boosts the hydrogel's mechanical strength and controls drug release [22]. For better response efficiency, pH-responsive fibers and nanoparticles are being used. Electrospun poly(styrene-co-maleic anhydride) and cellulose acetate composite fibers are strong and sensitive. These conditions cause carboxylic acid groups on the fibers to ionize, increasing their size and aqua absorption. Similar to pH-sensitive micro-/nanoparticles, their size swelling/shrinking depends on the surrounding pH. Polyaspartic acid-based nanoparticles can develop and rupture to disrupt lysosomal membranes in acidic circumstances, releasing encapsulated medicines and increasing therapeutic properties [23].

9.3.2.2 Reactive Oxygen Species (ROS)-Responsive Biomaterials

Targeting ROS high levels in ischemic brain tissue, these biomaterials are being considered for cerebrovascular disease treatment. These biomaterials improve and target drug release for oxidative stress illnesses like stroke and brain injury. Researchers have created sulfur, selenium, boric acid, and proline oligomer-containing ROS-responsive materials. These materials use ROS-induced scission, solubility changes that disintegrate carriers, and drug linker bond cleavage to control drug release [24]. For example, ROS accelerates the degradation of boronic esters, which increases therapeutic agent accumulation in the target tissue. In the presence of oxidizing agents, such as thioethers, some polymers convert hydrophilic to hydrophobic or vice versa, improving biocompatibility [25]. This characteristic helps build ROS-responsive nanocarriers, which improve medication delivery in ischemic zones. ROS-responsive biomaterials employ cerebrovascular diseases' oxidative stress to improve neuroprotective drug delivery and ischemic event outcomes.

9.3.2.3 Enzyme-Responsive Biomaterials

Nanoparticles are an enzyme-sensitive biomaterial with great potential for cerebrovascular disease medication delivery. Smart carriers can/should target increased proteases, phosphatases, and glycosidases in tumor or inflamed tissues to deliver drugs locally. Matrix metalloproteinases (MMPs), which are elevated in illnesses like myocardial infarction (MI), can target therapeutic delivery. Proteinases, or MMPs, overexpressed in sick brain tissue can release drugs from enzyme-sensitive carriers. These biomaterials can deliver site-specific drugs since they are sensitive to the enzyme concentration in wounded brain regions. Due to their high selectivity, particular substrate needs, and ability to act in mild circumstances (e.g., neutral pH and aqueous environments), enzymes can be useful triggers. It allows the development of regulated drug delivery systems at disease sites to reduce adverse effects and increase concentrations. However, several challenges remain regarding drug distribution to target tissues for activity. Some physical drug delivery systems have been evaluated in animal trials, but technological problems may limit their clinical use [26]. Therefore, enzyme-sensitive components in drug delivery systems can improve cerebrovascular disorder treatment outcomes by improving spatiotemporal drug release control.

9.3.2.4 Light-Responsive Biomaterials

Smart biomaterials that respond to light have been used to treat cerebrovascular problems and produce non-invasive drug delivery systems. These materials may also change conformation in response to UV, visible, or near-infrared (NIR) light. Photoisomerization, photodegradation of the polymer backbone, and photothermal action allow regulated medication release in sick brain tissue. An advantage of light-responsive systems is their localized medication administration and non-contact techniques, which allow for long-distance reaction. Photo-responsive hydrogels for encapsulating therapeutic agents and controlling their release on light exposure have been developed for treating damaged nerves and brains for cerebrovascular wound healing. Integrating chromophore molecules sensitive to different light sources enhances their applicability. UV light is employed because of its great energy, yet it damages tissue and penetrates shallowly. Thus, they are studying visible and near-infrared light as safer cancer treatments. Nanocarrier systems that release medications when exposed to visible or NIR light have superior tissue permeability and lower toxicity than other systems and may be beneficial for cardiovascular disease (CVD) treatment [27].

9.3.2.5 Magnetic-Responsive Biomaterials

Magnetic field-responsive smart materials may be applied in cerebrovascular diseases, including targeted medicine delivery and tissue engineering. Magnetic nanoparticles (MNPs) like Fe_3O_4 improve the mechanical and thermomechanical properties of bio-based polymers employed in the composite. Magnetic responsiveness allows controlled implantation and positioning inside the body using external magnetic fields to deliver medications directly to brain-sick areas. Polymers like hyperbranched polyurethane with Fe_3O_4 nanoparticles have improved shape memory performance when subjected to magnetic stimuli for usage in dynamic drug-delivering devices. Other experiments have combined MNPs with cobalt and copper ions to increase their functionalities. These composite materials feature magnetic field responsiveness and improved protein adsorption, which is important for medication delivery and tissue engineering. Collagen hydrogel with nickel beads can influence cellular response using mechanical cues and extracellular matrix (ECM) architecture [28]. Cerebrovascular diseases can be treated by coating MNPs with bio-based polymer or vice versa. Because these materials are pH sensitive, researchers can change therapeutic agent distribution, making treatment more effective and with fewer side effects.

9.3.2.6 Temperature-Responsive Biomaterials

Temperature-responsive polymers are efficient stimuli-responsive biomaterials for cerebral disorders. Polymers with a lower critical solution temperature (LCST) are hydrophilic and water-soluble. When the temperature exceeds the LCST, the polymers become hydrophobic and globular, causing substantial solubility fluctuations. This characteristic can release medications in inflammation and brain tumors with localized high temperatures. Polymers may produce micelles or self-organizing structures to encapsulate medicinal chemicals for cerebral diseases. When temperatures rise due to pathological processes or overheating, these structures may become unstable and release the entire drug deposit. The system could deliver therapeutic chemicals in response to disease-related cues using this technique. Several polymers have the upper critical solution temperatures (UCST) and can be utilized in systems that break down at high temperatures, the second technique to control drug release [29]. Copolymerization of the material that responds to physiological temperature fluctuations or external heat sources like infrared light or magnetic field oscillations may regulate the critical temperature. In conclusion, temperature-sensitive polymers can be designed to deliver drugs to cerebral disorders with temperature-sensitive release mechanisms that match pathological temperature changes.

9.3.2.7 Ultrasound-Responsive Biomaterials

Ultrasound drug delivery is novel, especially for brain diseases. Using standard physiotherapy equipment, ultrasound pulses can target tissue heating and generate bubble cavitation. This process enhances nanostructured drug carrier penetration into tissues and controls drug release. Ultrasound is focused and can reach deep into tissues to the exact spot, unlike other external stimulation. Most ultrasonic-mediated drug delivery has used polymeric micelles and layer-by-layer built structures that can be reversibly broken by acoustic cavitation. The frequency, power density, pulse duration, and pulse interval can be adjusted to maximize medication delivery, making the approach effective in therapeutic applications [28]. The enhanced permeability and retention (EPR) effect of ultrasound helps target micelle-entrapped medications to the tumor tissues, making it most useful in cancer treatment. The ultrasound is done after systemically administering the formulation to allow micelles to entrap in tumor tissue. This approach allows pulsatile drug administration and improves treatment efficiency through sonoporation, which increases cell membrane permeability and drug, micelle, and genetic material absorption [29].

9.3.3 Applications of Stimuli-Responsive Biomaterials in Cerebral Disorders

9.3.3.1 Targeted Drug Delivery in Neuroinflammation

Neuroinflammation, common after events like strokes and TBIs, can lead to additional damage in the brain if not controlled effectively. Stimuli-responsive biomaterials, especially pH-responsive nanoparticles, are engineered to release anti-inflammatory drugs specifically in inflamed brain areas, which tend to have a slightly more acidic environment than healthy tissue. This selective release is valuable for minimizing side effects, as it limits drug exposure to regions that need treatment, helping to control inflammation and preventing further neural damage [30]. Oxidative stress is a key factor in many neurodegenerative disorders, including Alzheimer's and Parkinson's diseases. Biomaterials that respond to ROS are being designed to release antioxidants at the site of oxidative stress. For example, nanoparticles carrying agents like N-acetylcysteine can respond directly to high ROS levels, providing neuroprotection where oxidative damage is high. This targeted approach reduces cell apoptosis and can slow the progression of neurodegeneration by protecting neurons from oxidative stress. Following a stroke, the brain's affected areas benefit from therapies promoting neuronal regeneration. Enzyme-sensitive hydrogels embedded with growth factors, such as brain-derived neurotrophic factors (BDNF) or vascular endothelial growth factor (VEGF), can foster neural repair. These hydrogels only release their therapeutic payload in the presence of enzymes produced by damaged brain tissue, encouraging cell growth and repair specifically where needed. This type of localized therapy is important in reducing complications and supporting brain recovery without affecting undamaged tissue [31].

For patients with TBI, long-term drug administration is often necessary to support recovery and minimize repeated drug delivery. Temperature-responsive or enzyme-sensitive biomaterials are useful for releasing therapeutic agents over extended periods. These biomaterials adjust their release based on body temperature or enzymatic activity, delivering neuroprotective or regenerative agents gradually, which supports sustained tissue repair, minimizes inflammation, and reduces the need for multiple interventions [32]. Magnetic-responsive biomaterials are particularly innovative for treating brain tumors, where crossing the BBB is a significant challenge. MNPs loaded with chemotherapeutic agents can be guided to the tumor site using external magnetic fields, enhancing drug concentration specifically at the tumor site. This technique minimizes systemic exposure to chemotherapeutics, reducing harmful side effects and improving efficacy. In recent studies, magnetic fields have successfully directed nanoparticles across the BBB and into brain tumors, showcasing a promising non-invasive strategy for targeted cancer therapy in the brain [33].

Neuromodulation treatments, like those for epilepsy or depression, often require precise control of neural stimulation. Emerging biomaterials that respond to electrical or magnetic stimuli can interface with neural tissues to either deliver drugs or modulate neuronal signals. For example, electrically responsive hydrogels and materials containing conductive polymers can respond to external electrical fields, releasing neurotransmitter-mimicking agents that influence neuron activity. Such applications open new avenues for managing epilepsy, chronic pain, or mood disorders through minimally invasive neural regulation [32]. The temperature-responsive materials are being explored to transiently open the BBB, allowing therapeutic agents to reach the brain more effectively. Mild, localized heating can enable BBB permeability, making it easier to deliver drugs directly to brain tissues. Thermosensitive hydrogels and liposomes respond to temperature changes by releasing their contents or changing their structure to improve drug diffusion, helping with conditions like brain tumors or neuroinfectious [31].

9.4 STIMULI-RESPONSIVE BIOMATERIALS FOR CARDIOVASCULAR DISORDERS

9.4.1 Pathophysiology of Cardiovascular Disorder

The process underlying CVDs, like atherosclerosis, Coronary artery disease (CAD), and HTN, involves multiple molecular and cellular signaling pathways and processes that lead to disease

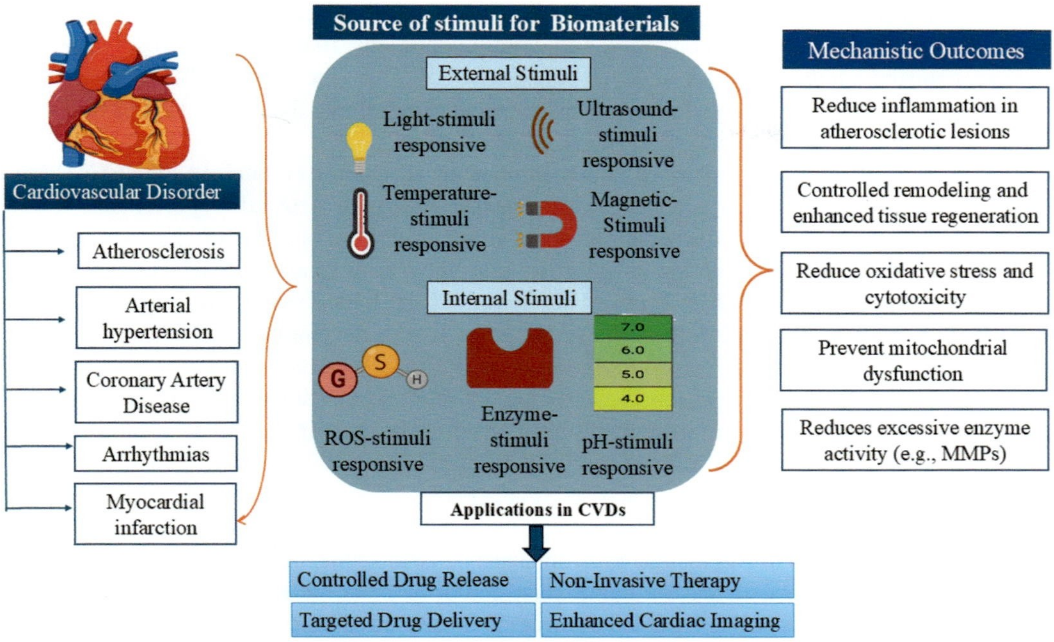

FIGURE 9.2 Role of stimuli-responsive biomaterials in cardiovascular disorders.

(Figure 9.2). Atherosclerosis has an essential role in the development and advancement of CVDs since it leads to the modification of arteries and vascular forms. It is characterized by the deposit of lipids, cholesterol, and other substances on the arterial walls, resulting in the formation of plaques called atherosclerosis. This plaque formation results in endothelial dysfunction, which is an important early feature of atherosclerosis [33]. When the endothelial cells are dysfunctional, they are unable to control the diameter of the blood vessels and to prevent clot formation, which has resulted in a reduction of nitric oxide (NO) and enhanced permeability for low-density lipoprotein (LDL) particles. The inflammatory response attracts other immune cells such as macrophages, which engulf oxidized LDL, change to foam cells, and accumulate to form fatty streaks [34]. Over time the plaques become complex with features of calcification and fibrosis that cause luminal narrowing and stenosis, which might lead to ischemic events such as MI or stroke. These plaques evolve and can destabilize, and when they rupture, they trigger thrombosis, which could lead to the blocking of the vessels, and this is very dangerous for life-threatening cardiovascular events. This complex process includes inflammatory mediators, oxidative stress, and genes that regulate lipid metabolism and immune responses that ultimately promote atherosclerosis progression. CAD is an important contributor to cardiovascular morbidity and mortality, which mainly arises from atherosclerotic lesions occurring in the coronary arteries and causing luminal stenosis. This reduces the amount of nutrients and oxygen supplied to the heart muscles and hence leads to conditions such as angina and MI (heart attack).

The pathophysiological process of CAD includes endothelial dysfunction, which means that endothelial cells – the inner lining of blood vessels – do not produce adequate amounts of NO, which is required for proper dilation of blood vessels and better inflammatory responses. High BP, high cholesterol levels, and smoking hinder the production of NO, which leads to atherosclerosis through plaque formation and narrowing of blood vessels [33, 35]. Chronic inflammation significantly contributes to CAD development, with immune cells entering the arterial walls, while ROS produced within the plaques harm cells, destabilizing plaques and worsening stenosis. In addition to reducing NO levels, oxidative stress produces an inflammatory environment suitable for plaque progression. These plaques over time become unstable, which may rupture and expose the inner vessel wall to the bloodstream and cause the formation of thrombi that may lead to blockage of the blood flow and result in acute coronary events such as heart attacks. Certain genetic traits, including polymorphism in LDL receptor genes, and certain conditions, like diet, smoking, and lack of exercise, contribute toward the risk of developing CAD [35]. Thus, these factors form a cascade of events from a multiple factorially driven process that tends to promote the progression of CAD and its related complications.

The MMPs are zinc-dependent enzymes implicated in tissue remodeling and ECM degradation that are involved in affecting blood vessel injury in arterial hypertension (AH). Overproduction of MMPs and decreased levels of tissue inhibitors of MMPs (TIMPs) cause the deterioration of endothelial function and fibrosis that may result in arterial stiffness and organ failure. High expression of MMP-2 and MMP-9 and TIMP-1 has been found in hypertensive patients, thus ascertaining the role of these enzymes in the development of the disease. For instance, MMP-2 processes the vasodilator adrenomedullin, which leads to increased BP, while MMP-9 has been linked to hypertensive-associated complications such as intracranial hemorrhage. Besides MMPs, there is immune system disruption as one of the most essential factors influencing AH [36].

The pro-inflammatory cytokines such as IL-6, TNF-a, and C-reactive protein (CRP) are increased in hypertensive patients, and CRP regulates endothelial dysfunction and HTN. Other cell types that also contribute to AH include macrophages, dendritic cells, and antigen-presenting cells whose effects are to either increase inflammation and/or activate the renin–angiotensin system. Moreover, oxidative stress is also regarded as an essential causative factor in AH due to ROS acting on the endothelium and leading to new vessel formation. NADPH oxidase (NOX), the major source of ROS in the vasculature, is overactivated in hypertensive disorders that promote oxidative stress and HTN. Consequently, MMPs, immune system activation, and oxidative stress are effective in the pathogenesis of AH; they might also be effective targets in the treatment of AH [37]. MMPs are zinc-dependent enzymes that play a significant role in tissue remodeling and ECM degradation, contributing to vascular damage in AH. An imbalance between MMPs and TIMPs exacerbates endothelial dysfunction and fibrosis, leading to complications such as arterial stiffness and organ failure. Elevated levels of MMP-2 and MMP-9, along with TIMP-1, are commonly observed in hypertensive patients, indicating their involvement in the progression of the disease. MMP-2, for instance, cleaves the vasodilator adrenomedullin, contributing to elevated BP, while MMP-9 is associated with hypertensive complications such as intracranial hemorrhage. In addition to MMPs, immune system dysregulation plays a critical role in AH [36].

Inflammatory markers like IL-6, TNF-α, and CRP are elevated in hypertensive individuals, with CRP contributing to endothelial dysfunction and increased BP. Immune cells, such as macrophages, dendritic cells, and antigen-presenting cells, further exacerbate AH by promoting inflammation and modulating the renin–angiotensin system. Furthermore, oxidative stress is a key factor in AH, with ROS damaging the endothelium and promoting vascular remodeling. NADPH oxidase (NOX), a major ROS source in the vasculature, is upregulated in hypertensive conditions, contributing to increased oxidative stress and BP elevation. Together, MMPs, immune system activation, and oxidative stress work synergistically in the pathogenesis of AH, highlighting their potential as therapeutic targets for managing the condition [37] (Figure 9.2).

9.4.2 Types of Biomaterials Used in Cardiovascular Disorders

Stimuli-responsive biomaterials for cardiovascular disorders refer to the types of biomaterials that are developed to respond to certain internal and external signals and are especially used to deliver controlled and localized therapy needed for heart tissue repair and in the management of CVDs. The types of stimuli-responsive biomaterials for cardiovascular disorders are specially designed to respond to specific internal and external triggers, allowing for controlled, localized therapeutic effects essential for heart tissue regeneration and disease management [38].

9.4.2.1 Temperature-Responsive Biomaterial

The temperature-responsive biomaterial commonly used is poly(N-isopropylacrylamide) or PNIPAAm. This material transitions around body temperature, and that makes it suitable for cardiac applications. For example, PNIPAAm can be grafted with single-walled carbon nanotubes (SWCNTs), subsequently forming a hydrogel with the ability to transport stem cells to an infarcted region and promote cell attachment/proliferation. The SWCNTs enhance the hydrogel's conductivity and biocompatibility to facilitate its incorporation into the cardiac tissue and support the survival of the cells within the hydrogel at the site of injury [39].

9.4.2.2 Light-Responsive Biomaterial

Collagen-polydopamine (Col-PDA)-based hydrogels are light-responsive biomaterials employed in cardiac tissue engineering. These hydrogels can regulate cardiomyocyte and neuron functions in response to light stimuli. The polydopamine component enables the hydrogel to change its mechanical properties when exposed to light and influences the cell function and proliferation [40]. This characteristic allows the Col-PDA hydrogels to provide accurate and specific cardiac repairs without having to undergo invasive procedures to promote myocardial regeneration.

9.4.2.2.1 Magnetic-Responsive Biomaterial

Smart magnetic hydrogels like chitosan–carbon nanotube (CH/CNT) contain magnetic particles like Fe_3O_4 for self-control of hydrogels. These hydrogels can be controlled using external magnetic fields to direct stem cells to the desired injury sites within the cardiac muscles and therefore increase the efficiency of stem cell therapy for cardiac tissue regeneration [38, 41]. Furthermore, the magnetic particles also improve the mechanical properties of the hydrogel in combination with cellular adhesion and mobility within the damaged heart tissue.

9.4.2.3 pH-Responsive Biomaterial

pH-sensitive hydrogels, such as poly(N-isopropyl-acrylamide)-butyl acrylate-propyl-acrylic acid (PNIPAAm-BA-PAA), respond to the changes in the pH of an infarcted myocardium. The structure of this hydrogel composite alters in response to acidic pH levels that are characteristic of the damaged cardiac tissue and releases encapsulated growth factors that stimulate angiogenesis and tissue repair. This eliminates the release of therapeutic agents in other areas within the body, leading to reduced side effects and furthering the regeneration process [42].

9.4.2.4 Enzyme-Responsive Biomaterial

MMP-responsive hydrogels, such as those composed of proline–leucine–glycine–leucine–alanine–glycine (PLGLAG) peptides, degrade in the presence of enzymes produced during MI. These hydrogels are activated in response to the increased levels of MMPs in the vicinity of cardiac injury and release incorporated therapeutic agents as a signal for cell proliferation and tissue repair. Such specificity renders MMP-responsive hydrogels useful for targeted cell therapy and reducing inflammation in the heart [43].

9.4.3 Applications of Stimuli-Responsive Biomaterials in Cardiovascular Disorders

9.4.3.1 Targeted Drug Delivery of Nanoparticles for Atherosclerosis

Stimuli-responsive biomaterials are proving to be potential therapeutic modalities in CVDs, especially in atherosclerosis. These materials include MNPs, light-responsive nanoparticles, and a pH-sensitive system that allows drug delivery to be initiated by distinct physiological conditions. MNPs, which are sensitive to magnetic fields, are employed for site-specific drug delivery and imaging of atherosclerotic plaques, while the possible cytotoxicity of MNPs is minimized with antioxidant approaches [1]. Light-responsive nanoparticles containing photodynamic agents induce cholesterol efflux from foam cells employing photodynamic therapy under the influence of NIR light. Moreover, pH-sensitive carriers, like cyclodextrin-based systems, have the capability to release the therapeutic agents, particularly in an acidic environment such as the inflamed regions, suitable for gene delivery and anti-inflammatory activity in atherosclerotic plaque [44].

9.4.3.2 Management of Inflammatory Responses and Ischemia-Reperfusion Injury

Inflammatory-responsive nanoparticles, including those targeting Toll-like receptor 4 (TLR4), can decrease the size of MI by alleviating inflammation. Likewise, the enzyme-sensitive nanocarriers, especially MMP-responsive nanoparticles, utilize the enzymes that are overexpressed in cardiac tissue remodeling to release encapsulated drugs at the injury site [45]. Stimuli-responsive biomaterials are also employed for the regulation of oxidative stress and ischemia-reperfusion (I/R) injury. ROS imbalance is the underlying cause of oxidative stress, which contributes to the development of heart diseases such as MI. At the physiological state, a low amount of ROS is involved in cardiac signaling, but at a high amount, ROS can disturb mitochondrial function, cell death, and tissue injury. Ischemia results in a profound reduction of tissue oxygen availability and a decline of ATP, creating an acidic milieu in MI, and reperfusion increases injury due to the generation of ROS. This oxidative burst leads to the activation of the mitochondrial permeability transition pore (MPTP), which thus enhances mitochondrial dysfunction and necrotic cell death. To overcome this damage, stimuli-responsive biomaterials including ROS-sensitive NPs can be used [46]. For example, poly(propylene sulfide) (PPS)-based nanoparticles that have been proven to switch solubility upon oxidation treatment can be applied for transporting ginsenoside Rg3 or celastrol. These agents have demonstrated anti-inflammatory and tissue-reparative effects in MI models [1].

9.4.3.3 Hydrogels for Cardiac Regeneration and Myocardial Infarction

Hydrogels are stimuli-responsive biomaterials that may help treat MI and other cardiac conditions, including remodeling and regeneration. In MI, left ventricular enlargement, fibrosis, hypertrophy, ventricular wall thinning, and heart failure occur. Stimuli-responsive hydrogels provide mechanical support, block proteases, and repair tissue through stem cells to reduce these effects. Sol–gel transition occurs at physiological temperature in hydrophilic polymer frameworks called thermoresponsive hydrogels. After MI, they can provide optimal mechanical support. A hydrogel called poly-N-isopropyl acrylamide-co-hydroxy ethyl methacrylate-methacrylate-polylactide (NIPAAm-co-HEMA-co-MAPLA) is injected into the myocardium and immediately solidifies to improve cardiac function. Ejection fraction, scar tissue development, and the renin–angiotensin system for heart regeneration are improved by these hydrogels. Encapsulated MMP-2 inhibitors in thermoresponsive hydrogels reduce ECM degradation, cardiac function, and fibrosis [47]. Stem cell or exosome-incorporated hydrogels such as iPS-CPCs and MSC-derived exosomes for cardiac tissue healing and neovascular creation are other discoveries. These hydrogels can alter cardiac morphology, reduce infarct size, and boost heart performance. For the infarcted zone, which has a lower pH than normal tissues, temperature and pH-responsive hydrogels have been produced. These hydrogels distribute and retain cells, facilitating differentiation and cardiac tissue remodeling. Stimuli-responsive hydrogels are a unique cardiotoxicity treatment because they increase myocardial structural support, prevent unfavorable remodeling processes, and stimulate regeneration to treat diseases of the heart [48].

9.4.3.4 Enhanced Imaging for Cardiovascular Disease Diagnosis

Imaging methods for CVDs such as atherosclerosis and IS use stimuli-responsive materials because these diseases are often asymptomatic and slow-progressing; early diagnosis is crucial. Stimuli-responsive imaging targets foam cell lipid droplets (LDs) and ROS for atherosclerosis. LDs and hypochlorous acid (HClO), an inflammatory marker, are targeted and responded to by the three-in-one fluorescence probe iSHERLOCK to detect atherosclerotic plaques. Using the probe, LDs increased fluorescence intensity, while HClO caused further alterations [4]. This dual-targeting technology showed that atherosclerotic plaques may be scanned in vivo for disease detection. Altering pH and ROS levels can be used to create imaging biomaterials for IS caused by atherosclerosis. Ischemia detection can use pH-sensitive materials like Fe_3O_4 micelles since ischemic tissues have a pH between 5.9 and 6.9. In mice injected with these micelles, magnetic resonance imaging (MRI) signals in the ischemic region were significantly reduced, demonstrating their use in pH-sensitive cerebral ischemia imaging [49]. Due to their tailored drug release, high lesion conjugation, and good bioavailability, stimuli-responsive nanoparticles have garnered attention in CVD theranostics, especially in atherosclerosis. These nanomaterials and imaging technologies can detect disease progression and medication targeting and accumulation, enhancing diagnostic and therapeutic efficiency [50]. Since real-time imaging can be used to evaluate biomarkers, LDs, ROS, and pH changes associated with diseases like atherosclerosis and IS, stimuli-responsive nanomaterials can improve CVD diagnosis and tracking [51].

9.5 DIAGNOSTIC AND IMAGING PLATFORMS USING STIMULI-RESPONSIVE BIOMATERIALS FOR CCVD

9.5.1 Diagnostic Technique and Imaging Platforms Using Stimuli-Responsive Biomaterials for Cardiac Vascular Disorders

9.5.1.1 Electrocardiography (ECG)

A non-invasive test, this diagnostic procedure maps the electrical activity of the heart through what has been attached to the skin. Biomaterials play a significant role in electrocardiography (ECG) by enabling accurate detection and monitoring of cardiovascular disorders. Conductive polymers, hydrogels, and graphene-based materials are mostly used for their flexibility and biocompatibility. These biomaterials improve the performance by minimizing the skin-electrode resistance and enhancing signal quality.

9.5.1.2 Echocardiography

This diagnostic method uses very short-wave sound waves (ultrasound) to create images of the heart at work. Biomaterial in echocardiography enhances the imaging and diagnosis of heart disorders. The biomaterial used in this technique is piezoelectric ceramics like lead zirconate titanate (PZT) for ultrasound transducers. These biomaterials provide high sensitivity and resolution for real-time imaging of heart structure and functions. Doppler echocardiography provides additional diagnostic information, particularly regarding the valvular disorders or structural abnormalities of the heart, including congenital heart disease or cardiomyopathies, and transesophageal echocardiography [52].

9.5.1.3 Cardiac Magnetic Resonance Imaging (MRI)

It is an advanced form of imaging that combines a strong magnetic field and radio waves to produce exquisitely clear images of the heart and adjacent structures. MRI of the heart offers almost full characterization of the myocardial tissue and blood flow and is very useful in the diagnosis of cardiomyopathies, myocardial viability, and congenital heart diseases. MRI with contrast agents can also be used in the detection of areas of fibrosis, infarction, or inflammation. Biomaterials like gadolinium-based contrast agents are commonly employed to enhance image quality and provide detailed tissue differentiation in cardiac MRI [53].

9.5.1.4 CT Coronary Angiography

This non-invasive test is a combination of the computed tomography (CT) scan and an injection with a contrast agent in the form of iodine. CT coronary angiography especially utilizes iodinated contrast agents for the visualization of coronary artery disease. It also offers CT for coronary artery calcium scoring, which speaks to the extent of atherosclerosis and so can assist in risk differentiation for further Cardiovascular incidents. These biomaterials aim to improve image quality while minimizing toxicity [54].

9.5.1.5 Nuclear Cardiology Tests

Myocardial perfusion imaging (MPI), positron emission tomography (PET) scans, and others are based on the injection of a small amount of radioactive material in the body, and their actions are directed to the investigation of the blood supply to the cardiac muscles. MPI, as part of stress and rest, in some cases can demonstrate zones of low perfusion that may mean ischemia. These tests are useful in determining the status of the myocardium, including viability, and are crucial for individuals with risk factors or documented. These tests, such as single-photon emission CT (SPECT) and PET, use radiotracers like Technetium-99m (Tc-99m) and Thallium-201. Biomaterials such as radiolabeled nanoparticles or contrast agents enhance image resolution and enable precise detection of cardiac conditions [55]. All diagnostic techniques and imaging platforms using stimulus-responsive biomaterials for cardiac vascular disorders are shown in Table 9.1.

TABLE 9.1
Diagnostic Technique and Imaging Platforms Using Stimuli-Responsive Biomaterials for Cardiac Vascular Disorders

Diagnostic/Imaging Technique	Type of Biomaterial	Stimuli-Responsiveness	Mechanism
Optical coherence tomography (OCT)	Polymer-based imaging agents	Photo-responsive	High-resolution visualization of coronary artery plaques and microstructure for precise diagnosis
Photoacoustic imaging (PAI)	Nanoparticles	Light-responsive	Combines laser-induced ultrasound for molecular imaging, enabling detection of blood flow dynamics and oxygenation
Fluorescence imaging (FLI)	Fluorescent nanodots	Molecular-targeting fluorescent properties	Allows real-time visualization of molecular markers like inflammation and fibrosis in cardiac tissues
Electrocardiography (ECG)	Conductive polymers	Conductivity-sensitive	Detects electrical activity changes in the heart, essential for arrhythmia or myocardial infarction diagnosis
Echocardiography	Ultrasound-responsive contrast agents	Pressure-sensitive	Enhances imaging of cardiac structure and blood flow in real time, aiding in valve and chamber evaluations
Cardiac magnetic resonance imaging (CMR)	Gadolinium-based agents	Magnetic field-responsive	Provides soft tissue contrast and functional analysis of myocardial health
Intravascular imaging (IVUS/OCT combo)	Lipid-sensitive optical probes	Lipid-responsive	High-resolution detection of atherosclerotic plaques with lipid profiling capabilities
Density-based spatial clustering imaging	Hybrid nanoparticles	Enzyme-responsive	Identifies and clusters cardiovascular anomalies based on tissue density and enzymatic activity
Afterglow imaging	Rare-earth-doped particles	Light/oxygen-responsive	Tracks oxygenation in ischemic tissues for advanced cardiovascular imaging

9.5.2 Diagnostic Technique and Imaging Platforms Using Stimuli-Responsive Biomaterials for Cerebral Vascular Disorders

9.5.2.1 Computed Tomography (CT)

CT is commonly the first imaging modality to be requested in cerebrovascular emergencies such as stroke. High-speed imaging allows the recognition of acute hemorrhages, calcifications, and large pathological formations. For example, gold nanoparticles containing scans are favored for CT scans due to the high atomic number of gold, enhancing the scan contrast. These biomaterials assist in enhanced documentation of tissues, facilitating enhanced determination of diseases. However, CT has limited ability to detect minor abnormalities of the white matter and the early signs of ischemic changes seen in CSVD, as seen with MRI.

9.5.2.2 Magnetic Resonance Imaging (MRI)

MRI is more elaborate than CT in CSVD. MRI scans such as FLAIR and T2 are applied to determine WMH, which indicates small vessel disease. Microbleeds are small, old hemorrhages that are markers of CSVD and are well depicted by using susceptibility-weighted imaging (SWI). In this MNPs like iron oxide (Fe_3O_4) enhance image resolution by selective localization in tissues and the desired region of the disease. These nanoparticles, sensitive to magnetic field interaction, are applied in accurate imaging modalities in CCVDs.

9.5.2.3 Fazekas Scale

The Fazekas scale is a widely applied MRI grading scale for WMH, with four levels, from 0 to 3, with correspondingly increasing severity. This scale assists in determining the level of white matter changes related to the severity of CSVD and the probability of disability and stroke [1].

9.5.2.4 Positron Emission Tomography (PET)

Molecular imaging technology PET tracks biomolecular processes such as metabolism and receptor activity in vivo. This requires biomaterials to provide improved sensitivity and specificity. To improve targeting and the resolution of PET imaging, nanomaterials are being developed as tracers. For example, metallic nanoparticles can be functionalized to bind specifically to tumor markers.

9.5.2.5 Ultrasound Imaging

A focused ultrasound treatment for targeted delivery beyond the BBB has been designed using biomaterials such as silica-coated gold nanorods. Cai and colleagues showed that these nanoparticles can improve the resolution and contrast of ultrasound imaging without disrupting tissue significantly.

9.5.2.6 Raman Imaging

They frequently use gold-based nanoparticles that exhibit surface-enhanced Raman scattering (SERS). The Raman signal is significantly enhanced by these biomaterials, allowing the imaging of molecular structures in brain tissue [56].

9.5.2.7 Photoacoustic Imaging

Nanoparticles such as silica-coated gold nanorods are used as contrast agents in photoacoustic imaging, which is an optical and ultrasound combined modality. Responding to one of many wavelengths of light, these materials enhance penetration depth and signal contrast.

9.5.2.8 Fluorescence Imaging

Fluorescence imaging uses fluorescent probes, including carbon-based nanomaterials and lanthanide-doped particles. The signal intensity and photobleaching of these materials are high enough for creating brain structures and pathologies. NIR fluorescent probes are particularly valuable in that they penetrate deep tissue and are free of much background noise (Table 9.2) [57].

TABLE 9.2
Diagnostic Technique and Imaging Platforms Using Stimuli-Responsive Biomaterials for Cerebrovascular Disorders

Diagnostic/Imaging Technique	Biomaterial	Nature of Biomaterial	MOA
MRI (magnetic resonance imaging)	Iron oxide nanoparticles	Magnetic nanoparticles	Used for imaging due to their magnetic properties which enhance contrast in MRI scans
PET (positron emission tomography)	Gold nanoparticles	Metallic nanoparticles	Serve as contrast agents for PET scans by targeting specific molecules and providing enhanced imaging resolution
CT (computed tomography)	Bismuth sulfide nanoparticles	Metallic nanoparticles	Enhanced contrast in CT scans due to their high atomic number, allowing better visualization of blood vessels and brain tissue
Ultrasound imaging	Perfluoropentane nanoparticles	Gas-filled nanoparticles	Used in ultrasound imaging due to their ability to form microbubbles under ultrasound stimulation, enhancing image contrast
Optical imaging	Quantum dots	Semiconductor nanoparticles	Provide high-resolution imaging due to their unique optical properties such as fluorescence
Photoacoustic imaging	Gold nanorods	Metallic nanoparticles	Convert absorbed light into heat, producing ultrasound waves that can be detected for imaging
Fluorescence imaging	Carbon dots	Carbon-based nanoparticles	Used for their strong fluorescence properties, allowing for detailed imaging of cellular
Raman imaging	Gold-silver alloy nanoparticles	Metallic nanoparticles	Enhance Raman scattering signals, providing detailed molecular information
Theranostic imaging (combines therapy and diagnosis)	Polymeric micelles loaded with drugs	Polymeric nanoparticles	Deliver therapeutic agents to targeted sites while simultaneously providing imaging capabilities

9.6 CHALLENGES AND LIMITATIONS

Stimuli-responsive nanotherapeutics for cerebrovascular and CVDs face major challenges in clinical translation. Advantageously small, their interaction with biological fluids and components like blood proteins and macrophages makes them susceptible to RES clearance. Because nanoparticles can enter the brain but flee, they cannot treat the disease target site, causing bioavailability issues. Several techniques to increase retention and reduce peripheral side effects, including ligand targeting and stimuli-addicted activation. Another drawback is cytotoxicity. The development is challenging since each nanoparticle type needs in vitro and in vivo testing to identify safe application conditions. Industrial manufacturing scale-up barriers modify particle size, drug encapsulation, and stability, periodically compromising therapeutic efficacy. Organic solvents for nanoparticle production may generate environmental waste, making lab-to-industry translation difficult. Regulations for nanomedicines are not specific enough to encompass future nanomedicines [4, 45].

9.7 FUTURE PERSPECTIVES

Targeted drug delivery and minimizing side effects represent the future of stimuli-responsive biomaterials for treating CCVDs. Researchers are trying to refine these materials so they will respond to particular pathological signals, such as ROS levels, pH, and enzymatic activity, thereby maximizing therapeutic efficacy while avoiding unnecessary damage to healthy cells. For example, leading to an endogenous drug release at the injury site by stimulus, e.g., thrombin and ROS within ischemic regions, improves drug precision and diminishes the need for high doses. Other attractive means of controlling drug release that do not require an invasive procedure are exogenous triggers such as magnetic fields and ultrasound. However, there are still important issues that need to be addressed concerning biocompatibility and safety questions for clinical application. Potential future work may entail the synthesis of hybrid structures that contain both organic and inorganic nanomaterials to obtain desired release profiles. Lastly, complicated nanomedicines will also have to pass through all phases of clinical trials to understand exactly how they affect the body in the long run and the possible complications they have for those taking the nanomedicine before they become an essential part of nanotherapeutic management.

9.8 CONCLUSION

Responsive hydrogels can be considered innovative platforms to manage CCVD challenges due to their capacity to respond to stimuli. These materials offer specific therapeutic or diagnostic answers employing depolarization, pH shift, oxidative stress, enzyme activity, light activation, or magnetic field sensitivity. Their accuracy makes it possible to deliver drugs and regenerative agents at the required rate and without side effects, as opposed to regular treatments. Some of the recent advancements include hydrogels for myocardial regeneration, nanoparticles for BBB targeting, and enzyme-responsive carriers for site-directed delivery. Although these materials possess great possibilities, some problems emerge when translating them into clinical use. Some problems used in the synthesis and preparation of scaffolds can be solved, but some pertinent questions are still out of control, including biocompatibility, large-scale production, and long-term biological safety. The development of hybrid biomaterials that combine both natural and synthetic parts should be a topic for further investigation. Also, the development of individualized medicine and theranostic approaches will probably increase their involvement in the differentiated treatment of CCVDs.

Declaration of AI and AI-Assisted technologies

During the preparation of this work, the authors used QuillBot AI in order to paraphrase the sentences. After using this tool, the authors reviewed and edited the content as needed and take full responsibility for the content of the publication.

REFERENCES

1. Tapeinos C, Gao H, Bauleth-Ramos T, Santos HA. Progress in stimuli-responsive biomaterials for treating cardiovascular and cerebrovascular diseases. Small. 2022 Sep;18(36):2200291.
2. Gelmi A, Schutt CE. Stimuli-responsive biomaterials: Scaffolds for stem cell control. Advanced Healthcare Materials. 2021 Jan;10(1):2001125.
3. Cicha I, Singh R, Garlichs CD, Alexiou C. Nano-biomaterials for cardiovascular applications: Clinical perspective. Journal of Controlled Release. 2016 May 10;229:23–36.
4. Chen X, Wu D, Chen Z. Biomedical applications of stimuli-responsive nanomaterials. MedComm. 2024 Aug;5(8):e643.
5. Di Cesare M, Perel P, Taylor S, Kabudula C, Bixby H, Gaziano TA, McGhie DV, Mwangi J, Pervan B, Narula J, Pineiro D. The heart of the world. Global Heart. 2024;19(1).
6. Song Y, Chen C, Li W. Ginsenoside Rb1 in cardiovascular and cerebrovascular diseases: A review of therapeutic potentials and molecular mechanisms. Chinese Herbal Medicines. 2024 Sep 16;16(4):489–504.
7. Iravani S, Varma RS. Advanced drug delivery micro-and nanosystems for cardiovascular diseases. Molecules. 2022 Sep 9;27(18):5843.
8. Benjamin EJ, Muntner P, Alonso A, Bittencourt MS, Callaway CW, Carson AP, Chamberlain AM, Chang AR, Cheng S, Das SR, Delling FN. Heart disease and stroke statistics—2019 update: A report from the American Heart Association. Circulation. 2019 Mar 5;139(10):e56–28.

9. Timmis A, Vardas P, Townsend N, Torbica A, Katus H, De Smedt D, Gale CP, Maggioni AP, Petersen SE, Huculeci R, Kazakiewicz D. European Society of Cardiology: Cardiovascular disease statistics 2021. European Heart Journal. 2022 Feb 21;43(8):716–99.
10. Sheikhy A, Fallahzadeh A, Aghaei Meybodi HR, Hasanzad M, Tajdini M, Hosseini K. Personalized medicine in cardiovascular disease: Review of literature. Journal of Diabetes & Metabolic Disorders. 2021 Dec;20(2):1793–805.
11. Lee MS, Flammer AJ, Lerman LO, Lerman A. Personalized medicine in cardiovascular diseases. Korean Circulation Journal. 2012 Sep 1;42(9):583–91.
12. Pardridge WM. Drug transport across the blood–brain barrier. Journal of Cerebral Blood Flow & Metabolism. 2012 Nov;32(11):1959–72.
13. Omidian H, Babanejad N, Cubeddu LX. Nanosystems in cardiovascular medicine: Advancements, applications, and future perspectives. Pharmaceutics. 2023 Jul 12;15(7):1935.
14. Badeau BA, DeForest CA. Programming stimuli-responsive behavior into biomaterials. Annual Review of Biomedical Engineering. 2019 Jun 4;21(1):241–65.
15. Anoop V, Cutinho LI, Mourya P, Maxwell A, Thomas G, Rajput BS. Approaches for encephalic drug delivery using nanomaterials: The current status. Brain Research Bulletin. 2020 Feb 1;155:184–90.
16. Salaudeen MA, Bello N, Danraka RN, Ammani ML. Understanding the pathophysiology of ischemic stroke: The basis of current therapies and opportunity for new ones. Biomolecules. 2024 Mar 4;14(3):305.
17. Woodruff TM, Thundyil J, Tang SC, Sobey CG, Taylor SM, Arumugam TV. Pathophysiology, treatment, and animal and cellular models of human ischemic stroke. Molecular Neurodegeneration. 2011 Dec;6:1–9.
18. Kuriakose D, Xiao Z. Pathophysiology and treatment of stroke: Present status and future perspectives. International Journal of Molecular Sciences. 2020 Oct 15;21(20):7609.
19. Testai FD, Aiyagari V. Acute hemorrhagic stroke pathophysiology and medical interventions: Blood pressure control, management of anticoagulant-associated brain hemorrhage and general management principles. Neurologic Clinics. 2008 Nov 1;26(4):963–85.
20. Werner C, Engelhard K. Pathophysiology of traumatic brain injury. British Journal of Anaesthesia. 2007 Jul 1;99(1):4–9.
21. Chu S, Shi X, Tian Y, Gao F. pH-responsive polymer nanomaterials for tumor therapy. Frontiers in Oncology. 2022 Mar 22;12:855019.
22. Ding H, Tan P, Fu S, Tian X, Zhang H, Ma X, Gu Z, Luo K. Preparation and application of pH-responsive drug delivery systems. Journal of Controlled Release. 2022 Aug 1;348:206–38.
23. Cui W, Qi M, Li X, Huang S, Zhou S, Weng J. Electrospun fibers of acid-labile biodegradable polymers with acetal groups as potential drug carriers. International Journal of Pharmaceutics. 2008 Sep 1;361(1–2):47–55.
24. Wu F, Zhang Z, Ma S, He Y, He Y, Ma L, Lei N, Deng W, Wang F. Microenvironment-responsive nanosystems for ischemic stroke therapy. Theranostics. 2024;14(14):5571.
25. Liu Y, Liu Y, Zang J, Abdullah AA, Li Y, Dong H. Design strategies and applications of ROS-responsive phenylborate ester-based nanomedicine. ACS Biomaterials Science & Engineering. 2020 Nov 17;6(12):6510–27.
26. Li M, Zhao G, Su WK, Shuai Q. Enzyme-responsive nanoparticles for anti-tumor drug delivery. Frontiers in Chemistry. 2020 Jul 30;8:647.
27. Ma W, Hua D, Xiong R, Huang C. Bio-based stimuli-responsive materials for biomedical applications. Materials Advances. 2023;4(2):458–75.
28. Pham SH, Choi Y, Choi J. Stimuli-responsive nanomaterials for application in antitumor therapy and drug delivery. Pharmaceutics. 2020 Jul 4;12(7):630.
29. Zhan Y, Dai Y, Ding Z, Lu M, He Z, Chen Z, Liu Y, Li Z, Cheng G, Peng S, Liu Y. Application of stimuli-responsive nanomedicines for the treatment of ischemic stroke. Frontiers in Bioengineering and Biotechnology. 2024 Feb 2;11:1329959.
30. Fan L, Jin L, Tang T, Zheng Y, Chen Z, Lin H, Ding C, Wang T, Chen H, Guo Y, Xu C. Neutrophil-like pH-responsive pro-efferocytic nanoparticles improve neurological recovery by promoting erythrophagocytosis after intracerebral hemorrhage. Theranostics. 2024;14(1):283.
31. Xie B, Xie H. Application of stimuli-responsive hydrogel in brain disease treatment. Frontiers in Bioengineering and Biotechnology. 2024 Jul 18;12:1450267.
32. Li X, Duan L, Kong M, Wen X, Guan F, Ma S. Applications and mechanisms of stimuli-responsive hydrogels in traumatic brain injury. Gels. 2022 Aug 1;8(8):482.
33. Frąk W, Wojtasińska A, Lisińska W, Młynarska E, Franczyk B, Rysz J. Pathophysiology of cardiovascular diseases: New insights into molecular mechanisms of atherosclerosis, arterial hypertension, and coronary artery disease. Biomedicines. 2022 Aug 10;10(8):1938.

34. Mussbacher M, Schossleitner K, Kral-Pointner JB, Salzmann M, Schrammel A, Schmid JA. More than just a monolayer: The multifaceted role of endothelial cells in the pathophysiology of atherosclerosis. Current Atherosclerosis Reports. 2022 Jun;24(6):483–92.
35. Mourouzis K, Siasos G, Oikonomou E, Zaromitidou M, Tsigkou V, Antonopoulos A, Bletsa E, Stampouloglou P, Vlasis K, Vavuranakis M, Tousoulis D. Lipoprotein-associated phospholipase A2 levels, endothelial dysfunction and arterial stiffness in patients with stable coronary artery disease. Lipids in Health and Disease. 2021 Dec;20:1–9.
36. Bisogni V, Cerasari A, Pucci G, Vaudo G. Matrix metalloproteinases and hypertension-mediated organ damage: Current insights. Integrated Blood Pressure Control. 2020 Nov; 2:157–69.
37. Mirhafez SR, Mohebati M, Disfani MF, Karimian MS, Ebrahimi M, Avan A, Eslami S, Pasdar A, Rooki H, Esmaeili H, Ferns GA. An imbalance in serum concentrations of inflammatory and anti-inflammatory cytokines in hypertension. Journal of the American Society of Hypertension. 2014 Sep 1;8(9):614–23.
38. El-Husseiny HM, Mady EA, El-Dakroury WA, Doghish AS, Tanaka R. Stimuli-responsive hydrogels: Smart state of-the-art platforms for cardiac tissue engineering. Frontiers in Bioengineering and Biotechnology. 2023 Jun 28;11:1174075.
39. Li X, Zhou J, Liu Z, Chen J, Lü S, Sun H, Li J, Lin Q, Yang B, Duan C, Xing MM. A PNIPAAm-based thermosensitive hydrogel containing SWCNTs for stem cell transplantation in myocardial repair. Biomaterials. 2014 Jul 1;35(22):5679–88.
40. Gholami Derami H, Gupta P, Weng KC, Seth A, Gupta R, Silva JR, Raman B, Singamaneni S. Reversible photothermal modulation of the electrical activity of excitable cells using polydopamine nanoparticles. Advanced Materials. 2021 Aug;33(32):2008809.
41. Martins AM, Eng G, Caridade SG, Mano JF, Reis RL, Vunjak-Novakovic G. Electrically conductive chitosan/carbon scaffolds for cardiac tissue engineering. Biomacromolecules. 2014 Feb 10;15(2):635–43.
42. Garbern JC, Minami E, Stayton PS, Murry CE. Delivery of basic fibroblast growth factor with a pH-responsive, injectable hydrogel to improve angiogenesis in infarcted myocardium. Biomaterials. 2011 Mar 1;32(9):2407–16.
43. Carlini AS, Gaetani R, Braden RL, Luo C, Christman KL, Gianneschi NC. Enzyme-responsive progelator cyclic peptides for minimally invasive delivery to the heart post-myocardial infarction. Nature Communications. 2019 Apr 15;10(1):1735.
44. Wang S, Fontana F, Shahbazi MA, Santos HA. Acetalated dextran-based nano-and microparticles: Synthesis, fabrication, and therapeutic applications. Chemical Communications. 2021;57(35):4212–29.
45. Battistella C, Liang Y, Gianneschi NC. Innovations in disease state responsive soft materials for targeting extracellular stimuli associated with cancer, cardiovascular disease, diabetes, and beyond. Advanced Materials. 2021 Nov;33(46):2007504.
46. Peoples JN, Saraf A, Ghazal N, Pham TT, Kwong JQ. Mitochondrial dysfunction and oxidative stress in heart disease. Experimental & Molecular Medicine. 2019 Dec;51(12):1–3.
47. Matsumura Y, Zhu Y, Jiang H, D'Amore A, Luketich SK, Charwat V, Yoshizumi T, Sato H, Yang B, Uchibori T, Healy KE. Intramyocardial injection of a fully synthetic hydrogel attenuates left ventricular remodeling post myocardial infarction. Biomaterials. 2019 Oct 1;217:119289.
48. Xu B, Li Y, Deng B, Liu X, Wang L, Zhu QL. Chitosan hydrogel improves mesenchymal stem cell transplant survival and cardiac function following myocardial infarction in rats. Experimental and Therapeutic Medicine. 2017 Feb;13(2):588–94.
49. Yang HY, Jang MS, Gao GH, Lee JH, Lee DS. pH-responsive biodegradable polymeric micelles with anchors to interface magnetic nanoparticles for MR imaging in detection of cerebral ischemic area. Nanoscale. 2016;8(25):12588–98.
50. Wang J, Lu B, Yin G, Liu L, Yang P, Huang N, Zhao A. Design and fabrication of environmentally responsive nanoparticles for the diagnosis and treatment of atherosclerosis. ACS Biomaterials Science & Engineering. 2024 Feb 12;10(3):1190–206.
51. Setia A, Mehata AK, Priya V, Pawde DM, Jain D, Mahto SK, Muthu MS. Current advances in nanotheranostics for molecular imaging and therapy of cardiovascular disorders. Molecular Pharmaceutics. 2023 Sep 12;20(10):4922–41.
52. Venkatesh C, Prasad BV, Khan M, Babu JC, Dasu MV. An automatic diagnostic model for the detection and classification of cardiovascular diseases based on swarm intelligence technique. Heliyon. 2024 Feb 15;10(3).
53. Liu Y, Zhang N. Gadolinium loaded nanoparticles in theranostic magnetic resonance imaging. Biomaterials. 2012 Jul 1;33(21):5363–75.

54. Liu G, Gu Y, Sollini M, Lazar A, Besson FL, Li S, Wu Z, Nardo L, Al-Ibraheem A, Zheng J, Kulkarni HR. Expert consensus on workflow of PET/CT with long axial field-of-view. European Journal of Nuclear Medicine and Molecular Imaging. 2024 Nov 9;52(3);1038–49.
55. Derdeyn CP, Powers WJ. Single-photon emission computed tomography (SPECT) and positron emission tomography (PET). In Transient Ischemic Attacks. 2004 Jan 1:137–61. https://doi.org/10.1002/9780470988442.ch6
56. Du W, Zhou L, Zhang Q, Liu X, Wei X, Li Y. Inorganic nanomaterials for biomedical imaging of brain diseases. Molecules. 2021 Dec 3;26(23):7340.
57. Fu Q, Zhu R, Song J, Yang H, Chen X. Photoacoustic imaging: Contrast agents and their biomedical applications. Advanced Materials. 2019 Feb;31(6):1805875.

10 Stimuli-Responsive Biomaterials for Inflammatory Autoimmune Disorders

Sonia Dangi
Jeffrey Cheah School of Medicine and Health Sciences, Monash University Malaysia, Subang Jaya, Selangor, Malaysia

Umama Shahid
School of Science, Monash University Malaysia, Subang Jaya, Selangor, Malaysia

Anand Krishnan
Precision Medicine and Integrated Nano-Diagnostics (P-MIND) Research Group, Office of the Dean, Faculty of Health Sciences, University of the Free State, Bloemfontein, South Africa

10.1 INTRODUCTION

10.1.1 Overview of Autoimmune Inflammatory Diseases

Autoimmune inflammatory disorders (AIDs) are chronic diseases that occur due to prolonged inflammation and damage. Most tissue inflammation is of autoimmune origin. Autoimmune diseases collectively refer to over 80 different conditions, with one of the most common being rheumatoid arthritis (RA), systemic lupus erythematosus (SLE), and inflammatory bowel disease (IBD), affecting 5%–8% of the world's human population [1], as depicted in Figure 10.1. These diseases result from losing immune tolerance regulated by genetic, environmental, and immunological determinants. Some factors, like major histocompatibility complex (MHC) alleles, show a strong connection between drug-induced RA development and diseases with specific regions of polymorphisms. Epstein–Barr virus infections, smoking, dietary salt, and vitamin D are other environmental factors adding to the complexity of immunological dysfunction, particularly between ethnic groups [2]. Overall, the IV MHC region is thought to be related to absent autoimmunity regulation. The hyper-response of proinflammatory cytokines such as tumor necrosis factor-alpha (TNF-α), IL-6, IL-1, and anti-citrullinated protein antibodies (ACPAs). Many cytokines can cause injury and damage to tissues and inflammation, which are typical for many diseases, including RA [3]. This development paves the way for remarkable development in AIDs management through devising new therapeutics through the implementation of specific biological medicines modulating inflammatory mediators [4]. Chronic treatment can help to achieve pain relief with traditional therapies, including corticosteroids, methotrexate, and NSAIDs, but long-term benefit leads to controlled treatment, which may further [5].

Advanced technologies such as stimuli-responsive biomaterials are also used in the treatment of AIDs, thus making nanoparticles a viable alternative [6]. These nanoparticles have a specific site behavior since they can change their structure or properties in response to external stimuli such as pH, temperature, and inflammatory markers. This may lead to the specific therapy at

DOI: 10.1201/9781003560203-10

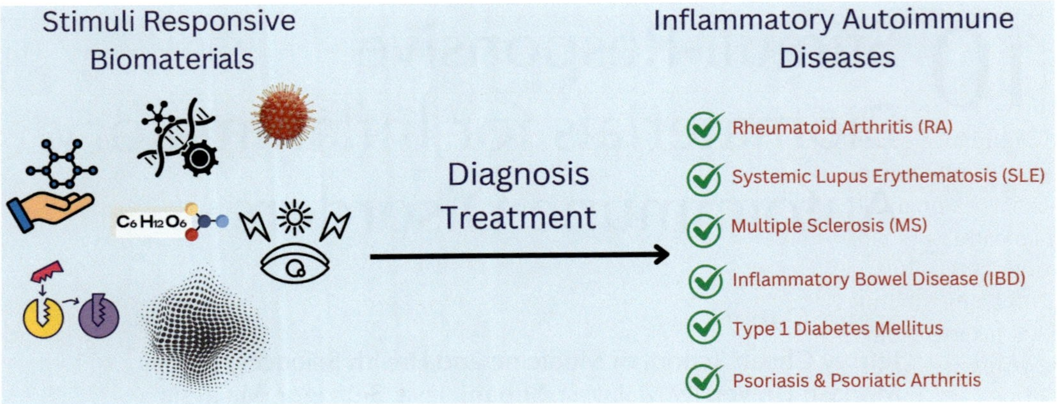

FIGURE 10.1 A diagram of stimuli-responsive biomaterials and a list of inflammatory autoimmune diseases imply them for diagnosis and treatment.

the specific site with better local effect and fewer side effects at the systemic level. For instance, pH-responsive nanocarriers that can deliver anti-inflammatory drugs to the inflamed tissues have been developed to avoid the side effects that are seen with conventional therapy [7]. The efficacy of thermosensitive hydrogels in the delivery of drugs for the treatment of RA joint inflammation has also been established [8]. The formation of therapeutic responses by responsive biomaterials improves treatment efficacy and dexterity, leads to improved patient results, and minimizes the costs of drug delivery [9]. However, there are still many issues to be solved, for instance, the medicines are economically viable and safe to manufacture. Such autoimmune disorders are generally relapsing-remitting in nature, which makes it quite a challenge from the treatment point of view, and thus rather demanding of a more flexible, consumer-centric perspective. Combining stimuli-responsive biomaterials with artificial intelligence (AI) or gene-editing innovations enables programmatic solutions to questions about the best ways to diagnose and manage AIDs. This training allows physicians and researchers to devise targeted and effective treatment strategies that consider not just the patient's physical health but their emotional and social well-being as well [10].

10.1.2 Current Challenges in Diagnosis and Treatment

The patient's complexity, the varied diseases, and the tracking of the progression are the main challenges in the management of autoimmune diseases. Despite the recent advances in biological therapy, many treatment plans that are developed today are not appropriate to the pathophysiology of many diseases [11]. At present, the treatments for patients with autoimmune disorders are inadequate due to several problems, including difficulties in accessing the treatment, high costs, and variability in the response to the treatment [12].

10.1.2.1 Review of Conventional Immunosuppressive Therapies

Several therapeutics, i.e., corticosteroids, methotrexate, and NSAIDs, are immunosuppressants used in the treatment of autoimmune disease. The underlying immunologic dysfunction is still not treated by these treatments, which merely reduce signs and symptoms of the disease. In the long term, they are therefore invariably ineffective in stopping the process to irreversible tissue and organ damage. Side effects of non-selective immunosuppressive drugs are numerous and include susceptibility to infection, osteoporosis, gastrointestinal abnormalities, hypertension, and cardiovascular illness. Corticosteroids represent a drug group: they are highly effective for treating acute inflammation, but long-term administration is complicated by metabolic adverse effects such as diabetes, obesity, and adrenal failure [13]. These side effects diminish the quality of patients' lives, particularly those needing treatment for an extended duration [14].

10.1.2.2 Barriers to Biologic Therapies

Autoimmune diseases have been managed with the help of biologic drugs that function on set pathways of inflammation. TNF inhibitors, such as infliximab and adalimumab, and IL-6 inhibitors, such as tocilizumab, have been very effective in RA and Crohn's disease, respectively [15]. But these medications are not without their problems. The biggest disadvantage of biologics is the patient-to-patient variability in response. Many of the patients are primary or secondary non-responders; they do not have an immediate response to the treatment or become non-responsive to the treatment [16]. This heterogeneity is attributed to the genetic, disease-specific factors, and the dynamic immune responses, which lead to different treatment responses that are often hard to predict. Patients who fail biologic therapy are usually managed by alternative monotherapies or combination regimens, which increase the complexity of management and the costs of care. An issue is the high costs of the biologic drugs which can be between $30,000 and $50,000 per patient per year. Patients will expect to get these medicines, but they will be beyond the reach of many people, especially those in low- and middle-income countries [17]. Treatment costs are a significant burden to healthcare systems and patients, and they limit the ability to access advanced therapy even in rich countries [18].

10.1.2.3 Interactions of Relapsing-Remitting Disease Courses

Most autoimmune diseases are characterized by relapsing remitting courses – exacerbations and remission periods, like multiple sclerosis (MS) and SLE [12]. These unexplained fluctuations make therapy planning difficult and worsen the long-term management of the disease [11]. Symptoms worsen, and tissue degradation increases rapidly during relapses, which are often treated more aggressively. However, although there are now disease-modifying medicines (DMTs) such as interferon β available, they are only modestly effective in preventing long-term disability or in slowing disease progression. The psychological burden for patients is also significant, with anxiety and depression, and a reduced quality of life due to the unpredictability of disease flares.

10.1.2.4 Therapy Resistance and Cumulative Toxicity

Another central concern is therapeutic resistance. For instance, patients receiving biologics may produce neutralizing antibodies that compromise the efficacy of the medicines and thus require higher doses or alternative therapy [19]. This increases the costs of treatment and subjects patients to more side effects and risk factors. Immunosuppressive and biological therapies also present a major problem regarding the cumulative toxicity of these drugs with prolonged use. These medicines have been found to have longer-term side effects, including liver failure, renal toxicity, and an increased cancer risk [20]. For example, hepatotoxicity is a long-term side effect of methotrexate, and biologics are associated with severe infections, including TB and opportunistic fungal infections [21]. This is still a key challenge in managing long-term injury in autoimmune diseases.

10.1.2.5 Data Preparation in Need of Personalized Medicine

The therapy of autoimmune disorders is also complicated by their diversity. Nevertheless, considerable heterogeneity in disease severity, clinical manifestations, and therapeutic response is observed in the same disease (e.g., RA or SLE). This heterogeneity is the result of the interplay of genetic and environmental factors and immunological factors in the pathogenesis of the illness [22]. However, the use of targeted treatment in autoimmune diseases is currently limited. There are no accurate biomarkers to guide the choice of medication or to predict the therapeutic response, and, therefore, the approach based on trial and error undermines the optimal disease control and brings disappointment to the patient. Autoimmune disease toxicity patients must be identified, and predictive algorithms are important for informing therapy selection for individual patients and predicting better outcomes.

This chapter aims to explore the existing international variation in access to healthcare for autoimmune diseases and the challenges that come with managing such illnesses. Many a time, biologics and Janus kinase inhibitors (JAK) inhibitors are unaffordable or unattainable in Low- and middle-income countries, and patients are left with poor-quality treatment with potential adverse effects [23]. For instance, in high-income countries, needy people may not be able to get sophisticated care because of cost, lack of insurance, and uneven access to healthcare.

10.1.2.6 Psycho-Social Implications of Autoimmune Diseases

Autoimmune diseases are not only a physical problem but also affect the mental state and life quality of patients. By chronic symptoms, relapses, and side effects of the treatment, depression, anxiety, and social isolation are quite usual. To address these psychosocial needs, a global approach that integrates medical, psychiatric, and social level management is needed [24].

10.1.2.7 New Treatments and a Look to the Future

New strategies are available because of the recent advancements in immunology and biotechnology, including small molecule inhibitors, cell-based therapeutic modalities, and gene-editing tools. For instance, JAK inhibitors have shown potential in the management of anti-RA by suppressing the signaling of inflammation. Likewise, regulatory T-cell therapy is designed to redefine the immune balance and avoid autoimmune attacks [25]. However, these experimental drugs are still in the early stages of clinical trials, and hence, there is uncertainty about safety, duration of effectiveness, and availability for mass production. Furthermore, a large research, infrastructure, and teaching effort would be required to guarantee that all patients have access to this treatment.

10.1.2.8 Why the Need for Developing New Strategies?

This chapter argues that it is important to develop new strategies to manage autoimmune diseases because the current diagnostic and treatment processes are inadequate. As a result, diagnosis is sometimes made based on poorly defined biomarkers or the clinical picture that is similar to that of other diseases, which results in a delay in diagnosis and treatment. Likewise, treatment options are also advancing but do not attack the immunological dysregulation and are also accompanied by adverse effects and/or high costs [26]. In this case, new strategies are crucial to improve the control of autoimmune diseases. One strategy that has been found to be very effective in addressing these challenges is personalized medicine, where the therapy is tailored to the patient's characteristics [27]. The integration of patients' genomic, genetic, and immunological data into treatment decision making is the concept of personalized medicine that may improve the therapy response and minimize the side effects [28]. It is possible that the cytokine spectrum of the patient's individual immune system may be characterized by its response to biologic therapy, whether this is by blocking TNF or IL-6, as the strong evidence suggests. Such accuracy can help eliminate the current method of selecting drugs on a trial-and-error basis, which can save time in the treatment of the disease. Moreover, the ongoing studies include the search for biomarkers that may help to predict the disease progression or the therapy response. ACPAs are well known to be biomarkers for severe RA. On the other hand, those associated with type I interferon signatures have been linked with lupus flares. Detection and validation of new markers may enhance risk assessment, early diagnosis, and treatment adjustment in most autoimmune pathologies [11].

10.2 GENE-EDITING TECHNOLOGIES HAVE ADVANCED THE TREATMENT STRATEGIES FOR AUTOIMMUNE DISEASES

As such, CRISPR-Cas9 is leading the way to unparalleled autoimmune disease treatments. The stability of CRISPR technology that allows for the precise alteration of the genome can be used to repair genetic mutations that put the individual at risk of autoimmunity. For instance, previous studies have indicated that genes such as FOXP3 that regulate the development and function of regulatory T cells can be edited using the CRISPR system [29]. Mutations of FOXP3 are linked to autoimmune poly-endocrinopathy syndrome, and preliminary studies imply that in these scenarios, one could use gene editing to improve immunological tolerance [30]. However, the following are the possible options that can be explored in relation to the management of autoimmune diseases: replacement of the single gene mutation, alteration of cytokines, or the cells that produce cytokines that are involved in the pathogenesis of the autoimmune diseases. Gene-editing medicines are in the early phases of investigation, but they have significant potential, and safety, delivery systems, and ethical questions remain to be addressed. Although these approaches remain experimental, they suggest a novel, possibly less invasive approach to autoimmune management [31]. The application of advanced technologies for the treatment of autoimmune diseases is not limited to gene therapy and microbiome-based therapy. AI and machine learning (ML) are currently being applied to large data sets and patterns that can be used in clinical decision making [32].

These technologies are particularly useful for discovering new biomarkers, predicting the disease trajectory, and optimizing the treatment plans. For instance, AI algorithms may sort through the expression of hundreds of genes to identify those that are most related to disease activity that may lead to the identification of new treatment targets [31]. Likewise, ML models may combine information from different sources, including electronic health records, imaging scans, and genetic tests, to predict which patients will gain the most from certain drugs [33]. As these techniques advance, they can change the diagnosis and treatment of autoimmune disorders by allowing for hitherto impossible levels of accuracy and efficiency [32]. However, there are several difficulties in implementing new methods in clinical practice. The side effects, the immune response to the delivery systems, and the ethical concerns of the gene-editing tools, such as CRISPR, are some of the issues that are still present [34]. The same applies to microbiome-based therapies, which need further understanding of the mutual influence between microbiota and the host immune system and the establishment of standardized approaches for procedures like Fecal Microbiota Transplantation (FMT) [24]. Nevertheless, the cost of many of these new technologies is an issue of concern in terms of equity and accessibility, particularly in low-resource settings. To ensure the safety and efficacy of novel medicines, further research, a multiprofessional approach, and proper regulatory mechanisms will be required [32].

10.3 SIGNIFICANCE OF AUTOIMMUNE DISORDER MANAGEMENT: GAPS AND PROSPECTS

Autoimmune diseases are numerous and chronic and are among the most significant disorders in the healthcare systems. Immune dysregulation and related diseases affect millions of people. Nevertheless, immunology and biotechnology have progressed, but the therapy of such diseases is still based on the symptoms rather than the diseases. For instance, proinflammatory cytokines (TNF-α and IL-6) or T cells are used in the management of RA or Crohn's disease. The biologic medications have improved the treatment of many patients but are not always potent and can be associated with serious long-term side effects, e.g., an increased risk of infection and malignancy [16, 35]. These limitations reveal the failure of the current treatment models, which are usually designed to be general for many people and are quite insensitive to the varied etiologic factors that are characteristic of most autoimmune diseases. In addition, the management of these disorders in the long term is a major problem. Many diseases including MS and SLE have a relapsing-remitting course, with episodes of worsening and improvement. Current treatments can help to reduce the severity of relapses, but they are rarely able to prevent disease progression, leading to progressive disability and a significant deterioration in the quality of life over a lifetime [36].

The developing field of precision medicine opens the door to possible solutions for the gaps. Precision medicine is an effective strategy that aims to individualize the management of a given disease based on the person's genetic, molecular, and environmental factors. This is possible because of the progress in high-throughput sequencing and bioinformatics to have patient-specific biomarkers identified to predict the outcome of treatment, the likely course of the disease, and even the likelihood of complications. The hope is that this targeted strategy can improve treatment outcomes by targeting pathogenic pathways and reducing side effects or improving the therapeutic index. For instance, molecular profiling in SLE has shown potential to help in the identification of early treatment goals to avoid organ failure; however, this has not yet been implemented in the clinic [37].

In addition, the gene therapies such as CRISPR-Cas9 and RNA-based therapeutic agents are stoked with potential. For instance, in preclinical studies, CRISPR has been employed to edit mutations in genes essential for regulatory T-cell function, for instance, FOXP3. Nevertheless, each of these therapies is still riddled with several safety, delivery, and ethical issues that remain unresolved and must be solved before they can be adopted for routine use [34]. But the cell treatments are also certain to be the new moniker of the game in treating autoimmune disorders as well. CAR T-cell treatment is an immunotherapy that genetically modifies the patient's T cells to make them express chimeric antigen receptors that enable the T cells to recognize particular antigens. It is showing promising phase I/II clinical trial findings in autoimmune diseases like lupus and MS. It is hence perhaps the onset of a new therapy for their immune dysregulation in a small number of patients. Other immunomodulatory stem cells, such as regulatory T cells and mesenchymal stromal cells, have also been shown to possess the capacity to modulate immune responses and may therefore be of value in the therapy of systemic autoimmune diseases. Nevertheless, the major drawbacks include the following: the durability issue, the safety issue, and the technical issue in the scaling up of the production process [23].

The advancement in the field of computation and epigenetics is also impacting the practice of autoimmune diseases. If trained properly, these algorithms can give a comprehensive view of the DNA methylation changes and the probability of the drug being significant or causing autoimmunity. They can assist investigators in the assessment of new druggable targets in patients or in the assessment of the likelihood of response to a particular treatment, for instance, in RA [6]. These epigenetic analyses revealed the common regulatory mechanisms in various autoimmune diseases and the possibility of applying precision medicine to develop new treatment strategies. However, application of these advanced therapies like CAR-T cells is limited by their high cost and ethical, genetic, and molecular profiling issues. To enable these therapies to reach more patients, simplification of the manufacturing processes, reduction of the costs, and resolution of the ethical issues are necessary [36].

10.4 STIMULI-RESPONSIVE BIOMATERIALS: VITAL FOR TARGETING AUTOIMMUNE DISORDERS

A major concern in the management of autoimmune diseases is establishing antigen tolerance in patients. These smart, stimuli-responsive materials show high precision in targeted drug delivery and therapeutic activity as they respond to very specific stimuli like pH, temperature, light, and enzymes, as shown in Figure 10.2. Such biomaterials have huge potential in autoimmune conditions where inflammation is restricted to a specific tissue, as observed in RA and IBD. Leveraging this property, stimuli-responsive biomaterials enable stimulus dependent, spatially localized delivery of loading of therapeutic agents with minimal systemic exposure and off-target side effects [15]. The main advantage of stimuli-responsive biomaterials is that they can selectively accumulate at the inflamed sites. pH-sensitive hydrogels have been investigated for the administration of anti-inflammatory drugs since inflamed tissues have an acidic microenvironment that can lead to the discharge of these types of drugs [14]. The hydrogel will be stable in the normal physiological condition, but it will decompose and release its therapeutic payload at the inflamed tissues for site-specific delivery, as shown in Figure 10.2. In addition, both structural and biochemical changes are also capable of activating biomaterials, resulting in the improved delivery of biologic therapies, including monoclonal antibodies and cytokine inhibitors essential in the treatment of autoimmune diseases. The encapsulation of biologics in responsive nanocarriers, in addition to improving their stability (for

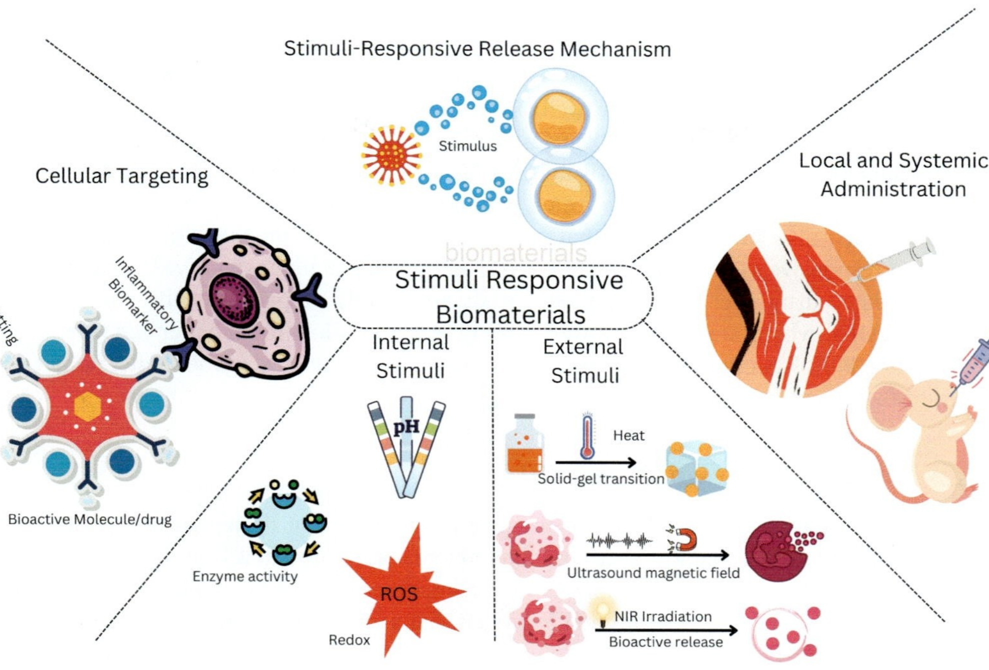

FIGURE 10.2 Schematic illustration of stimuli-responsive biomaterials that adapt to physiological triggers for targeted drug delivery and immune modulation in autoimmune disorders, enhancing therapeutic precision and minimizing side effects.

example, by preventing denaturation or aggregation), permits their controlled release in response to disease-specific stimuli that, in turn, result in optimal therapeutic outcome with low associated risk [38]. Some of these innovations may help change the treatment of diseases such as SLE and MS, which require precise immune modulation for a favorable outcome.

Enzyme-responsive nanomaterials have emerged as a promising category of stimuli-responsive biomaterials for auto-immune diseases. The majority of autoimmune diseases, like RA, are characterized by the excess expression of enzymes, like matrix metalloproteinases (MMPs), which cause breakdown of tissue and inflammation. Such medications ensure the drug delivery to the site of tissue damage by formulating biomaterials that induce drug release on exposure to excessive MMPs. This not only increases the therapeutic effect but also reduces the possibility of unwanted effects and systemic toxicity. The potential of these technologies is immense, and current research is aimed at combining several stimuli-responsive mechanisms to achieve higher sophistication. For instance, dual responsive materials that can respond to both pH and enzyme can provide better control over drug delivery [39]. These innovations are expected to change the way of treating autoimmune disease by providing highly personalized and effective therapeutic choices.

10.5 APPLICATIONS OF SMART BIOMATERIALS IN INFLAMMATORY AUTOIMMUNE DISEASES

10.5.1 Rheumatoid Arthritis (RA)

RA is a prototype of a chronic autoimmune disease with inflammatory joint tissue, immune deregulation, and heightened inflammatory cytokines, including TNF-α and IL-6. Although the outstanding success of patient improvement with the systematic treatment, including biologics, the treatment is usually followed by severe side effects and non-responsiveness in some patients [25].

This is because, for instance, certain stimuli-sensitive hydrogels have been designed to capitalize on the acidic disease microenvironment of inflammatory conditions like an inflamed joint. pH-responsive polymers facilitate the pH-initiated release of TNF-α inhibitors or methotrexate to inflammation sites in an attempt to evade systemic toxicity [10]. In addition, anti-inflammatory drugs can also be encapsulated and delivered via nanocarriers like liposomes and polymeric nanoparticles. Very small amounts of tumor-associated antigens (TAAs) lead to immune tolerance mechanisms such as immunosuppression, depletion of effector lymphocytes, and the ability of the tumor cells to self-renew, which also involve TAAs that are antigens derived from the self-antigen. Recently, dual-stimuli-responsive systems have been developed that enable pH-responsive drug delivery and enzyme-mediated drug release. These biomaterials are mainly prepared for the purpose of sensitivity to MMPs, which are produced in excess in RA and allow for a better schedule of drug administration [40]. RA management has already made significant strides with better adherence to medications and long-term disease control.

10.5.2 Inflammatory Bowel Disease (IBD)

There have been successful treatments for the past half-century but do not sustain remission and induce systemic side effects in most instances. Smart biomaterials are a novel approach to site-specific delivery of therapeutics to the inflamed region of the intestines. One of the most used methods is the synthesis of pH-sensitive nanoparticles and hydrogels that are released in the inflamed intestine and adjust the pH values. Drugs such as monoclonal antibodies or corticosteroids are released only in areas of inflammation to enhance the effectiveness while lessening the side effects. A good example is amine functionalized mesoporous silica nanoparticles that target low pH regions where inflammation has occurred and have been shown to have a better therapeutic effect in model experiments for IBD [15]. Another potential approach is the development of enzyme-responsive biomaterials. These materials use the presence of high levels of enzymes such as proteases or phosphatases in the inflamed tissues [41]. For instance, the therapeutic peptides released from enzyme-sensitive dextran-based hydrogels that are cross-linked with enzyme-sensitive linkers led to reduced incidence of IBD in animal models [28]. Along with the current development of oral drug delivery systems, these strategies may be applied to enhance the patient's compliance and the convenience of use.

10.5.3 Multiple Sclerosis (MS)

MS is an autoimmune disorder of the central nervous system (CNS) due to immune assault on the myelin sheath, leading to neurologic deterioration. Conventional treatments are aimed at immunological activation but are non-specific and generally followed by severe side effects and incomplete efficacy. These include the development of intelligent biomaterials to control the release of neuroprotective and immunosuppressive therapeutic agents to the injury site in the brain. Fingolimod-loaded injectable hydrogels have been developed for local and controlled delivery in the CNS. These hydrogels can be designed responsive to particular biochemical markers like oxidative stress or inflammatory cytokines, which are typically elevated in MS relapses [42]. Lipid-based nanoparticles and exosomes have also been shown to cross the blood-brain barrier in MS treatment. For this purpose, curcumin exosome-mimetic vesicles have been shown to be anti-inflammatory and neuroprotective in preclinical models of MS. For the improvement of MS treatment efficacy, targeting, drug delivery of the therapeutic drug, and imaging must be further studied with the help of multifunctional biomaterials [43].

10.5.4 Type 1 Diabetes (T1D)

Type 1 diabetes (T1D) is a condition where autoimmunity-based destruction of the insulin-producing beta cells of the pancreas occurs. There exists, besides employment of the exogenous insulin treatment, despite that they are lifesaving and they cannot replicate the glucose-modulating effects of the pancreas. Glucose-sensitive insulin delivery systems and smart biomaterials are expected to enhance the management of T1D significantly. For instance, glucose-sensitive hydrogels are intended to provide insulin in a manner similar to the way the pancreas secretes insulin in relation to the variations in blood glucose levels. These hydrogels are usually cross-linked with glucose oxidase or phenylboronic acid derivatives to obtain glucose sensitivity. Their potential to maintain glycemic control with low risk of hypoglycemia has been shown in preclinical studies [44]. Smart biomaterials are also being developed for the purpose of beta cell replacement therapy and insulin delivery. The same way encapsulation is used to protect the transplanted beta cells from immune system attacks while allowing nutrients and oxygen to pass through [15]. In this direction, nanoengineering developments will make these encapsulation systems better and longer-lasting, and drive the systems nearer to the clinic.

10.5.5 Systemic Lupus Erythematosus (SLE) and Psoriasis

SLE and psoriasis are systemic inflammation and immune dysregulation-associated autoimmune diseases. However, biologic application in the majority of diseases has been associated with delivery-related adverse effects of a systemic nature. Efforts are also made in the development of stimuli-responsive nanoparticles that home to the immune cells that contribute to lupus nephritis in SLE. Mycophenolate mofetil encapsulated in polymeric nanoparticles has been developed to release the drug in the event of cytokine inflammatory activation and to prevent kidney damage [41]. Similarly, there is a hydrogel-based system that releases corticosteroids upon enzymatic stimulation to possibly decrease the disease activity while sparing the normal tissue. In the case of psoriasis, however, smart biomaterials have been explored for the development of topical formulations that can deliver anti-inflammatory drugs to the affected areas of the skin. An example would be nanostructured lipid carriers (NLC) of IL-17 inhibitors that had improved skin penetration and prolonged drug residence time for a better and patient-compliant treatment. Advances in microneedle technology also allow for site-specific delivery with minimal invasion for a better drug delivery system [45].

10.6 CASE STUDIES, PATENTS, AND CLINICAL TRIALS

Autoimmune diseases represent a new field where the research on smart biomaterials has been on the rise in recent years, and there is more information about their ability to change the treatment of these diseases. The efficacy, safety, and translation issues are described in case studies, patents, and clinical trials of these sophisticated materials and their therapeutic potential. While these developments are suggestive of the potential to bring preclinical science to the clinic, they also highlight some gaps that must be addressed. Smart biomaterials have also been synthesized with prospective uses in the treatment of autoimmune disorders through drug targeting by injections, immune system modulation, and healing of tissue. Their applications for the treatment of RA, MS, and SLE have been validated by previous studies. For instance, injectable hydrogels have promised novel immune modulation in RA through reducing inflammation and joint damage [3]. Likewise, drug delivery systems on the basis of nanoparticles have been designed to make drug delivery into the targeted area in MS with improved efficacy and reduced side effects). Another excellent practice is biomimetic scaffold engineering for SLE therapy. The scaffolds are extracellular matrix bio-mimicry aimed at enhancing drug delivery and immunological tolerance [16].

In addition, thermosensitive polymers and pH-sensitive nanoparticles have been developed to administer immunosuppressive drugs to the inflamed area precisely, which can avoid the side effects in other parts of the body and improve the overall health of the patient. Several patents are available that highlight the implications of smart biomaterials (Table 10.1). For instance, the stability and efficacy of self-assembling nanostructures for regulated immunosuppressive drug delivery have been patentable (US Patent 10,654,321, 2022). Similarly, thermosensitive polymers with site-specific

TABLE 10.1
Key Examples of Case Studies and Patents in This Domain

Category	Examples	Key Features	Outcomes	References
Case study 1	Injectable hydrogels for rheumatoid arthritis	Localized immune modulation	Reduced inflammation and joint damage	[3]
Case study 2	Dendritic polymer carriers for lupus nephritis	High drug loading capacity	Prolonged drug release	[6]
Case study 3	pH-responsive nanoparticles for psoriasis	Stimuli-responsive drug release	Minimized off-target effects	[7]
Case study 4	Nanoparticles for multiple sclerosis	Targeted drug delivery	Enhanced drug efficacy and reduced side effects	[15]
Case study 5	Biomimetic scaffolds for systemic lupus erythematosus	Extracellular matrix mimicry	Improved immune tolerance	[16]
Case study 6	Injectable microgels for lupus nephritis	Localized delivery and controlled release	Reduced renal inflammation	[21]
Case study 7	Alginate-based hydrogels for type 1 diabetes	Immune shielding of transplanted islets	Enhanced islet survival and function	[23]
Case study 8	Liposome-based therapies for Crohn's disease	Lipid bilayer encapsulation	Enhanced bioavailability	[46]
Patent 1	Self-assembling nanostructures for immunosuppressive drug delivery	Controlled and sustained release	Improved drug stability and efficacy	US Patent 10,654,321, 2022
Patent 2	Thermosensitive polymers for site-specific drug release	Temperature-sensitive delivery	Precise targeting and minimized systemic risks	EU Patent 202034567, 2021
Patent 3	Multi-responsive biomaterials for autoimmune therapies	Multi-stimuli responsiveness	Enhanced specificity in drug release	JP Patent 201920456, 2019
Patent 4	Bioengineered hydrogels for RA treatment	Biocompatible and biodegradable	Localized and sustained therapeutic effects	CN Patent 34562107, 2020
Patent 5	Nanocarriers for crossing the blood–brain barrier in MS therapies	Brain-targeted delivery	Improved drug delivery to the central nervous system	CN Patent 34562107, 2020
Patent 6	Gene-activated scaffolds for RA	Stimulated regenerative pathways	Enhanced tissue repair	JP Patent 201920789, 2019
Patent 7	Light-activated nanoparticles for MS therapies	External light-triggered drug release	Spatial and temporal precision in drug delivery	US Patent 11,789,654, 2022
Patent 8	Smart coatings for autoimmune implantable	Anti-inflammatory surface properties	Reduced immune rejection	US Patent 12,345,678, 2021
Patent 9	pH-sensitive vesicles for ulcerative colitis	Site-specific release in the colon	Improved treatment efficacy	JP Patent 201920456, 2019
Patent 10	Biodegradable nanoparticles for systemic autoimmunity	Enhanced drug stability and bioavailability	Reduced systemic immune activation	EU Patent 202034567, 2021

release characteristics have been patented for controlled drug delivery with minimal systemic toxicity (EU Patent 202034567, 2021). Another area of interest is the development of patents on multi-responsive biomaterials, which can be designed to release drugs in response to various stimuli, including temperature, pH, or enzymatic activity (JP Patent 201920456, 2019). As listed in Table 10.1, bioengineered hydrogels for the treatment of RA and nanocarriers to cross the blood–brain barrier for MS treatment are other significant breakthroughs (CN Patent 34562107, 2020).

Clinical studies have established the effectiveness of smart biomaterials in autoimmune diseases. A Phase II clinical trial of hydrogel-based SLE treatment showed notable enhancements in disease markers and patient global assessment (ClinicalTrials.gov ID: NCT04567890). For instance, a randomized controlled trial of nanoparticle-based vaccination for autoimmune diabetes had promising results in terms of altering the immune response (ClinicalTrials.gov ID: NCT04234567). Other studies are ongoing to examine the use of bioengineered scaffolds for tissue regeneration in RA, pH-responsive nanoparticles for psoriasis treatment, and multifunctional drug delivery systems for MS [40]. Hence, the translational potential of smart biomaterials can be stated based on this research, with the exception of some aspects such as regulatory approval, scalability of manufacturing, and long-term safety) (Table 10.1).

10.7 CHALLENGES AND OPPORTUNITIES

Although encouraging discoveries have been made, there are still considerable difficulties in bringing normal clinical usage of smart biomaterials. The barriers include regulatory approval, repeatability, scalability, and cost-effectiveness. For example, having consistent manufacturing procedures that fulfill regulatory criteria is critical to commercialization [46]. Furthermore, these materials' long-term biocompatibility and safety must be proven in human trials. Multidisciplinary cooperation provides opportunities to tackle these challenges. Advances in three-dimensional (3D) printing, computational modeling, and synthetic biology may assist in overcoming biomaterial design and scalability issues. Furthermore, integrating patient-specific techniques and real-time monitoring technologies may enhance the clinical utility of these novel medicines. The expanding collection of data from case studies, patents, and clinical trials shows the revolutionary potential of smart biomaterials in the treatment of autoimmune diseases. These materials are a paradigm change in treatment techniques: accurate, effective, and flexible. Preliminary results of the clinical trials of the application of smart biomaterials in autoimmune diseases are quite promising. For example, a glucose-sensitive hydrogel for T1D. Large-scale phase II clinical trials were used to test a glucose-sensitive hydrogel capable of releasing insulin in response to the fluctuation of blood glucose levels. Initial findings were that glycemic control was enhanced and hypoglycemia occurred less often compared to the control insulin therapy Several researches are ongoing to evaluate the enzyme-sensitive nanoparticles that selectively target immunomodulatory drugs based on the measurement of MMPs that are usually elevated during the active phases of MS [12].

Preliminary findings of the study suggest that these enzyme-sensitive materials have the potential to decrease the rate of relapse and the rate of progression of neurological symptoms in MS patients. As the interest in the application of smart biomaterials for autoimmune disease management continues to rise, the number of patent applications has also increased [15, 16]. European Patent on NKT Cell Modulators: In the Philippines, GRI Bio was able to obtain a European patent (EPO Patent No. 19,166,502) for GRI-0803 and over 500 other chemicals that act on autoimmune diseases, such as SLE (Patent Review, 2020). Preclinical studies also showed that these compounds have the ability to inhibit iNKT cells, and when given orally, they were able to improve lupus nephritis and survival (Patent Review, 2020). Investigators at the University of Florida have created a copyrighted product that improves the effectiveness of adoptive T-cell (Treg) treatment of autoimmune diseases, which may also help enhance the efficacy of Treg therapy (Patent Review, 2020). The National Institutes of Health is planning to grant an exclusive patent license for dimethyl synaptamide, a molecule under investigation for the treatment of autoimmune and inflammatory diseases, which is another ongoing effort to create new treatments for autoimmune diseases (Patent Review, 2020). These recent patents show the possibility that smart biomaterials can offer better patient results in autoimmune diseases.

10.8 BIOMEDICAL IMAGING TECHNIQUES AND DIAGNOSTIC METHODS USING SMART MATERIALS

Combining the latest developments in biomedical imaging with the new smart biomaterials may completely change the current approaches to the autoimmune disease's diagnosis and management (Figure 10.3). The combination of imaging modalities and stimuli-response materials can provide temporal in vivo information on the disease evolution and treatment effects and may even predict the flares of autoimmune diseases [17]. Theragnostic nanoparticles have been developed to recognize alterations in the microenvironment of the inflamed tissue (pH, enzymatic activity) and provide feedback signals to imaging modalities (MRI, PET, fluorescence imaging). These particles can be used for diagnosis and treatment at the same time and deliver medicines that give a real-time image of inflammation. Inflammatory cytokines such as TNF-α can be used to detect MRI-inflamed joints over time to help identify new disease onset and treatment response in RA and osteoarthritis. Likewise, in MS, nanoparticles that can selectively accumulate at the sites of neuroinflammation are being developed to increase the sensitivity of detecting active lesions, which are often not well seen on conventional imaging [14]. Aside from imaging, various smart materials are being studied for the diagnostic sector in autoimmune disorders. For example, as illustrated in Figure 10.3, biosensors based on smart materials may detect extremely slight changes in biochemical markers associated with autoimmune

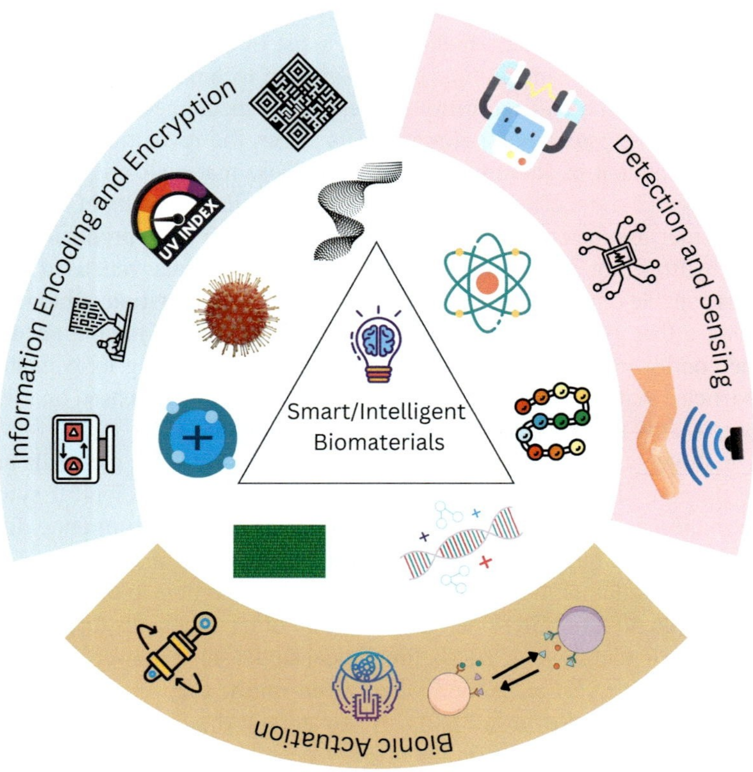

FIGURE 10.3 Schematic illustration of diverse smart biomaterials, highlighting their stimuli-responsive properties in imaging, diagnosis, and key biomedical applications.

disorders. For example, biosensors combined with smart hydrogels are being utilized to detect autoantibodies in lupus and RA, enabling earlier and more precise diagnosis [2]. These technologies can potentially reduce diagnostic delays, which are a significant issue in several autoimmune illnesses.

10.9 FUTURE DIRECTIONS AND EMERGING TRENDS

10.9.1 A Future Prospect for Autoimmune Disorder Treatment

The future of treating autoimmune disorders is found in the combination of intelligent biomaterials and personalized medicine. Autoimmune disorders are characterized by this variability – with a diversity of symptoms and unique responses to therapy in different patients. Conventional therapeutic approaches are often based on a 'one-size fits all' principle and may lead to suboptimal results or even adverse effects. On the other hand, personalized medicine, which modifies treatment methods based on an individual's unique characteristics/traits, may revolutionize the control of these complex diseases [22]. This personalized approach is enabled by the smart biomaterials developed in this research focus. These materials could be programmed to react to the specific needs of each patient through the addition of sensitive elements and incorporation with existing technology to ensure the best possible outcomes.

10.9.2 Disease-Specific Biomarker-Responsive Biomaterials

One key element of personalized medicine is adapting therapy delivery based on real-time information on the patient's disease condition. These smart biomaterials have the advantage of high affinity to the specific biomarkers in the patient's elegant sequence (known as the inflammatory cytokine, autoantibody, disease-specific protein, etc.). In particular, biomaterials can be designed to deliver therapeutic compounds only when certain biomarkers rise above a certain level, so that treatment is given only when and where it is required. Using this strategy, it is possible to improve the therapeutic efficacy without increasing the risk of systemic drug exposure and associated adverse effects [47].

10.9.3 Adaptive and Dynamic Therapies Biomaterials

Autoimmune disorders are highly dynamic and, therefore, demand adaptive therapy strategies that can be adjusted in real time in response to patient condition changes. Feedback systems that can keep on observing the therapy administration and making changes to it can be incorporated into the smart biomaterials to make the treatment better [15]. Biomaterials can be incorporated with sensors that can sense alterations in the patient's physiology, like inflammation or immune cell activity. The latter could be employed to initiate the delivery of more drugs or to modify the characteristics of the biomaterial to a rapidly changing disease condition.

10.9.4 Predictive Modeling Using Bioinformatics and Machine Learning

Novel bioinformatics approaches and ML enable the development of predictive models of disease trajectories in autoimmune diseases. Big databases of patient information, including genetic, epigenetic, and environmental variables, may be analyzed to identify patterns and predict disease trajectory and therapeutic response. Such information can be used for patient-specific treatment programming and the selection of optimal biomaterials [28].

10.9.5 Wearable Technology Integration

Integration of wearable technology, like smartwatches and fitness trackers, with smart biomaterials offers continuous patient health monitoring, and adjustments can thus be made with real-time momentum. Wearable devices, for instance, can monitor vital signs, physical activity levels, and environmental conditions, providing essential insights into a patient's overall health [28]. Such data can be wirelessly transferred via a central database or the biomaterial, enabling the system to personalize therapy delivery according to real-time adjustments in patient needs. Translating personalized medicine and intelligent biomaterials to the clinic has several hurdles in spite of their promise. These are building robust biomarkers. Biomarker discovery and qualification are at the core of personalized medicine that accurately reflects disease activity and treatment response. Long-term safety and efficacy of responsive biomaterials must be established. Furthermore, further safety and efficacy in vivo testing will be required, and extensive preclinical and clinical studies will be necessary. Data privacy, equity of access, and the potential for unanticipated effects all warrant close examination. To surpass these limitations will require more research and development and collaboration among the sciences, engineering, medicine, and ethics. Customized medicine, with intelligent biomaterials, makes possible a paradigm shift in the management of autoimmune disease. The promise of these new technologies has the ability to lead us to the future where treatments are customized to each patient's unique needs, improving our outcomes and health.

10.9.6 New Material Science Breakthroughs

The function and reactivity of smart biomaterials are going to be drastically altered by a revolution in material sciences. Far more complex drug release regulation mechanisms have been made possible by recent advances in nanotechnology that have led to the generation of materials that can respond to many stimuli (pH, temperature, enzyme activity, etc.). These multifunctional materials are also particularly interesting for multiple autoimmune diseases, where it is often necessary to target multimodalities of the damaged pathways. Smart polymer enzymes degradable to the extent of the enzyme activity specific to inflammation are being developed for inflammatory diseases like Crohn's disease and lupus [15]. In addition, concrete is also becoming a trend in the construction of bioinspired structured and functional materials originating from biological systems. These materials hold promise to induce biocompatibility and reduce immunogenicity, which are needed for their application in clinical scenarios in chronic autoimmune diseases. Hydrogels mimicking the extracellular matrix, for example, are investigated to repair tissue injury in autoimmune disorders like MS, a degenerative disease of the nervous system [3].

A possible future of treating autoimmune disorders is presented, combining intelligent biomaterials with personalized medicine. The variety of symptoms and the diverse responses to therapy in each patient make autoimmune disorders different. Traditional therapy techniques are based on a single approach and hence produce poor results along with severe side effects. In contrast, customized medicine, which tailors treatment techniques to each patient's unique traits, can change the management of these complicated conditions [27]. Smart biomaterials play an essential role in allowing this personalized approach. By adding responsive features and integrating with current technology, these materials may be tailored to respond to each patient's demands, assuring optimal therapy outcomes. Autoimmune disorders are dynamic, adaptive therapy techniques that can be altered in real time to reflect the patient's changing status. Smart biomaterials can be created with feedback systems that enable continuous monitoring and modification of therapy administration [9]. For example, biomaterials can be combined with sensors that monitor changes in the patient's physiology, such as inflammation levels or immune cell activity. This information can initiate the release of more therapeutic drugs or modify the biomaterial's characteristics in response to a changing illness [39]. Advances in bioinformatics and ML are allowing the creation of predictive models of disease trajectories in autoimmune disorders. Large databases of patient information, including genetic, epigenetic, and environmental variables, may be analyzed to detect patterns and predict illness progression and therapy response. This information may be utilized to create tailored treatment programs and choose the best biomaterials for each patient [33]. Wearable devices such as smartwatches and fitness trackers may be integrated with intelligent biomaterials to enable constant monitoring of patient health and timely modification of treatment strategies. Wearable devices, for example, can track vital signs, physical activity, and environmental conditions, and these valuable pieces of information about a patient's overall health [28]. This data can be remotely loaded into a central database or the biomaterial, allowing the system to adapt treatment delivery based on the patient's changing needs.

10.10 CHALLENGES AND FUTURE DIRECTIONS

Even with its enormous potential, transitioning customized medicine and smart biomaterials into the clinic is fraught with several challenges. These include the development of reliable biomarkers. Personalized medicine relies primarily on the identification and verification of biomarkers that mirror disease activity and therapeutic response. For long-term safe and effective function of responsive biomaterials to be assured, extensive preclinical and clinical testing must be done in order to assess their safety and effectiveness within a living organism. A study of the ethics of personalized medicine, privacy of information, equity of access, and possible unforeseen effects must be thoroughly debated. Submission of these challenges will require sustained research and development and interdisciplinary collaboration between scientists, engineers, physicians, and ethicists [16].

The development of smart biomaterials for autoimmune diseases is still an emerging field that is reliant on developing cutting-edge technologies. The future generation of innovative materials, 3D bioprinting, gene editing, and AI is likely to shape this next wave of material innovation and make more personalized and effective treatments possible. 3D bioprinting is a powerful tool for the production of patient-specific replicas of disease-defective tissues. It allows investigators to create 3D structures highly similar to the complex organization and cellular content of autoimmune disease-blasted tissues, such as MS and RA [47]. The patient-derived replicas allow new smart biomaterials and medications to be assessed within a personalized context. We hope scientists will be able to work with these materials and learn how they act in the patient's tissues and cells and thus select the most hopeful candidates for clinical translation. Moreover, 3D bioprinting has been employed to develop patient-specific scaffolds and implants for the tissue replacement of the damaged tissue. To this end, patient-derived cell-seeded 3D-printed scaffolds can facilitate reconstruction of the damaged cartilage and bone in RA, thereby enhancing the tissue healing process as well as articular movement [48].

Gene-editing tools like CRISPR-Cas9 are changing the way, or can alter, genomic material with a precision that was heretofore unattainable. These technologies are able to modify immune cells and restore function in autoimmune diseases. For instance, CRISPR-Cas9 can repair a genetic defect that results in autoimmune disease or design immune cells to recognize and attack particular disease-targeted molecules. Smart biomaterials may be crucial for transporting gene-editing tools to the right tissues and cells. Biodegradable nanoparticles and hydrogels could be created to carry the CRISPR-Cas9 system and administer it to the inflammatory site or immune target cells. This approach allows for more powerful and targeted delivery of the gene-editing tool with reduced off-target effects and improved therapeutic index [49]. For example, in T1D, CRISPR-Cas9 controls immune cells to stop them from attacking pancreatic insulin-producing cells. Combined gene editing and smart biomaterial delivery systems can restore enough tolerance to stop disease progression.

AI and ML algorithms are revolutionizing biomaterial design. AI systems trained on big data can discover the implicit connections and patterns in experimental and clinical data, which might be otherwise unnoticed by human investigators. This data can be used to predict the properties of potential materials, optimize the development of those in a design cycle, or accelerate the discovery of better therapeutic biomaterials. For instance, biomaterial's biocompatibility, biodegradability, and immunomodulatory properties can be predicted by AI algorithms from the chemical structure and structural features of the material. This information helps produce materials with distinct properties tailored to every patient's needs. ML may also be utilized to analyze patient data including genetic profiles, disease progression, and therapy response to identify biomarkers predicting treatment outcomes. Such data can be used to design individualized treatment strategies and select the optimal biomaterial for each person [50].

All such new technologies collectively will make an extraordinary impact on innovative smart biomaterials for their applications in autoimmune diseases [51]. Utilizing 3D bioprinting, gene editing, and AI, the investigators can provide patient-specific therapy to such advanced and long-lasting ailments. The 3D bioprinting is capable of bioprinting the patient-specific model of the afflicted tissue, which also assists in the precise screening of the new drug. Gene-editing tools like CRISPR-Cas9 will be used to cure genetic diseases and modulate immune functions, and AI will assist in the identification and optimization of new biomaterials. Thanks to recent developments, it is expected that in the coming few years, biomaterials with multifunctionality, such as drug delivery, immunomodulation, and tissue regeneration, will be produced. These new materials will facilitate the creation of more selective, target-oriented, and less invasive personalized medications than the current treatments [52].

10.11 CONCLUSION

As a result, the advent of smart biomaterials has heralded a transformative paradigm shift in treating autoimmune disorders, paving the way for the departure from traditional therapeutic strategies to an era of precise medicine. These multifunctional new materials, which integrate functions like localized drug delivery, sustained release, immune modulation, and tissue restoration, can revolutionize our ability to diagnose, treat, and monitor these complex diseases. By tailoring the therapy to individual patient characteristics, smart biomaterials provide personalized medicine, leading to greater therapeutic efficacy with reduced systemic side effects. A growing body of research, including case studies and clinical trials, shows how these new tools are implemented in clinical practice. In one example, biocompatible implants with embedded biomaterials can be used to locally deliver drugs and promote the healing of joints in inflammatory arthritis. Likewise, biomaterials-based vaccines have also been studied for autoimmune diseases through either the immune system's orientation or disease activity regulation. These initial successes have foundations on which to build further research and innovation in this field. However, there are still many barriers that prevent smart biomaterials from moving from the bench to the bedside. This could be arduous and time-consuming for innovative biomaterials to go through the regulatory environment. The production process for complex biomaterials is difficult and expensive to scale up. Safekeeping of biomaterials in vivo for an extended period for clinical use remains challenging.

Research and production costs of new biomaterials may also be costly, which can be unfeasible for the patient to afford. These challenges, however, demand a multidisciplinary approach by different scientists, engineers, physicians, and regulatory agencies. In addition, there is a need for further R&D on the biomaterials' design, production processes, and clinical trials to support the current regulatory approval of such complex technologies. Overall, the vast potential of innovative biomaterials will be available in treating autoimmune diseases only after better engineering in future studies. Understanding the interactions between biomaterials and the immune system is one of the key study interests because it is crucial for patient safety and optimal treatment results, especially in predicting and avoiding long-term adverse effects. Biodegradable and biocompatible biomaterials: The key is to minimize the environmental impact and to reach complete degradation in vivo, which is consistent with long-term healthcare sustainability and patient safety. The prospect of integrating biomaterials with other emerging technologies like gene editing, immunotherapy, and AI opens a possibility to create more sophisticated and specific therapies. Moreover, ethical implications and social consequences must be well considered. Equitable access to these new technologies, minimizing potential risks, and considering the social impact of personalized medicine, is all necessary to promote responsible and ethical adoption. There is also great potential for applying AI and ML in designing and developing biomaterials. These technologies enable the rapid identification and optimization of new biomaterials to develop tailored therapeutics to meet the specific needs of patients. Nanobiomaterials make use of nanotechnology for biological/biomedical applications. Its potential for creating multifunctional biomaterials with unique capabilities, such as real-time disease monitoring, adaptive drug delivery, and regenerative medicine applications, will lead the field in the future. The medical use of innovative biomaterials represents a new paradigm in autoimmune disease therapy. These novel materials promise to bring the day when autoimmune disease will be safely controlled, and the patient's quality of life maximized. However, turning this promise into reality requires continued research, development, and collaboration.

Declaration of AI and AI-Assisted Technologies

During the preparation of this work, the authors used QuillBot AI in order to paraphrase the sentences. After using this tool, the authors reviewed and edited the content as needed and take full responsibility for the content of the publication.

REFERENCES

1. Shaheen WA, Quraishi MN, Iqbal TH. Gut microbiome and autoimmune disorders. Clinical and Experimental Immunology. 2022 Aug 1;209(2):161–74.
2. Kremers HM, Nicola P, Crowson CS, O'Fallon WM, Gabriel SE. Therapeutic strategies in rheumatoid arthritis over a 40-year period. The Journal of Rheumatology. 2004 Dec 1;31(12):2366–73.
3. Kumar A, Ali A, Kanika, Vyawahare A, Ahmad A, Mishra RK, Ansari MM, Nadeem A, Siddiqui N, Raza SS, Khan R. Highly biocompatible smart injectable hydrogel for the management of rheumatoid arthritis. ACS Biomaterials Science & Engineering. 2023 Aug 18;9(9):5312–21.
4. Imboden JB. The immunopathogenesis of rheumatoid arthritis. Annual Review of Pathology: Mechanisms of Disease. 2009 Feb 28;4(1):417–34.
5. Maese J, Del Campo PD, Seoane-Mato D, Guerra M, Cañete JD. Effectiveness of conventional disease-modifying antirheumatic drugs in psoriatic arthritis: A systematic review. Reumatología Clínica (English Edition). 2018 Mar 1;14(2):81–9.
6. Parvin N, Joo SW, Mandal TK. Biodegradable and stimuli-responsive nanomaterials for targeted drug delivery in autoimmune diseases. Journal of Functional Biomaterials. 2025 Jan 14;16(1):24.
7. Beloqui A, Coco R, Memvanga PB, Ucakar B, des Rieux A, Préat V. pH-sensitive nanoparticles for colonic delivery of curcumin in inflammatory bowel disease. International Journal of Pharmaceutics. 2014 Oct 1;473(1–2):203–12.
8. Wu H, Wang K, Wang H, Chen F, Huang W, Chen Y, Chen J, Tao J, Wen X, Xiong S. Novel self-assembled tacrolimus nanoparticles cross-linking thermosensitive hydrogels for local rheumatoid arthritis therapy. Colloids and Surfaces B: Biointerfaces 2017 Jan 1;149:97–104.
9. Fenton OS, Olafson KN, Pillai PS, Mitchell MJ, Langer R. Advances in biomaterials for drug delivery. Advanced Materials. 2018 Jul;30(29):1705328.
10. Siddiqui F, Aslam D, Tanveer K, Soudy M. The role of artificial intelligence and machine learning in autoimmune disorders. In Artificial intelligence and autoimmune diseases: Applications in the diagnosis, prognosis, and therapeutics 2024 Feb 14 (pp. 61–75). Singapore: Springer Nature Singapore.
11. Park Y, Kwok SK. Recent advances in cell therapeutics for systemic autoimmune diseases. Immune Network. 2022 Feb 11;22(1):e10.
12. Rudick RA. Disease-modifying drugs for relapsing-remitting multiple sclerosis and future directions for multiple sclerosis therapeutics. Archives of Neurology. 1999 Sep 1;56(9):1079–84.
13. Patel JP, Srinivasa NK, Gande A, Anusha M, Dar H, Baji DB. The role of biologics in rheumatoid arthritis: A narrative review. Cureus. 2023 Jan 3;15(1):e33293.
14. Song Y, Li J, Wu Y. Evolving understanding of autoimmune mechanisms and new therapeutic strategies of autoimmune disorders. Signal Transduction and Targeted Therapy. 2024 Oct 4;9(1):263.
15. Ali I. The development of targeted therapies for autoimmune diseases: Current status and future prospects. Frontiers in Healthcare Technology. 2024 Dec 31;1(2):108–13.
16. Rosman Z, Shoenfeld Y, Zandman-Goddard G. Biologic therapy for autoimmune diseases: An update. BMC Medicine. 2013 Apr 4;11(1):88.
17. Baumgart DC, Misery L, Naeyaert S, Taylor PC. Biological therapies in immune-mediated inflammatory diseases: Can biosimilars reduce access inequities? Frontiers in pharmacology. 2019 Mar 28;10:279.

18. Genchi GG, Marino A, Tapeinos C, Ciofani G. Smart materials meet multifunctional biomedical devices: Current and prospective implications for nanomedicine. Frontiers in Bioengineering and Biotechnology. 2017 Dec 18;5:80.
19. Wu B, Chung S, Jiang XR, McNally J, Pedras-Vasconcelos J, Pillutla R, White JT, Xu Y, Gupta S. Strategies to determine assay format for the assessment of neutralizing antibody responses to biotherapeutics. The AAPS Journal. 2016 Nov;18(6):1335–50.
20. Chan KK, Bass AR. Autoimmune complications of immunotherapy: Pathophysiology and management. BMJ. 2020 Apr 6;369:m736.
21. Rathee P, Chaudhary H, Rathee S, Rathee D, Kumar V. Immunosuppressants: A review. The Pharma Innovation. 2013 Feb 1;1(12):90–101.
22. Tavakolpour S. Towards personalized medicine for patients with autoimmune diseases: Opportunities and challenges. Immunology Letters. 2017 Oct 1;190:130–8.
23. Rathore AS, Gardner PJ, Chhabra H, Raman R. Global outlook on affordability of biotherapeutic drugs. Annals of the New York Academy of Sciences. 2024 Jul;1537(1):168–78.
24. Askari G, Ghavami A, Shahdadian F, Moravejolahkami AR. Effect of synbiotics and probiotics supplementation on autoimmune diseases: A systematic review and meta-analysis of clinical trials. Clinical Nutrition. 2021 May 1;40(5):3221–34.
25. Fraenkel L, Bathon JM, England BR, St., Clair EW, Arayssi T, Carandang K, Deane KD, Genovese M, Huston KK, Kerr G, Kremer J. 2021 American College of Rheumatology guideline for the treatment of rheumatoid arthritis. Arthritis & Rheumatology. 2021 Jul;73(7):1108–23.
26. De Mattos AM, Olyaei AJ, Bennett WM. Nephrotoxicity of immunosuppressive drugs: Long-term consequences and challenges for the future. American Journal of Kidney Diseases. 2000 Feb 1;35(2):333–46.
27. Holdsworth SR, Gan PY, Kitching AR. Biologics for the treatment of autoimmune renal diseases. Nature Reviews Nephrology. 2016 Apr;12(4):217–31.
28. Laigle L, Chadli L, Moingeon P. Biomarker-driven development of new therapies for autoimmune diseases: Current status and future promises. Expert Review of Clinical Immunology. 2023 Mar 4;19(3):305–14.
29. Li H, Yang Y, Hong W, Huang M, Wu M, Zhao X. Applications of genome editing technology in the targeted therapy of human diseases: Mechanisms, advances and prospects. Signal Transduction and Targeted Therapy. 2020 Jan 3;5(1):1.
30. Wu Y, Borde M, Heissmeyer V, Feuerer M, Lapan AD, Stroud JC, Bates DL, Guo L, Han A, Ziegler SF, Mathis D. FOXP3 controls regulatory T cell function through cooperation with NFAT. Cell. 2006 Jul 28;126(2):375–87.
31. Israr J, Kumar A. Current progress in CRISPR-Cas systems for autoimmune diseases. Progress in Molecular Biology and Translational Science. 2024 Jan 1;208:231–59.
32. Mane DV, Deshmukh AN, Ambare RH, Solankar AA, Madane CS. AI in autoimmune diseases: Transforming diagnosis and treatment. Journal of Pharmaceutical and Biological Sciences. 2024;12(2):109–18.
33. Mehta J, Singla I, Mehra T, Garg H, Yadav N, Goyal AK. Leveraging Machine Learning for Biomarker Discovery and Risk Prediction in Autoimmune Disease Genetics. In 2025 10th International Conference on Signal Processing and Communication (ICSC) 2025 Feb 20 (pp. 464–469). IEEE.
34. Brokowski C, Adli M. CRISPR ethics: Moral considerations for applications of a powerful tool. Journal of Molecular Biology. 2019 Jan 4;431(1):88–101.
35. Kedra J, Davergne T, Braithwaite B, Servy H, Gossec L. Machine learning approaches to improve disease management of patients with rheumatoid arthritis: Review and future directions. Expert Review of Clinical Immunology. 2021 Dec 2;17(12):1311–21.
36. Sindhu RK, Madaan P, Chandel P, Akter R, Adilakshmi G, Rahman MH. Therapeutic approaches for the management of autoimmune disorders via gene therapy: Prospects, challenges and opportunities. Current Gene Therapy. 2022 Jun 1;22(3):245–61.
37. Barrat FJ, Crow MK, Ivashkiv LB. Interferon target-gene expression and epigenomic signatures in health and disease. Nature Immunology. 2019 Dec;20(12):1574–83.
38. Prosperi D, Colombo M, Zanoni I, Granucci F. Drug nanocarriers to treat autoimmunity and chronic inflammatory diseases. Seminars in Immunology 2017 Dec 1;34:61–67.
39. Laurano R, Boffito M, Abrami M, Grassi M, Zoso A, Chiono V, Ciardelli G. Dual stimuli-responsive polyurethane-based hydrogels as smart drug delivery carriers for the advanced treatment of chronic skin wounds. Bioactive Materials. 2021 Sep 1;6(9):3013–24.
40. Woessner Jr JF. Matrix metalloproteinases and their inhibitors in connective tissue remodeling. The FASEB Journal. 1991 May;5(8):2145–54.

41. Liu Y, Huang J, Li S, Li Z, Chen C, Qu G, Chen K, Teng Y, Ma R, Wu X, Ren J. Advancements in hydrogel-based drug delivery systems for the treatment of inflammatory bowel disease: A review. Biomaterials Science. 2024;12(4):837–62.
42. Schreiner TG, Romanescu C, Popescu BO. The blood–brain barrier—A key player in multiple sclerosis disease mechanisms. Biomolecules. 2022 Apr 2;12(4):538.
43. Nguyen TL, Choi Y, Im J, Shin H, Phan NM, Kim MK, Choi SW, Kim J. Immunosuppressive biomaterial-based therapeutic vaccine to treat multiple sclerosis via re-establishing immune tolerance. Nature Communications. 2022 Dec 2;13(1):7449.
44. Li Y, Feng G, Liu J, Yang T, Hou R, Liu J, Wang X. Progress in glucose-sensitive hydrogels for biomedical applications. Macromolecular Chemistry and Physics. 2023 Dec;224(23):2300257.
45. Park CO, Kim HL, Park JW. Microneedle transdermal drug delivery systems for allergen-specific immunotherapy, skin disease treatment, and vaccine development. Yonsei Medical Journal. 2022 Sep 7;63(10):881.
46. Albarbar B, Aga H. A review on autoimmune diseases: Recent advances and future perspectives. AlQalam Journal of Medical and Applied Sciences. 2024 Aug 5;7(3):718–29.
47. Fu Y, Feng C, Qin S, Xing Z, Liu C, Liu Z, Yu H. Breaking barriers: Advancing cellular therapies in autoimmune disease management. Frontiers in Immunology. 2024 Nov 29;15:1503099.
48. Desvaux E, Aussy A, Hubert S, Keime-Guibert F, Blesius A, Soret P, et al. Model-based computational precision medicine to develop combination therapies for autoimmune diseases. Expert Review of Clinical Immunology. 2021 Nov 29;18(1):47–56.
49. Li Y, Wu X, Fang D, Luo Y. Informing immunotherapy with multi-omics driven machine learning. NPJ Digital Medicine. 2024 Mar 14;7(1):67.
50. Nag S, Mohanto S, Ahmed MG, Subramaniyan V. "Smart" stimuli-responsive biomaterials revolutionizing the theranostic landscape of inflammatory arthritis. Materials Today Chemistry. 2024 Jul 1;39:102178.
51. Devadasu VR, Alshammari TM, Aljofan M. Current advances in the utilization of nanotechnology for the diagnosis and treatment of diabetes. International Journal of Diabetes in Developing Countries. 2017 Apr 28;38(1):11–9.
52. Baglaenko Y, Wagner C, Bhoj VG, Brodin P, Gershwin, ME, Graham D, et al. Making inroads to precision medicine for the treatment of autoimmune diseases: Harnessing genomic studies to better diagnose and treat complex disorders. Cambridge Prisms Precision Medicine. 2023 Jan 1;1:e25.

11 Stimuli-Responsive Biomaterials for Chronic and Diabetic Inflammatory Wounds

Fiza SH
Department of Pharmacy Practice,
Rajeev College of Pharmacy, Hassan, Karnataka, India

Sanjana A
Department of Pharmaceutics, Rajeev College of Pharmacy,
Hassan, Karnataka, India

Mohammed Gulzar Ahmed
Department of Pharmaceutics,
Yenepoya Pharmacy College & Research Centre,
Mangalore, Karnataka, India

11.1 INTRODUCTION

The largest organ in the human body is the skin. There are several factors for the causes of wounds, such as mechanical, thermal, chemical, or radiogenic integrity of the skin or organs [1]. An interruption of the continuity of the skin's epithelial lining is called a wound, and it can spread to muscles, tendons, other subcutaneous tissue, and even the bone [2]. Depending on how they develop, they are classified as either acute or chronic wounds, or as open or closed wounds [3]. The mechanical injuries that result from external factors, such as abrasions and tears, which are brought on by frictional contact between the skin and hard surfaces, are included in acute wounds [2]. The presence of polymicrobial communities in chronic wounds, on the other hand, usually presents as an ambiguous and protracted situation that might produce biofilms, leading to excessive inflammation and infection [4]. In order to prevent infection and inflammation, wounds should be managed to heal quickly and completely. Two distinct elements make up the process: the interior and exterior microenvironments [4]. While the second refers to the external surface in touch with the wound, the first refers to the skin area surrounding the wound [1]. Although the external and interior microenvironments have very distinct environmental conditions, including temperature, pressure, hydration, pH, O_2, and CO_2 levels, the two microenvironments are constantly interacting and influencing one another [1]. Depending on the kind, extent, and nature of the injury, acute wounds can usually heal without any problems in a predictable amount of issue [3]. In contrast to acute wounds, chronic wounds are complex tissue injuries that take longer than three months to heal and do not follow a structured healing process [4]. Elderly individuals, patients with diabetes mellitus (DM), chronic venous insufficiency, peripheral artery occlusive disease, pressure injury, vascular disease, obesity, malnutrition, and chronic mechanical stress, or a combination of these factors, are more likely to sustain chronic wounds [4].

One of the biggest public health concerns of this century is DM, a metabolic condition marked by persistent hyperglycemia. Serious problems, including blindness, cardiovascular disease, neuropathy, renal damage, and diabetic wounds, are linked to diabetes as it worsens [5]. Diabetic wounds

DOI: 10.1201/9781003560203-11

are one of the most common types of disease; about 20% of them develop diabetic wounds worldwide [3]. Compared with acute wounds, more than half of diabetic wounds develop into chronic wounds; this is due to a decline in the metabolism of glucose levels resulting in hyperglycemic conditions [6]. They exhibit prolonged infection, such as cellulitis, abscess, osteomyelitis, gangrene, septicemia, aberrant angiogenesis, delayed re-epithelialization, and protracted infection, like walking difficulties. These result in increased risks of psychiatric stress, depression, amputation, and death [7]. Although the primary goals of wound healing are to stop infections from happening and to clean the area, understanding and managing wound healing is still exceedingly difficult from a clinical standpoint [8]. Diabetic wounds cannot be adequately treated by standard treatments that only clean the wounds [8]. Controlling blood glucose levels, surgical debridement, skin transplantation, and changing wound dressings are some of the approaches; nonetheless, infections can quickly arise since the skin layer's unique barrier is lost [4]. Thus, new biomaterials and bioactive compounds are needed to further diabetic wound care in order to prevent wound infection and bacterial infection [6]. By stimulating angiogenesis, improving collagen deposition, and encouraging cell proliferation, interactive wound dressings and scaffolds that operate as a barrier to prevent bacteria from entering diabetic wounds can be created. These include, but are not limited to, films, hydrogels, hydrocolloids, alginates, and foams [6]. In order to improve the wound healing property, growth factors (GFs) and antimicrobials are frequently added to the bioactive dressing, which is made from biomaterials like collagen, hyaluronic acid, and chitosan [8]. This chapter provides a thorough overview of the stimuli-responsive biomaterials in the form of conductive wound dressings' recent enormous success and enormous potential for skin tissue engineering and wound healing for chronic diabetic wounds.

11.2 PATHOPHYSIOLOGY AND MECHANISM OF DIABETIC AND CHRONIC WOUNDS

Diabetic wounds are more common in diabetic patients due to the combined effects of several contributing factors, including peripheral neuropathy, peripheral vascular disease, impaired infection response, and, in many cases, concurrent peripheral artery occlusive disease [9]. The most prevalent uncontrollable consequence of diabetes is peripheral neuropathy, which affects over 66% of people with the disease; patients with type 1 and type 2 diabetes are similarly impacted [10]. Neuropathy is caused by a number of causes, including myoinositol, protein kinase-C pathway activation, fatty acid metabolic problems, prediabetes neuropathy, and the production of glycated end products [9]. Not surprisingly, underlying neuropathy is the primary cause of foot ulcers in almost 60% of diabetes patients [9]. The polyol route has been described as one of the more often used mechanisms of action. When neuropathy develops, the hyperglycemic condition causes sorbitol dehydrogenase and aldose reductase to function more actively [9]. This causes intracellular glucose to be converted to fructose and sorbitol. Myoinositol production in nerve cells, which is necessary for regular neuron conduction, is reduced as a result of the buildup of these sugar products [9]. Furthermore, the chemical conversion of glucose causes the stocks of nicotinamide adenine dinucleotide phosphate to be depleted [9]. These stores are essential for the production of the vasodilator nitric oxide and for the detoxification of reactive oxygen species (ROS). As a result, the nerve cell experiences more oxidative stress and vasoconstriction, which will cause ischemia and further damage and death of the nerve cell. Inappropriate activation of protein kinase C and aberrant glycation of nerve cell proteins are also caused by hyperglycemia and oxidative stress, which further impair neuronal function and cause ischemia [9]. Neuropathy-affected diabetics display the nerve system's motor, sensory, and autonomic divisions. Involvement of the motor nerve: An imbalance of the long flexor and extensor tendons results from a loss of neural supply to the foot's intrinsic muscles [10]. Autonomic neuropathy: When diabetic neuropathy causes autonomic dysfunction in the foot, perspiration and oil gland function are lost [10]. Sensory neuropathy: Without the accompanying loss of protective sensation in the foot, the effects of the motor and autonomic neurological abnormalities would be much less pronounced [10].

Fifty percent of diabetic patients develop foot ulcers as a result of peripheral arterial disease (PAD), a chronic arterial occlusive atherosclerotic condition of the lower extremities that ranges in severity [10]. Sometimes ulcers begin with rest pain, tissue loss, and intermittent claudication. They can quickly develop into gangrene, which results in insufficient blood supply [9]. Vasodilators generated from the endothelium are reduced as a result, which causes constriction. Additionally, thromboxane A2, a vasoconstrictor and platelet aggregation agonist, rises in response to hyperglycemia in diabetes, increasing the risk of plasma hypercoagulability [9]. Stenosis of the arterial lumen may also result from changes in the vascular extracellular matrix (ECM) [9].

Around 15%–20% of foot ulcers are primarily ischemic ulcers with little to no accompanying neuropathy, and another 15%–20% have a mixed neuropathic–vascular etiology [10]. Endothelial damage, hyperlipidemia, elevated platelet viscosity and activity, and eventually the onset of atherosclerosis are all caused by hyperglycemia and related alterations in glucose metabolism [11]. Diabetics have a different distribution of lower extremity atherosclerotic disease than non-diabetics. It primarily affects the infra-geniculate leg arteries (posterior and anterior tibial arteries), with less frequent involvement of the femoropopliteal arterial segment (superficial femoral, popliteal). The aortoiliac artery segment is frequently spared with the development of diffuse tibial artery occlusive disease or more proximal arterial occlusion, and the foot's perfusion is below a level sufficient to preserve skin [11].

The main cause of morbidity and death in diabetic foot ulcers is infection [11], as summarized in Figure 11.1. Although diabetic foot infections can be caused by a variety of organisms, including simple cellulitis or limb infections, the most common cause of pathogenic and potentially fatal necrotizing fasciitis is Gram-positive cocci, particularly staphylococci (*Staphylococcus aureus*) [12]. Invasive tissue infection is facilitated by immunologic dysfunction brought on by periods of inadequate glycemic management, which also decreases leukocyte and complement function. A foot-threatening infection and sepsis can result from bacteria quickly penetrating deep into fascia when there is injured or inadequately perfused skin and soft tissues [11].

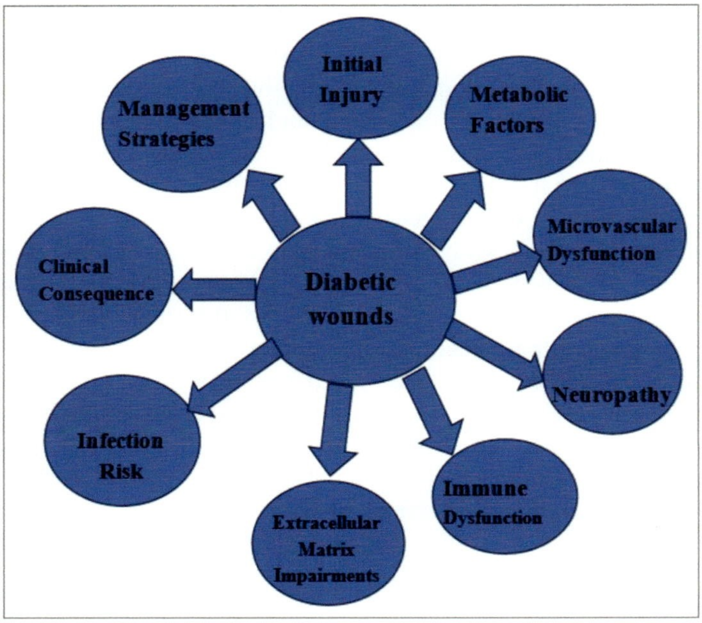

FIGURE 11.1 Various factors responsible for the diabetic wound progression [1, 7].

11.3 CAUSES, RISK FACTORS, CHARACTERISTICS, AND MONITORING OF DIABETIC AND CHRONIC WOUNDS

11.3.1 Causes of Diabetic and Chronic Wounds

The chronic process of wound healing is a complicated mechanism. The cellular and molecular impairment levels are poorly understood in diabetic wounds [3]. The endless efforts from the researchers to find the solitary therapeutic agent as a magic bullet for healing are still evolving. The causes of chronic wounds, such as hyperglycemia, peripheral sensory neuropathy, peripheral vascular ischemia, coronary artery disease, cerebrovascular disease, and obstructive vascular disease, are the primary factors of trauma [4, 7].

11.3.2 Risk Factors of Chronic and Diabetic Wound

Numerous risk factors, including co-morbidities such as cardiovascular illnesses, diabetic retinopathy, renal disease, nerve and/or vascular damage, and diabetic foot complications [5], impair the general health and well-being of each patient with DM. Chronic inflammation, hypoxia, peripheral neuropathy, PAD, poor angiogenesis, persistent hyperglycemia, and trouble battling infections are among the conditions unique to diabetic foot [5]. Defective foot structure and biomechanics, including high arch, subluxed metatarsophalangeal joints, and toe clawing, which results in excessive pressure, callus development, and ulcers [2]. Insufficient protective feeling that results in tiny injuries that go unnoticed due to excessive pressure, mechanical damage, or heat damage [1]. Atypical anatomy and biomechanics result in excessive pressure, particularly in the midplantar region [4]. Vascular insufficiency (arterial): deterioration of neutrophil delivery, wound healing, and tissue viability [4]. Hyperglycemia and other metabolic abnormalities: impaired fasting glucose and impaired glucose tolerance, high blood pressure, dyslipidemia, overweight and obesity, high waist circumference, excessive collagen cross-linking, impaired immunological activity, particularly neutrophil function, and wound healing [13]. The other risk factors include prior amputation of the lower extremities, an ulcer on the foot earlier, anatomical foot abnormality, inadequate glycemic management, obesity, the use of alcoholic beverages, and smoking [4].

11.3.3 Characteristics of Chronic and Diabetic Wound

The multiple factors in the chronic wound can delay the diabetic wound healing process in patients, making it extremely difficult to cure.

11.3.3.1 Hyperglycemia

The most common symptom of diabetes is hyperglycemia. In addition, the physiological environment of elevated glucose levels causes decreased levels of vascular endothelial GF (VEGF) and hypoxia-inducible factor 1α (HIF-1α), which in turn trigger the non-enzymatic glycosylation reaction of biological macromolecules, leading to the production of glycation end products [14].

11.3.3.2 Hypoxia

Due to peripheral vascular dysfunction, the diabetic wound does not receive enough oxygen, and the immune cells at the wound site consume a lot of oxygen during the inflammatory phase. The oxygen-deficient environment is made worse [14].

11.3.3.3 High ROS Level

Glycolytic metabolic disorders are characterized by the production of excessive ROS by the mitochondria of endothelial cells, which are hyperglycemia-sensitive cells. By interfering with proteins, phospholipids, and genetic materials, ROS also contributes to mitochondrial dysfunction and damage to cells [14].

11.3.3.4 pH

The hasty bacterial growth or the anaerobic environment is the cause of anaerobic glycolysis leading to the acidic diabetic wound, including biofilm [14].

11.3.4 Monitoring of Diabetic Wounds

The process of wound healing is dynamic, and ongoing wound diagnosis and monitoring, particularly for chronic wounds, are crucial. The four overlay stages of the wound healing process include temperature, humidity, pH, and glucose level fluctuations [6]. However, for long-time surveillance of diabetic patients, hospitalization is required with spontaneous screening and monitoring [15]. Numerous electrochemical sensors have been created for wound diagnostics; nevertheless, therapy and wound dressing cannot be completed simultaneously [15]. A significant advantage of contemporary wound care is the conductive dressing's ability to recognize changes in the wound and convert them into signals, allowing for synchronized wound treatment and monitoring. Thus, it has been possible to track the wound healing in real time by keeping an eye on changes in the indicators, including physiological signals [16].

11.4 IMMUNE SYSTEM MODULATED BY BIOMATERIALS

According to a 2021 International Diabetes Federation report, 463 million people worldwide will have diabetes, and by 2045, it's predicted that the number of diabetics could reach 700 million [5]. In that 19%–34% of the diabetic patients had shown a very poor wound healing process [5]. It is highly harmonized and precisely regulated for the preservation of skin barrier function, but the wound healing process has several complications like functional limitation and infections like cellulitis, abscess, gangrene, and 85% of them underwent amputation [11]. These injuries can significantly lower a patient's quality of life and death rate in comparison to a cancer patient [6]. These chronic wounds that don't heal are caused by a number of factors, such as age, diabetes, obesity, metabolic disorders, sensory neuropathies, autoimmune diseases, and cardiovascular issues. Gauze, bandages, and cotton wool are examples of classic wound dressings that barely fit open wounds and have ineffective wound healing properties [6].

Bacteria-infected wounds pose a serious threat to patients' lives and significantly lower their quality of life. They also place a significant financial strain on healthcare systems worldwide. Therefore, the development of biomaterials to treat bacterially infected wounds is urgently needed [17]. After several attempts from the researcher, an approach to treatment that has increasing promise because of the development of immunomodulatory biomaterials for macro and micro wound healing and clinical applications for the diabetic wound has been initiated [5]. An appropriate substance that would cover the wound to avoid infection has always been necessary for efficient wound healing. It is demonstrated that the biomaterials modulate immune responses, eliminate the risk of infection in the affected tissue, and restore the structure and function of the skin [8]. Nowadays, there are many different uses for biomaterials in the medical industry, including medication delivery systems, tissue engineering, and medical implants [8]. Their unique property of triggering the foreign body reaction in the inflammatory reaction upon implantation activates the immune system for integration and performance [6]. Modulating immune responses, controlling or accomplishing inflammation, and enhancing the overall biocompatibility, biodegradability, and hydrophilicity of implanted biomaterials are all possible through the proper selection of biomaterials with precise characteristics that are the ideal candidates for therapeutic applications [5].

Because of their comparable conductivity to human skin, strong antioxidant and antibacterial properties, electrically controlled drug delivery, and photothermal effect, conductive biomaterials based on conductive polymers, carbon nanomaterials, or conductive inorganic nanomaterials show great promise in wound healing and skin tissue engineering [8]. For tissue regeneration and repair, a variety of biomaterials, including hydrogels, scaffolds, and nanoparticles, have been widely employed. Despite playing distinct roles, they will only interact with the immune system, which affects their biological processes [18].

Biomaterials for wound healing might be synthetic, natural, or a mix of the two. A particular biomaterial serves as a framework for skin regeneration after it has been chosen. The scaffold enables the upregulation of specific molecular signaling pathways crucial for skin restoration when it is applied to a wound. Even though tissue engineering has advanced significantly, further study is required to validate the application of biomaterials for wound healing in clinical settings [5]. The ideal characteristic of the biomaterials for the management of diabetic wounds is shown below. First, it should exhibit superior biocompatibility and biodegradability to safeguard tissue restoration [5]. Second, it must produce a warm and humid atmosphere that promotes tissue repair [5]. Third, the dressing should prevent polymicrobial infections to ensure appropriate wound healing [5]. Finally, it should have sufficient porosity to facilitate gas exchange and promote neovascularization, cell migration, and proliferation [5]. In order to integrate multifunctionality, many natural and synthetic polymeric materials—such as chitosan, fibrin, gelatin, hyaluronic acid, alginate, cellulose, silk fibroin, polyethylene glycol, polycaprolactone, poly (lactic acid), poly (glycolic acid), polyvinyl alcohol, and polyurethane—are combined either by straightforward blending or cross-linking. These biomaterials exhibit a range of characteristics that are inherent to their constituents [6]. In addition to offering a strong platform for regulating and stimulating angiogenesis at the site of damage, biomaterials' physical and chemical characteristics also enable the regulation of temporal dynamics. Films, membranes, and fibers with a two-dimensional structure typically feature robust mechanical qualities, high oxygen permeability, and water resistance. Sponge, foam, and hydrogel with their 3D network and porous structure could absorb a lot of exudates, keep the air humid, and transport cells and bioactive substances [5]. Table 11.1 displays the claims made about various biomaterials and their function in the human body.

11.4.1 Type of Biomaterials

The components of biomaterials can be broadly divided into three categories: synthetic polymers, natural bioactive polymers, and natural inert polymers.

11.4.1.1 Natural Inert Polymers

Biomedical applications have made extensive use of natural polymers derived from plant, bacterial, fungal, or animal sources due to their biological characteristics, such as biocompatibility, biodegradability, and resemblance to macromolecules that cells recognize for biomedical purposes [19]. Microporosity, biodegradability, hemocompatibility, and biocompatibility make them one of the most widely utilized natural polymeric materials for wound healing because of their exceptional mechanical [19].

11.4.1.2 Natural Bioactive Polymers

Most notably, bioactive polymers actively treat one or more phases of wound healing. The most often used natural bioactive polymers in the wound healing process include collagen (including gelatin), hyaluronic acid, chitosan, and sodium alginate due to their biocompatibility and biodegradability [2].

11.4.1.3 Synthetic Polymers

The primary benefits of synthetic polymers are their adaptability to certain uses and characteristics by modifying their molecular weight, copolymerization, chemical composition, and crystallinity of polymers [2]. The synthetic polymers have found widespread usage in biomedical applications due to their adjustable properties like mechanical strength, non-toxic degradation, and processability [19]. The aliphatic polyesters have found widespread usage in the biomedical treatment due to their biodegradability [19].

TABLE 11.1
Biomaterials Classification with Their Roles in the Human Body, Advantages, Disadvantages, and Applications

Sl. No	Materials	Advantages	Disadvantages	Applications	References
1.	Metals and alloys (cobalt, steel, titanium, gold, platinum, and chromium)	High mechanical strength and suitability for load-bearing applications; good resistance to corrosion; and compatibility with imaging methods like X-rays	• Could result in stress shielding, which causes bone loss by absorbing stress on the implant rather than the surrounding bone • Limited capacity to encourage tissue repair	Plates, screws, pins, and orthopedic implants	[5, 6, 19]
2.	Composites (methyl methacrylate bone cement reinforced with carbon fiber, dental filling composites, and ultra-high molecular weight polyethylene)	Capable of simulating the characteristics of real tissues; adaptable mechanical qualities that combine the advantages of various materials. Compared to metals, it is more biocompatible and has the capacity to encourage tissue-regeneration	• Difficult fabrication procedures • Limited supply of biocompatible composite materials • Potential for matrix and reinforcement • Delamination or interface failure	Dental fillings, porous orthopedic implants, and rubber gloves and catheters	[5, 6, 19]
3.	Ceramics (glass, titanium and aluminum oxides, calcium phosphate salts, etc.)	Improved biocompatibility High hardness and strength Chemical stability and wear resistance Able to encourage bone regrowth	• Low tensile strength and poor toughness • Challenging to form a link with the surrounding tissues	Dental implants, bioactive orthopedic implants, and artificial hearing aids	[5, 6, 19]
4.	Polymers [PMMA, PLA, polycarbonates, polycaprolactone (PCL), and polyurethanes]	Easily fabricated and versatile; able to be customized to replicate the characteristics of genuine tissues Flexible and lightweight Tissue integration has strong biocompatibility	• Limited resistance to wear and deterioration; lower mechanical strength in comparison to metals and ceramics • The possibility of chemical leakage or degradation byproducts • In certain situations, it may result in immunological	Scaffolds for tissue engineering; drug delivery systems; and orthopedic and dental implants	[5, 6, 19]

11.4.2 Stimuli-Responsive Materials and Their Types for Diabetic Wound Healing

Nanotechnology has emerged as one of the most concentrated research topics for the treatment of diabetic patient, because of their tuned physicochemical properties, regulated size, and larger surface area for encapsulation of more active compounds to accelerate cell regeneration [20]. The nanoparticles can increase the accumulation of active substances and accelerate wound healing, making them the perfect and promising topical delivery for chronic diabetic wounds [18]. Drugs in nanotechnology-based drug delivery systems are either covalently bonded to the surface matrix of the nanoparticles or are absorbed, disseminated, or dissolved around the nanoparticle and confined in an aqueous core with shell-like surroundings. Diffusion, dissolution, reduction, and distension will all release the medications contained in the nanoparticles within the biological system [20]. There are many different kinds of biomaterials based on nanotechnology, including hydrogels, scaffolds, and nanoparticles. Nanofibers, foams, films, and nanocrystals found in nanoparticles have been widely exploited for tissue regeneration and repair [18].

11.4.3 Metal Nanoparticles and Applications

Compared to normal wound healing, the healing process of diabetic wounds is described as being more complicated and delayed. The development of a nanomaterial that can effectively stimulate the quick and full healing of diabetic wounds is therefore required. Furthermore, the material should be biocompatible, extremely non-toxic, and conducive to a humid climate [8]. The progression in nanobiotechnology leads to the development of metal nanoparticles (MNPs). These MNPs offer a number of benefits, including high purity, the appropriate shape, and structure and exhibit significant effects on diabetic wounds healing, due to their unique physical and chemical properties [8].

11.4.3.1 Gold Nanoparticles (AuNPs)

Small gold particles with dimensions ranging from 1 to 100 nm are known as gold nanoparticles, or AuNPs. They range in color from red to purple, depending on the size. Green AuNPs are made from an aqueous extract of *Acalypha indica* at low pressures, temperatures, and pH levels in order to avoid many negative effects and to function as a carrier [9]. At 100 µg/mL, it has strong antioxidant and antibacterial properties. Together, these have been used to provide GFs to the cells or even the nucleus of the wound site, promoting normal wound healing and lowering the risk of diabetic wound infection [21].

11.4.3.2 Silver Nanoparticles (AgNPs)

Silver nanoparticles (AgNPs), which are the most often utilized MNPs, are silver particles with a size range of 1–100 nm. They are antibacterial, anti-inflammatory, and free radical scavengers [10]. When AgNPs coordinate with electron-donating groups like amine, thiol, hydroxyl, etc., they can damage microbial cell membranes and stop enzyme, RNA, and DNA function, which kills the bacterium [22]. The mechanism of AgNPs' antibacterial activity is established by explaining their fallow ionic and colloidal forms. (1) The interaction of released $Ag+$ ions with the cell membrane disrupts membrane function, and (2) the production of ROS damages the cell membrane extensively, ultimately leading to oxidative stress-induced cell damage [23].

11.4.3.3 Copper Nanoparticles (CuNPs)

Since ancient times, copper and its complexes have been used as disinfectants to treat wounds and infections. Copper oxide nanoparticles (CuNPs) are a more affordable and accessible form of copper [1]. By decreasing cell–cell aggregation and matrix instability, CuNPs support the rehabilitation of bacterial lipopolysaccharides and enhance antibacterial membrane activity. More direct interactions between CuNPs and bacterial strains may result in increased membrane rupture and infiltration [2].

11.4.3.4 Zinc Nanoparticles (ZnNPs)

Zinc oxide nanoparticles (ZnONPs) are a metal oxide with n-type semiconducting properties. They have a number of properties, including high catalytic activity, semi-conductivity, optical activity, UV filtration, anti-inflammatory, antimicrobial, and wound healing qualities [8]. Zinc is an essential element that humans need for growth. ZnONPs affect healing by two mechanisms: (1) keratinocyte migration, which is aided by an enzyme complex cofactor, and (2) the formation of bacterial cell membrane perforations. It is therefore regarded as a promising metal oxide for the process of wound healing [8].

11.4.3.5 Titanium Dioxide Nanoparticles (TiNPs)

Unlike other MNPs, titanium dioxide nanoparticles (TiNPs) are not very harmful to healthy cells. The antibacterial properties of TiNPs are primarily attributed to TiO_2, which produces ROS that completely eradicates microorganisms [18]. When exposed to UV light, TiNPs photocatalyze and encourage platelets to proliferate in order to eradicate bacteria [18]. Additionally, through changes in their permeability, positively charged nanoparticles affect the growth and viability of bacteria [8].

11.4.3.6 Iron Nanoparticles (FeNPs)

The fourth most common element in MNPs is iron nanoparticles (FeNPs). Due to their small size, volumetric extent, and large surface area, FeNPs act as both independent antibacterial agents and as carriers and mediators of antibiotics [24]. They also have antibacterial effects on both Gram-positive and Gram-negative bacteria, produce ROS, and interfere with electron transport, which leads to the production of superoxide [8].

11.4.3.7 Cerium Oxide Nanoparticles (CeO_2NPs)

Recently, it has been discovered that ceria nanoparticles, for instance, in the form of colloid solutions, are effective at shielding living things from free radicals and ROS [25]. All biological activities, but especially those related to bacterial etiology, are known to involve ROS and free radicals [25]. Similar to other MNPs, cesium oxide nanoparticles (CeO_2NPs) exhibit broad-spectrum antibacterial activity [8].

11.4.4 2D or 3D Nanoparticles and Their Applications

11.4.4.1 2D Conductive Biomaterials for Wound Healing

Nanomaterials are categorized according to their dimensions, such as zero (0D), one (1D), two (2D), and three (3D). Recently, there has been a lot of interest in the biomedical application of 2D metallic nanomaterials [6]. It is the thinnest nanomaterial due to its thickness and dimensions on the nanoscale. It is recognized as one of the thinnest nanomaterials, a unique property. Their strong mechanical stability, large surface area, excellent electrical conductivity, and ideal photothermal response are inherent to their unique structural and interatomic layer interactions [13]. Even under intense stress circumstances, it can change shape, such as bending, in response to certain external forces without breaking [13]. In particular, 2DNMs are becoming more and more popular because of their strong antibacterial qualities, good biocompatibility, and effective photothermal conversion. Due to their ability to provide anti-inflammatory, antibacterial, antioxidative, angiogenic, and epithelialization-promoting properties, 2DNMs are extremely helpful in applications involving wound repair [26].

11.4.4.2 Film

Films are semipermeable, which allow water vapor and oxygen to flow through but inhibit a massive amount of liquids and bacteria from flowing through [6]. Film-based wound dressings are appropriate for thin wounds with slight exudates and sensitive skin because they are lightweight, flexible, and have a low capacity to absorb water [6]. Additionally, conductive materials and other bioactive chemicals can activate thin films as a matrix. In addition to being widely utilized to study how conductive materials alter cell activity in both in vitro and in vivo settings, conductive thin films also make it easier for them to be used in other, more elegant forms in the future [6].

11.4.4.3 Polypyrrole (PPy)

Polypyrrole (PPy) is synthesized using various oxidizing agents by chemical oxidative polymerization. Extra ion-doping capacity is desirable to load a clinically adequate number of medicines into PPy [27]. ES-free or ES-containing human cutaneous fibroblasts may be able to adhere, spread, and proliferate. Additionally, cell survival was considerably increased when the composite film was subjected to a direct electrical field strength of 100 mV/mm. They further investigated the network process by which PPy/PLLA Poly (l-lactic acid) film promotes wound healing [13]. By altering cytokines like IL-6 and IL-8, under ES mediation, human cutaneous fibroblast survival may be enhanced by the conductive PPy/PLLA film [13]. Additionally, PPy can be used to develop electronically controlled medication delivery and controlled drug delivery systems based on conductive polymer film, which facilitates wound healing by reacting to electrical impulses [27]. Conductive composite films based on PPy will promote wound healing without ES. Without the inclusion of PPy, numerous studies have shown that conductive film is an excellent way to enhance wound healing [6].

11.4.4.4 Poly (3,4-Ethylenedioxythiophene) (PEDOT)

One polythiophene derivative that improves cell adherence and proliferation is poly (3,4-ethylenedioxythiophene) (PEDOT) [6]. It also has greater thermal stability and stronger conductivity than PPy [8]. With a strong affinity for proteins like bovine serum albumin, PEDOT film demonstrated good electro-compatibility and electroactivity [28]. PEDOT–TOS film can be used as a wound dressing to improve and manage the persistence period of bovine aortic endothelial cells. It can also be improved by mixing it with PEDOT–TOS [26].

11.4.4.5 Polyaniline (PANI) and Aniline Oligomers

The most popular conducting polymer is polyaniline (PANI); however, because of its poor solubility and high infusibility, pure PANI-based conductive films were rarely used as wound dressing materials [6]. There are several attempts to get rid of this limitation, such as doping approaches with additives or forming a composite with another polymer matrix. The polymer matrix is a frequently used technique for of sustain drug delivery system [29]. Recently, the chitosan blends with PANI polymer matrix were prepared, due to its biodegradable, hemostatic, antimicrobial, and film-forming property. The optimized PANI was selected based on their conductivity for wound healing [29].

11.4.4.6 3D Conductive Biomaterials for Wound Healing

Although 2D conductive biomaterials have achieved remarkable success in wound healing by utilizing cell attachment, proliferation, differentiation, and a variety of other functions, there are still various structures, compositions, and interactions in wound healing that cannot be demonstrated in real life [6]. As a result, 3D biomaterials have drawn increased attention from researchers looking into the process of wound healing [6]. By combining the fields of cell biology and materials science, 3D biomaterials are being deposited layer by layer, enabling the production of new biological tools such as patient-specific scaffolds, cell-mimicking tissue-engineered 3D scaffolds, and communication-imitating ECM products [30]. In the context of wound care, 3D porous structures derived from bioresorbable, biodegradable, bioactive, and mechanically robust biomaterials that promote cell growth and proliferation, allow nutrients and oxygen to pass through, and encourage the formation of new tissue have emerged as a highly promising tool [31]. The 3D biomaterials with a highly interconnected porous structure show a number of benefits over 2D biomaterials, including sustained release profiles that can aid in healing [30].

11.4.4.7 Hydrogel

Hydrogel, is a gel substance that swell in aquatic scenery and has a high-water absorption capacity, a promising technique with enormous potential in the area of wound care [6], because of their three-dimensional network structure and high-water absorption, hydrogels can keep the site wet by reducing the rate of infection and accelerating the healing of wounds [32]. The main mechanisms of wound healing include moisturizing, absorption and drainage, promotion of healing, protection, and inflammation regulation [18]. First, in terms of moisturizing, hydrogel successfully maintains a moist environment on the wound surface moist, which helps to prevent dry skin by elevated blood sugar and encourage the development and revival of epithelial cells [32]. Second, in terms of drainage and absorption, hydrogel quickly takes up wound exudate and trap it inside the gel, lowering the chance of infection and preventing the recommendation of the wound surface [32]. Lastly, the active components in hydrogel have the ability to regulate inflammatory responses, lessening the intensity of inflammation and promoting wound healing and repair [18]. Additionally, hydrogel works to promote healing by containing a variety of active chemicals including GFs and antimicrobials, which prevent infection and inflammation while accelerating wound healing and supporting the repair of generation of new tissue [1]. Furthermore, hydrogel creates a gentle barrier that effectively blocks stimuli and contaminants, falling bacterial and viral raid, relives the pressure and friction surrounding the wound, and shields it from further damage [33]. In chronic wound by introducing the functional polymers or bioactive substances to hydrogels can precisely legalize the microenvironment [18].

11.4.4.8 pH-Responsive Polysaccharide Hydrogels

The hydrogel exhibits swelling based on the pH, with greatest amount of edema at pH 7 neutrality, which declines both in acidic and alkaline environment [1]. Furthermore, the composite hydrogel's young modulus was higher than that of actual human skin, according to the stress-strain curves, material stress concentration enhanced it tensile strength. Consequently, the finished composite material outperformed the normal human skin in terms of mechanical qualities [1]. The oscillation of pH is dependent on various factors like bacteria and their toxicity, tissue type, existence of proteases, angiogenesis procedure, release of oxygen, and the stage of the healing process [33]. The pH has impact on the healing process, it usually fluctuates between pH 4 and 6 as a result of growth of common bacteria like Both acute and chronic wounds require a pH of 7–9, and the presence of *Escherichia coli* and *S. aureus* [1]. The use of stimuli-responsive hydrogel in the hydrogel matrix for wound healing has increased interest. Imine, hydrazine, and arylhydrazone linkages are examples of Schiff bases that are frequently used in the manufacturing of pH-sensitive wound dressings [1].

11.4.4.9 Redox-Responsive Polysaccharide Hydrogels

Non-healing ulcers like chronic wound exhibit sever oxidative stress leads to the increased ROS level and diminished reduced redox potential and antioxidant content in the cells [1]. In the damaged and infected skin area, there is fluctuation of redox potential during healing progression. Disulfide bonds are frequently utilized, due to its reversible synthesis under oxidative and reductive circumstances, in the production of redox-responsive materials [5]. Redox-responsive hydrogel is created when amide bonds are formed between the amino groups of AED and the carboxylic acid groups of HA [34]. The resulting hydrogels were biocompatible and encouraged fibroblast growth and multiplication for seven days; however, in the presence of GSH, the hydrogels gradually disintegrated due to the fragmentation of disulfide connections at the cross-link junction [35]. Another ROS-responsive injectable hydrogel was developed for use as a wound dressing. The sodium alginate and pectin network hydrogels, which were crosslinked with calcium chloride, were combined with the zeolite imidazole framework-8 (ZIF-8) nanoparticles [1]. Applying the 10-aminoacid neuro peptide (substance P, SP) to ZIF-8 nanoparticles has been shown to promote the mobilization of CD29(+) stromal cells into the bloodstream, which speeds up wound healing and controls inflammation [1].

11.4.4.10 Photo-Responsive Polysaccharide Hydrogels

Photo-responsive hydrogels are a viable treatment option for bacterial infections throughout the wound-healing process [1]. The applied stimulus's spatiotemporal control, which in turn affects the hydrogels' mechanical characteristics and release profiles of encapsulated actives [12]. As a biomedical instrument, near infrared (NIR) light has several advantages, such as deep tissue penetration, minimal phototoxicity, and non-invasive treatment. In one technique, light may be transformed into heat, which could cause bacterial lysis in the targeted location [12]. In the in vitro method the *S. aureus* bacteria are repressed completely in the illuminated nanocomposite, and in vivo it shown effective of 95% of wound recovery. Additionally, the substance demonstrated injectability, adhesion, hemostatic, antioxidant, and self-healing qualities [12].

11.5 DUAL RESPONSIVE HYDROGELS PH AND TEMPERATURE-RESPONSIVE HYDROGELS OF POLYSACCHARIDES

Thermally responsive hydrogels have gained interest in the thermoresponsive drug-releasing system by triggering temperature change, there will be change in the gelation and swelling in the hydrogels [32]. This can be achieved in biomedical applications by raising the temperature from ambient to physiological [32]. However, scientist is also trying to measure temperature and pH simultaneously on a single hydrogel dressing [36]. Utilizing temperature and pH fluctuation to activate the thermoresponsive drug-releasing mechanism, the dressing not only tracks temperature change (35.0–40.0°C) and pH change (3.0–7.0), but it also demonstrates expectational antibacterial qualities based on test against *E. coli* and *S. aureus* [36]. The hybrid gel formulation utilized HPCH polysaccharide for the humid environment for the tissue regeneration and tannic acid (TA) for antimicrobial activity [37]. The above strategies were utilized in the formulation of in situ hydrogel, where they can be delivered in the solution form in minimally invasive manner, they instantly start the gelation when the temperature or pH is attained [37].

11.5.1 pH- and ROS-Responsive Polysaccharide Hydrogels

The Infected wound has acidic condition and high ROS concentration, for the management of infected wound formulated the dual responsive hydrogel like pH and ROS hydrogel [38]. The breaking of the boronic ester linkages caused the hydrogel to disassociate at high ROS concentrations and acidic conditions, which increased the release of the antibacterial and anti-inflammatory medication [33].

11.5.2 Polysaccharide Hydrogels that Respond to pH and Electricity

Recently, electric impulses have become a more appealing option for treating chronic wound. Electrical fields may be applied easily and precisely, making them a useful tool for wireless implant and medication delivery system [1]. The intelligent dual pH and electro-responsive polysaccharide hydrogel is based on a chitosan-g-polyaniline (CP) graft copolymer called as electro responsive material that combine intrinsic antibacterial capabilities and superior biocompatibility, among other advantage [39].

11.5.3 Scaffolds for Tissue Engineering

The term scaffold system generally refers to materials that can be implanted into various tissues and integrate with living tissues and cells [40]. A scaffold composed of biological materials that act as an artificial ECM is required to promote the growth and differentiation of seed cells [19]. The impact of the scaffold biomaterials on the immune system is currently thought to be the primary factor for tissue regeneration [18]. The development of biologically responsive scaffold that are accompanied by cells and multiple biomolecules that mimic the novel techniques used in skin regenerating treatments are primarily focused on the structure and biochemical cues of the natural ECM [19]. The scaffold facilitates cell adhesion, proliferation, and differentiation, scaffold biomaterials offer an appropriate environment. Their application in tissue engineering has been widely used [18]. For cells sown within or on the matrix, the biomaterial or matrix is essential for transmitting or transducing environmental stimuli [19]. In essence, the atmosphere helps to create physiologically viable, functioning tissue by serving as a translator between the mechanical environment and the growing tissue [19]. When the matrix decomposes into biocompatible fragments or monomers that the host cells can metabolize, it is usually advantageous, nevertheless, that rate of disintegration must be equal to or lower than the rate at which the tissue grows and develops [41]. In an effort to regenerate various body tissues and organs, a wide range of scaffolds made from diverse biomaterial and constructed using a multitude of fabrication technique have been employed in the field [10]. Regardless of the type of tissue, a number of important considerations must be made while developing or evaluating the scaffold's potential for use in tissue engineering [10]. Biocompatibility is the first and foremost, any scaffolds used in tissue engineering needs to be biocompatible; cells must adhere, function normally, migrate onto the scaffolds surface, eventually pass through it, and start to multiply before lying down new matrix [40]. Biodegradability is eventually, the implanted scaffold or tissue-engineered product should eventually be replaced by the body's own cells, which is the aim of tissue engineering [42].

Ideally speaking, the scaffold should be strong enough to permit surgical handling during implantation and ideally have mechanical characteristics compatible with the anatomical site into which it is to be placed [40]. This is significant for all tissues, but it presents some difficulties for cardiovascular and orthopedic applications specifically [40]. When trying to manufacture tissue to cartilage, one of the biggest hurdles is creating scaffold with sufficient mechanical characteristics [43]. In order for these tissues to operate from the moment of implantation until the remodeling process is finished, the scaffold implanted must possess adequate mechanical integrity [43]. The three main type of biomaterials utilized in scaffold application are natural, ceramics, and synthetic [44]. Porous scaffolds can be created by processing these naturally existing biomaterials after they have been extracted from their natural sources [44]. Due to their better biological response than synthetic scaffolds, biomimetic natural biopolymer scaffolds have recently gained importance for tissue scaffolds for tissue regeneration [45].

Fibrous scaffold also referred to as nanofibrous scaffolds (NFSs), fibrous scaffold is one of the adjuvant treatment modalities that has the highest potential to accelerate wound healing [6]. Although electrospun scaffolds are thought to be potential prospects for tissue engineering, several factors, including pore size and pore interconnectivity, still limit their use [40]. These factors have an impact on ingrowth of tissue and cellular infiltration into the scaffold. The use of nanofibers as wound dressing was not hampered by their small pore size, although their surface may have limited cell adhesion and growth [6]. Fibrous scaffolds are made from both natural and artificial biomaterials. Examples of these biomaterials include collagen, gelatin, hyaluronic, chitosan, silk, PLGA, PCL, PEVA, and PLA [44]. One popular method for functionalizing nanofibrous materials is the mixing process. Particularly for diabetics, the addition of several bioactive substances to polymer-based dressings has demonstrated encouraging outcomes in wound care and healing [46]. The most popular method for wound healing is electrospinning, which may be used to create NFS with pore structures that are linked. This strategy has the capacity to be used in cartilage tissue engineering [44].

11.5.3.1 Porous Scaffold

3D porous scaffolds with homogenous linked pore networks and high porosities have been frequently used in tissue engineering [44]. In tissue engineering applications, such as organ vascularization, host tissue development, and home regeneration, the spongy or foam porous form has been used [44]. Every cell and tissue had a varied pore size. Microsphere sintering, solvent casting, gas foaming, melt molding, and salt leaching (pyrogen leaching), are some of the fabrication techniques that can be used to create a porous scaffold. Recently advanced in electrospinning have produced a new technique that uses nano- and micro-scale biodegradable fibers to (1) establish a place for the cells' ECM. (2) improve nutrient transport to the center by using the porous interconnecting network channel (3) maintain cell cluster sizes within the foam's pore size to aid in preventing the formation of necrotic centers.

11.5.3.2 Rapid Prototyping Scaffold

Customized scaffolding, is another name for rapid prototyping scaffold. It is made utilizing a design methodology known as computer-aided design (CAD) [44]. The computer system typically helps with design conception, analysis, optimization, and modification. A variety of fabrication techniques, including stereolithography, membrane lamination, organ printing, 3D printing, selective laser sintering, and fused deposition modelling, can be utilized to create rapid prototyping scaffolds [44]. The 3D printing technique has been applied to bone marrow stem cells using PLA and PGA. Cell infiltration of the scaffold and high cellular compatibility were noted in the study [47]. Additionally, the study demonstrated how the technique might be used to fix abnormalities in the craniomaxillofacial bones [47].

11.5.3.3 Hydrogel Scaffold

Hydrogels are made of chains of polymers that swell in an aqueous solution and can be either natural or artificial [44]. Because of their high-water content, they are generally biocompatible because they don't trigger inflammation or an immunological reaction [5]. Hydrogel scaffolds are manufactured using a variety of fabrication processes, including solvent casting, gas foaming, microfluidics, copolymerization/crosslinking, and freeze drying. Injectable hydrogels are also useful for cosmetic surgery and the treatment of irregularly shaped deformities [5]. The hydrogel scaffolds have properties that are comparable to those of natural tissues, their usage in tissues has drawn attention [44]. Their composition consists of both synthetic biomaterials like PLA and PEG and their variations and natural biomaterials like collagen, alginate, gelatin, chitosan, fibrinogen, and hyaluronic acid [46]. On the whole; hydrogel scaffold dressings are intended to ameliorate a number of characteristics of infected diabetic wounds. The majority of hydrogel scaffolds administered several components simultaneously for wound healing rather than in a precisely timed sequential manner [46].

11.6 STIMULI-RESPONSIVE DRUG DELIVERY STRATEGIES

11.6.1 Endogenous Systems Respond to Stimuli pH-Responsive Therapeutic Systems

Wound infection is one of the most common problems in diabetes people. Because of the pathogen's interaction with the host tissue, an acidic microenvironment develops in the infected wound [14]. Numerous acid-sensitive systems were created for the treatment of infected wounds by utilizing this trait [14]. Because of their viscosity, the hydrogel therapeutic systems can stick to the wound's surface, making it easier to apply medications. In order to prevent secondary wound infection, a hydrogel simultaneously serves as an artificial skin. Consequently, majority of acid-responsive medicinal formulations are hydrogels [48].

11.6.2 Redox Stress-Responsive Therapeutic Systems

The primary cause of persistent wounds that do not heal, is an imbalance in tissue redox homeostasis brought on by excessive oxidative stress and malfunctioning antioxidant systems [16]. Several stages of wound healing are significantly regulated by ROS. In fact, preventing external damage necessitates low ROS levels [16]. Chronic diabetes wounds are found in a physiological milieu that is highly oxidized, according to current findings. To restructure the severely oxidized wound, antibacterial nano enzyme agents with ROS-scavenging capabilities were added [14].

11.6.3 Hypoxia-Responsive Therapeutic Systems

Diabetic wounds and solid tumors both exhibit a hypoxic environment. Currently, the majority of hypoxia-responsive therapeutic systems are designed to treat cancer [14]. To load hypoxia-activated antimicrobial metronidazole, for instance, hyaluronic acid nanocarriers are used [16]. The carriers in infected wounds were broken down to release metronidazole, which was subsequently further activated by hypoxic diabetic wounds. Additionally, photodynamic therapy may make the hypoxic situation worse [16].

11.6.4 Enzyme-Responsive Therapeutic Systems

The enzyme-responsive therapeutic systems include gelatinase-responsive therapeutic system, hyaluronidase-responsive therapeutic system, and matrix metalloproteinase (MMP)-responsive therapeutic systems [14].

11.6.5 Enzyme-Responsive Therapeutic Systems

Methicillin-intolerant diabetic wound infections can be caused by *S. aureus* (MRSA), a common and persistent bacterium in the clinic [14]. According to recent studies, MRSA may oversecrete gelatinase. This occurrence led to the development of AuNS-Apt-Cy, a gelatinase-responsive photo-thermostatic nano reagent, for the management of diabetic wounds with MRSA infections [49]. The catalytic treatment can be used to eliminate germs by turning H_2O_2 into a more toxic form by using the peroxidase-like activity of nanozymes [14]. However, the alkaline environment and minimal H_2O_2 in the diabetic infected tissue site did not support the catalytic process that resembled an enzyme. In order to address these issues, a bacterial sterilization triggerable nanozyme capsule for hyaluronidase (APGH) was created [14]. MMPs are a family of enzymes that are involved in many processes, including cancer, and are often used as therapeutic targets and cancer biomarkers. As ECM hydrolases, MMPs are essential for controlling cell migration, proliferation, and ECM reconstruction [14].

11.6.6 Exogenous Stimuli-Responsive Systems

11.6.6.1 Photo-Responsive Medical Devices

The last ten years have seen a significant increase in interest in the fight against bacterial infections due to the high controllability and potent antibacterial activity of photo-antimicrobial therapy, which encompasses photothermal and photodynamic antibacterial approaches, against drug-resistant bacteria [14]. The practice of producing physical heat with photothermal agents upon light irradiation, known as photothermal treatment (PTT), offers the most alluring substitute for existing antibiotic therapy in terms of bacterial elimination [49]. Using photothermal antibacterial therapy, which is a non-invasive and selective therapeutic approach. Pathogen integrity can be destroyed by transforming photoenergy into heat [15]. More importantly, photothermal antibacterial therapy has been extensively used in the eradication of bacterial biofilms because it may destroy the proteins, polysaccharides, and nucleic acids that are biofilm active in order to upset the structure of mature biofilms [15]. In addition to their antibacterial properties, photothermal agents can be used as carriers to control how harmful substances are released. Nanocomposites of silver and photothermal agents are now being researched for bimodal antibacterial therapy [14]. Potential therapeutic strategy for the inactivation of infections, the photodynamic antimicrobial therapy has been used to destroy bacterial biofilms due to its strong antibacterial activity and low drug resistance. Nevertheless, have matching drawbacks that keep them from being used further [14]. A popular technique for eliminating bacterial biofilms was established, photodynamic treatment (PDT) is based on photosensitizers (PS) and offers several benefits, such as remote control, optimal precision, and deeper tissue penetration depth [50]. Benign gold-silver core-shell nanoparticles (TBO-chit-Au-Ag NPs) co-functionalized with toluidine blue and chitosan were created as a PDT for infected diabetic foot ulcers [5]. Addition of 5.4-octyl itaconate (4OI) to the surface of BP nanosheets gave them anti-inflammatory and antioxidant characteristics. A gelatin methacryloyl (GelMA) hydrogel was then modified to contain 4OI functionalized black phosphorus for the treatment of diabetic wound infection [14].

11.6.6.2 Magnetic-Responsive Therapeutic Systems

The development of biofilm at the wound site enhances the pathogens' resistance to antibacterial agents and the body's immune system because of the extracellular polymeric matrix's shielding qualities, which further fuels chronic infection. Therefore, it is imperative to employ innovative treatment strategies. Recently, the hydrogel with adjustable bioactive activity was found to have promising potential for use in the removal of infections and biofilms [50]. For example, to eradicate biofilms, for instance, a magnetite iron oxide (Fe_3O_4)/chitin gel nanocomposite was created [27].

11.6.6.3 Dual-Responsive Therapeutic Systems

11.6.6.3.1 Redox-Responsive and pH-Responsive Therapeutic Systems

The pair of most prevalent elements that promote wound healing are pH and redox, as the infected diabetic lesion has an acidic and oxidative environment [14]. To achieve tailored medication release, redox-activated antibacterial systems, also known as pH systems, have been extensively studied [51]. By combining these features, a pH or H_2O_2-responsive hydrogel system was created that produces oxygen (O_2), manages hyperglycemia, eliminates pathogens, and scavenges ROS to change the unfavorable diabetic wounds' microenvironment [51].

11.6.6.3.2 pH or Photo-Responsive Therapeutic Systems

Many studies have looked into using pH or photo-activated therapeutic systems to treat bacterial infections and cancers. Several theragnostic systems with pH or photo-responsive activity are produced by combining a pH-activated section with phototherapeutic chemicals [51]. They function by inhibiting the development of *Pseudomonas aeruginosa* and *S. aureus* biofilms, and by reducing pro-inflammatory cytokine levels, they hasten the healing of diabetic wounds. For instance, TNF-α, IL-6, and IL-1β [14].

11.6.6.3.3 Photo/Magnetic-Responsive Therapeutic Systems

The magnetic field is another external stimulus that is used in conjunction with the light stimulus. Recently, some photo- or magnetic dual-responsive devices have been used as targeted therapeutic agents to treat deep diabetic infected wounds [14].

11.6.6.3.4 Enzyme/Thermo-Responsive Therapeutic Systems

In order to cure cancer and bacterial infections, enzyme or thermoresponsive therapy methods have been employed. Curcumin was applied to diabetic wounds using the MMP9/thermo dual-stimuli hydrogel [14]. This therapeutic approach was developed by coating curcumin nanoparticles (CNPs) with gelatin to enhance their bioavailability and multifunctional bioactivity, which would enable CNPs@GMs to react to MMP9. Following that, CNPs@GMs were incorporated [40]. The experiment's findings demonstrated that CNPs@GMs or hydrogel with enhanced antioxidant and cell migration activity might significantly speed up the healing of diabetic wounds. Additionally, due to curcumin's antibacterial properties, the CNPs@GMs/hydrogel can be used to treat diabetic wounds [40].

11.7 CLINICAL RESPONSES OF BIOMATERIALS

Applying biomaterials as wound dressings is one promising therapeutic strategy for addressing the challenging macro and micro wound environment of individuals with DM [5]. Biomaterials have long been linked to unique hydrophilicity, biodegradability, biocompatibility, and flexibility, making them ideal for therapeutic uses in the context of wound healing [5]. All things considered, these GFs aid in coordinating and accelerating the healing process. Synthetic biomaterial scaffolds may help deliver GFs to wounds, promoting tissue regeneration [45]. A variety of applications for synthetic polymers have been found in wound healing, including scaffolds that efficiently speed up the healing process, drug delivery, and GF delivery systems, coils for aneurysms, and suture material [52]. Because they can keep the wound bed wet and provide protection, biomaterials are being used in clinical settings to treat wounds as wound dressings [53]. The possibility of treating human wounds with natural-based biomaterial solutions has been bolstered by a few clinical investigations [52]. As stated earlier, naturally derived biomaterials have demonstrated potential for use as biological wound dressings because of their inherent qualities, such as hemostatic control and biocompatibility, as well as their capacity to be functionalized or altered to incorporate into medications to produce a bioactive dressing [54]. Prolonged infections are a sign that a wound has entered the chronic phase. However, it is not advised to use antibiotics topically until severe bacterial colonization is discovered, as a result of delayed allergic reactions, poor healing, high levels of antibiotic resistance, and superinfection [13]. The development of artificial skin grafts and wound dressing solutions utilizing natural biomaterial matrices supplemented with medication particles (antibacterial and antimicrobial) is an emerging trend in biomaterial engineering because it is impractical to include antibiotics into the biomaterial structure [53].

11.8 CONCLUSION

Numerous studies have been conducted recently on biomaterials and their natural qualities as wound dressings for chronic diabetic lesions. Although many materials are being investigated in pre- and clinical trials, only a small number of biomaterial-based treatment approaches have effectively made it to the market. Multidisciplinary teams must work together to provide more effective treatment alternatives in order to close the gap between research and clinical application. Furthermore, to effectively demonstrate the effectiveness of innovative biomaterial-based therapy techniques, future research must incorporate more precise models of non-healing diabetic foot ulcers. In order to improve diabetic wound repair and skin reconstruction, the majority of documented bioactive dressings primarily rely on the activity of loaded biologic agents; the intrinsic pro-healing qualities of biomaterials are comparatively underemphasized. The creation of potent bioactive biomaterials for novel treatments of persistent diabetic ulcers is desperately needed. Together with the rapid advancement of biomaterial technology, the analysis in this paper raises cautious hopes for a breakthrough that could allow diabetic wounds to mend regeneratively and offer a much-needed remedy for persistent diabetic ulcers.

Declaration of AI and AI-Assisted Technologies

During the preparation of this work, the authors used QuillBot AI and Grammarly in order to paraphrase the sentences. After using this tool, the authors reviewed and edited the content as needed and take full responsibility for the content of the publication.

REFERENCES

1. Psarrou M, Mitraki A, Vamvakaki M, Kokotidou C. Stimuli-responsive polysaccharide hydrogels and their composites for wound healing applications. Polymers. 2023 Feb 16;15(4):986.
2. Boateng J, Catanzano O. Advanced therapeutic dressings for effective wound healing—A review. Journal of Pharmaceutical Sciences. 2015 Nov 1;104(11):3653–80.
3. Patel S, Srivastava S, Singh MR, Singh D. Mechanistic insight into diabetic wounds: Pathogenesis, molecular targets and treatment strategies to pace wound healing. Biomedicine & Pharmacotherapy. 2019 Apr 1;112:108615.
4. Dissemond J, Romanelli M. Inflammatory skin diseases and wounds. British Journal of Dermatology. 2022 Aug 1;187(2):167–77.
5. Da Silva J, Leal EC, Carvalho E, Silva EA. Innovative functional biomaterials as therapeutic wound dressings for chronic diabetic foot ulcers. International Journal of Molecular Sciences. 2023 Jun 8;24(12):9900.
6. Yu R, Zhang H, Guo B. Conductive biomaterials as bioactive wound dressing for wound healing and skin tissue engineering. Nano-Micro Letters. 2022 Dec;14(1):1.
7. Gupta S, Andersen C, Black J, de Leon J, Fife C, Lantis Ii JC, Niezgoda J, Snyder R, Sumpio B, Tettelbach W, Treadwell T, Weir D, Silverman RP. Management of chronic wounds: Diagnosis, preparation, treatment, and follow-up. Wounds: A Compendium of Clinical Research and Practice. 2017;29(9):S19–S36.

8. Zheng Q, Chen C, Liu Y, Gao J, Li L, Yin C, Yuan X. Metal nanoparticles: Advanced and promising technology in diabetic wound therapy. International Journal of Nanomedicine. 2024 Dec 31:965–92.
9. Clayton W Jr, Elasy TA. A review of the pathophysiology, classification, and treatment of foot ulcers in diabetic patients. Clinical Diabetes. 2009 Apr 1;27(2):52–8.
10. Bowering CK. Diabetic foot ulcers. Pathophysiology, assessment, and therapy. Canadian Family Physician. 2001 May 1;47(5):1007–16.
11. Bandyk DF. The diabetic foot: Pathophysiology, evaluation, and treatment. Seminars in vascular surgery 2018 Jun 1 (Vol. 31, No. 2–4, pp. 43–48). WB Saunders.
12. Yang N, Zhu M, Xu G, Liu N, Yu C. A near-infrared light-responsive multifunctional nanocomposite hydrogel for efficient and synergistic antibacterial wound therapy and healing promotion. Journal of Materials Chemistry B. 2020;8(17):3908–17.
13. Fadilah NI, Maarof M, Motta A, Tabata Y, Fauzi MB. The discovery and development of natural-based biomaterials with demonstrated wound healing properties: A reliable approach in clinical trials. Biomedicines. 2022 Sep 8;10(9):2226.
14. Hu Y, Li H, Lv X, Xu Y, Xie Y, Yuwen L, Song Y, Li S, Shao J, Yang D. Stimuli-responsive therapeutic systems for the treatment of diabetic infected wounds. Nanoscale. 2022;14(36):12967–83.
15. McLister A, McHugh J, Cundell J, Davis J. New developments in smart bandage technologies for wound diagnostics. Advanced Materials. 2016 Jul;28(27):5732–7.
16. Jia Z, Gong J, Zeng Y, Ran J, Liu J, Wang K, Xie C, Lu X, Wang J. Bioinspired conductive silk microfiber integrated bioelectronic for diagnosis and wound healing in diabetes. Advanced Functional Materials. 2021 May;31(19):2010461.
17. Gaumet M, Vargas A, Gurny R, Delie F. Nanoparticles for drug delivery: The need for precision in reporting particle size parameters. European Journal of Pharmaceutics and Biopharmaceutics. 2008 May 1;69(1):1–9.
18. Nakkala JR, Li Z, Ahmad W, Wang K, Gao C. Immunomodulatory biomaterials and their application in therapies for chronic inflammation-related diseases. Acta Biomaterialia. 2021 Mar 15;123:1–30.
19. Norouzi M, Boroujeni SM, Omidvarkordshouli N, Soleimani M. Advances in skin regeneration: Application of electrospun scaffolds. Advanced Healthcare Materials. 2015 Jun;4(8):1114–33.
20. Haldorai Y, Shim JJ. Novel chitosan-TiO2 nanohybrid: Preparation, characterization, antibacterial, and photocatalytic properties. Polymer Composites. 2014 Feb;35(2):327–33.
21. Boomi P, Ganesan R, Prabu Poorani G, Jegatheeswaran S, Balakumar C, Gurumallesh Prabu H, Anand K, Marimuthu Prabhu N, Jeyakanthan J, Saravanan M. Phyto-engineered gold nanoparticles (AuNPs) with potential antibacterial, antioxidant, and wound healing activities under in vitro and in vivo conditions. International Journal of Nanomedicine. 2020 Oct 7;15:7553–68.
22. Shi G, Chen W, Zhang Y, Dai X, Zhang X, Wu Z. An antifouling hydrogel containing silver nanoparticles for modulating the therapeutic immune response in chronic wound healing. Langmuir. 2018 Aug 7;35(5):1837–45.
23. Vimbela GV, Ngo SM, Fraze C, Yang L, Stout DA. Antibacterial properties and toxicity from metallic nanomaterials. International Journal of Nanomedicine. 2017 May 24:3941–65.
24. Li X, Wei J, Aifantis KE, Fan Y, Feng Q, Cui FZ, Watari F. Current investigations into magnetic nanoparticles for biomedical applications. Journal of Biomedical Materials Research Part A. 2016 May;104(5):1285–96.
25. Zholobak NM, Ivanov VK, Shcherbakov AB. Interaction of nanoceria with microorganisms. In Nanobiomaterials in antimicrobial therapy 2016 Jan 1 (pp. 419–450). William Andrew Publishing.
26. Gumus A, Califano JP, Wan AM, Huynh J, Reinhart-King CA, Malliaras GG. Control of cell migration using a conducting polymer device. Soft Matter. 2010;6(20):5138–42.
27. Shi G, Zhang Z, Rouabhia M. The regulation of cell functions electrically using biodegradable polypyrrole–polylactide conductors. Biomaterials. 2008 Oct 1;29(28):3792–8.
28. Del Valle LJ, Aradilla D, Oliver R, Sepulcre F, Gamez A, Armelin E, Alemán C, Estrany F. Cellular adhesion and proliferation on poly (3, 4-ethylenedioxythiophene): Benefits in the electroactivity of the conducting polymer. European Polymer Journal. 2007 Jun 1;43(6):2342–9.
29. Dong R, Ma PX, Guo B. Conductive biomaterials for muscle tissue engineering. Biomaterials. 2020 Jan 1;229:119584.
30. He J, Shi M, Liang Y, Guo B. Conductive adhesive self-healing nanocomposite hydrogel wound dressing for photothermal therapy of infected full-thickness skin wounds. Chemical Engineering Journal. 2020 Aug 15;394:124888.
31. Mir M, Ali MN, Barakullah A, Gulzar A, Arshad M, Fatima S, Asad M. Synthetic polymeric biomaterials for wound healing: A review. Progress in Biomaterials. 2018 Mar;7(1):1–21.

32. Klouda L. Thermoresponsive hydrogels in biomedical applications: A seven-year update. European Journal of Pharmaceutics and Biopharmaceutics. 2015 Nov 1;97:338–49.
33. Hu C, Zhang F, Long L, Kong Q, Luo R, Wang Y. Dual-responsive injectable hydrogels encapsulating drug-loaded micelles for on-demand antimicrobial activity and accelerated wound healing. Journal of Controlled Release. 2020 Aug 10;324:204–17.
34. Gao Z, Golland B, Tronci G, Thornton PD. A redox-responsive hyaluronic acid-based hydrogel for chronic wound management. Journal of Materials Chemistry B. 2019;7(47):7494–501.
35. Wu C, Belenda C, Leroux JC, Gauthier MA. Interplay of chemical microenvironment and redox environment on thiol–disulfide exchange kinetics. Chemistry–A European Journal. 2011 Aug 29;17(36):10064–70.
36. Wang S, Zheng H, Zhou L, Cheng F, Liu Z, Zhang H, Wang L, Zhang Q. Nanoenzyme-reinforced injectable hydrogel for healing diabetic wounds infected with multidrug resistant bacteria. Nano Letters. 2020 Jun 23;20(7):5149–58.
37. Kaczmarek B. Tannic acid with antiviral and antibacterial activity as a promising component of biomaterials—A minireview. Materials. 2020 Jul 20;13(14):3224.
38. Li Y, Ding X, Hu H, Xu F-J. Stimulus-responsive polysaccharide-based hydrogels: From design to biomedical applications. Precision Medicine and Engineering. 2024;1(1): 100001
39. Aghajani M, Garshasbi HR, Naghib SM, Mozafari MR. 3D printing of hydrogel polysaccharides for biomedical applications: A review. Biomedicines. 2025;13(3):731.
40. Zhao Y, Li Z, Song S, Yang K, Liu H, Yang Z, Wang J, Yang B, Lin Q. Skin-inspired antibacterial conductive hydrogels for epidermal sensors and diabetic foot wound dressings. Advanced Functional Materials. 2019 Aug;29(31):1901474.
41. Qu J, Zhao X, Ma PX, Guo B. Injectable antibacterial conductive hydrogels with dual response to an electric field and pH for localized “smart” drug release. Acta Biomaterialia. 2018 May 1;72:55–69.
42. O’brien FJ. Biomaterials & scaffolds for tissue engineering. Materials Today. 2011 Mar 1;14(3):88–95.
43. Altman GH, Diaz F, Jakuba C, Calabro T, Horan RL, Chen J, Lu H, Richmond J, Kaplan DL. Silk-based biomaterials. Biomaterials. 2003 Feb 1;24(3):401–16.
44. Babensee JE, Anderson JM, McIntire LV, Mikos AG. Host response to tissue engineered devices. Advanced drug delivery reviews. 1998 Aug 3;33(1–2):111–39.
45. Hutmacher DW. Scaffolds in tissue engineering bone and cartilage. Biomaterials. 2000 Dec 15; 21(24):2529–43.
46. Alaribe FN, Manoto SL, Motaung SC. Scaffolds from biomaterials: Advantages and limitations in bone and tissue engineering. Biologia. 2016;71(4):353–66.
47. Berkland C, King M, Cox A, Kim KK, Pack DW. Precise control of PLG microsphere size provides enhanced control of drug release rate. Journal of Controlled Release. 2002 Jul 18;82(1):137–47.
48. Tran RT, Naseri E, Kolasnikov A, Bai X, Yang J. A new generation of sodium chloride porogen for tissue engineering. Biotechnology and Applied Biochemistry. 2011 Sep;58(5):335–44.
49. Kaihara S, Matsumura S, Fisher JP. Synthesis and characterization of cyclic acetal based degradable hydrogels. European Journal of Pharmaceutics and Biopharmaceutics. 2008 Jan 1;68(1):67–73.
50. Khafajah Y, Shaheen M, El Natour D, Merheb M, Matar R, Borjac J. Neuroprotective effects of zinc oxide nanoparticles in a rotenone-induced mouse model of Parkinson’s disease. Nanotheranostics. 2024 Jun 8;8(4):497.
51. Du X, Wang W, Wu C, Jia B, Li W, Qiu L, Jiang P, Wang J, Li YQ. Enzyme-responsive turn-on nanoprobes for in situ fluorescence imaging and localized photothermal treatment of multidrug-resistant bacterial infections. Journal of Materials Chemistry B. 2020;8(33):7403–12.
52. Zou L, Hu D, Wang F, Jin Q, Ji J. The relief of hypoxic microenvironment using an O2 self-sufficient fluorinated nanoplatform for enhanced photodynamic eradication of bacterial biofilms. Nano Research. 2022 Feb;15(2):1636–44.
53. Korupalli C, Li H, Nguyen N, Mi FL, Chang Y, Lin YJ, Sung HW. Conductive materials for healing wounds: Their incorporation in electroactive wound dressings, characterization, and perspectives. Advanced Healthcare Materials. 2021 Mar;10(6):2001384.
54. Schneider A, Garlick JA, Egles C. Self-assembling peptide nanofiber scaffolds accelerate wound healing. PLoS One. 2008 Jan 9;3(1):e1410.

12 Stimuli-Responsive Biomaterials for Imaging Modalities and Diagnosing Inflammatory Disorders

Aathira Sujathan Nair, and Amrita Muralikrishnan
School of Pharmacy, Monash University Malaysia,
Subang Jaya, Selangor, Malaysia

Sunil Kumar Sah
Department of Pharmaceutics,
National Institute of Pharmaceutical Education and Research (NIPER),
Kolkata, West Bengal, India

Bijo Mathew
Department of Pharmaceutical Chemistry, Amrita School of Pharmacy,
Amrita Vishwa Vidyapeetham, AIMS Health Science Campus, Kochi, India

12.1 INTRODUCTION

Acute inflammatory conditions like sepsis and autoimmune diseases like rheumatoid arthritis and inflammatory bowel disease are examples of inflammatory disorders that frequently involve complex biochemical and physiological changes, such as changes in pH, enzyme activity, temperature, and oxidative stress [1]. While effective, traditional imaging and diagnostic approaches often lack the specificity and responsiveness necessary to detect dynamic changes in the inflammatory microenvironment. Early and accurate diagnosis of inflammation is essential to improving patient outcomes and halting the progression of the disease [2]. A novel class of materials known as stimuli-responsive biomaterials has been developed to react to biochemical signals in the body. These materials are ideal for diagnostic imaging applications because they dynamically alter their chemical or physical characteristics in response to internal or external stimuli. These materials allow for targeted, non-invasive, real-time monitoring of inflammatory processes by integrating with many imaging modalities, including fluorescence imaging, positron emission tomography (PET), and magnetic resonance imaging (MRI). Smart materials, often referred to as stimulus-responsive biomaterials, are designed to alter in a regulated and reversible way in response to stimuli [3]. These stimuli fall into the following categories:

- *Internal stimuli*: pH, temperature, enzyme activity, oxidative stress, hypoxia, and biomolecular interactions which involve both protein–protein and protein–DNA interactions.
- *External stimuli*: Light, ultrasound, magnetic fields, and electric fields.

These biomaterials are extremely useful for imaging and diagnostics because of their capacity to respond to the biochemical environment. For instance, inflammatory tissues, which usually

DOI: 10.1201/9781003560203-12

have acidic microenvironments, can be seen with the use of pH-responsive materials. Likewise, disease-specific enzymatic activity may be detected using enzyme-sensitive materials, allowing for accurate inflammatory localization [4]. Early uses of stimuli-responsive biomaterials were centered on medication delivery devices, and the idea came from the larger subject of biomaterials engineering. These materials growth into the fields of imaging and diagnostics has been accelerated by advancements in bioengineering, polymer chemistry, and nanotechnology. With advancements in material science and imaging technology, the integration of stimuli-responsive biomaterials into imaging modalities has opened new possibilities for early disease detection, real-time monitoring, and personalized medicine [5]. Localized biochemical and physiological alterations are common features of inflammatory illnesses, and they can be difficult to identify using standard imaging methods. In this regard, stimuli-responsive biomaterials provide the following benefits: improved sensitivity and specificity of drug delivery in controlled manner and minimize the side effects by maintain the healthy tissues. These substances react to biomarkers unique to an illness, increasing the precision of diagnosis [6]. Targeted imaging: They reduce background noise and off-target effects by concentrating just at inflammatory areas. Real-time monitoring: Variations in biomaterial characteristics over time reveal information on how inflammation develops [7]. Non-invasive diagnostics: By enabling non-invasive imaging, several of these materials lessen the need for invasive treatments like biopsies [8]. The MRI contrast compounds can be used to detect inflammatory tissues in diseases like arthritis because they activate in acidic environments. Likewise, fluorescence-based sensors that react to reactive oxygen species (ROS) shed light on the inflammation linked to oxidative stress in neurodegenerative illnesses [9].

The integration of stimuli-responsive biomaterials with advanced imaging modalities represents a paradigm shift in the diagnosis of inflammatory disorders. These materials have the potential to transform clinical practice by enabling precise, real-time, and non-invasive disease monitoring [10]. As research

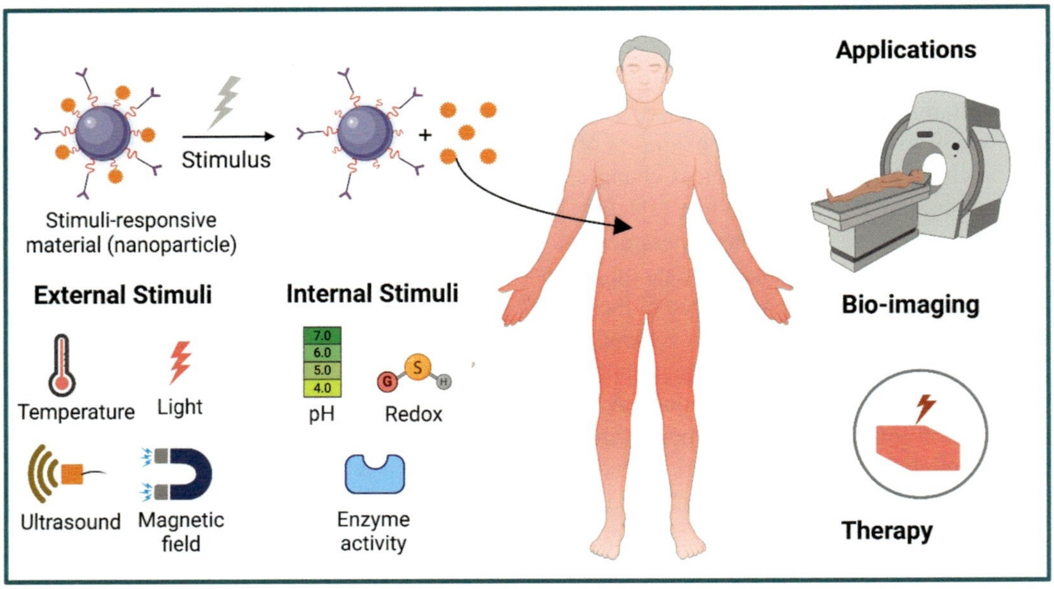

FIGURE 12.1 Stimuli-responsive biomaterials and their applications. The schematic representation depicts a concept that refers to stimuli-responsive materials, particularly nanoparticles, activated by external and internal stimuli. External stimuli include temperature, light, ultrasound, and magnetic fields, while internal triggers include the slight modifications in pH, redox conditions, or enzyme action. These materials activate the release of therapeutic agents that can be applied in various biomedical contexts such as bio-imaging and therapy. On the right side of the figure, a selection of major applications is highlighted, which includes MRI-based imaging and intervention therapy.

progresses, the development of more sophisticated biomaterials and hybrid imaging approaches will further enhance the accuracy and efficiency of inflammatory disease diagnostics, ultimately improving patient care and treatment outcomes [11]. In this chapter, the fascinating topic of stimuli-responsive biomaterials is examined, along with how they might be used in sophisticated imaging techniques to identify inflammatory diseases. Significant diagnostic difficulties arise from inflammatory ailments, which can range from acute infections and sepsis to chronic illnesses like rheumatoid arthritis and inflammatory bowel disease. Conventional imaging methods sometimes don't have the precision to identify minute metabolic alterations linked to inflammation. By dynamically changing their characteristics in response to internal or external stimuli, such as pH, temperature, enzyme activity, oxidative stress, or external signals, such as light and magnetic fields, stimulus-responsive biomaterials also referred to as smart materials fill this gap. By improving sensitivity, specificity, and focused visualization of disease locations, these materials have completely changed in medical imaging (Figure 12.1).

12.2 TYPES OF STIMULI-RESPONSIVE BIOMATERIALS

12.2.1 pH-Responsive Biomaterials

A type of smart materials known as pH-responsive materials responds to pH changes by altering their chemical, mechanical, or physical characteristics. pH-sensitive polymers are classified as either cationic or anionic based on the protonation/ionization mechanism, which is based on their charge at physiological pH. Ionizable polyamines found in cationic polymers are typically hydrophobic at physiological pH and turn hydrophilic when protonated in acidic environments while anionic polymers become hydrophobic when the pH falls under the pKa. This shift in hydrophilic properties causes the remodeling of the polymeric nanocarrier structure made up of these polymer materials and results in drug's eventual discharge. Low-pH-responsive nanoparticles have been used in cancer therapy because they can release the encapsulated chemotherapeutic agents when they come into contact with the acidic tumor microenvironment. This is for the reason that cancer cells are known to have enhanced glucose intake to support explosive growth and occasionally insufficient vasculature to provide enough oxygen. As a result, cancerous cells prefer the oxygen deprived route for breakdown of glucose, resulting in lactic acid as a result of incomplete oxidation [12]. The capacity of pH-responsive materials, like PEGylated nanogels, to selectively react to the acidic environment commonly present in tumors has drawn a lot of interest in the field of tumor imaging. The volume phase transition of these nanogels, which were developed from a copolymer of EAMA and TFEMA, occurs in the pH range of 6.5–7.0, which is the same as the extracellular pH of tumor tissues. The nanogels remain hydrophobic and exhibit a weak 19F MR signal at normal pH (7.4); however, they swell and produce a strong 19F MR signal at the acidic pH of the tumor environment. Tumor-specific imaging agents can be developed attributable to this pH-dependent activity, which improves contrast in magnetic resonance spectroscopy (MRS/I) and makes it possible to detect individual tumors with less background noise [13]. Nwe et al. identified a pH-responsive MRI contrast agent for neoplastic tumor imaging. The main components of the contrast agent, glycol chitosan (GC)–NH_2–GdDOTA, are a Gd-chelating molecule (DOTA) and a water-soluble GC that contains a primary amine (a pH-responsive moiety). As GC–NH_2–GdDOTA is positively charged in tumor environments, it has a tendency to bond with the negatively charged cell membrane through electrostatic charges. This lengthened the time spent in these areas of interest. GC–NH_2–GdDOTA exhibited a noticeable improvement in MRI images (~2 hours post-injection), reducing the usual time required in the clinic (~24 hours) [14].

12.2.2 Temperature-Responsive Biomaterials

One of the most commonly used external stimuli-responsive biomaterials is temperature-responsive biomaterials. Since human body temperatures are always maintained between 35 and 37°C, despite of the functioning of the cells, tissues, and organs, a thermo-responsive material is the most efficient activation mechanism. Specifically, in biomedical and biomaterial purposes, a temperature-responsive material does not require consideration for the target organs, tissues, or cells, unlike other stimuli systems. One of its distinguishing characteristics is a phase transition that can be changed reversibly in reaction to temperature variations. The above feature enables special control over these materials through "on-demand" remote management and "on–off" temperature-based adjustable regulation.

A Poly(N-isopropylacrylamide)-based nanogel with a pendant fluorescent moiety (DBThD-AA) was developed by Uchiyama et al. At lower temperatures, water molecules quench the DBThD-AA molecules and cause pNIPAm-based nanogels to swell significantly. As the temperature rises, the nanogels contract, intensifying the fluorescence. The nanogels were pushed to pass through the cell membrane and enter the cytoplasm by endocytosis and positive chemical potential (caused by the cationic initiator). Fundamentally, nanogels' exceptional non-cytotoxicity makes them appropriate for employing fluorescence signals to measure intracellular temperature [15]. For in vivo photoacoustic imaging (PAI) of a tumor-bearing mouse, Chen et al. developed pNIPAm-based nanogels loaded with Au nanorods (AuNRs). It was discovered that the photoacoustic (PA) intensity produced by pNIPAm–AuNR solutions is significantly higher than that of pure AuNR solutions. This results from the thermal profiles' irregular overlaps, which raise the temperature gradient. The pNIPAm–AuNR solution displayed a dramatic rise in PAI intensity when the temperature surpassed the nanogel's lower critical solution temperature (LCST) [16].

A category of biomaterials known as thermos responsive hydrogels experience a reversible sol–gel phase, which facilitates the integration and encapsulation of different therapeutic substances, such as proteins, peptides, nucleic acids, and small molecules, inside the matrix of hydrogel. The delivery of drugs can be confined and extended by loading the drug molecules into the sol state and releasing them in a controlled way when the gel forms. Furthermore, external stimuli, such as targeted heating or infrared irradiation, can be used to initiate the gelation process at specific locations or inside particular tissues. This characteristic makes site-specific drug administration possible, which lowers overall adverse effects and enhances treatment results [15].

12.2.3 Enzyme-Responsive Materials

Enzyme-responsive materials are responded to the stimuli that can change macroscopically due to altered intramolecular or intermolecular interactions when activated by an enzyme. There are several advantages to using enzymes as biological stimuli: (a) enzymes have chemo-, regio-, and enantioselectivity; (b) they naturally function in mild environments (aqueous, pH 5–8); and (c) several enzymes are important specific biocatalysts to cell pathways in medical conditions. In general, an enzyme-sensitive substrate along with an additional component that guides or regulates interactions that result in macroscopic alterations makes up enzyme-responsive materials. Changes in supramolecular structures, gel expansion or collapse, or surface property modification can result from the enzyme's catalytic action on the substrate. Endonucleases, proteases, phosphatases, kinases, esterase, and oxidoreductases are the enzyme types that are most frequently mentioned as stimuli. Endonucleases and proteases are commonly employed to cleave oligonucleotides and peptides, respectively, in order to break down or deconstruct materials that are sensitive to enzymes. On the other hand, covalent bonds, which are formed by enzymes like transglutaminases, improve the structural strength of materials that are receptive to enzymes by forming crosslinks. Furthermore, it is well recognized that kinases and phosphatases have complimentary catalytic activities. In the presence of adenosine 5′-triphosphate, kinases can phosphorylate molecules, whereas phosphatases can catalyze dephosphorylation [16].

12.3 OTHER STIMULI-RESPONSIVE BIOMATERIALS

12.3.1 Light-Responsive Biomaterials

A developing group of materials for biomedical engineering uses, such as drug delivery, regenerative medicine, photothermal, and photodynamic treatment, are light-responsive biomaterials. In addition to allowing for the spatiotemporal tunability of biomaterial ink, light-responsive biomaterials additionally offer biological triggers that have a major impact on cellular behavior and function. The light-responsive substances in photodynamic therapy (PDT) remain harmless and may be stimulated spatiotemporally, which is a substantial benefit over conventional chemotherapy. This is in contrast to chemotherapy medications, which may induce systemic toxicity to the neighboring normal cells. Furthermore, due to their reusable nature, photosensitizers can improve patients' quality of life with minimal invasiveness [17]. Cell regulation is possible with light-responsive nanomaterials, particularly for neurons and heart cells. Inorganic nanoparticles can be used to modify a single cell by photothermal or photoelectric stimulation using advanced light-controlled platforms. Single-cell methods of this kind enable the detection or immediate activation of cellular functions. Numerous disorders can be treated by extracellular activation of excitatory cellular types, including brain cells, cardiac cells as well as cells of the skeletal muscle. In this regard, by replacing light-sensing tissue, photovoltaic retinal prostheses may help reduce the indications of retinitis, which is brought on by a loss of the capacity to convert light into electrical impulses. The light-guided nanovehicle is another promising method for achieving active distribution in the physiological microenvironment. Furthermore, by precisely adjusting light strength, rate, polarization, and path in both space and time, light can offer more degrees of freedom for manipulating light-responsive materials. In order to produce an electrochemical or temperature gradient, light-responsive substances, including photoelectrochemical cells or thermal substances, can take in photon energy in a physiologic setting devoid of fuel [18].

12.3.2 Electrically Responsive Biomaterials

In recent years, research on neural interface, medication or chemical discharge via designed systems, and mechanical activation working upon cells has focused on the incorporation of conductive biomaterials. One of the most popular biomaterials for interacting with cells is conductive polymers [19]. This kind of polymer offers various benefits over traditional conductive materials (like metals) and is utilized both as a biomaterial as well as in the fields of tissue engineering. In "organ-on-a-chip" systems, conductive polymers are utilized to mechanically stimulate cells. They can cause the intracellular calcium content of stimulated cells to be electrically activated. Additionally, research has been performed on the activation characteristics of conductive materials within three-dimensional (3D) architectures. For instance, when an electrical signal was supplied to the tissue structure, PPy-coated poly(lactic-co-glycolic acid) (PLGA) fibers underwent recurrent swelling as well as shrinkage. It caused directional contraction and moved to the seeded cells through the structure's pore spaces. Recent research has demonstrated that electrical signals may initiate rapid, specific, receptive, and controllable release of drugs, facilitating localized rapid release that is suitable for over-time implants. This makes targeted burst release possible, which is suitable for implants that are left in place for a long time. Furthermore, a number of medications and growth factors, such as dopamine, naproxen, heparin, nerve growth factor (NGF), and dexamethasone, are included into conductive polymers for regulated release [20]. Some examples of electrically responsive biomaterials in diagnostics are given as follows:

- *Neural Interfaces and Neuroelectronic Diagnostics*: Neuronal prosthetics and brain–computer interfaces (BCIs) have made extensive use of electrically sensitive biomaterials. In order to improve signal sensitivity for diagnostic applications, conductive polymers, including polypyrrole (PPy) and poly(3,4-ethylenedioxythiophene) (PEDOT) have been used as coatings for neural electrodes. These resources make it possible to track neural activity in real time and identify anomalies in brain activity, including epilepsy, Parkinson's disease, and neurodegenerative diseases [20].
- *Smart Wound Monitoring and Infection Detection*: Biomaterials that conduct electricity have been created to measure temperature changes, bacterial infections, and pH levels in

order to follow the healing of wounds. Medical practitioners are notified in real time when infections occur using electroactive hydrogels embedded with graphene or carbon nanotubes (CNTs), which give continuous data on wound conditions. By combining biosensing and diagnostics, these smart dressings lower risks and enhance patient outcomes [21].

- *Electrically Controlled Biosensing for Disease Detection*: Biosensing for disease diagnosis is one of the most exciting uses of electrically sensitive biomaterials. Biomarkers including glucose, lactate, and inflammatory cytokines may now be detected in real time using conductive polymer films, such as PPy-based biosensors. These materials enable quick and non-invasive testing by providing extremely sensitive diagnostic instruments for illnesses, including diabetes and cardiovascular disorders [22].
- *Cardiac Health Monitoring*: The potential of conductive biomaterials in cardiac diagnostics is being investigated. PEDOT-PSS (poly(styrenesulfonate)) or CNT-integrated hydrogels have been used to create electrically sensitive scaffolds that can operate as biosensors to identify electrophysiological activity in individuals recuperating from myocardial infarctions. These resources allow for the early identification of arrhythmias and other cardiac conditions by offering real-time data on heart rhythms, which may lower the risk of unexpected cardiac events [23].

12.3.3 Magnetically Responsive Biomaterials

In biomedicine, magnetically responsive biomaterials are used to enhance physiological activities of organs, tissues as well as cells. Their sensitivity to external magnetic fields is the main reason for this. The biochemical, physical, and mechanical characteristics of bodily tissues and organs are remotely controlled by this stimulation. Magnetic biomaterial inks have been shown in a number of results to be efficient drug release and targeted systems. A magnetized bio material ink designed around ferromagnetic vertex domain iron oxide was created by Gao et al. The outcome showed that the developed magnetic ink can effectively prevent breast cancers from recurring locally [24]. Using crosslinked superparamagnetic iron oxide nanoparticles attached to an NO-sensitive cleavable linker, Lu et al. developed NO-responsive magnetic probes for extremely sensitive and specific NO-MRI in vivo. With the help of these probes, NO can be detected at concentrations as low as 0.147 μM. NO can also be imaged and measured in mouse tumor models, its effects on tumor development and immunity can be studied, and the response of tumor-associated macrophages to cancer immunotherapeutic agents can be evaluated. Furthermore, they enable simultaneous molecular and anatomical imaging of organs, which aids in the detection of disease changes in the liver [25]. Likewise, Li et al. designed a pH-responsive magnetic resonance tuning (MRET) probe for precise in situ MRI of bacterial infections in vivo. This probe's T1-weighted signal is triggered in the acid microenvironment infected by bacteria. The MRET probe (MDVG-1) is a combination of the precursor of the superparamagnetic quencher (DNA and vancomycin-modified magnetic nanoparticle, or MDV) and the paramagnetic enhancer (gadolinium-modified i-motif DNA3, or Gd-DNA3-Gd). After MDVG-1 was developed, the Gd-DNA3-Gd T1-weighted signal was quenched (MRET ON). In the acidic environment caused by bacteria, the MDVG-1 probe broke down into the monomers of Gd-DNA3-Gd and MDV, leading to a markedly increased T1-weighted signal at the infected region (MRET OFF). This pH-responsive MRET probe improved MRI signal and bacteria targeting, which greatly improved the differentiation between bacterial-infected regions and sterile inflamed tissues [26].

12.3.4 Ultrasound Stimulation

For 3D constructions, controlled remote stimuli in the form of ultrasonic pressure waves with frequencies higher than 20 kHz are employed. Many tissue engineering applications, such as regulating the ejection through acoustically reactive carriers, increasing transcutaneous permeation in compounds via sonophoresis, and reshaping cells *in vitro* into specific geometrical groups, have made extensive use of the pressure generated through vibration and the resulting mechanical impacts. Because ultrasound waves may easily pass through tissue-like structures and manufactured tissues, materials and cells can be manipulated *in situ*. Integrating acoustic-responsive delivery components to the biomaterial ink is one method for producing ultrasound-responsive biomaterial inks. Crosslinks in a biomaterial ink can be controlled by ultrasound stimulation, which may affect the release profile. Xu et al. reported the development of organic nanoparticles producing ultrasound-induced afterglow. A sonosensitizer serves as the activator for the production of singlet oxygen (1O2) under ultrasonic conditions in sonoafterglow nanoparticles (SNAPs). The sonosensitizer then transforms a sonoafterglow substrate into active dioxetane substrates, which have a long-lasting luminescence that can return to the sonosensitizer. Sonoafterglow induction via deep-seated nanoparticles is guaranteed by the ultrasonic initiation method. They created a sonoafterglow cancer nanoimmunotheranostic probe (SCAN) by encapsulating a macrophage-polarization prodrug into the nanoparticle. Only when ultrasound is applied does SCAN initiate immunotherapeutic activity, producing a sonoafterglow signal that can be linked to the tumor immunomicroenvironment's pro-inflammatory levels (as shown by the presence of M1 macrophages). Therefore, SNAP functioned as a modular system for cancer theranostics and deep-tissue high-contrast biomarker imaging [27].

12.3.5 Integration with Imaging Modalities

The integration of stimuli-responsive biomaterials with imaging modalities has revolutionized disease diagnosis, particularly for inflammatory disorders. Traditional imaging techniques are useful, but occasionally they lack the accuracy required to detect inflammation at the molecular level. Through their interactions with disease-specific indicators like pH changes, enzyme activity, oxidative stress, or temperature fluctuations, stimuli-responsive biomaterials offer a real-time, dynamic, and tailored approach. To show how these materials can improve the sensitivity, specificity, and accuracy of inflammation detection, this section examines their use in MRI, PET, fluorescence imaging, and other cutting-edge methods [28].

12.4 MAGNETIC RESONANCE IMAGING (MRI) AND STIMULI-RESPONSIVE BIOMATERIALS

12.4.1 Overview of MRI for Inflammatory Disorders

High-resolution anatomical and functional pictures of tissues may be obtained using MRI, a potent non-invasive medical imaging method. It is especially useful for identifying inflammatory diseases, since traditional imaging methods like computed tomography (CT) scans or X-rays might not offer enough contrast or molecular-level details [29]. In clinical and research contexts, MRI is widely used to assess inflammation in conditions such as autoimmune illnesses, cardiovascular problems, neuroinflammation, and musculoskeletal ailments.

12.4.2 MRI for Diagnosing Inflammatory Disorders

Because MRI may identify tissue edema, increased vascular permeability, and immune cell infiltration, it is essential for the diagnosis and ongoing surveillance of disorders linked to inflammation. The following are some important inflammatory conditions for which MRI is used: MRI can identify joint erosion, cartilage deterioration, and synovial inflammation before serious harm is done [30]. MRI aids in the early detection of brain tissue destruction and disruption of the blood–brain barrier in conditions such as multiple sclerosis (MS), Alzheimer's disease, and Parkinson's disease [31]. In diseases including Crohn's disease and ulcerative colitis, MRI offers a non-invasive way to evaluate intestinal wall thickness, ulceration, and inflammation [32]. MRI is utilized to assess myocardial inflammation in cardiovascular disorders and identify inflammatory atherosclerotic plaques [33].

12.4.3 Limitations of Conventional MRI in Inflammation Detection

Conventional MRI has limits in identifying molecular-level alterations linked to inflammation, despite its advantages. While MRI can identify structural and physiological alterations, it is unable to distinguish between distinct inflammatory indicators or kinds of inflammation. It may be difficult to identify inflammation in some soft tissues due to their natural lack of contrast. Conventional MRI scans are mainly used to detect macroscopic tissue changes; however, early-stage inflammatory processes take place at the molecular level and are difficult to see with conventional MRI scans. Stimuli-responsive biomaterials have been created as sophisticated contrast agents to address these issues and allow for precise and focused imaging of inflammation [34].

12.4.4 Role of Stimuli-Responsive Biomaterials in MRI

Stimuli-responsive contrast agents (SRCA) improve the specificity of MRI for inflammation detection by activating signal enhancement only at disease sites. These materials can respond to pH, enzymes, or oxidative stress associated with inflamed tissues. Because of metabolic alterations, inflammation sites frequently have an acidic microenvironment (pH 6.5–6.8). For instance, pH-sensitive polymers added to gadolinium-based nanoprobes only improve MRI contrast in acidic environments, lowering background signals in healthy tissues [35]. Inflammation causes the upregulation of several enzymes, including cathepsins and matrix metalloproteinases (MMPs). When enzyme-cleavable ligand-coated nanoparticles are activated, contrast agents are released, enabling targeted imaging [36]. Inflamed tissues create excessive amounts of ROS. High ROS levels cause manganese- or iron oxide-based nanoparticles to oxidize, enhancing their ability to detect inflammation by activating their paramagnetic characteristics [37].

12.4.5 Positron Emission Tomography (PET) and Stimuli-Responsive Biomaterials

PET is a very sensitive molecular imaging method that uses biomolecules labeled with radiotracer to identify changes in metabolism and biochemistry. PET scans are frequently used to identify inflammation in illnesses such cancer-associated inflammation, autoimmune disorders, and infectious diseases. However, conventional PET imaging agents can provide false-positive findings and frequently lack specificity. Stimuli-responsive biomaterials improve PET imaging by enabling targeted tracer release, ensuring better localization of inflammation sites. Protonation or structural alterations in PET tracers can be triggered by acidic pH at inflammatory areas, which enhances their accumulation at the illness site. For instance, in acidic settings, fluorine-18 labeled nanocarriers change structurally, allowing for the regulated release of the tracer, while remaining inactive at normal physiological pH. This guarantees improved contrast and specificity while imaging inflammatory areas [38]. Enzymes linked to inflammation, such as caspases and MMPs, are essential for immunological responses and tissue remodeling. Only in sick tissues can these enzymes activate the imaging signal by cleaving PET probe linkers. In inflammatory arthritis, for instance, MMPs selectively activate 64Cu-labeled peptide-based probes. This focused activation improves diagnostic accuracy by enabling more accurate imaging of inflammatory joints [39]. ROS levels rise as a result of oxidative stress, which is a defining feature of inflammation. This property is taken advantage of by redox-responsive PET probes, which increase tracer absorption in inflammatory tissues by causing oxidative cleavage of probe coatings due to elevated ROS levels. The PET tracers based on nitroimidazole, which preferentially accumulate in inflammatory hypoxic tissues, are one prominent example. Important information on inflammatory microenvironments and their development is provided by this selective uptake [40].

Particularly in diseases like Crohn's disease, enzyme-activated PET probes have shown great promise in the early identification of intestinal inflammation. These probes allow for accurate visualization of disease activity by focusing on inflammation-related enzymes, which promotes prompt intervention and better disease management [41, 42]. ROS-responsive PET tracers have become useful instruments for locating susceptible plaques linked to inflammation in the cardiovascular system. These imaging tools support risk assessment and early intervention tactics by identifying oxidative stress in atherosclerotic lesions, which may help avoid serious cardiovascular events [43]. By taking use of the acidic milieu frequently present in diseased tissues, pH-sensitive PET tracers offer accurate localization of infection-related inflammation. By differentiating between bacterial or viral infections and sterile inflammation, these tracers improve the precision of infection diagnosis and therapy planning [44].

12.4.5.1 Fluorescence Imaging and Stimuli-Responsive Biomaterials

Light-emitting fluorescent probes are the foundation of fluorescence imaging, which allows for high-resolution, real-time observation of biological processes. Preclinical research, intraoperative imaging, and biomarker tracking in disorders linked to inflammation all make extensive use of it [45]. Fluorescence imaging has gained popularity as a useful technique for observing molecular alterations in a range of inflammatory diseases due to its exceptional sensitivity and specificity. Stimuli-responsive fluorescent probes provide superior spatiotemporal resolution, allowing targeted inflammation detection. Some common types include the following:

- *pH-Responsive Fluorescent Probes*: Fluorophores coupled with pH-sensitive dyes are perfect for identifying inflammation-related acidosis because they boost fluorescence in acidic conditions. Coumarin-based probes, which are made to glow strongly in acidic environments frequently present in inflammatory locations like arthritis and tumor microenvironments, are one example of this strategy [46]. By reducing background signal in healthy tissues, this selective fluorescence activation increases the specificity of imaging inflammation.
- *Enzyme-Activated Fluorescent Probes*: Only in inflammatory tissues do fluorescent dyes attached to enzyme-cleavable peptides become fluorescent after undergoing enzymatic cleavage. Caspases-3-activated near-infrared (NIR) fluorophores are a prominent example; they function as markers of apoptosis in inflammatory diseases [47]. By precisely monitoring cell death in inflammatory tissues, these probes offer vital information about the course of the illness and the effectiveness of treatment.
- *ROS-Responsive Fluorescent Sensors*: Since inflammation is greatly influenced by ROS, ROS-sensitive molecular probes take advantage of this characteristic to increase fluorescence under oxidative stress conditions. Boronic acid-based probes are one example; when ROS are present, they oxidize and provide a fluorescence signal that emphasizes neuroinflammation [48]. This method makes it possible to monitor oxidative stress in real time, which helps with the early detection of neurodegenerative diseases linked to inflammation.

12.4.6 Other Imaging Techniques and Stimuli-Responsive Biomaterials

12.4.6.1 Photoacoustic Imaging (PAI)

The basis of PAI is the photoacoustic phenomenon, in which biological tissues absorb short-pulsed laser light, producing ultrasonic vibrations in the process. High-resolution imaging of biological structures is made possible by the multi-step PAI method, which includes optical excitation and acoustic detection. PAI leverages the photoacoustic effect, in which pulsed laser light is absorbed by biological tissues, causing localized thermal expansion and the subsequent generation of ultrasonic waves [49–51]. These ultrasonic signals are then detected and reconstructed to form high-resolution images of the tissue's structure and composition. The multi-step PAI process involves optical excitation followed by acoustic detection. The technique is particularly advantageous because it merges the high contrast of optical imaging with the deep penetration of ultrasound imaging, enabling researchers and clinicians to obtain detailed insights into the biological micro-environment [52]. Due to this combination, PAI is a new biomedical imaging technique that has uses in vascular medicine, neurology, cardiology, and cancer. The photoacoustic effect, initially explained by Alexander Graham Bell in 1880, is the basis for PAI's operation. This effect occurs when biological tissues' inherent chromophores—like hemoglobin, melanin, or lipids—or exogenous contrast agents—like dyes or nanoparticles—absorb short-pulsed laser light. Acoustic waves are produced when the absorbed light energy is transformed into heat through a process known as transient thermoelastic expansion. Ultrasound transducers pick up these acoustic waves as they travel through tissues and use them to rebuild a picture. The capacity of PAI to offer good spatial resolution at different tissue depths is one of its main benefits. The medium's optical and auditory characteristics affect PAI's resolution. The penetrating depth of optical resolution photoacoustic microscopy (OR-PAM) is only around 1 mm, yet it achieves excellent resolution (on the order of microns). Acoustic resolution photoacoustic microscopy (AR-PAM), on the other hand, offers slightly lower resolution but deeper tissue penetration (up to several centimeters). PAI has attracted substantial interest in oncology because of its capacity to detect cancers at an early stage by seeing aberrant vasculature, angiogenesis, and hypoxia levels. PAI can offer endogenous contrast to distinguish between healthy and cancerous cells since hemoglobin is a naturally occurring chromophore. Additionally, PAI can be used to track how well cancer treatments, including immunotherapy, chemotherapy, and photothermal therapy are working.

It has demonstrated potential in neuroimaging applications, making it possible to see brain activity, oxygenation levels, and cerebral blood flow. It may be applied to the research of traumatic brain damage, Alzheimer's disease, and stroke. For long-term neurological research, PAI is a safer option because it doesn't use ionizing radiation. Additionally, vascular structure imaging, blood flow dynamics assessment, and atherosclerotic plaque detection are performed. The method can offer microcirculation imaging in real time, which is useful for identifying cardiovascular conditions, including hypertension and peripheral artery disease. Compared to more conventional optical imaging methods like diffuse optical tomography and fluorescence, PAI offers superior spatial resolution. It uses ultrasonic sensing to get deeper penetrations than simply optical imaging techniques. Additionally, it can evaluate molecular biomarkers, metabolism, and tissue oxygenation without the need of external contrast agents [53].

12.4.6.2 Computed Tomography (CT) and Stimuli-Responsive Biomaterials

Based on X-ray attenuation, CT is a popular medical imaging method that offers high-resolution 3D anatomical imaging. But because of its limitations in functional imaging, traditional CT imaging is less useful for identifying physiological and biochemical alterations such inflammation, oxidative stress, and changes in the tumor microenvironment. Stimuli-responsive biomaterials have become novel contrast agents to improve CT imaging, allowing for molecular-level, tailored, and very sensitive imaging. These substances enable accurate imaging of sick tissues by reacting to certain biological stimuli, including pH variations, ROS, temperature, enzymes, and light [53].

12.4.6.3 Ultrasound- and Stimuli-Responsive Contrast Agents

Ultrasound imaging is a real-time, non-invasive imaging method that is often employed in clinical diagnostics because of its great temporal resolution, cheap cost, and safety. However, because of its poor tissue contrast, its application in identifying specific pathological alterations (such as inflammation, tumors, or early-stage illnesses) has been restricted. SRCA) are designed to improve ultrasonic imaging's sensitivity and specificity. These substances are designed to respond to certain physiological or pathological stimuli, such temperature, enzyme activity, pH shifts, or ROS, which amplify ultrasonic signals at the target location [54].

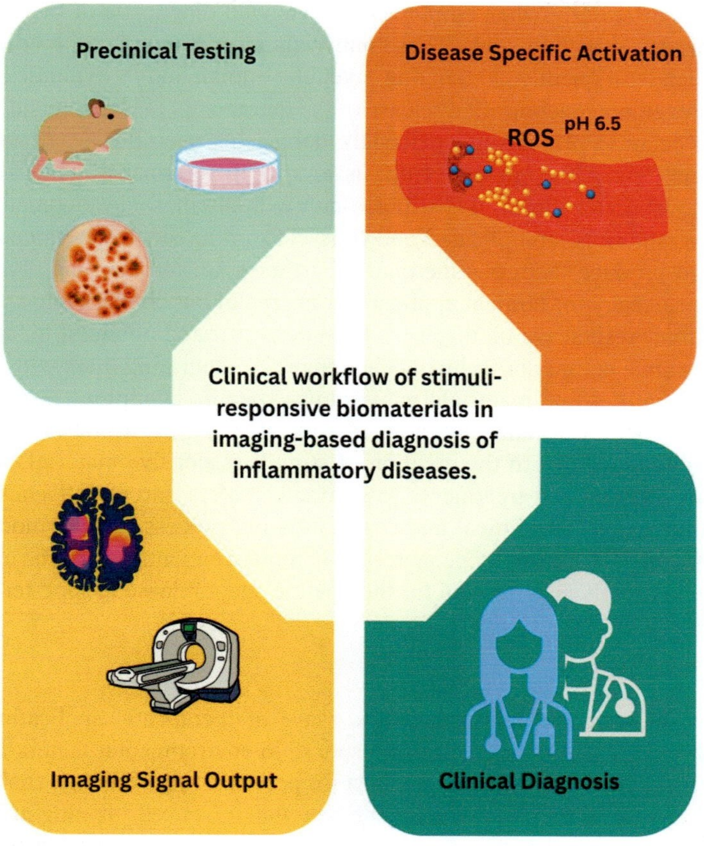

FIGURE 12.2 Clinical workflow of stimuli-responsive biomaterials in imaging-based diagnosis of inflammatory diseases.

12.4.6.4 Hybrid Imaging Approaches

Compared to individual imaging techniques alone, hybrid imaging approaches offer improved sensitivity, specificity, and functional insights by combining the characteristics of numerous imaging modalities to produce superior diagnostic accuracy. By combining several technologies, it is possible to see diseases in many dimensions and obtain both functional and anatomical information in a single imaging session. These methods are especially helpful in neurological conditions, cardiovascular illnesses, and cancer imaging, where it's necessary to assess both structure and function. Several imaging modalities' complementing qualities are used in hybrid imaging (Figure 12.2) [54].

12.5 LIMITATIONS AND FUTURE PERSPECTIVES

Despite the tremendous potential of stimuli-responsive biomaterials, several challenges remain that need to be addressed to fully realize their clinical and diagnostic applications. Biocompatibility is a major issue with stimuli-responsive biomaterials, especially when they are utilized in vivo. The materials must be safe for long-term exposure within the body in addition to reacting to external stimuli. The practical application of some materials may be limited due to immunological reactions, toxicity, or undesirable interactions with adjacent tissues. The difficulty is in creating biocompatible and responsive materials without triggering negative immune reactions or causing long-term injury [55]. The stability of stimuli-responsive materials under physiological settings is another difficulty. Particularly when employed for extended diagnostic or therapeutic purposes, these materials must continue to work. These materials must respond in a predictable and regulated manner, which is frequently challenging given the human body's dynamic and complicated environment. For example, uncontrolled release of the therapeutic payload outside of the intended environment may occur in pH-sensitive materials, decreasing overall efficacy and perhaps causing adverse effects [56]. Although the synthesis of stimuli-responsive materials has advanced significantly at the laboratory level, it is still difficult to apply these developments to large-scale production. These materials' complicated and time-consuming synthesis procedures may make it more difficult to produce them commercially. Furthermore, maintaining quality control and batch-to-batch consistency for clinical applications is crucial but challenging with existing techniques. While stimuli-responsive biomaterials have demonstrated potential for improving imaging methods, there are a number of technical challenges in integrating them with current imaging modalities. Additionally, some materials may require specific conditions (such as temperature changes or the presence of certain enzymes) that are difficult to mimic in real-world clinical settings. Strict regulations govern the creation of stimuli-responsive materials for use in medicine, especially in imaging and treatment. To guarantee safety and effectiveness, the materials must go through a rigorous preclinical and clinical testing process. Furthermore, ethical issues surrounding the use of such cutting-edge materials in human patients need to be considered, especially when those materials may be used for therapeutic agent release or long-term monitoring.

12.6 CONCLUSIONS

Stimuli-responsive biomaterials represent a new wave of therapeutic applications and medical diagnostics. Their unique ability to change in response to environmental factors such as pH, temperature, or enzymes offers a fascinating prospect for personalized medicine, enabling more accurate imaging and targeted therapies. When combined with advanced imaging methods, including MRI, fluorescence imaging, and PET, these materials allow improved treatment monitoring and early detection, marking a significant breakthrough in non-invasive diagnostics. The application of stimuli-responsive materials has already shown great promise in raising the sensitivity and specificity of imaging techniques. For instance, pH-responsive nanoparticles have demonstrated potential in cancer imaging by taking advantage of the acidic milieu commonly seen in tumors. Similarly, temperature-responsive hydrogels and enzyme-sensitive nanoparticles have opened new avenues for multimodal imaging and targeted drug delivery, leading to more comprehensive methods to diagnosis and therapy. These advancements demonstrate that stimuli-responsive materials are not only enhancing current imaging techniques but also contributing to the creation of new, more effective disease detection approaches. As with any novel technology, however, difficulties must be overcome before these materials may be widely employed in therapies. Three enduring problems that require improvement are stability, controlled response in vivo, and biocompatibility. The materials' scalability for mass production and seamless integration with existing imaging techniques are technical issues that must be resolved. Despite these challenges, stimuli-responsive biomaterials are unquestionably capable of revolutionizing medical imaging and therapy, and more research is likely to yield solutions in the near future. Biomaterials that respond to stimuli seem to have a promising future. Due to continuous improvements in material synthesis, a deeper understanding of biological interactions, and the development of complex manufacturing techniques, the gap between laboratory research and clinical application is progressively closing. One of the future approaches is the development of multi-stimuli-responsive systems, which may respond to many external stimuli simultaneously and allow for more precise and customized diagnostics. Combining therapeutic and diagnostic skills into a single "theranostic" platform that offers real-time imaging and the ability to provide localized treatments or release drugs as required is another intriguing field. Furthermore, stimuli-responsive materials will probably be essential in customizing therapies for each patient according to their unique biological surroundings as personalized medicine gains traction. The stimuli-responsive biomaterials have enormous promise for use in medical diagnostics and imaging as well as in the larger field of personalized medicine. Even if there are still obstacles to overcome, the speed at which this sector is developing indicates that these materials will have a significant impact on healthcare in the future. With sustained multidisciplinary cooperation and innovation, the promise of smarter, more focused diagnoses and treatments is within grasp, providing hope for better patient care and results globally.

Declaration of AI and AI-Assisted Technologies

During the preparation of this work, the authors used QuillBot AI and Grammarly in order to paraphrase the sentences. After using this tool, the authors reviewed and edited the content as needed and take full responsibility for the content of the publication.

REFERENCES

1. Wei F, Yang W, Wang H, Song S, Ji Y, Chen Z, Zhuang Y, Dai J, Shen H. Reactive oxygen species-scavenging biomaterials for neural regenerative medicine. Biomaterials Science 2025;14:343–63.
2. Liu CH, Abrams ND, Carrick DM, Chander P, Dwyer J, Hamlet MR, Kindzelski AL, PrabhuDas M, Tsai SY, Vedamony MM, Wang C. Imaging inflammation and its resolution in health and disease: Current status, clinical needs, challenges, and opportunities. The FASEB Journal 2019 Dec;33(12):13085.
3. Zare EN, Makvandi P, Sumera K. Stimuli-responsive materials for biomedical applications. Washington, DC: American Chemical Society; 2023.
4. Nag S, Mohanto S, Ahmed MG, Subramaniyan V. "Smart" stimuli-responsive biomaterials revolutionizing the theranostic landscape of inflammatory arthritis. Materials Today Chemistry 2024 Jul 1;39:102178.
5. El-Husseiny HM, Mady EA, Hamabe L, Abugomaa A, Shimada K, Yoshida T, Tanaka T, Yokoi A, Elbadawy M, Tanaka R. Smart/stimuli-responsive hydrogels: Cutting-edge platforms for tissue engineering and other biomedical applications. Materials Today Bio 2022 Jan 1;13:100186.
6. Kruczkowska W, Gałęziewska J, Grabowska K, Liese G, Buczek P, Kłosiński KK, Kciuk M, Pasieka Z, Kałuzińska-Kołat Ż, Kołat D. Biomedical trends in stimuli-responsive hydrogels with emphasis on chitosan-based formulations. Gels 2024 Apr 25;10(5):295.
7. Liu Y, Lin Z, Wang Y, Chen L, Wang Y, Luo C. Nanotechnology in inflammation: Cutting-edge advances in diagnostics, therapeutics and theranostics. Theranostics 2024;14(6):2490.
8. Romano A, Di Stasio D, Petruzzi M, Fiori F, Lajolo C, Santarelli A, Lucchese A, Serpico R, Contaldo M. Noninvasive imaging methods to improve the diagnosis of oral carcinoma and its precursors: State of the art and proposal of a three-step diagnostic process. Cancers 2021 Jun 8;13(12):2864.
9. Lee MY, Lee D, Choi D, Kim KS, Kang PM. Targeting reactive oxygen species for diagnosis of various diseases. Journal of Functional Biomaterials 2024 Dec 15;15(12):378.
10. Municoy S, Alvarez Echazu MI, Antezana PE, Galdopórpora JM, Olivetti C, Mebert AM, Foglia ML, Tuttolomondo MV, Alvarez GS, Hardy JG, Desimone MF. Stimuli-responsive materials for tissue engineering and drug delivery. International Journal of Molecular Sciences 2020 Jul 2;21(13):4724.
11. Liu L, Chen H, Zhao X, Han Q, Xu Y, Liu Y, Zhang A, Li Y, Zhang W, Chen B, Wang J. Advances in the application and research of biomaterials in promoting bone repair and regeneration through immune modulation. Materials Today Bio 2024 Dec 16;30:101410.
12. Brooks GA. Lactate as a fulcrum of metabolism. Redox Biology 2020 Aug 1;35:101454.
13. Oishi M, Nagasaki Y. Stimuli-responsive smart nanogels for cancer diagnostics and therapy. Nanomedicine 2010 Apr 1;5(3):451–68.
14. Nwe K, Huang CH, Tsourkas A. Gd-labeled glycol chitosan as a pH-responsive magnetic resonance imaging agent for detecting acidic tumor microenvironments. Journal of Medicinal Chemistry 2013 Oct 24;56(20):7862–9.
15. Uchiyama S, Tsuji T, Kawamoto K, et al. A cell-targeted non-cytotoxic fluorescent nanogel thermometer created with an imidazolium-containing cationic radical initiator. Angewandte Chemie International Edition in English 2018 May 4;57(19):5413–7.
16. Chen YS, Yoon SJ, Frey W, Dockery M, Emelianov S. Dynamic contrast-enhanced photoacoustic imaging using photothermal stimuli-responsive composite nanomodulators. Nature Communications 2017 Jun 8;8(1):15782.

17. Kolouchova K, Sedlacek O, Jirak D, et al. Self-assembled thermoresponsive polymeric nanogels for 19F MR imaging. Biomacromolecules 2018 Jul 16;19(8):3515–24.
18. Wang M, Gao B, Wang X, Li W, Feng Y. Enzyme-responsive strategy as a prospective cue to construct intelligent biomaterials for disease diagnosis and therapy. Biomaterials Science 2022;10(8):1883–903.
19. Li Y, Qian Y, Liu T, Zhang G, Liu S. Light-triggered concomitant enhancement of magnetic resonance imaging contrast performance and drug release rate of functionalized amphiphilic diblock copolymer micelles. Biomacromolecules 2012 Nov 12;13(11):3877–86.
20. Green R, Abidian MR. Conducting polymers for neural prosthetic and neural interface applications. Advanced Materials 2015 Dec;27(46):7620–37.
21. Shirzaei Sani E, Xu C, Wang C, Song Y, Min J, Tu J, Solomon SA, Li J, Banks JL, Armstrong DG, Gao W. A stretchable wireless wearable bioelectronic system for multiplexed monitoring and combination treatment of infected chronic wounds. Science Advances 2023 Mar 24;9(12):eadf7388.
22. Khaksarinejad R, Arabpour Z, RezaKhani L, Parvizpour F, Rasmi Y. Biomarker based biosensors: An opportunity for diagnosis of COVID-19. Reviews in Medical Virology 2022 Sep;32(5):e2356.
23. Roshanbinfar K, Schiffer M, Carls E, et al. Electrically conductive collagen-PEDOT:PSS hydrogel prevents post-infarct cardiac arrhythmia and supports hiPSC-cardiomyocyte function. Advanced Materials 2024 Jul;36(28):2403642.
24. Gao B, Yang Q, Zhao X, Jin G, Ma Y, Xu F. 4D bioprinting for biomedical applications. Trends in Biotechnology 2016 Sep 1;34(9):746–56.
25. Lu C, Liao S, Chen B, Xu L, Wu N, Lu D, Kang H, Zhang XB, Song G. Responsive probes for in vivo magnetic resonance imaging of nitric oxide. Nature Materials 2024 Nov 25;24:133–42.
26. Li L, Liu M, Deng S, et al. A pH-responsive magnetic resonance tuning probe for precise imaging of bacterial infection in vivo. Acta Biomater 2023 Jul 1;164:487–95.
27. Xu C, Huang J, Jiang Y, He S, Zhang C, Pu K. Nanoparticles with ultrasound-induced afterglow luminescence for tumour-specific theranostics. Nature Biomedical Engineering 2023 Mar;7(3):298–312.
28. Aili T, Zong JB, Zhou YF, Liu YX, Yang XL, Hu B, Wu JH. Recent advances of self-assembled nanoparticles in the diagnosis and treatment of atherosclerosis. Theranostics 2024 Nov 4;14(19):7505.
29. Hussain S, Mubeen I, Ullah N, Shah SS, Khan BA, Zahoor M, Ullah R, Khan FA, Sultan MA. Modern diagnostic imaging technique applications and risk factors in the medical field: A review. BioMed Research International 2022;2022(1):5164970.
30. Burke CJ, Alizai H, Beltran LS, Regatte RR. MRI of synovitis and joint fluid. Journal of Magnetic Resonance Imaging 2019 Jun;49(6):1512–27.
31. Moyaert P, Padrela BE, Morgan CA, Petr J, Versijpt J, Barkhof F, Jurkiewicz MT, Shao X, Oyeniran O, Manson T, Wang DJ. Imaging blood-brain barrier dysfunction: A state-of-the-art review from a clinical perspective. Frontiers in Aging Neuroscience 2023 Apr 17;15:1132077.
32. Rimola J, Torres J, Kumar S, et al. Recent advances in clinical practice: Advances in cross-sectional imaging in inflammatory bowel disease. Gut 2022 Dec 1;71(12):2587–97.
33. Lewis AJ, Burrage MK, Ferreira VM. Cardiovascular magnetic resonance imaging for inflammatory heart diseases. Cardiovascular Diagnosis and Therapy 2020 Jun;10(3):598.
34. Møller-Bisgaard S, Hørslev-Petersen K, Ejbjerg B, Hetland ML, Ørnbjerg LM, Glinatsi D, Møller J, Boesen M, Christensen R, Stengaard-Pedersen K, Madsen OR. Effect of magnetic resonance imaging vs conventional treat-to-target strategies on disease activity remission and radiographic progression in rheumatoid arthritis: The IMAGINE-RA randomized clinical trial. JAMA 2019;321(5):461–472.
35. Palanikumar L, Kalmouni M, Houhou T, et al. pH-responsive upconversion mesoporous silica nanospheres for combined multimodal diagnostic imaging and targeted photodynamic and photothermal cancer therapy. ACS Nano 2023 Sep 13;17(19):18979–99.
36. Gonzalez-Avila G, Sommer B, García-Hernandez AA, Ramos C, Flores-Soto E. Nanotechnology and matrix metalloproteinases in cancer diagnosis and treatment. Frontiers in Molecular Biosciences 2022 Jun 1;9:918789.
37. Rizwan S, ReddySekhar P, MalikAsrar B. Reactive oxygen species in inflammation and tissue injury. Antioxid Redox Signal. 2014 Feb 12;20(7):1126–67.
38. Nasrallah I, Dubroff J. An overview of PET neuroimaging. Seminars in Nuclear Medicine 2013 Nov 1;43(6):449–461.
39. Born DVD, Pees A, Poot AJ, Orru RVA, Windhorst AD, Vugts DJ. Fluorine-18 labelled building blocks for PET tracer synthesis. Chemical Society Reviews 2017 Jun 13;46:4709–73.
40. Crişan G, Moldovean-Cioroianu NS, Timaru DG, Andrieş G, Căinap C, Chiş V. Radiopharmaceuticals for PET and SPECT imaging: A literature review over the last decade. International Journal of Molecular Sciences 2022 Apr 30;23(9):5023.

41. Tada T, Mizuno Y, Shibata Y, Yasui H, Kuge Y. Application of copper (I) selective ligands for PET imaging of reactive oxygen species through metabolic trapping. Nuclear Medicine and Biology 2024 Jul 1;134:108914.
42. Rezazadeh F, Kilcline AP, Viola NT. Imaging agents for PET of inflammatory bowel disease: A review. Journal of Nuclear Medicine 2023 Dec 1;64(12):1858–64.
43. Vogiatzi G, Tousoulis D, Stefanadis C. The role of oxidative stress in atherosclerosis. Hellenic Journal of Cardiology 2009 Sep 1;50(5):402–9.
44. Calabria FF, Guadagnino G, Cimini A, Leporace M. PET/CT imaging of infectious diseases: Overview of novel radiopharmaceuticals. Diagnostics 2024 May 17;14(10):1043.
45. Wang X, Ding Q, Groleau RR, Wu L, Mao Y, Che F, Kotova O, Scanlan EM, Lewis SE, Li P, Tang B. Fluorescent probes for disease diagnosis. Chemical Reviews 2024 May 17;124(11):7106–64.
46. Vasylevska AS, Karasyov AA, Borisov SM, Krause C. Novel coumarin-based fluorescent pH indicators, probes and membranes covering a broad pH range. Analytical and Bioanalytical Chemistry 2007 Mar;387:2131–41.
47. Weng J, Wang Y, Zhang Y, Ye D. An activatable near-infrared fluorescence probe for in vivo imaging of acute kidney injury by targeting phosphatidylserine and caspase-3. Journal of the American Chemical Society. 2021 Oct 21;143(43):18294–304.
48. Wang R, Bian Z, Zhan D, Wu Z, Yao Q, Zhang G. Boronic acid-based sensors for small-molecule reactive species: A review. Dyes and Pigments 2021 Feb 1;185:108885.
49. Wu J, Xia W, Lu Y, et al. Construction of a dual "off-on" near-infrared fluorescent probe for bioimaging of HClO in rheumatoid arthritis. Talanta 2024 Dec 1;280:126721.
50. Geng Y, Zhang H, Zhang G, Zhou J, Zhu M, Ma L, Wang X, James TD, Wang Z. Near-infrared fluorescent probe for the in situ visualization of oxidative stress in the brains of neuroinflammatory and schizophrenic mice. Analytical Chemistry 2023 Aug 1;95(32):11943–52.
51. Hosseinaee Z, Le M, Bell K, Reza PH. Towards non-contact photoacoustic imaging. Photoacoustics 2020;20:100207.
52. Sun L, Li Q, Zhang L, Chai H, Yu L, Xu Z, Kang Y, Xue P. Stimuli responsive PEGylated bismuth selenide hollow nanocapsules for fluorescence/CT imaging and light-driven multimodal tumor therapy. Biomaterials Science 2019;7(7):3025–40.
53. Rix A, Lederle W, Theek B, Lammers T, Moonen C, Schmitz G, Kiessling F Advanced ultrasound technologies for diagnosis and therapy. Journal of Nuclear Medicine 2018 May 1;59(5):740–6.
54. Goodwin AP, Nakatsuka MA, Mattrey RF. Stimulus–responsive ultrasound contrast agents for clinical imaging: Motivations, demonstrations, and future directions. Wiley Interdisciplinary Reviews: Nanomedicine and Nanobiotechnology 2015 Jan;7(1):111–23.
55. Kyriakides TR, Raj A, Tseng TH, Xiao H, Nguyen R, Mohammed FS, Halder S, Xu M, Wu MJ, Bao S, Sheu WC. Biocompatibility of nanomaterials and their immunological properties. Biomedical Materials 2021 Mar 11;16(4):042005.
56. Wang Y, Shim MS, Levinson NS, Sung HW, Xia Y. Stimuli-responsive materials for controlled release of theranostic agents. Advanced Functional Materials 2014 Jul;24(27):4206–20.

13 Smart Programmed Drug Delivery Systems

An Ode to AI and ML Technology

Gatadi Srikanth and Rakesh Barik
GITAM School of Pharmacy, GITAM Deemed to be University, Hyderabad, India

Bhima Sridevi
KL College of Pharmacy, KL Deemed to be University, Guntur, Andhra Pradesh, India

Santosha Chandra Rao Karanam
GITAM School of Technology, GITAM Deemed to be University, Hyderabad, India

Bappaditya Chatterjee
GITAM School of Pharmacy, GITAM Deemed to be University, Hyderabad, India

13.1 INTRODUCTION

Unwanted adverse events in patients are the major concern for traditional drug delivery systems. Uncontrolled drug release and ineffective targeting are two main causes. Conventional systems frequently exhibit low or poor bioavailability. As a result of all these problems, controlled and long-lasting drug delivery systems were created. After a zero-order drug release, controlled drug delivery systems deliver the medication to the intended location of the body at a pre-established rate [1]. Conversely, sustained drug delivery systems provide the medication for an extended period of action, though not in zero order. Over time, both systems aid in sustaining the intended therapeutic concentration. In general, targeted drug delivery systems are those that can deliver medication to the intended site of action. These systems, which are especially helpful in treating neurological disorders, cancers, etc., get around the problem of unwanted side effects. As a result, the need for precise and regulated drug delivery methods grows daily. Active targeting and passive targeting are the two main tactics used to direct the medication to the intended site of action [2]. Active targeting involves conjugating a particular component, called a ligand, with the system to help direct it to a particular receptor or location within the human body. Conversely, passive targeting releases the drug at a specific location based on the biological or biochemical environment of tissues. Maintaining effectiveness in targeting and producing repeatable outcomes across various patient populations, despite genetic or anatomical variations, is the main challenge of such systems. Such a problem does not exist with implants or inserts. Implants that release the medication at a regulated rate over an extended period of time, occasionally a few months to years, are positioned in deep tissue layers or inside bodily cavities or organs, such as the brain, heart, or beneath the skin [3–5].

 DOI: 10.1201/9781003560203-13

However, it is not possible to regulate the release of drugs from implants or inserts according to the patient's needs. The drug is released based on the biological environment and built-in mechanism after it is implanted. This is where electromechanically operated or programmed devices that can be managed and observed *via* applications come in. An electromechanical implant is a device that uses an electrical battery to power a mechanical pump that delivers the medication. For instance, the Medtronic® Synchromed® pump, which is positioned over the abdomen, can administer medication to the brain through a catheter that travels through the spinal cord to the nervous system [6]. When necessary, the medication can be refilled into the device, and the rate of delivery can be externally adjusted. The Vibrant® capsule is another non-medicated electromechanical system, although it is not an implant [7]. It is operated by a battery device for treating irregular bowel movements. This device encourages a smooth bowel movement by vibrating as soon as it enters the colon after ingestion. In all of these systems, mechanical, electrical, and occasionally artificial intelligence (AI)-based techniques are integrated.

The need for electromechanical drug delivery systems has grown over the past few decades, with the goal of controlling drug release externally and individually. A system's drug release could be need-driven, which would mean the drug would only be given when the body needed it. Moreover, AI can be used to pre-program or regulate the entire system. This is where externally controlled or programmed drug delivery systems come in. The creation of programmed (smart) drug delivery systems has benefited from the development of AI and machine learning (ML). Although they are not the same, the well-known terms AI and ML are frequently used interchangeably. AI is a more general term for a method of using a machine to mimic the cognitive processes of the human brain. Similar to the human brain, ML is a branch of AI that focuses specifically on data and algorithms to support AI's ongoing learning [8]. ML algorithms typically assist in decision-making by estimating or predicting a pattern in the data. AI and ML have significantly improved the drug development process. Beginning with the discovery of new targets, AI and ML greatly advance our knowledge of disease and its related targets, as well as the design of molecular compounds, the prediction of 3D protein structures, the investigation of complex disease mechanisms, and more [8, 9]. In particular, the creation of intelligent or programmed drug delivery systems has made extensive use of AI and artificial neural networks (ANNs) during the past 20 years. New delivery systems that are intended for precise and personalized drug release in the human body are being introduced by the use of AI and the emergence of nanotechnology. The cargo (drug) may be delivered to the intended locations by AI-controlled nanobots. Consequently, the risk of toxicity and overdosing is reduced [10].

13.2 OVERVIEW OF AI–ML IN DRUG DELIVERY SYSTEMS

In recent times, AI and ML have become fundamental to drug discovery. Drug development time, cost, and failure risk have all significantly decreased since the advent of AI-based molecule library creation, novel drug candidate and target identification, and protein structure prediction. AI and ML constitute a vital tool for predicting drug loading, release, or targeting efficiency of nanoparticles and for minimizing the number of trials in the design of delivery systems [11]. AI-driven nanorobots with integrated circuits, compatible power storage units, sensors, data backup, and effective data transfer mechanisms are being developed for the smart drug delivery industry [12]. The aforementioned nanorobots are monitored and controlled by AI-based technologies. Table 13.1 summarizes the role of AI in the development of drug delivery systems.

AI-based models are primarily utilized in the computational simulation of the formulation. Extensive testing and comprehension of key delivery system components, including excipient selection, solubility estimation, formulation efficacy, drug release mechanism, and absorption process, are necessary for the simulation. Understanding the shortcomings of complex formulations is aided by a variety of algorithm techniques, such as QSAR, molecular physics, molecular dynamics, and computational fluid mechanics. Electronically controlled smart delivery systems are based on those understandings [13]. Additionally, the formulation and process parameters are correlated with in

TABLE 13.1
The Role of AI in Formulation Development and Drug Delivery System Design

- Data-driven prediction of dose and performance of delivery systems
- Fast recognition of bioactive and monitoring of drug release
- Computation simulation of drug formulation
- Development of an in vitro–in vivo correlation (IVIVC) model
- Optimizing drug loading in nanoparticles
- Optimization and prediction of drug release from sustained-release drug delivery systems
- Correlating formulation factors and process parameters to the drug release profile
- Controlling drug release based on the biological feedback mechanism

vitro drug release by the computational model, which subsequently correlates this with in vivo studies. AI-powered tools help forecast formulation behavior in relation to compositional changes. Such a prediction lowers the risk of failure in the later stages of drug development and cuts down on development time and expense. Excipient selection and preliminary testing for a variety of delivery systems, including oral, transdermal, tablet, and nanoparticle forms, are also aided by computational tools [14].

AI is essential for comprehending the biological environment, which helps with drug modifications to lower the risk of toxicity and allow for dose adjustment. The development of therapies based on nanocarriers and nanoparticles is greatly aided by AI and ML. These nanoparticles serve as diagnostic tools in addition to delivering medications to the intended site of action. One cutting-edge method for achieving controlled and programmed drug release is the design of implantable microchips using microfabrication techniques [15]. AI-enabled microchips gather and send data to external devices in addition to controlling drug release through a sensor-controlled feedback mechanism. Drug reservoirs of different sizes and shapes are found in microfabricated devices, which can be programmed to start or stop the release of drugs. Such a system guarantees pulsatile or precisely regulated drug delivery. It might also be motivated by need. Depending on the therapeutic need, electromechanical implants with AI-driven controls can adjust the drug's plasma concentration [16]. These electronic devices improve medication efficacy and patient safety while marking a significant breakthrough in AI-driven smart delivery systems. Through extensive searching in the minimized period, model evolution, algorithm recoding, and analysis refinement, a mechanized framework supports systemic modeling and parameter evaluation in delivery systems. In drug development, AI-driven models focus on the cycle of trying, failing, analyzing what went wrong, and improving the model. This type of in silico testing frequently handles large amounts of data and reports a reliable result.

As smart delivery systems, AI-driven feedback-regulated delivery systems are progressively far more popular. Depending on the therapeutic need, the feedback-regulated system releases the medication. One significant benefit of AI-controlled smart systems over traditional controlled drug delivery systems is the need-driven release. Let's look at an illustration. For patients with type II insulin-dependent diabetes, insulin is a necessary treatment that regulates the blood glucose level. Insulin must be taken by the patients either on a regular basis or as needed. Blood glucose levels are drastically lowered by excess insulin, which is undesirable. Therefore, the issue might be resolved by simultaneous insulin administration and continuous glucose monitoring. This is where intelligent delivery systems emerge. An insulin pump that connects to the body through an infusion system receives a signal from a sensor that continuously measures the body's glucose level. An AI algorithm is used to program the pump so that, without human assistance, insulin is automatically infused into the system when the glucose level rises above a predetermined point. These kinds of AI-driven, feedback-regulated systems may be the way of the future for chronic illnesses that need ongoing care [17].

AI has significantly advanced the robotics industry by enabling the automated completion of a variety of tasks without the need for human intervention. AI-driven microbots or nanobots were

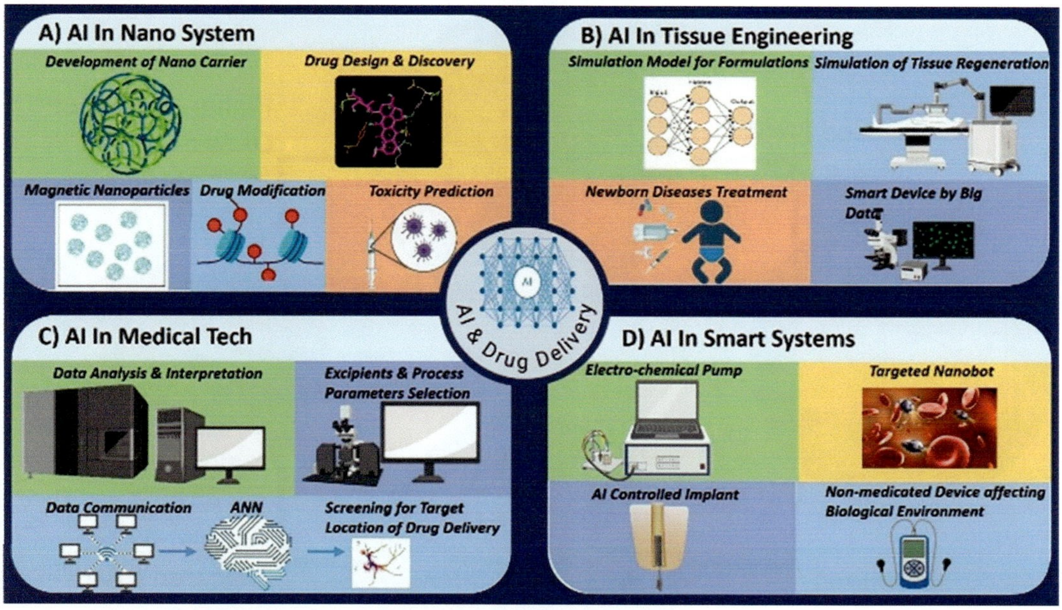

FIGURE 13.1 Overview of the application of AI and ML in drug delivery systems and theranostic applications.

created after the breakthrough, and they have the potential to transform the field of controlled drug delivery and diagnostics. After the dose is administered, microbots and nanobots can be successfully converted into intelligently controlled machines that can follow external instructions to the intended location of the body. Several researchers have reported using AI-based micro and nanobots to improve targeting and reduce adverse effects [18, 19]. ANNs are the most widely used ML-based algorithm in drug delivery. One of the most well-liked and effective ML tools that replicates the neuronal architecture of the human central nervous system is the ANN. The most popular ML-driven method for creating drug delivery systems is most likely ANN-based prediction and system optimization. The dissolution profiles of various drug formulation and delivery systems, including tablets, pellets, solid dispersions, hydrogel, and nanoparticles, are being modeled using both dynamic and static ANNs [20–22]. The ideal dosage form composition in relation to the desired drug release profile can be accurately predicted by a trained ANN model, both in vitro and in vivo. The drug release profile can be predicted using an ANN model, an ALP network, and a self-organizing map to assess the interactions between the independent and dependent variables. A common tenet of the "Quality by Design (QbD) concept" is that such prediction shortens development time and delivers a deeper comprehension of the correlation between variables. Analyzing datasets produced by extensive pharmacokinetic or pharmacodynamic studies or clinical trials is another possible use of AI and ML. The AI algorithm is trained using the available datasets, and it is then used for in vivo response prediction, adverse reaction assessment, dose modification, and drug safety analysis in large populations. The design of the delivery system is also aided by these skilled AI algorithms. An overview of the application of AI and ML in drug delivery systems development and working is presented in Figure 13.1.

13.3 MECHANISM OF AI-DRIVEN SMART PROGRAMMED DRUG DELIVERY SYSTEMS

Often referred to as non-feedback regulated systems, conventional controlled drug delivery systems operate on an "open loop" basis. Drug delivery in these systems is independent of biological feedback. On the other hand, intelligently programmed drug delivery systems operate via a "closed loop" mechanism. Drug delivery in these systems is managed or regulated in accordance

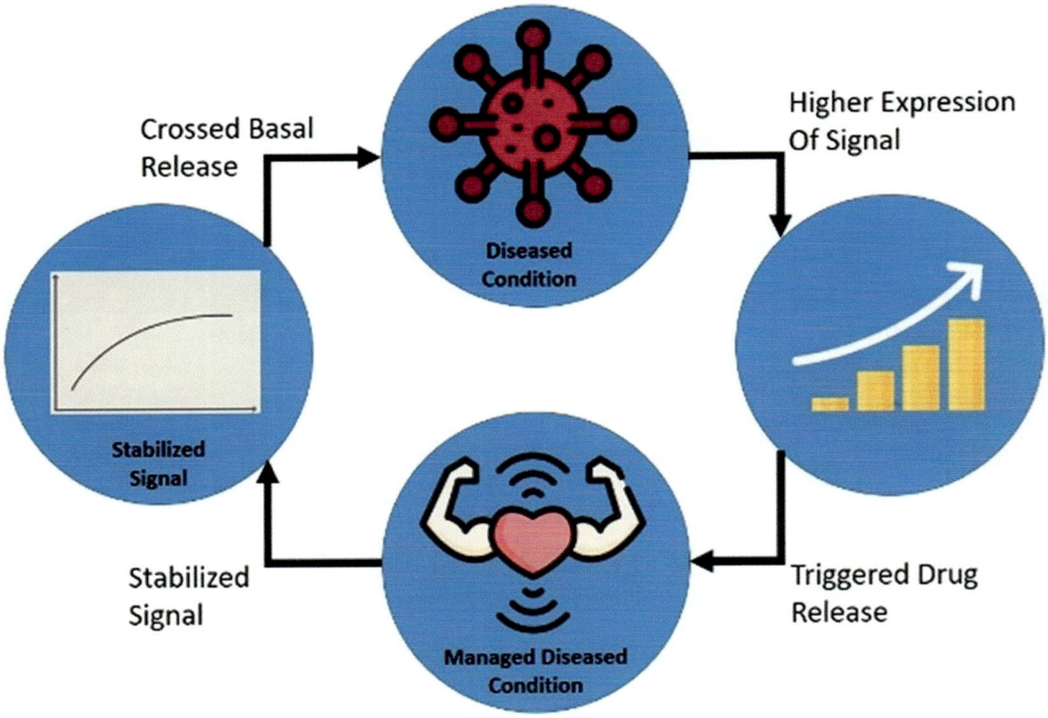

FIGURE 13.2 Closed-loop mechanism of smart drug delivery systems.

with the biological reaction or feedback. The primary distinction between "open loop" and "closed loop" systems is that the former release drugs at a predefined rate, while the latter adjusts release based on pharmacodynamics or kinetic response. The closed-loop system is connected to a sensor and monitoring component that ascertains the physiological state of the environment and an actuator device that, in response to the signal provided by the sensor, initiates the drug's release [23]. Digital connectivity is an additional component made possible by AI for closed-loop systems (Figure 13.2). The actuator can automatically modify and release the dose, or the patient can use a smartphone or other interface to change the dosage, thanks to the connectivity. To regulate drug release, intelligently programmed systems with closed loops require precise algorithms and strong mathematical models.

13.3.1 Mechanism of Implantable Microchip for Programmed Drug Delivery

Drug-loaded microfabricated devices known as implantable microchips are surgically inserted into various physiological locations. Surgery is required to remove those microchips following the duration of action, which may range from a few months to a few years. They can be placed beneath the skin, in the bone marrow, in the heart, in the vitreous portion of the eye, etc. [24]. These microchips are common reservoir-type devices, in which a reservoir cap permits drug release and a membrane encloses the core containing the active ingredient or drug. These chips use an electrochemical or electrothermal mechanism to release the drug. When a voltage is applied through an electrode in an active electrothermal mechanism, the drug is delivered by dissolving the reservoir cap. The drug is released through the gradual dissolution of a biodegradable polymer in the passive method. Devices with smartly programmed microfabricated chips operate on the active drug delivery mechanism. Human parathyroid hormone (h-PTH) was used in the first clinical trial of externally controlled drug delivery enabled by microchips [25]. Eight postmenopausal women with osteoarthritis received implants of microfabricated chips loaded with particular dosages of h-PTH as part of the trial. During the four months that the chips were implanted, they were programmed to deliver discrete doses of h-PTH once a day for three weeks. The chips created a bidirectional wireless link that allowed the programmer and clinicians to use a computer to monitor the external functioning and control the dosage. When compared to multiple injections, the results of the pharmacokinetic, safety, and bioequivalence analyses demonstrated comparable therapeutic benefits.

AI-enabled microchips, also known as biochips, can be effectively used to monitor diabetes and administer insulin to patients with insulin-dependent diabetes. The detection of glucose in bodily fluids has improved over the past few decades thanks to a number of biochemical techniques. Glucose oxidase is most frequently used to generate detectable electrical signals that correlate with the amount of glucose in different bodily fluids, including blood, sweat, tears, and saliva [26]. Significant progress has been made in wearable or implantable biochips that constantly or frequently measure intestinal fluid glucose levels and give patients real-time feedback so they can modify their insulin dosage or eating habits. If a device with an actuator is connected to the system, AI and ML-based algorithms can quickly analyze the feedback (glucose level) gathered by the biochips and either trigger or inhibit the release of insulin. These gadgets work via a closed-loop system. AI can help healthcare providers create individualized treatment plans for each patient by spotting trends and patterns in glucose data gathered over an extended period of time.

13.3.2 Hybrid Closed-Loop Systems of Programmed Drug Delivery

In insulin therapy and diabetes management, hybrid closed-loop systems are becoming more and more popular. By using a computerized algorithm, these systems help to keep the glucose level within a target range and reduce variations in the level (hyperglycemia or hypoglycemia). The algorithm helps determine the appropriate bolus doses and modifies the basal insulin level. Unlike closed-loop systems, which require the user to manually modify diets and bolus insulin dosages, these systems are referred to as hybrid [27].

The first commercially available hybrid closed-loop system for managing hyperglycemia or hypoglycemia was the MiniMed 670G, which was unveiled by Medtronic Inc. in 2016. Figure 13.3 illustrates the fundamental workings of a hybrid closed-loop insulin pump. In recent years, a

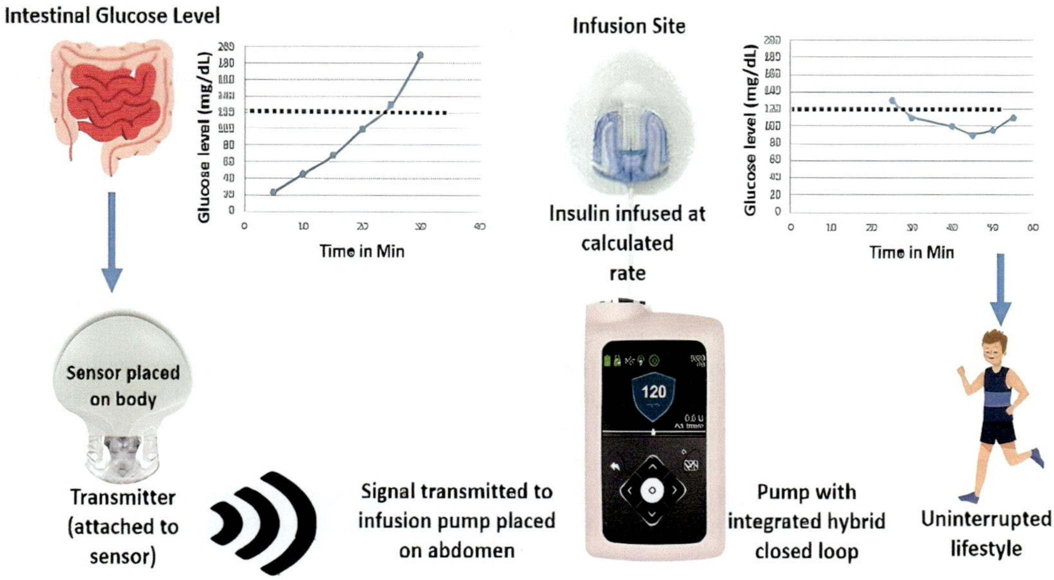

FIGURE 13.3 Hybrid closed-loop-based insulin pump for monitoring and maintaining blood glucose level.

number of other comparable system types have received approval. The MiniMed 780G (Medtronic), t: Slim X2 with Control-IQ (Tandem), and CamAPS FX (CamDiab, Cambridge, UK) are among the devices on the list [28]. These available systems are usually based on three main algorithms: fuzzy logic, proportional-integral-derivative (PID), and model predictive control (MPC). To predict the future glucose level, the MPC algorithm uses a mathematical model of the patient's glucose control systems. After determining the insulin sensitivity, the insulin delivery level is changed to balance the hyperglycemia to the intended basal level.

As a result, this algorithm can be referred to as predictive. The three components of PID, on the other hand, are as follows: (a) the proportional component, which is the difference between the target basal glucose level and the measured glucose level at a specific time point; (b) the integral component, which is the area under the curve derived using the measured and target glucose levels; and (c) the derivative component, which is the change in glucose concentration measured over a discrete period. Being a little out of the ordinary, fuzzy logic functions under a set of circumstances that mimic the expertise and analysis of a clinician who has been treating diabetes for years [29]. The first authorized smart programmed hybrid loop system, MiniMed 670G, uses Smart Guard TM technology, a modified PID algorithm [30]. Every 5 minutes, it automatically regulates the release of insulin through the MiniMed pump by either increasing, decreasing, or inhibiting it.

13.3.3 AI-Enabled Nanobots/Microbots

Nanobots are engineered microscopic devices that range in size from 1 to 100 nm. Targeted therapy and disease diagnosis have benefited greatly from the use of nanobot technology in recent decades. They are composed of a variety of nanomaterials, including carbon nanotubes, lipids, polymers, and polymer composites [31]. Sensing, measurement, and computation components are connected to sophisticated nanobots. These integrated nanobots have the ability to move through biological systems, reach the intended tissues, and perform the required function. Nanobots can deliver "cargo" (drugs), track biomarkers, deliver biochemical elements, create imaging, and alter the biochemical makeup of tissues in the least invasive ways possible at the cellular level. For a variety of theragnostic applications, targeting these microscopic robots, or nanobots, to a specific in vivo tissue microenvironment has become increasingly popular. Device modeling, feedback-controlled systems (open loop or closed loop), and regulating fields (magnetic, optical, etc.) are necessary to control the movement of nanobots and guide them toward the intended target. One of the nanobots' successful maneuvers involved the use of a magnetic field during the MRI procedure.

According to published clinical trials, AI-enabled nanobots have demonstrated notable advantages in smart drug delivery. Nanobots are being trained to identify diseased tissues using ML algorithms [32], and they direct the drug delivery system to the intended disease site. AI-based regulation, either at a discrete dose (open loop) or relying on biochemical regulation/feedback (closed loop), initiates the drug release in the cellular microenvironment once the system reaches the target and regulates its rate and duration. These targeted nanobots with AI capabilities are especially helpful in the treatment of neurological conditions and cancer. Conventional therapy for neurological disorders faces difficulties in crossing the blood–brain barrier, and anticancer medications must be delivered to the targeted tissues to prevent severe side effects.

AI-enabled nanobots have demonstrated their effectiveness in both situations. According to a Johns Hopkins University clinical study, nanobots can target lung tissues affected by cancer with 95% accuracy in about 1000 patients [33]. AI facilitates remote monitoring of nanobots so they can find the intended target tissues and release the medication in a regulated way. To target the nanobots with extreme precision, however, a suitable algorithm is required. AI-enabled nanobots' fundamental function is data collection, analysis, and predictive modeling. Once injected, nanobots use external controls (either magnetic or optical) to navigate through bodily systems and arrive at the desired locations. It gathers the required data while travelling through the microenvironment and transmits it to the ML model. The model directs nanobots to modify drug release and forecasts potential changes in biochemical regulation in the targeted disease state [34, 35].

13.4 AI-DRIVEN DESIGN

Using AI to design nanocarriers is a novel approach in the pharmaceutical industry. Specifically, nanocarriers are nanoscale, precision-based media that are used to deliver genes, medications, or imaging agents to particular bodily targets. The most popular AI technologies, ML and deep learning (DL), have significantly improved the efficacy and patient specificity of nanocarriers while also streamlining their design [36].

13.4.1 Nanocarriers and Their Design Challenges

In addition to being time-consuming, traditional hit-and-trial methods of designing nanocarriers require a thorough research-based approach. AI offers appropriate substitutes to lessen the difficulties associated with the high dimensions and multiscale nature of nanocarrier design [36]. AI has been used to design a variety of nanocarriers, including dendrimers, liposomes, and micelles, with streamlined procedures and increased efficiency [37].

13.4.2 Nanocarrier Design Using Artificial Intelligence

AI uses a variety of techniques to simplify the intricate design of nanocarriers, including data-driven decision making, predictive modeling, and parameter optimization. AI can recognize large databases and analyze intricate patterns to determine the ideal nanocarrier properties [38].

13.4.3 Machine Learning Algorithms

The creation of algorithms that forecast the optimal nanocarrier design for specific therapeutic applications is aided by ML. It is also possible to know the physicochemical characteristics and in vivo behavior of nanocarriers. To train models on expected features and outcomes, it can be used extensively [39].

13.4.4 Deep Learning Models

Novel nanocarrier designs based on input features with well-defined specificity have been made possible by DL techniques such as generative adversarial networks (GANs) and variational autoencoders (VAEs) [40]. Images of nanoparticles have been analyzed using other widely used techniques, such as recurrent neural networks (RNNs) and convolutional neural networks (CNNs), to identify surface features that affect cellular uptake. Predicting interactions, particularly with biological membranes, is another use for these.

13.4.5 Reinforcement Learning (RL)

By using trial-and-error techniques, this method allows learning to take place in a simulated environment. It has been widely applied to improve drug release profiles and target specificity. To choose the precise makeup of a nanocarrier for achieving controlled release in a fixed physiological environment, studies have been conducted using RL [41].

13.4.6 Applications of AI in Nanocarrier Design

13.4.6.1 Predicting Drug Encapsulation Efficiency and Release Profiles

When designing an effective nanocarrier, the two most crucial factors are controlled release and encapsulation efficiency. AI models aid in making precise predictions about these factors. Using regression models to analyze drug properties such as molecular weight and solubility, and then analyzing the surface charge and material type of the nanocarrier, research studies have demonstrated that encapsulation chances can be predicted [42]. Moreover, techniques like RNNs can accurately predict drug release and other processes. RNNs can forecast how a specific nanocarrier will release its payload over time by examining historical release profiles. While establishing treatments that call for sustained or pulsed release, this information is extremely helpful.

13.4.6.2 Optimizing Targeting and Biodistribution

One major benefit of nanocarriers is their ability to deliver therapeutic agents directly to diseased tissues while reducing side effects. By meticulously investigating ligand attachment, surface alterations, and particle size, AI algorithms maximize targeting. Certain modifications to the surface structure can have a major impact on the accumulation of a nanocarrier's surface in a particular organ or tissue. ML models trained on biodistribution data can forecast such changes [43].

13.4.6.3 Toxicity Prediction and Safety Optimization

The biggest obstacle in designing nanocarriers has always been toxicity, which is caused by accidental interactions with healthy cells. AI, on the other hand, offers predictive models that can evaluate anticipated toxicity by taking into account the size, shape, charge, and material composition of the nanocarrier. In order to categorize nanoparticles according to their cytotoxicity profiles, AI techniques such as support vector machines (SVMs) have been thoroughly researched. As a result, it is frequently utilized for safety standards and regulatory compliance [44].

13.5 OPTIMIZATION: PATIENT-SPECIFIC TREATMENT

The health care system is moving toward a more accurate and data-driven therapy that takes into account individual differences in drug metabolism, disease progression, and therapeutic response as a result of the integration of AI with drug delivery techniques. Combining AI with creative and programmable drug delivery methods greatly optimizes patient-specific treatment [45].

13.5.1 Role of AI in Personalized Medicine

AI algorithms, particularly ML and DL, have enabled patient-specific treatment options. These algorithms assist researchers in drawing data-supported conclusions about drug types by analyzing information from real-time biomarkers, genomic databases, and electronic health records [46], dosages, and schedules. AI integration has made it possible to evaluate differences in a patient's response to various treatment regimens as well as genetic, phenotypic, and past treatment data [47].

13.5.2 Smart Drug Delivery Systems (SDDS)

These are specially made devices that release medications in response to more precise physiological cues in the body, such as changes in pH, temperature, and disease-related enzymes. When AI and smart drug delivery systems (SDDS) are used together, drug release becomes more dynamic, allowing treatment plans to be modified in response to disease progression and available health data. AI-controlled implantable drug delivery systems are one example, which also offers the benefit of real-time data analysis [48, 49].

13.5.3 Applications in Oncology and Chronic Disease Management

Cancer treatment is one of the main fields that has experienced revolutionary change among all the treatments that have greatly benefited from AI integration, particularly through the use of AI-enabled SDDS. AI has enabled individualized cancer treatment that takes into account the tumor profile and immune response of the patient. AI algorithms that forecast individual responses and modify drug release rates to correspond with disease regression or progression handle the complexity and high variability involved [50, 51]. Additionally, AI-powered medication delivery systems have proven successful in the treatment of long-term illnesses like diabetes, cardiovascular disease, and neurodegenerative diseases. This is mostly accomplished by using AI-integrated systems to monitor biomarkers and modify drug intake to maintain therapeutic levels and lessen the burden of daily medication for patients [52, 53].

13.6 LARGE LANGUAGE MODELS AND COMPUTATIONAL TOOLS

These offer cutting-edge techniques for handling, analyzing, and responding to massive amounts of data. They can generate human-like responses in a variety of themes and styles that are contextually relevant [54, 55]. Because of their ability to generate coherent texts, code, analyze data, and change intricate linguistic patterns, they have significantly decreased the workload of humans [56]. Furthermore, AI has the ability to evolve from conversational agents into powerful, interactive tools with computational capabilities for problem-solving. Together with computational tools like data analysis libraries, visualization frameworks, and real-time information retrieval capabilities, LLMs may develop from conversational agents into powerful, interactive problem-solving tools. Because of this combination, the models are able to perform tasks that help users with analysis, decision-making, creativity, and insight production. Real-time online access enables models to retrieve recent data on events or quickly evolving areas [57].

13.7 APPLICATIONS

AI-powered insulin pumps automatically modify insulin dosages based on data from continuous glucose monitoring to forecast blood sugar trends. Designing nanoparticles that transport medications across the blood–brain barrier, a significant obstacle in the treatment of neurological conditions like Parkinson's and Alzheimer's, can be accomplished using ML models [58]. The structure and function of nanoparticles can be optimized by AI algorithms to target particular brain regions, increasing efficacy and lowering systemic side effects. Smart bandages with embedded sensors can track temperature, humidity, and pH levels to aid in wound healing [59]. In order to speed up healing and reduce the risk of infection, AI algorithms can process this data and regulate the release of antibiotics or painkillers only when required.

AI may mitigate bacterial resistance and guarantee successful treatment by optimizing the type, dosage, and timing of antimicrobial agents. When fighting resistant bacteria in severe infections, smart systems' ability to modify drug release in response to real-time infection marker detection is particularly helpful. Based on biomarker information or patient-reported pain levels, smart pain management devices, like implanted pumps, can administer opioids or other painkillers. Because ML algorithms are able to anticipate pain patterns, these devices can release the least amount of medication necessary to manage pain without leading to tolerance or addiction [60]. When necessary, AI-driven drug delivery systems for diseases like hypertension or arrhythmia can release medications to stabilize heart function based on real-time blood pressure and heart rhythm monitoring.

Patients with varying conditions who need quick treatment modifications will particularly benefit from these systems. In order to improve asthma or COPD treatments, AI-enabled inhalers can monitor usage trends and environmental triggers. By adapting to the patient's breathing patterns and warning them of potential environmental hazards or problems with medication adherence, smart inhalers with ML algorithms can administer medications more efficiently. SDDS in hormone replacement therapy are able to release hormones like testosterone or estrogen when necessary and track hormone levels in real time. By doing this, the negative effects of conventional, fixed-dose hormone treatments are reduced [61, 62]. Wearable technology can be integrated with AI-powered drug delivery systems to remotely monitor physiological markers in patients and modify dosages based on predictive models. For the treatment of long-term illnesses like thyroid issues, epilepsy, or hypertension, this app is especially helpful [63]. The effectiveness, safety, and personalization of drug delivery can all be transformed by AI and ML, as demonstrated by each of these applications, which will drive healthcare toward improved, patient-oriented solutions [64].

One of the biggest obstacles to AI-integrated drug delivery is creating accurate algorithms that manage the variability of complex patient responses, which would necessitate a large amount of high-quality, diverse data that is difficult to integrate. Other challenges include ensuring privacy and data security [65]. Translating such technology from lab to clinic requires regulatory approvals. Sensor accuracy, battery life, and device miniaturization are additional technical constraints. Therefore, there are few opportunities for broad adoption, particularly in environments with limited resources [66, 67].

13.8 CONCLUSIONS

Allegedly, the groundbreaking potential of SDDS, some contend that the use of AI and ML in healthcare presents moral and practical issues. Because certain algorithms are opaque and frequently referred to as "black boxes," it can be challenging for patients and clinicians to comprehend or question automated decisions. This could have an effect on patient accountability and trust. Furthermore, biases in training data can exacerbate healthcare disparities by producing inconsistent results across diverse populations. Concerns that these technologies might put profit ahead of patient welfare by concentrating on conditions that yield the highest revenue rather than addressing more general health needs are also fueled by elevated expenses and commercial interests. Subsequently, the focus on technologically advanced solutions may obscure crucial facets of care that prioritize patients, where human discernment and compassion are indispensable for efficacious therapy.

Individualized treatment adjustments will be possible thanks to more adaptive and sophisticated algorithms made possible by extensive research and developments in AI and ML. By continuously monitoring vital signs, biochemical markers, and environmental factors, future developments such as seamless integration with wearable and implantable sensors will provide a comprehensive perspective of healthcare. To guarantee the greatest possible benefits of such innovations among a variety of patient populations, simplified designs, cost-effectiveness, and democratized access will be essential. Potential partnerships between healthcare professionals, technology developers, and regulatory bodies can impact ethical considerations and rigorous norms for preserving patient safety and trust.

DECLARATION OF AI AND AI-ASSISTED TECHNOLOGIES

During the preparation of this work, the authors used QuillBot AI and Grammarly in order to paraphrase the sentences. After using this tool, the authors reviewed and edited the content as needed and take full responsibility for the content of the publication.

REFERENCES

1. Laracuente M-L, Yu MH, McHugh KJ. Zero-order drug delivery: State of the art and future prospects. J Control Release. 2020 Nov;327:834–856. doi: 10.1016/j.jconrel.2020.09.020.
2. Torchilin VP. Passive and active drug targeting: Drug delivery to tumors as an example. In: Drug Delivery. Berlin, Heidelberg: Springer; 2010. p. 3–53. doi:10.1007/978-3-642-00477-3_1.
3. Wang PP, Frazier J, Brem H. Local drug delivery to the brain. Adv Drug Deliv Rev. 2002 Oct;54(7):987–1013. doi: 10.1016/S0169-409X(02)00054-6.
4. Mostafa M, Al Fatease A, Alany RG, Abdelkader H. Recent advances of ocular drug delivery systems: Prominence of ocular implants for chronic eye diseases. Pharmaceutics. 2023 Jun;15(6):1746. doi: 10.3390/pharmaceutics15061746.
5. Magill E, et al. Solid implantable devices for sustained drug delivery. Adv Drug Deliv Rev. 2023 Aug;199:114950. doi: 10.1016/j.addr.2023.114950.

6. Chappel E. Implantable drug delivery devices. In: Drug Delivery Devices and Therapeutic Systems. 1st ed. Elsevier; 2021. p. 129–156. doi:10.1016/B978-0-12-819838-4.00001-8.
7. Lembo A, et al. Clinical trial: Effects of treatment with a vibrating capsule in patients with severe chronic constipation. Aliment Pharmacol Ther. 2024 Oct;60(7):855–862. doi: 10.1111/apt.18198.
8. Bannigan P, Aldeghi M, Bao Z, Häse F, Aspuru-Guzik A, Allen C. Machine learning directed drug formulation development. Adv Drug Deliv Rev. 2021 Aug;175:113806. doi: 10.1016/j.addr.2021.05.016.
9. Bonetta R, Valentino G. Machine learning techniques for protein function prediction. Proteins. 2020 Mar;88(3):397–413. doi: 10.1002/prot.25832.
10. Vatansever S, et al. Artificial intelligence and machine learning-aided drug discovery in central nervous system diseases: State-of-the-art and future directions. Med Res Rev. 2021 May;41(3):1427–1473. doi: 10.1002/med.21764.
11. Alshawwa SZ, Kassem AA, Farid RM, Mostafa SK, Labib GS. Nanocarrier drug delivery systems: Characterization, limitations, future perspectives and implementation of artificial intelligence. Pharmaceutics. 2022 Apr;14(4):883. doi: 10.3390/pharmaceutics14040883.
12. Rai A, Shah K, Dewangan HK. Review on the artificial intelligence-based nanorobotics targeted drug delivery system for brain-specific targeting. Curr Pharm Des. 2023 Dec;29(44):3519–3531. doi: 10.2174/0113816128279248231210172053.
13. Muñiz Castro B, et al. Machine learning predicts 3D printing performance of over 900 drug delivery systems. J Control Release. 2021 Sep;337:530–545. doi: 10.1016/j.jconrel.2021.07.046.
14. Wang W, Ye Z, Gao H, Ouyang D. Computational pharmaceutics – A new paradigm of drug delivery. J Control Release. 2021 Oct;338:119–136. doi: 10.1016/j.jconrel.2021.08.030.
15. Rodoplu Solovchuk D. Advances in AI-assisted biochip technology for biomedicine. Biomed Pharmacother. 2024 Aug;177:116997. doi: 10.1016/j.biopha.2024.116997.
16. Anandhakrishnan A, Hussain S. Automating insulin delivery through pump and continuous glucose monitoring connectivity: Maximizing opportunities to improve outcomes. Diabetes Obes Metab. 2024 Sep. doi: 10.1111/dom.15920.
17. Wang X, Si J, Li Y, Tse P, Zhang G, Wang X, et al. Effectiveness and safety of AI-driven closed-loop systems in diabetes management: A systematic review and meta-analysis. Diabetol Metab Syndr [Internet]. 2025;17(1):238. doi: 10.1186/s13098-025-01819-0.
18. Li J, Dekanovsky L, Khezri B, Wu B, Zhou H, Sofer Z. Biohybrid micro- and nanorobots for intelligent drug delivery. Cyborg Bionic Syst. 2022 Jan;2022:9824057. doi: 10.34133/2022/9824057.
19. Hu M, Ge X, Chen X, Mao W, Qian X, Yuan W-E. Micro/nanorobot: A promising targeted drug delivery system. Pharmaceutics. 2020 Jul;12(7):665. doi: 10.3390/pharmaceutics12070665.
20. Khan AM, et al. Artificial neural network (ANN) approach to predict an optimized pH-dependent mesalamine matrix tablet. Drug Des Devel Ther. 2020 Jun;14:2435–2448. doi: 10.2147/DDDT.S244016.
21. Obeid S, Madžarević M, Krkobabić M, Ibrić S. Predicting drug release from diazepam FDM printed tablets using deep learning approach: Influence of process parameters and tablet surface/volume ratio. Int J Pharm. 2021 May;601:120507. doi: 10.1016/j.ijpharm.2021.120507.
22. Boztepe C, Künkül A, Yüceer M. Application of artificial intelligence in modeling of the doxorubicin release behavior of pH and temperature responsive poly (NIPAAm-co-AAc)-PEG IPN hydrogel. J Drug Deliv Sci Technol. 2020Jun;57:101603. doi: 10.1016/j.jddst.2020.101603.
23. Paci MM, Saha T, Djassemi O, Wu S, Chua CYX, Wang J, et al. Smart closed-loop drug delivery systems. Nat Rev Bioeng [Internet]. 2025 [cited 2025 Jul 20]. doi: 10.1038/s44222-025-00328-z.
24. Kar A, Ahamad N, Dewani M, Awasthi L, Patil R, Banerjee R. Wearable and implantable devices for drug delivery: Applications and challenges. Biomaterials. 2022 Apr;283:121435. doi: 10.1016/j.biomaterials.2022.121435.
25. Farra R, et al. First-in-human testing of a wirelessly controlled drug delivery microchip. Sci Transl Med. 2012 Feb;4(122):122ra21. doi: 10.1126/scitranslmed.3003276.
26. Naveen Prasad S, Mahasivam S, Ramanathan R, Bansal V. Silver-based bimetallic nanozyme fabrics with peroxidase-mimic activity for urinary glucose detection. Anal Bioanal Chem. 2024 Nov;416(27):6149–6159. doi: 10.1007/s00216-024-05483-7.
27. Templer S. Closed-loop insulin delivery systems: Past, present, and future directions. Front Endocrinol (Lausanne). 2022 Jun;13:919942. doi: 10.3389/fendo.2022.919942.
28. Hartnell S, Fuchs J, Boughton CK, Hovorka R. Closed-loop technology: A practical guide. Pract Diabetes. 2021 Jul;38(4):33–39. doi: 10.1002/pdi.2350.
29. Boughton CK, Hovorka R. Automated insulin delivery in adults. Endocrinol Metab Clin North Am. 2020 Mar;49(1):167–178. doi: 10.1016/j.ecl.2019.10.007.

30. Stone MP, et al. Retrospective analysis of 3-month real-world glucose data after the MiniMed 670G system commercial launch. Diabetes Technol Ther. 2018 Oct;20(10):689–692. doi: 10.1089/dia.2018.0202.
31. Singh AV, et al. Emerging application of nanorobotics and artificial intelligence to cross the BBB: Advances in design, controlled maneuvering, and targeting of the barriers. ACS Chem Neurosci. 2021 Jun;12(11):1835–1853. doi: 10.1021/acschemneuro.1c00087.
32. Yang L, et al. Machine learning for micro- and nanorobots. Nat Mach Intell. 2024 Jun;6(6):605–618. doi: 10.1038/s42256-024-00859-x.
33. Jiang F, et al. Artificial intelligence in healthcare: Past, present, and future. Stroke Vasc Neurol. 2017;2(4):230–243.
34. Mitchell R, et al. AI and smart drug delivery systems: Revolutionizing personalized medicine. J Control Release. 2021;333:226–244.
35. Yu KH, Beam AL, Kohane IS. Artificial intelligence in healthcare. Nat Biomed Eng. 2018;2(10):719–731.
36. Tian T, et al. Smart nanoparticles for multi-modality cancer treatment: Bio-responsive and dynamic targeting, penetration, and transport. Adv Drug Deliv Rev. 2020;163:54–67.
37. Sharma A, et al. Machine learning for predicting pharmacokinetics and pharmacodynamics in precision medicine. Clin Pharmacol Ther. 2022;112(2):333–345.
38. Kapoor DU, Sharma JB, Gandhi SM, Prajapati BG, Thanawuth K, Limmatvapirat S, Sriamornsak P. AI-driven design and optimization of nanoparticle-based drug delivery systems. Sci Eng Health Stud. 2024;18:24010003. doi: 10.69598/sehs.18.24010003.
39. Zhang L, Wang S, Li Z. Prediction of drug encapsulation efficiency in polymeric nanoparticles using machine learning algorithms. J Nanomedicine. 2021;12(4):315–328.
40. Chen J, Zhang X, Wang Y. Applications of machine learning in nanomedicine design: A review. Nano Today. 2020;30:100789.
41. López Díaz D., Escobar A., Torres G. Deep learning approaches for predicting nanoparticle cell interactions. Biomed Nanotechnol. 2022;18(6):9871002.
42. Lu Y, Tang H, Zhang W. Application of reinforcement learning in drug delivery systems. Pharmaceutics. 2021;13(5):619.
43. Patel M, Kumar R, Gupta S. Machine learning in drug delivery: Optimization of drug loaded nanocarriers. Curr Pharm Des. 2022;28(3):210–220.
44. Rao K, Bhat P, Rao S. Machine learning in targeted nanomedicine: A comprehensive review. Adv Drug Deliv Rev. 2023;123:112–125.
45. Li F, Xu Z, Yang C. Predicting cytotoxicity of nanoparticles with support vector machines. NanoImpact. 2020;18:100227.
46. Huang Y, Li S, Zhang H. Deep learning in drug delivery systems: Optimizing enzyme sensitive release profiles. Adv Drug Deliv Rev. 2022;191:114486.
47. Kim M, Choi J, Lee S. Deep learning enabled design of enzyme responsive hydrogels for targeted drug delivery. Nano Today. 2020;35:100946.
48. Lee T, Jung K, Kim Y. AI driven bio-responsive material development: A comprehensive review. J Biomed Nanotechnol. 2021;17(4):663–678.
49. Li Z, Huang C, Lin Y. Machine learning optimization of temperature sensitive hydrogels for tissue engineering. Mater Sci Eng C. 2022;134:112528.
50. Patel A, Ramesh R, Kumar P. ML-based optimization of pH sensitive nanocarriers for targeted cancer therapy. J Control Release. 2021;335:456–467.
51. Smith J, Xu T, Wang D. Predictive modeling of hydrogel behavior using machine learning for drug delivery applications. Bioeng Transl Med. 2022;7(1):e10214.
52. Wang Q, Li L, Chen T. Machine learning enhanced bioresponsive glucose biosensors for diabetes management. Biosens Bioelectron. 2021;176:112925.
53. Xu Z, Liu Y, Zhou G. Deep learning in tissue engineering: Scaffold design for stem cell differentiation. Biomaterials. 2023;295:121914.
54. Yang M, Zhao X, Yu R. Multi analyte biosensors using AI optimized bio-responsive materials. Anal Chem. 2023;95(3):456–465.
55. Zhao L, Liu Q, Chen Y. Reinforcement learning for temperature sensitive materials in smart bandages. IEEE Trans Biomed Eng. 2023;70(2):601–609.
56. Ekins S, Puhl AC, Zorn KM, et al. Exploiting machine learning for end-to-end drug discovery and development. Nat Mater. 2019;18(5):435–441.
57. LeCun Y, Bengio Y, Hinton G. Deep learning. Nature. 2015;521(7553):436–444.
58. Topol EJ. High-performance medicine: The convergence of human and artificial intelligence. Nat Med. 2019;25(1):44–56.

59. Trasande L, Attina TM, Blustein J. Association between urinary bisphenol A concentration and obesity prevalence in children and adolescents. JAMA. 2012;308(11):1113–1121.
60. Vehik K, Ajami NJ, Hadley D, Petrosino JF, Burkhardt AR. The changing landscape of type 1 diabetes: Recent developments and future frontiers. Curr Diab Rep. 2013;13:642–650.
61. Viollet B, Mounier R, Leclerc J, Yazigi A, Foretz M, Andreelli F. Targeting AMP-activated protein kinase as a novel therapeutic approach for the treatment of metabolic disorders. Diabetes Metab. 2007;33(6):395–402.
62. Volkow ND, Wang GJ, Tomasi D, Baler RD. Obesity and addiction: Neurobiological overlaps. Obes Rev. 2013;14(1):2–18.
63. Waalen J. The genetics of human obesity. Transl Res. 2014;164(4):293–301.
64. Wild S, Roglic G, Green A, Sicree R, King H. Global prevalence of diabetes: Estimates for the year 2000 and projections for 2030. Diabetes Care. 2004;27(5):1047–1053.
65. Yadav U, Rani V, Deep G, Singh RK, Palle K. Oxidative stress in metabolic disorders: Pathogenesis, prevention, and therapeutics. Oxid Med Cell Longev. 2016;148:183–193.
66. Younossi ZM, Koenig AB, Abdelatif D, Fazel Y, Henry L, Wymer M. Global epidemiology of nonalcoholic fatty liver disease: Meta-analytic assessment of prevalence, incidence, and outcomes. Hepatology. 2016;64(1):73–84.
67. Zakir F, Mohapatra S, Farooq U, Mirza MA, Iqbal Z. Introduction to metabolic disorders. In: Drug Delivery Systems for Metabolic Disorders. Academic Press; 2022. p. 1–20.

14 Advances in 3D and 4D Bioprinting for Fabrication of Stimuli-Responsive Biomaterials

Amrita Muralikrishnan and Aathira Sujathan Nair
School of Pharmacy, Monash University Malaysia,
Bandar Sunway, Subang Jaya, Selangor, Malaysia

Saumya Bansal
Manipal College of Pharmaceutical Sciences, Manipal
Academy of Higher Education, Manipal, Karnataka, India

Mahendran Sekar
School of Pharmacy, Monash University Malaysia,
Bandar Sunway, Subang Jaya, Selangor, Malaysia

14.1 INTRODUCTION

Bioprinting is a field dedicated to overcoming the engineering challenges associated with tissue fabrication. It is a combination of polymers, cells, and other biological molecules to form a three- (3D) or four-dimensional (4D) material that mimics the biological environment of the organ and tissue. The limitation of conventional tissue engineering is the inability to develop the complex tissue structure, while bioprinting overcomes the challenge and also stands with the requirement of the fabrication of the ideal scaffold. The advancement in bioprinting has led to the development of intricate, complex microarchitectures with multiple cell types to mimic the ideal tissue structure [1]. 3D and 4D are the next-generation fabrication technologies making printing complex materials easy and intricate to print layer by layer with precision. One of the major differences between 3D and 4D bioprinting is the choice of raw materials. For 3D/additive manufacturing (AM), the materials are polymers, bioactive glass, ceramics, etc., but for 4D bioprinting it is the X, Y, and Z dimensions and the stimuli-responsive materials or commonly known as smart polymers. In 4D bioprinting, the smart polymers/stimuli-responsive materials are time-dependent and tune themselves accordingly, while 3D printing is static. Some applications that widely use 3D- and 4D-printed biomaterials are surgical and diagnostic tools, tissue engineering, implants and prosthetics, and drug delivery [1].

The foundation of bioprinting began with cell theory and the discovery of stem cells in the 1990s. In 1984, Charles Hull developed and patented the first bioprinter which used the stereolithographic method and later came to the market by the name of stereolithography (SLA) apparatus. In the late 1990s, Sachs used metals, plastics, and ceramics for printing and coined the term 3D printer. In 1996, Forgacs's observation of a single cellular aggregate to form the tissue complex and tissue regeneration was also one of the remarkable achievements in the history of bioprinting. Further, the researchers at Wake Forest Institute printed a full lab-grown bladder and implanted it in the patient. In 2000 the field of medicine started adopting printing technologies, and the first

 DOI: 10.1201/9781003560203-14

commercial 3D bio-plotter was made available. In 2003, Thomas Boland developed a new method for printing high-viability cells in the shape of an organ and later patented it as the inkjet printing technique. This invention of the Boland led to the shift to bioprinting in the field of tissue engineering. Later in 2004 Forgacs also engineered a tissue with cells, but scaffolds were not used. In 2009, NovoGen MMX, the commercial bioprinter, was invented. Also, in that year cell encapsulation in the hydrogels was achieved, and organoids with the first printed blood vessel were developed. In the past ten years, some of the recent advancements in the history of bioprinting are the development of scaffold-free vascular constructs, bioprinted articular cartilage, heart valve, and ExVive liver as a functional organ model for research studies and transplantation. Extrusion-based bioprinting was used to develop the artificial liver and skin constructs. In 2018, Poieskin, a full-thickness human tissue model, was 4D printed in response to external stimuli, making the first lab-grown printed skin. Further, in 2019, a complete heart with an intricate blood vessel network was printed by researchers at Tel Aviv University. Apart from that M3DIMAKER is the first 3D printer to manufacture personalized medicine [2].

Stimuli-responsive biomaterials are also known as smart biomaterials. Biomaterials have been used for developing the regenerative tissue of damaged body parts for several years. Over the years, biomaterial was defined on the nature of its bio-inertness, biocompatibility, and bioactiveness of the material. The degree of interaction of the material with the body defines its nature. Smart biomaterial was first defined in 2004, when the response to specific cellular signals was also taken into consideration for the development of the biomaterial. As the increase in technology and advancement happens, the current smart polymers will become dumb in the next 40 years. Currently, the level of smartness for biomaterials is in the increasing order of inert (i.e., no toxic reaction in or to the body), active, responsive (it can sense the external and internal stimuli to release the therapeutics) and, fourth and last, autonomous [3, 4].

14.2 FOUNDATIONS OF 3D BIOPRINTING

14.2.1 Basic Principles of 3D Bioprinting

3D bioprinting focuses upon three basic methods: (i) autonomous self-assembly, (ii) biomimicry or biomimetics, and (iii) mini-tissue building components. For generating an advanced 3D biological structure containing numerous mechanicals, structural as well as functional elements and qualities, an association of the aforementioned strategies tends to be generally essential. Understanding the way nature functions to develop fresh approaches to human issues is known as biomimicry. 3D bioprinting is the process of creating exact replicas of the cellular and extracellular components of an organ or tissue. The microscale duplication of biological tissues is required for this strategy to be successful. Therefore, it is necessary to comprehend the microenvironment, specifically, precise positioning of supporting as well as active varieties of cells, concentrations for insoluble or soluble substances, the extracellular matrix (ECM) makeup, and the characteristics of the biological forces present. The success of this strategy will depend on the creation of this knowledge base, which can be derived from fundamental studies in domains like engineering, imaging, biomaterials, cellular biology, biophysics, as well as medicine [5]. Using the development of embryonic organs as a guide is another method for reproducing biological tissues. To achieve the intended biological microarchitecture and function, the initial cellular elements within a maturing tissue generate distinct ECM components and suitable cell signaling, along with independent arrangement and patterning. A scaffold-free variant of this method mimics emerging tissues by using self-contained cellular spheroids that endure fusion and cellular organization. As the main force behind histogenesis, autonomous self-assembling depends on the cell to control the tissue's composition, location, and structural, functional, and other characteristics [6].

Both of the aforementioned 3D bioprinting methods capitalize on the idea of mini-tissues. Both tissues and organs are composed of mini-tissues, which are smaller, functional building fragments.

Using self-assembly, conceptual design, or a combination of the two, mini-tissues can be created and put together to form the bigger construct. There are two main approaches: first, using biologically influenced design and organization, self-assembled cell spheres are combined into a macro-tissue; second, precise, high-quality replicas of a tissue section are created and subsequently permitted to self-construct into an efficient macro-tissue [6].

14.2.2 Steps in 3D Bioprinting

14.2.2.1 Pre-Bioprinting

The characteristics of bioprinted structures are greatly influenced by the pre-bioprinting phase. Proper processes must be followed during the pre-bioprinting stage in order to guarantee that the right grade of cells is obtained together with anatomically accurate tissue models and suitable process design for bioprinting. Acquiring an organ biopsy to take a cell sample is one of the initial steps. Magnetic resonance imaging (MRI) and computed tomography (CT) are typical bioprinting technologies. These images undergo tomographic reconstruction in order to print using a layer-by-layer method. These 2D images are then processed by the printer to reconstruct a 3D model. Some cells are isolated and multiplied after the image is formed. These cells are combined with a unique liquid substance that gives them oxygen along with additional nutrients to remain viable. For procedures like extrusion, this cell aggregation is necessary for placement in the tubular-like tissue fusion, but it does not require a scaffold [7].

14.2.2.2 Bioprinting

The three main stages of the bioprinting stage are the bioprinting process, the bioprinter, and the bioink. This phase involves employing the patients' medical scans to deposit the bioinks—liquid combinations of cells, matrix, and nutrients—into a printer cartridge. Cell-based pre-tissue that has been bioprinted develops into a tissue when it is placed in an incubator. When creating biological constructs by 3D bioprinting, cells are usually dispensed onto a biocompatible substrate layer by layer to create 3D structures that resemble tissue. It has been demonstrated that 3D-bioprinted artificial organs, such as livers and kidneys, lack vital components that have an impact on the body, like functional blood arteries, urine collection tubules, and the development of billions of cells needed for these organs. The body cannot obtain the vital nutrition and oxygen it needs from deep within without these elements. Every tissue in the body is naturally made up of various cell types; hence, the capacity of various printing methods to maintain the stability and survival of the cells during the production process varies [7].

14.2.2.3 Post-Bioprinting

For the biological material to form a stable structure, post-bioprinting is required. The 3D-printed object's functionality and structural stability are in jeopardy if this procedure is not properly maintained. Both chemical-based and mechanical stimulations are required to keep the object in place. The cells get signals from these stimulations that regulate tissue growth and remodeling. Furthermore, recent advancements in bioreactor technologies have made it possible for tissues to vascularize, mature, and survive transplants [7].

14.3 BIOINK MATERIALS USED IN 3D BIOPRINTING

Bioinks are essential parts of bioprinting since they are biomaterial solutions that contain living cells. The components of the biomaterial solution must shield each cell from external stresses while the printing procedure is underway. To be compatible with biological organisms, printable, and able to maintain the survivability and activity of cells, biological inks need to meet defined standards. Advances in bioink technique help 3D bioprinting become more accurate and versatile, which advances our goal of creating therapeutically useful biological tissues and organs that can be implanted [8]. Figure 14.1 illustrates several commonly used bioinks.

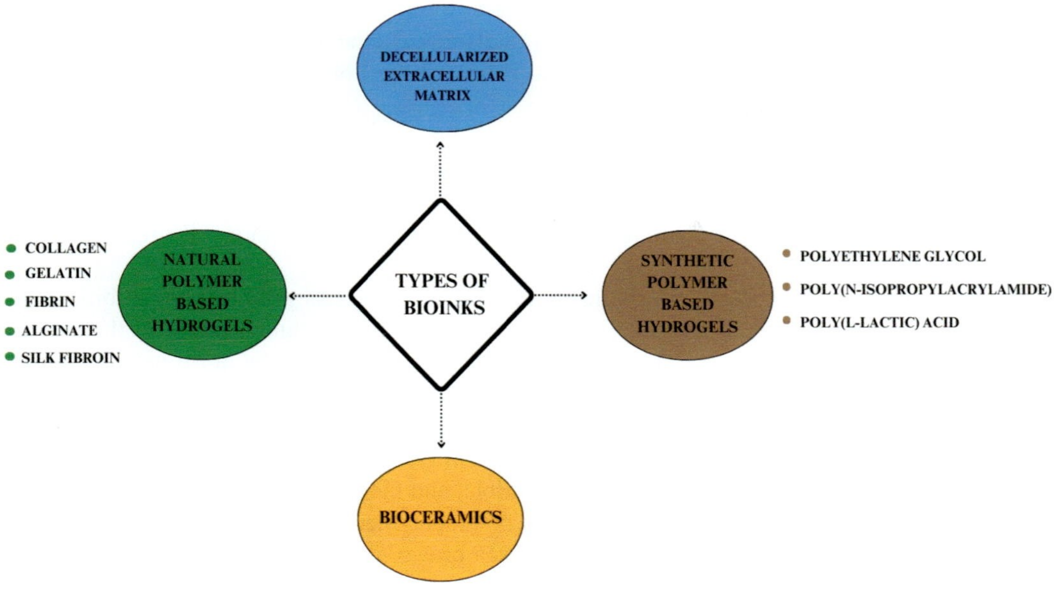

FIGURE 14.1 Types of bioink materials. This image illustrates the several types of bioinks—natural, synthetic, and hybrid—that are employed in 3D and 4D bioprinting. It demonstrates ways the bioink materials can be optimized for particular purposes in drug testing, tissue engineering, and regenerative medicine.

14.3.1 Polymer-Based Hydrogels

Hydrogels, which are hydrated systems of bonded organic or artificial polymers, are frequently used materials for bioinks. Hydrogel materials can also be greatly biocompatible and biodegradable, which is essential for in vivo uses. Additionally, when the hydrogel undergoes gelation, cells can be encapsulated in three dimensions. Typical hydrogel constituents include hyaluronic acid (HA), gelatin, agarose, and alginate. In the course of the printing procedure, such components enable the successive distribution of cells and offer a favorable environment for proliferation of cells. The complex structure of living organisms is well suited to these interconnected, aqueous-based polymer structures as they have an elevated water content and exhibit viscoelastic properties [9]. Hydrogels also can be converted to contain sustainable materials, like bioactive substances, so as to enhance their potential to influence cells and remodel tissues. Particularly, thermoplastic and injection-molded hydrogels preserve the unique biological activity traits that make those biomaterials vital for 3D biofabrication processes. They enable the development of intricate, biomimetic architectures that are utilized in tissue engineering, regenerative medicine, and personalized medicine [10]. However, hydrogels do have a disadvantage: they may be hard to keep their shape and often have poor mechanical properties. Hydrogels come in two primary varieties: synthetic and natural.

Among the most significant natural components in human cells' ECM is collagen type I. It exhibits exceptional biological compatibility and is frequently used in biomedical applications. A noteworthy study was created by Yoon and colleagues. They employed pure (single-component) collagen bioinks to produce 3D skin substitutes. Cell-rich 3D scaffolds were created using primary human epidermal keratinocytes (HEK) and HDF. The study's findings indicate that cell-loaded 3D scaffolds have effectively shown their effectiveness in a 1×1 cm^2 full-thickness excision animal model [11]. The damaged skin almost entirely and visibly recovered after a week. Similarly, a structure facilitating osteochondral tissue repair in the rabbit knee joint was printed by Shim et al. A preprinted polycaprolactone (PCL) scaffold was printed with pure collagen bioink made of atelocollagen, human turbinate-derived mesenchymal stromal cells (hTMSCs), and recombinant human bone morphogenetic protein-2 (rhBMP-2) [12].

Gelatin is an environmentally friendly, denatured protein that is produced by acid and alkaline denaturation of collagen, which modifies the electrical charge distribution of collagen to produce a different isoelectric point of gelatin. Gelatin-based bioinks have been used with a variety of encapsulated cell types and bioprinting strategies (extrusion, droplet, and light/laser-based). It has a comparable molecular makeup to collagen, but it has a less organized macromolecular framework, maintains crucial bonding groups for cell attachment, and includes sequences of peptide that can be broken down by the matrix metalloproteinases (MMPs) enzymes. Additionally, gelatin exhibits viscoelastic features that promote cell migration, differentiation, and growth [13].

Fibrin is a hemostatic substance that enhances cell attachment, has good biocompatibility, and produces few foreign body reactions and inflammation. A thrombin solution catalyzes the polymerization of fibrinogen monomers, which results in fibrin gels. Because the fibrin network facilitates blood clotting through a cross-linking mechanism that stops blood loss, fibrin can be used to treat wounds. Although fibrin's cell attachment feature encourages homogeneous cell distribution and great cell seeding efficiency, it has long-term stability issues. Alginate is a naturally existing polymer that is mild in toxic effects, biocompatible, and biodegradable. Marine algae (brown algae) and bacteria are the two primary sources of biopolymer alginate. This naturally occurring polysaccharide is present in the cell walls of sea brown algae (Phaeophyceae) as structural elements, and in certain bacteria (*Azotobacter* and *Pseudomonas*) as capsular polysaccharides. Alginate hydrogels are frequently employed as biomaterials in drug delivery, tissue engineering, and fundamental biological research as ECM models. Without the use of chemicals, alginate treated with cell attachment ligands can interact together with cells to create a recoverable, long-distance network [14].

Silk fibroin (SF), a fibrous protein, and sericin, a glue-like protein that envelops the fibroin strands, combine to form silk, considered one of nature's toughest fibrous proteins with biocompatible and recyclable qualities. A repeating polypeptide sequence of Gly–Ala–Gly–Ala–Gly–Ser and Gly–Ala/Ser/Tyr dipeptides can form sustained antiparallel β-sheet crystallites in the hydrophobic regions (H-chain) of SF [15]. Because SF may cause the sol-to-gel transition without the need of hazardous organic solvents or high temperatures, its application as a material for drug delivery systems is especially interesting. By varying the ink rheology with parameters like pH and ionic strength, SF-based bioinks are amphiphilic and can be utilized to produce protein droplets or extruded filaments for inkjet or extrusion printing, respectively [16].

Polyethylene glycol (PEG) is an artificial polyether that is inexpensive, soluble in water-based or organic solvents, and highly biocompatible. It can be used to make hydrogels and can be modified with diacrylate or dimethacrylate groups to produce a photocrosslinkable polymer. PEG-alginate-nanoclay hydrogels with cell survival rates in the range of 75.5%–86.0% over a seven-daytime culture period were created by Hong et al. using PEG in conjunction with nanoclay. Each component's characteristics produced a very tough and flexible hydrogel that could be utilized to build intricate 3D structures [17]. With a gelation temperature of 30–37°C, poly(N-isopropylacrylamide) (PNIPAAm) is another kind of artificial polymer utilized in 3D bioprinting process. The PNIPAAm networks go through a coil–globule transformation and become hydrophobic in this temperature range; these chains' hydrophobic interactions cause gelation. PNIPAAm is often mixed with alginate to increase biocompatibility [18]. Lactic acid made from sustainable sugarcane or corn starch sources is the raw material for poly(l-lactic) acid (PLA), an aliphatic and recyclable polyester. The cyclization and oligomerization processes combine to form PLA. PLA is a biocompatible polymer that is frequently utilized in biomedical applications since it does not cause cancer or harm local tissue [19]. Because of its flexible mechanical qualities, biodegradability, biocompatibility, and wide range of erosion times, poly(lactic-co-glycolic) acid (PLGA) is a different polymer that is frequently utilized in tissue engineering and drug administration. The FDA has authorized this polymer since it is widely used in several investigations due to its physical strength and biocompatibility [20].

14.3.2 Bioceramics

Bioceramics plays a major role in the advancement of 3D bioprinting techniques, particularly in the fields of tissue engineering and regenerative healthcare. One popular option is hydroxyapatite, a form of bioceramic, because of its chemical structure, which is incredibly identical to the mineral content present in bone. Through integrating bioceramics to the bioinks used in 3D bioprinting, printed structures' mechanical and architectural characteristics are improved, making them ideal for use in bone tissue engineering purposes. By simulating the rigidity of natural bone, the scaffold created by the incorporation of bioceramics into the bioinks has a substantial compressive strength and adds to the general stability of the printed construct. While developing replacements for bones and implants, where the goal is to generate structures that effectively aid in the procedure of regeneration while also offering structural support to the tissues nearby, the incorporation of bioceramics into bioinks is especially beneficial. By providing individualized implants that fit the complex anatomical and mechanical characteristics of natural bone tissue, as well as tailored remedies for bone deformities and fractures, the use of bioceramics in 3D bioprinting demonstrates the possibility to completely reinvent orthopedic interventions [21].

14.3.3 DECELLULARIZED EXTRACELLULAR MATRIX (dECM)

Decellularized ECM (dECM) can be converted into a bioink, which produces an environment tailored to a particular tissue to which seeded cells can be introduced. The dECM eliminates cell components while preserving the complex architecture of the ECM through a rigorous decellularization process. As a basic bioink, this acellular matrix acts as an organic scaffold to enable the accurate placement of live cells throughout the bioprinting procedure. When bioprinted components undergo transplantation, the immune-modulating qualities of dECM further reduce the possibility of immunological reactions. Furthermore, the proteins included in the dECM give the printed structures structural durability and rigidity, which is crucial for uses employing tissues that can support loads. Overall, using dECM in 3D bioprinting improves the biomimicry of bioprinted materials while also strengthening their practicality, solidity of structure, and likelihood of integrating successfully into host tissues [22].

14.4 3D BIOPRINTING TYPES

A variety of bioprinting methods have been developed to address a range of material characteristics, resolution requirements, and biological applications as the demand for producing organs and modified tissues increases. Table 14.1 offers comprehensive details on several bioprinting methods, pointing out both their benefits and drawbacks.

14.4.1 Inkjet Bioprinting

Inkjet bioprinting is a noncontact printing technique where a few picoliter to nanoliter drops of bioink are deposited onto a "biopaper" in a digitally controlled pattern. Since it is a straightforward modification of the traditional inkjet printing technique, most inkjet bioprinting operations still use commercial desktop inkjet printers that have been partially modified. Inkjet printing can be approached in two basic ways: drop-on-demand (DOD) and continuous inkjet (CIJ). Inkjet printing is superior to other methods of 3D printing techniques because it can print overhanging structures and channels utilizing sacrificial materials, improve surface quality with microdroplets, and be used for structural components and microfluidics. This technique, nonetheless, has a number of drawbacks. One of the main restrictions, for instance, is that the substance must be liquid and low viscous in order to facilitate the development of droplets and avoid nozzle obstruction. This implies that an additional cross-linking phase is required to improve the mechanical strength of the structure

TABLE 14.1
Summarization of Several Bioprinting Techniques, Advantages, Disadvantages, and Applications in Drug Delivery Technology

Bioprinting Techniques	Advantages	Disadvantage	Applications	References
Inkjet bioprinting	• Effective for microfluidics and structural components • Allow printing of overhanging structures and enhance surface quality with microdroplets.	• Require low-viscosity, liquid bioinks • More cross-linking could damage biomolecules • Resolution can be decreased by satellite droplets.	Structural components, microfluidics, and tissue scaffolds.	[30]
Vat photopolymerization	• High quality • Fast printing • Customized material design.	• Structural integrity requires post-processing • Resin separation presents difficulties.	Medication delivery systems, soft robotics, dental implants, medical devices, and microfluidics.	[30, 31]
Pressure-assisted bioprinting (PAB)	• Can precisely manage the printing of a range of biomaterials, making it suitable for cell-laden structures.	• Material viscosity limits • Structural stability often requires post-processing.	Printing tissue constructs, hybrid biomaterial structures, and medical research applications.	[32]
Laser-assisted bioprinting (LAB)	• High precision for cell patterning • Noncontact exchange of sensitive biologic substances.	• Requires specialized equipment • Post-processing may be necessary for stability.	Cell patterning, tissue engineering, and biological material deposition.	[33]
Solenoid valve-based printing	• Suitable for live cell printing • Can distribute a broad range of biomaterials without heating.	• Limited by viscosity of materials • Temperature control may be needed for specific bioinks.	Skin healing, diagnostic applications, micro-dispensing, and live cell printing.	[31]

in order to effectively generate 3D components utilizing inkjet. This procedure could lengthen the duration needed to fabricate the components and could be harmful to the cells or biomolecules that are a part of the bioink. Satellite droplets, which are tiny secondary drops that can appear among the bigger main droplets and reduce total accuracy and resolution, are another potential problem that inkjet bioprinting may encounter [23].

14.4.2 Vat Photopolymerization

Photopolymerization, which generally refers to the fixing of photo-reactive polymers using a laser, light, or ultraviolet (UV), is the primary 3D printing technology that is most commonly utilized [24]. Vat photopolymerization is a chemical-based 3D printing method with several impressive benefits, including rapid printing, high print resolution, variable material design, and a clean print surface. SLA alongside digital light processing (DLP) are the most widely used vat photopolymerization techniques. They have demonstrated great promise in the tailored construction of tissue scaffolds, medical devices, soft robots, dental implants, microfluidic devices, and drug delivery systems [25]. A concentrated laser beam serves as the light source in SLA. The printing surface is usually submerged slightly below the solution layer to start the procedure. The process of polymerization is commenced by scanning the material's cross-section with the laser beam. The building sheet is further dropped once a layer has been printed, and the procedure continues until the 3D structure is finished. A similar procedure is employed in DLP; however, a UV or blue light projector instantly projects the cross-section picture to polymerize a complete layer at a time unlike employing a focused laser. Due to this, DLP prints at far faster speeds than SLA. The untreated resin is separated from an object at the last stage of the print procedure for both SLA and DLP, and a post-processing step is typically performed to improve the mechanical characteristics of the printed construct [26].

14.4.3 Pressure-Assisted Bioprinting

The term "pressure-assisted bioprinting" (PAB) describes a group of layered fabrication techniques based on extrusion that may produce digitally controlled 3D patterns and structures. PAB can be used to print biomaterials such as polymers and ceramics, proteins and biological molecules, growth factors, viable cells, and their hybrid structures [26]. The biomaterials employed in printing are typically pastes, solutions, or dispersions that are extruded onto an immobile substrate by directing the movement of a continuous filament of pneumatic pressure or pressure based on a plunger or screw through a microscale nozzle aperture or a microneedle. Detailed 3D patterns and constructions are eventually created after layer-by-layer application [27].

14.4.4 Laser-Assisted Bioprinting

A series of noncontact linear printing methods known as laser-assisted bioprinting (LAB) use a pulsed laser beam to place biological components—such as cells—over substrates. It uses UV/laser for photopolymerizing the biomaterials. The bioink deposition through the nozzle layer by layer yields a structure; also, liquid bioink absorbs the laser and polymerizes the ink to form the determined pattern. The majority of LAB systems consist of three essential parts: a receptive substrate, a bioink-coated "ribbon," along with a pulsed laser source. The ribbon is exposed to laser radiation, which causes the liquid biological components to vaporize and fall as droplets onto the receiving substrate. Following the transfer of cells from the ribbon, the receiving substrate contains a biopolymer or cell culture medium to maintain adhesion of cells and further multiplication. It is widely used in the development of nerve tissues that require high cell viability in delicate structures [28].

14.4.5 Solenoid Valve-Based Printing

Applications for micro-dispensing with solenoid valves include the application of biomolecules like proteins, DNA, and diagnostic reagents. The technology has demonstrated the ability to print structures in a monitored environment, mesenchymal stem cells over tissue well plates as well as live biological cells for skin healing. A liquid reservoir, a solenoid-based dispensing mechanism, heating components to regulate the temperature of the nozzle head, interfaces to the pneumatic controller, and an inert gas make up a full system. The solenoid valve system can dispense viscous polymers like collagen and sodium alginate (12%) without requiring heat. To create a complicated heterogeneous build, the robotic stage can be equipped with several nozzles that can print different materials [29].

3D bioprinting's stimuli-responsive mechanism improves the functionality of printed structures in biomedical applications by enabling them to adapt and respond to external stimuli like temperature, light, or pH. Static, inflexible structures have given way to dynamic, morphing structures that react to environmental cues in the field of 3D bioprinting. Developments in cellular engineering, biomaterial science, and biofabrication methods are propelling this shift by making it possible to create structures that can change post-printing to resemble the behavior of genuine tissues. Researchers may create dynamic tissue models, biohybrid robots, and implantable medical devices that adjust to physiological changes by programming shape morphing into bioprinted constructions. The differential swelling of hydrogels, cell-mediated remodeling, and pre-strained biomaterials that experience regulated deformation upon activation are important processes behind shape morphing. Hydrogel-based biological inks stand as essential components in this process because they absorb water which leads to substantial volume alterations that produce flexing, folding, and expansion when exposed to external stimuli. Scientists develop complex but manageable shape-changing structures through the integration of temperature-sensitive polymers with photopolymerizable biological inks and ionic cross-linking agents. Additionally, because live cells exert stresses and release ECM components that drive self-morphing behavior, including biological activities into bioprinted structures adds another layer of flexibility. Since synthetic tissues must adapt to the body's changing biomechanical environment, these advancements have important ramifications for regenerative medicine [34].

The design of self-expanding vascular transplants together with shape-adaptive cartilage implants enables these medical devices to replicate both the mechanical features and functional adaptability found in natural tissues. The path toward clinical application of shape-morphing bioprinted structures remains promising despite ongoing difficulties in validating the biological compatibility along with scalable production methods and consistent material quality of these novel biomaterials. In order to create next-generation bioprinted tissues and organs, research is now concentrated on improving biofabrication methods to get exact control over morphing dynamics while preserving cell viability and function [35].

3D bioprinting achieves higher adaptability through its capability to establish immediate interactions between printed constructions and environmental stimuli. These technologies prove highly beneficial for drug delivery and soft robotics applications because they depend on external signals, including temperature and pH levels as well as light and electrical impulses to produce reversible and irreversible shape transformations. Poly(N-isopropylacrylamide) (PNIPAM) along with similar temperature-sensitive materials enable structures to expand or contract by undergoing phase transitions when exposed to body temperature. The swelling behavior of pH-responsive hydrogels allows them to function as targeted medication release systems and smart wound dressings because they respond to environmental acidity levels. Light-activated bioinks utilize photochemical reactions to enable precise control of morphing which benefits applications such as responsive implants and guided tissue creation. The creation of biohybrid actuators and functionalized implants that dynamically adjust to physiological signals is made easier by materials that respond to electrical and magnetic fields, which provide new opportunities for remote actuation of bioprinted structures [36].

In addition to increasing the number of possible uses, the incorporation of these stimulus-responsive components with bioprinting methods also creates new difficulties for responsiveness, durability, and biocompatibility optimization. Making sure that the stimulus-triggered changes don't eventually jeopardize the construct's cellular functioning or mechanical integrity is one of the main challenges. In order to overcome this, scientists are looking at hybrid bioinks, which combine a number of responsive qualities to provide multifunctional behavior that can be tailored for certain biomedical uses. Our capacity to anticipate and regulate these changes can be further enhanced by upcoming developments in computational modeling and material design, opening the door to the creation of extremely complex, adaptable bioprinted structures. As 3D bioprinting continues to advance, the combination of stimulus-responsive mechanisms and shape-morphing effects will transform tissue engineering, personalized medicine, and bio-integrated devices, advancing the creation of truly intelligent and self-governing biomedical structures [37].

14.5 FUTURE FRONTIERS OF 4D BIOPRINTING

14.5.1 4D Bioprinting Development

The need for more intricate and useful tissue engineering techniques led to the development of 4D bioprinting. It reveals a substantial development over traditional 3D bioprinting through combining the ability to alternate form when exposed to environmental cues [38]. Applying AM, 3D bioprinting creates living components layer after layer. Nevertheless, it is frequently impractical for 3D-printed systems to have interaction dynamically with their surroundings. To address this issue, 4D bioprinting was created.

It includes time-dependent changes in shape, function, or properties [39]. Components that could self-assemble and alternate shape, specifically in soft robotics and smart substances, served as early suggestion for 4D bioprinting. Researchers were hoping to apply those properties for biological applications with the aid of using incorporating stimulus-responsive biomaterials, additionally known as smart biomaterials. When exposed to outside signals which include temperature, pH, hydration, or light, those substances permit printed structures to extrude in managed ways [40]. The viability of 4D bioprinting has been similarly more desirable with the aid of using developments in biofabrication technologies, such as inkjet, extrusion-based, and SLA. Furthermore, the prediction and optimization of shape-changing behavior have benefited significantly from computer modeling and simulation. 4D bioprinting is now broadly utilized in tissue engineering, regenerative medicine, and personalized healthcare because of the aggregate of recent biomaterials, state-of-the-art printing methods, and computational tools [41]. The foundation for comprehending shape transformation concepts was established by early research on self-folding structures in the 1990s. The field was further driven toward dynamic biological applications in the early 2000s with the development of programmable materials and soft actuators. The first effective applications of 4D bioprinting in regenerative medicine, specifically in the creation of tissue scaffolds with controlled shape morphing, were seen in the 2010s [42]. Recent studies have concentrated on combining multi-material bioinks, improving printing accuracy, and refining computer models to precisely forecast shape transformation in light of the ongoing developments in biofabrication. With uses extending beyond tissue engineering to encompass medication delivery systems, biosensors, and soft robotics, these advancements portend a bright future for 4D bioprinting [43].

14.5.2 Shape-Morphing Effects and Stimulus-Responsive Mechanism of 4D Bioprinting

The core principle of 4D bioprinting lies in the ability of printed constructs to undergo programmed transformations. These transformations are dictated by various shape-morphing effects and stimulus-responsive mechanisms [44]. In 4D bioprinting, shape morphing is initiated using various methods, including self-unfolding and folding, expansion and contraction, and helical transformations.

14.5.2.1 Self-Unfolding and Folding

Bioprinted components guided by origami have the ability to unfold or self-fold in response to outside stimuli. For example, when hydrogels are exposed to moisture, their differential swelling characteristics enable controlled folding. This phenomenon can be precisely controlled to create complex structures that go through predesigned changes in applications, including tissue engineering and drug delivery where high structural control is essential [44].

14.5.2.2 Expansion and Contraction

Shape-memory polymer (SMP) substances and hydrogels can extend and reduce primarily based on modifications in pH, water content, or temperature. It is a highly desirable effect when designing soft actuators and dynamic tissue scaffolds, when the dimension and shape that can be controlled in relation to physiological conditions is desirable. For instance, the expansion or contraction can control the release of therapeutics in a controlled way when developing responsive drug delivery systems [44].

14.5.2.3 Helical Transformations

The potential uses in soft robotics and bio-actuated implants benefit from the ability to create 4D bioprinted elements that can twist helically, mimicking biological helices. Bioprinted materials can mimic the twisting motion of muscles or tendons by employing helical transformations, offering more flexible and adaptive solutions for bioengineering and medical devices. This technique is particularly powerful for growing systems that want to reply actively and in a managed manner to mechanical forces or modifications within the environment [44].

14.6 MECHANISMS THAT RESPOND TO STIMULI

In 4D bioprinting, stimulus-responsive systems mostly control the shape change. Temperature is another significant parameter as thermoresponsive polymer materials like poly(N-isopropylacrylamide) (PNIPAAm) exhibit a phase transition upon temperature variation. This allows for shape-morphing functionality. pH-sensitive hydrogels can swell or shrink based on the acidity or basicity of the environment. This property renders them appealing for drug release and wound healing. Some biopolymers find applications in wound dressings and self-healing scaffolds. They swell when they take up water, which is similar to the response of biological tissues. Shape changes are thus also determined by humidity and moisture. Photo-reversible polymers can undergo changes in shape when irradiated with specific wavelengths, enabling one to have high control over the transformation process. As materials that react to electric fields can be used, and given that bioprinted structures with magnetic nanoparticles enable remote-controlled actuation, magnetic and electric fields help enhance bioelectronics and artificial muscles [45]. Researchers may create dynamic biological constructions that react to physiological and environmental stimuli by using these pathways, opening the door to highly functioning biomedical gadgets. Several factors influence the effectiveness and efficiency of 4D bioprinting. These factors can be broadly categorized into material considerations, printing techniques, computational modeling, and biological integration. For 4D bioprinting to be implemented successfully, the selection of biomaterials is essential. Reversible shape changes, biocompatibility, and biodegradability are essential properties of smart biomaterials. When subjected to external stimuli, materials known as SMPs may maintain a distorted shape and regain its original shape. The effectiveness of 4D bioprinting depends on the printing technique employed. Among the popular techniques is extrusion-based bioprinting, which is perfect for producing huge, intricate structures and permits the use of extremely viscous bioinks. Bioprinting using inkjet allows for the exact deposition of biomaterials and is suitable for high-resolution printing. SLA is a technique that is effective for printing photopolymerizable materials since it employs light-based curing to create intricate structures. LAB uses laser energy to direct the placement of bioink, ensuring great precision and cell survival [46].

14.7 PERSPECTIVES IN 3D AND 4D BIOPRINTING

Here we highlight some of the major areas in which 3D- and 4D bioprinting strategies are anticipated to rapidly impact humankind: organ transplantation, disease modeling, and personalized medicine (Figure 14.2). The rise of 3D and 4D printing has been pivotal in transforming the fields of biomedical engineering, tissue engineering, and regenerative medicine. The progress of the bioprinting technology is expected to offer brighter opportunities in the future.

14.7.1 Organ and Tissue Engineering

4D bioprinting can incorporate dynamic tissue behavior, and this could make printed organs more similar to the natural response in human tissues. Fully functional human prints are among the most anticipated breakthroughs in bioprinting, and with the decline in organ donation globally, 3D bioprinting has been regarded as a potential solution. While 3D-printed organs are still experimental, the next decade will probably see advancements that make these bioprinted organs available for transplant [13, 47].

14.7.2 Personalized Medicine and Drug Testing

Pharmaceutical companies already use 3D bioprinting for high-throughput drug screening, and the technology is predicted to be used in preclinical studies as standard as it matures. Scientists will be

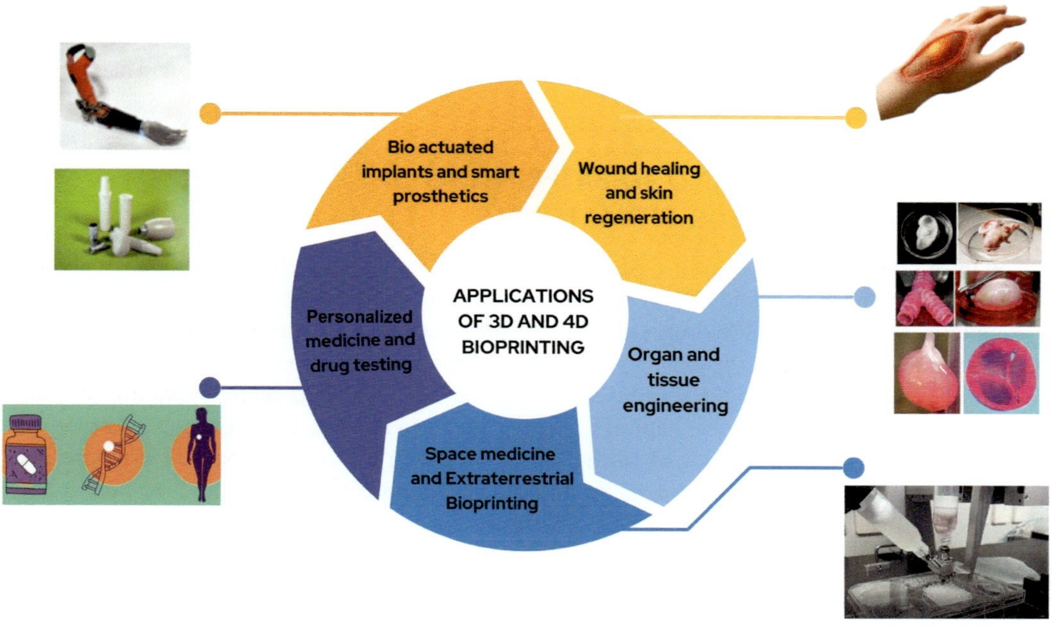

FIGURE 14.2 Applications of 3D and 4D bioprinting. The many potential uses of 3D and 4D bioprinting technologies in the medical domain are depicted in this figure. These include the fabrication of bio-actuated implants and prosthetics, dynamic, organ models for surgical planning, personalized medicine, and regenerative medicine. The development of adaptive 4D systems from static 3D models presents pioneering possibilities for the production of bioactive, functional organs and tissues for medical use.

able to test the effectiveness of medications on realistic tissues prior to human treatment thanks to the ability to bioprint patient-specific tissues and organ models. This will increase treatment efficacy, decrease adverse drug responses, and lessen the need for animal testing [48].

14.7.3 Skin Regeneration and Wound Healing

The utilization of 3D and 4D bioprinting in skin regeneration and wound healing is yet another fascinating application. Bioprinted skin grafts tailored to the individual needs of burn patients and patients with persistent wounds may be beneficial. Multilayered skin tissue, including the epidermis, dermis, and even hair follicles, is being bioprinted by researchers. Bioprinted skin may eventually be able to cover wounds and become a part of the patient's body, lowering the possibility of infection and rejection [49].

14.7.4 Bio-Actuated Implants and Smart Prosthetics

It is anticipated that the development of bio-actuated implants and prosthetics would be revolutionized by the combination of 4D bioprinting with smart materials. 4D-bioprinted implants have the potential to dynamically adjust to the physiological parameters of the patient, in contrast to traditional implants that stay fixed. Shape-morphing bone grafts or self-expanding heart valves, for instance, may improve surgical results and lower risks. These developments will open the door for less invasive medical devices tailored to each patient [50].

14.7.5 Extraterrestrial Bioprinting and Space Treatment

Yet another exciting prospect is the application of bioprinting in space healthcare. As space exploration continues, astronauts may require medical care that is not dependent on resources from Earth.

On-demand manufacturing of tissues, medicinal patches, and even bone transplants in space may be made possible via 3D and 4D bioprinting. Printing biomaterials in microgravity has the potential to revolutionize medical assistance for extended space missions, including those aimed at exploring Mars [51].

14.8 ADVANCES IN 3D AND 4D BIOPRINTING OF STIMULI-RESPONSIVE BIOMATERIALS

Although 3D bioprinting is a cutting-edge technique that combines cells and biologically active compounds into one bioscaffold, 3D bioprinting is unable to adapt, change, or expand to a changing surrounding. A new phase of hydrogels and smart polymers has just surfaced, which can address some of the shortcomings of the existing methods by adding a new dimension, such as time to 3D bioprinting. 4D bioprinting is the term used to describe this idea. This method could help create tissue-like structures that resemble natural tissue in both form and function. Although 4D bioprinting is currently in its early years and further work is needed to improve it, these structures can adapt and reconfigure when the tissue is modified with the potential of specific drugs or biological molecules distributed for different biological uses, covering biological sensing, wound repair, soft robotics, drug delivery, and tissue engineering. The current biomaterials used for biomedical devices are being prepared with the help of 3D and 4D bioprinting.

14.8.1 Tissue Engineering

For a material to be qualified for the use of tissue engineering, it has to be biocompatible, biodegradable, and have high mechanical support. Recently it was reported that composite of alginate and polylactic acid (PLA) showed high mechanical and cell attachment support for osteosarcoma cells, as previously alginate hydrogels were not compatible for the development of the 3D-printed inks due to reduced cell proliferation and mechanical support. Extrusion-based method was used to develop HA, nanofibrillated cellulose (NC), and alginate hydrogel, showing higher cyto- and biocompatibility for cartilage constructs [52]. Further, using direct ink writing (DIW) method, Cu-doped composite scaffolds, 45S5 scaffolds, and Ag-doped scaffold ceramics were also prepared for several applications in the field. For the field of 4D printing, Payno et al. developed a two-layer-based hydrogel with alginate and HA. The composite acquired a unique property of differential swelling in the zones and resemblance to the natural structure of the cartilage tissue. Another study revealed that alginate-dialdehyde (ADA)/gelatin (Gel) and GelMA/PEGDM, when 4D bioprinted, depicted a shape-morphing and increased cell survivability in the scaffolds, making them an ideal candidate for precision-based therapy by the development of the fully functional system for the organ and tissue transplantation [53].

14.8.2 Drug Delivery

The main reason for which the polymers are being used for the drug delivery is to do precision-based therapeutic targeting of the drug to the site of target. Multiple polymers such as PLA, alginate, ceramics, polylactide glycolic acid (PLGA), and PCL are being used in this field. Currently the focus is on the advancements of the calcium phosphate (CaP) ceramic polymer systems. One of the major reasons is that the CaP-based scaffolds can be flexible with multiple polymers, change in temperature conditions, addition of antibiotics, heat-labile molecules, and flexible physical and mechanical properties with change in conditions; it can also maintain the pharmacokinetic drug release control. In multiple studies it has been reported that the CaP scaffolds printed with extrusion-based method have successfully delivered vancomycin in in-vitro assays, with higher mechanical strength and increased biocompatibility of the mesenchymal stem cells. One of the challenges with increased temperature fabrication of the CaP is the uneven printing, lack of uniform cell density, and increased pre- and post-processing modifications. Some of the major limitations held by 3D printing in drug delivery are lack of treatment outcomes, specific delivery, precision-patient based dosing, and controlled release that are overcome by the 4D-printed materials. In a study it was reported that these 4D-printed biomaterials can control the release and delivery of the drug based on the stimuli response such as change in pH, temperature, electric, magnetic, or even water. It was observed that the drug will only be released by the stimuli-responsive hydrogel when it's in stomach pH, hence minimizing the drug dosage and side effects. Also, currently implants are also being made for target delivery to cancer cells which only respond in the change in pH or in the presence of cancer-associated factors [54].

14.8.3 Diagnostic and Surgical Tools

The requirement of the polymers is not limited to the biological aspects but also includes the development of the surgical and diagnostic tools. The easy and precise development of the tools has not only helped in the biological but also in the hospitals in third-world environment and combat zones. Multiple studies have reported the development of tools such as 3D-printed Ag scaffolds for wound dressing and faster healing of the infection, surgical retractors for army-navy with same mechanical strength as the conventional ones and rapid development of the sterile surgical tool kits to eradicate the supply chain issue. Some of the diagnostics are also being fabricated using advanced printing technologies. Recently, in a study by Cardoso et al., fabricated amperometric biosensor which can detect the glucose level in biofluids was used [54]. Also, multiple researchers have developed biosensors which can detect both hydrogen peroxide and glucose in the fluid simultaneously making them advantageous for both environmental and biological applications. These 3D-printed biosensors are also being used in the detection of the cancer biomarkers; one such study by Ren et al. demonstrated the development of a device for the detection of cervical cancer biomarkers [55]. The 4D printing technology has made smart biomaterials which can adapt to external stimuli and can tailor the therapeutic release of the drug as well as control the surgical procedures. These materials can also change their stiffness and shape based on the specific stimuli. A tool by Ge et al. changed its shape in response to the minute stimulus change in the body by enabling specific grip and controlling soft tissues with minimum damage [56]. Another device by Zhou et al. was developed which can acquire the shape of the wound for providing the wound closure with reduced scar and maximum closure [57]. These devices have multiple advantages over 3D-printed ones such as reduced risk of damage to the biological samples, better precise-patient therapies, effective wound management, and adaptation to several surgical scenarios.

14.8.4 Implants and Prosthetics

Generally, implants are developed for the missing parts or to replace the damaged body part. They are also being used for the internal delivery of the medicines, providing support, and for monitoring the body functions of the tissues and organs. Some of the recent advancements in 3D-printed medical implants are the use of titanium (Ti) and its alloys to increase the mechanical strength. The surface modifications with PLGA, chitosan, and antibiotics help in increasing the biocompatibility and antimicrobial activity of the implant. The magnesium (Mg) implants are being used for increasing the X-ray transparency and increased biological degradation. Further, bioceramics are also being used for bone regeneration and treatment of osteosarcoma. Some of the other applications are the development of dental implants, facial and other reconstruction implants. Although the 3D-printed implants have better compatibility, reduced cost and easy development, the 4D-printed implants can also respond to stimuli such as temperature, light, electrochemical, moisture, and magnetic fields. Some of the applications for which the 4D-printed implants are being developed are in orthopedic for precise healing, shape-memory spinal, and biomimetic stents for providing support during the time of recovery. Ti implants are being used for the developments of dental and maxillofacial surgery to reduce the risk of complications and better adaptive fit [53].

The recent advances in printing technology are the development of the stimuli-responsive hydrogel, self-healing capacity scaffolds, and the environmental adaptability of the scaffold. The 3D-printed materials are being used in the development of wearable electronics for wound management in the food industry to determine the granule size, texture, cost-effectiveness, etc. Some of the major challenges faced by the 3D bioprinting industry are inadequate optimization of the structural design, internal moisture, cross-link density, pore size, and insufficient mechanical strength. The 4D bioprinting integrates the fourth dimension—time—to enable structures to change shape or function in response to internal or external stimuli. The 4D-printed stimulus-responsive polymers are engineered for controlled growth factor delivery based on the tissue needs, using the graphene-based system for the drug and gene delivery. Additionally, electrical simulations are being used for influencing neural differentiation, vascular regeneration through stem cells, and also the development of self-adjusting stents. 4D bioprinting helps in facilitating the regeneration of the tissue by the creation of high-resolution scaffolds. These scaffolds undergo dynamic and morphological changes over time leading to therapeutic response based on the stimulus and resulting in precision medicine and therapeutic interventions [58].

14.9 CONCLUSIONS

Many naturally occurring materials have been used for the development of medical devices for almost 100 years, but recently, technological advances in the material have resulted in smart biomaterials. These engineered materials have inert, active, responsive, and autonomous properties to tune them to provide a better material. The advancement in fabrication techniques and printing technologies has produced tailor-made materials that have resulted in the manufacturing of different stimuli-responsive biomaterials based on the personalized approach. Stimuli-responsive biomaterials are being explored for clinical translation in biomedical applications, but they hold certain challenges; some of them are material limitations as it is not able to completely mimic the properties of natural tissue and also the mechanical properties. Another limitation is the sample size, limited number of experiments, unavailability of multiple stimulation-responsive materials, and replication of the tissue complexity. In the 4D system, one of the major limitations is the control response over the dynamic approach as the material cannot predict the external stimuli and respond to them. Some of the technical challenges to overcome over the period are the printing quality control of the various batches and maintaining the consistency also optimization of the post-processing requirements to achieve the desired properties. Despite challenges in clinical translation, the advancement of stimuli-responsive materials holds significant potential for biomedical applications and the development of regenerative tissues.

Declaration of AI and AI-Assisted Technologies

During the preparation of this work, the authors used QuillBot AI and Grammarly in order to paraphrase the sentences. After using this tool, the authors reviewed and edited the content as needed and take full responsibility for the content of the publication.

REFERENCES

1. Wu CA, Zhu Y, Woo YJ. Advances in 3D bioprinting: Techniques, applications, and future directions for cardiac tissue engineering. Bioengineering 2023;10(7):842.
2. Karzyński K, Kosowska K, Ambrożkiewicz F, Berman A, Cichoń J, Klak M, Serwańska-Świętek M, Wszoła M. Use of 3D bioprinting in biomedical engineering for clinical application. Medical Studies/Studia Medyczne 2018;34(1):93.

3. Montoya C, Du Y, Gianforcaro AL, Orrego S, Yang M, Lelkes PI. On the road to smart biomaterials for bone research: Definitions, concepts, advances, and outlook. Bone Research 2021;9(1):12.
4. Yang K, Wu Z, Zhang K, Weir MD, Xu HH, Cheng L, Huang X, Zhou W. Unlocking the potential of stimuli-responsive biomaterials for bone regeneration. Frontiers in Pharmacology 2024;15:1437457.
5. Murphy SV, Atala A. 3D bioprinting of tissues and organs. Nature Biotechnology 2014;32(8):773.
6. Papaioannou TG, Manolesou D, Dimakakos E, Tsoucalas G, Vavuranakis M, Tousoulis D. 3D bioprinting methods and techniques: Applications on artificial blood vessel fabrication. Acta Cardiologica Sinica 2019;35(3):284.
7. Datta P, Barui A, Wu Y, Ozbolat V, Moncal KK, Ozbolat IT. Essential steps in bioprinting: From pre-to post-bioprinting. Biotechnology Advances 2018;36(5):1481.
8. Gungor-Ozkerim PS, Inci I, Zhang YS, Khademhosseini A, Dokmeci MR. Bioinks for 3D bioprinting: An overview. Biomaterials Science 2018;6(5):915.
9. Fatimi A, Okoro OV, Podstawczyk D, Siminska-Stanny J, Shavandi A. Natural hydrogel-based bio-inks for 3D bioprinting in tissue engineering: A review. Gels 2022;8(3):179.
10. Unagolla JM, Jayasuriya AC. Hydrogel-based 3D bioprinting: A comprehensive review on cell-laden hydrogels, bioink formulations, and future perspectives. Applied Materials Today 2020;18:100479.
11. Yoon H, Lee JS, Yim H, Kim G, Chun W. Development of cell-laden 3D scaffolds for efficient engineered skin substitutes by collagen gelation. RSC Advances 2016;6(26):21439.
12. Shim JH, Jang KM, Hahn SK, Park JY, Jung H, Oh K, Park KM, Yeom J, Park SH, Kim SW, Wang JH. Three-dimensional bioprinting of multilayered constructs containing human mesenchymal stromal cells for osteochondral tissue regeneration in the rabbit knee joint. Biofabrication 2016;8(1):014102.
13. Caliari SR, Burdick JA. A practical guide to hydrogels for cell culture. Nature Methods 2016;13(5):405.
14. Kim SH, Hong H, Ajiteru O, Sultan MT, Lee YJ, Lee JS, Lee OJ, Lee H, Park HS, Choi KY, Lee JS. 3D bioprinted silk fibroin hydrogels for tissue engineering. Nature Protocols 2021;16(12):5484.
15. Khosropanah MH, Rajabi M, Behboodi Tanourlouee S, Azimzadeh A, Alizadeh Vaghasloo M, Hassannejad Z. Silk as a promising biomaterial for 3D bioprinting: A comprehensive review of *Bombyx mori* silk's biomedical applications. International Journal of Polymeric Materials and Polymeric Biomaterials 2024;74(6):538.
16. Kumar S, Tharayil A, Thomas S. 3D bioprinting of nature-inspired hydrogel inks based on synthetic polymers. ACS Applied Polymer Materials 2021;3(8):3685.
17. Alexander A, Khan J, Saraf S, Saraf S. Polyethylene glycol (PEG)–Poly (N-isopropylacrylamide) (PNIPAAm) based thermosensitive injectable hydrogels for biomedical applications. European Journal of Pharmaceutics and Biopharmaceutics 2014;88(3):575.
18. Ilyas RA, Zuhri MY, Aisyah HA, Asyraf MR, Hassan SA, Zainudin ES, Sapuan SM, Sharma S, Bangar SP, Jumaidin R, Nawab Y. Natural fiber-reinforced polylactic acid, polylactic acid blends and their composites for advanced applications. Polymers 2022;14(1):202.
19. Ko YG, Kwon OH. Reinforced gelatin-methacrylate hydrogels containing poly (lactic-co-glycolic acid) nanofiber fragments for 3D bioprinting. Journal of Industrial and Engineering Chemistry 2020;89:147.
20. Salah M, Naini FB, Tayebi L. 3D printing and bioprinting of biomaterials and bioceramic scaffolds: Clinical outcomes and implications in bone tissue engineering and maxillofacial reconstructive surgery. Innovative Bioceramics in Translational Medicine II: Surgical Applications 2022;18:15.
21. Dzobo K, Motaung KS, Adesida A. Recent trends in decellularized extracellular matrix bioinks for 3D printing: An updated review. International Journal of Molecular Sciences 2019;20(18):4628.
22. Kačarević ŽP, Rider PM, Alkildani S, Retnasingh S, Smeets R, Jung O, Ivanišević Z, Barbeck M. An introduction to 3D bioprinting: Possibilities, challenges and future aspects. Materials 2018;11(11):2199.
23. Seol YJ, Kang HW, Lee SJ, Atala A, Yoo JJ. Bioprinting technology and its applications. European Journal of Cardio-Thoracic Surgery 2014;46(3):342.
24. Shahrubudin N, Lee TC, Ramlan RJ. An overview on 3D printing technology: Technological, materials, and applications. Procedia Manufacturing 2019;35:1286.
25. Bao Y. Recent trends in advanced photoinitiators for vat photopolymerization 3D printing. Macromolecular Rapid Communications 2022;43(14):2200202.
26. Wubneh A, Tsekoura EK, Ayranci C, Uludağ H. Current state of fabrication technologies and materials for bone tissue engineering. Acta Biomaterialia 2018;80:1.
27. Li J, Chen M, Fan X, Zhou H. Recent advances in bioprinting techniques: Approaches, applications and future prospects. Journal of Translational Medicine 2016;14(271):1.
28. Dou C, Perez V, Qu J, Tsin A, Xu B, Li J. A state-of-the-art review of laser-assisted bioprinting and its future research trends. ChemBioEng Reviews 2021;8(5):517.

29. Woods P, Smith C, Clark S, Habib A. Integrating pneumatic and thermal control in 3D bioprinting for improved bio-ink handling. Designs 2024;8(4):83.
30. Tan B, Gan S, Wang X, Liu W, Li X. Applications of 3D bioprinting in tissue engineering: Advantages, deficiencies, improvements, and future perspectives. Journal of Materials Chemistry B 2021;9(27):5385.
31. Pagac M, Hajnys J, Ma QP, Jancar L, Jansa J, Stefek P, Mesicek J. A review of vat photopolymerization technology: Materials, applications, challenges, and future trends of 3D printing. Polymers 2021;13(4):598.
32. Kong Z, Wang X. Bioprinting technologies and bioinks for vascular model establishment. International Journal of Molecular Sciences 2023;24(1):891.
33. Ventura RD. An overview of laser-assisted bioprinting (LAB) in tissue engineering applications. Medical Lasers; Engineering, Basic Research, and Clinical Application 2021;10(2):76.
34. Elkhoury K, Morsink M, Sanchez-Gonzalez L, Kahn C, Tamayol A, Arab-Tehrany E. Biofabrication of natural hydrogels for cardiac, neural, and bone tissue engineering applications. Bioactive Materials 2021;6(11):3904.
35. Choi J, Lee EJ, Jang WB, Kwon SM. Development of biocompatible 3D-printed artificial blood vessels through multidimensional approaches. Journal of Functional Biomaterials 2023;14(10):497.
36. Haidari H, Kopecki Z, Sutton AT, Garg S, Cowin AJ, Vasilev K. pH-responsive "smart" hydrogel for controlled delivery of silver nanoparticles to infected wounds. Antibiotics 2021;10(1):49.
37. Osouli-Bostanabad K, Masalehdan T, Kapsa RM, Quigley A, Lalatsa A, Bruggeman KF, Franks SJ, Williams RJ, Nisbet DR. Traction of 3D and 4D printing in the healthcare industry: From drug delivery and analysis to regenerative medicine. ACS Biomaterials Science & Engineering 2022;8(7):2764.
38. Lai J, Liu Y, Lu G, Yung P, Wang X, Tuan RS, Li ZA. 4D bioprinting of programmed dynamic tissues. Bioactive Materials 2024;37:348.
39. Mirshafiei M, Rashedi H, Yazdian F, Rahdar A, Baino F. Advancements in tissue and organ 3D bioprinting: Current techniques, applications, and future perspectives. Materials & Design 2024;240:112853.
40. Kim J, Gouripriya DA, Debnath P, Saha P. Smart multi-responsive biomaterials and their applications for 4D bioprinting. Biomimetics 2024;9(8):484.
41. Ghilan A, Chiriac AP, Nita LE, Rusu AG, Neamtu I, Chiriac VM. Trends in 3D printing processes for biomedical field: Opportunities and challenges. Journal of Polymers and the Environment 2020;28:1345.
42. Kalogeropoulou M, Díaz-Payno PJ, Mirzaali MJ, van Osch GJ, Fratila-Apachitei LE, Zadpoor AA. 4D printed shape-shifting biomaterials for tissue engineering and regenerative medicine applications. Biofabrication 2024;16(2):022002.
43. Zhang Z, Zhou X, Fang Y, Xiong Z, Zhang T. AI-driven 3D bioprinting for regenerative medicine: From bench to bedside. Bioactive Materials 2025;45:201.
44. Morouço P, Azimi B, Milazzo M, Mokhtari F, Fernandes C, Reis D, Danti S. Four-dimensional (bio-) printing: A review on stimuli-responsive mechanisms and their biomedical suitability. Applied Sciences 2020;10(24):9143.
45. Arif ZU, Khalid MY, Zolfagharian A, Bodaghi M. 4D bioprinting of smart polymers for biomedical applications: Recent progress, challenges, and future perspectives. Reactive and Functional Polymers 2022;179:105374.
46. Abolhassani S, Fattahi R, Safshekan F, Saremi J, Hasanzadeh E. Advances in 4D bioprinting: The next frontier in regenerative medicine and tissue engineering applications. Advanced Healthcare Materials 2024;14(4):2403065.
47. Zhan Y, Jiang W, Liu Z, Wang Z, Guo K, Sun J. Utilizing bioprinting to engineer spatially organized tissues from the bottom-up. Stem Cell Research & Therapy 2024;15(1):101.
48. Faber L, Yau A, Chen Y. Translational biomaterials of four-dimensional bioprinting for tissue regeneration. Biofabrication 2023;16(1):012001.
49. Wallace ER, Yue Z, Dottori M, Wood FM, Fear M, Wallace GG, Beirne S. Point of care approaches to 3D bioprinting for wound healing applications. Progress in Biomedical Engineering 2023;5(2):023002.
50. Qu G, Huang J, Gu G, Li Z, Wu X, Ren J. Smart implants: 4D-printed shape-morphing scaffolds for medical implantation. International Journal of Bioprinting 2023;9(5):764.
51. Wu YF, Wen YT, Salamanca E, Aung LM, Chao YQ, Chen CY, Sun YS, Chang WJ. 3D-bioprinted alginate-based bioink scaffolds with β-tricalcium phosphate for bone regeneration applications. Journal of Dental Sciences 2024;19(2):1116.
52. Appuhamillage GA, Ambagaspitiya SS, Dassanayake RS, Wijenayake A. 3D and 4D printing of biomedical materials: Current trends, challenges, and future outlook. Exploration of Medicine 2024;5(1):17.

53. Ishack S, Mediero A, Wilder T, Ricci JL, Cronstein BN. Bone regeneration in critical bone defects using three-dimensionally printed β-tricalcium phosphate/hydroxyapatite scaffolds is enhanced by coating scaffolds with either dipyridamole or BMP-2. Journal of Biomedical Materials Research Part B: Applied Biomaterials 2017;105(2):366.
54. Cardoso RM, Silva PR, Lima AP, Rocha DP, Oliveira TC, do, Prado TM, Fava EL, Fatibello-Filho O, Richter EM, Muñoz RA. 3D-printed graphene/polylactic acid electrode for bioanalysis: Biosensing of glucose and simultaneous determination of uric acid and nitrite in biological fluids. Sensors and Actuators B: Chemical 2020;307:127621.
55. Ren W, Mohammed SI, Wereley S, Irudayaraj J. Magnetic focus lateral flow sensor for detection of cervical cancer biomarkers. Analytical Chemistry 2019;91(4):2876.
56. Ge Q, Sakhaei AH, Lee H, Dunn CK, Fang NX, Dunn ML. Multimaterial 4D printing with tailorable shape memory polymers. Scientific Reports 2016;6(1):31110.
57. Zhou L, Min T, Bian X, Dong Y, Zhang P, Wen Y. Rational design of intelligent and multifunctional dressing to promote acute/chronic wound healing. ACS Applied Bio Materials 2022;5(9):4055.
58. Rahimnejad M, Jahangiri S, Hassan Kiadeh ZS, Rezvaninejad S, Ahmadi Z, Ahmadi S, Safarkhani M, Rabiee N. Stimuli-responsive biomaterials: Smart avenue toward 4D bioprinting. Critical Reviews in Biotechnology 2024;44(5):860.

Index

Note: Locators in *italics* represent figures and **bold** indicate tables in the text.

B

C

D

E

L

M

R

S

T

U

V

W

Z

For Product Safety Concerns and Information please contact our EU representative GPSR@taylorandfrancis.com Taylor & Francis Verlag GmbH, Kaufingerstraße 24, 80331 München, Germany